Practical Approach to the
Neurological Patient

A Clinician's Guide

Practical Approach to the Neurological Patient

to the

A Clinician's Guide

William J. Mullally, MD
Associate Neurologist
Department of Neurology
Brigham and Women's Hospital;
Associate Chief of Clinical Neurology
Department of Neurology
Brigham and Women's Faulkner Hospital
Boston, Massachusetts

ELSEVIER

Elsevier
1600 John F. Kennedy Blvd.
Ste 1800
Philadelphia, PA 19103-2899

PRACTICAL APPROACH TO THE NEUROLOGICAL PATIENT:
A CLINICIAN'S GUIDE

ISBN: 978-0-443-12642-0

Notice

Practitioners and researchers must always rely on their own experience and knowledge in evaluating and using any information, methods, compounds or experiments described herein. Because of rapid advances in the medical sciences, in particular, independent verification of diagnoses and drug dosages should be made. To the fullest extent of the law, no responsibility is assumed by Elsevier, authors, editors or contributors for any injury and/or damage to persons or property as a matter of products liability, negligence or otherwise, or from any use or operation of any methods, products, instructions, or ideas contained in the material herein.

Senior Content Strategist: Lauren Boyle
Senior Content Development Specialist: Sneha Kashyap
Publishing Services Manager: Deepthi Unni
Senior Project Manager: Beula Christopher
Senior Book Designer: Patrick C. Ferguson

Printed in India

Last digit is the print number: 9 8 7 6 5 4 3 2 1

CONTRIBUTORS

Jessica M. Baker, MD
Assistant Professor
Department of Neurology
University of Wisconsin School of Medicine and Public
   Health
Madison, Wisconsin

Elizabeth Benge, MD
Clinical Sleep Medicine Fellow
Department of Neurology
Brigham and Women's Faulkner Hospital
Boston, Massachusetts

Aaron L. Berkowitz, MD, PhD
Professor of Clinical Neurology
Department of Neurology
University of California, San Francisco
San Francisco, California

Shamik Bhattacharyya, MD, MS, FAAN
Neurologist
Department of Neurology
Brigham and Women's Hospital;
Assistant Professor
Harvard Medical School
Boston, Massachusetts

Anderson Chen, MD
Physician
Department of Psychiatry
Massachusetts General Hospital
Boston, Massachusetts

Kirk R. Daffner, MD
J David and Virginia Wimberly Professor of Neurology
Department of Neurology
Harvard Medical School;
Chief
Division of Cognitive and Behavioural Neurology,
Stephen Muss Clinical Director of the Alzheimer Center
Department of Neurology
Brigham and Women's Hospital
Boston, Massachusetts

Melissa Darsey, MPAS, PA-C
Physician Assistant III
Department of Neurology
Brigham and Woman's Hospital
Boston, Massachusetts

Christopher T. Doughty, MD
Assistant Professor
Department of Neurology
Harvard Medical School;
Clinical Director
Division of Neuromuscular Medicine
Department of Neurology
Brigham and Women's Hospital;
Associate Program Director, MGB Neurology Residency
Department of Neurology
Mass General Brigham
Boston, Massachusetts

Michael Erkkinen, MD
Associate Neurologist
Department of Neurology
Brigham and Women's Hospital
Boston, Massachusetts

Steven Feske, MD
Chief, Stroke Division
Department of Neurology
Boston Medical Center, Boston University School of
   Medicine;
Vice-Chair of Education
Department of Neurology
Boston Medical Center
Boston, Massachusetts

Seth A. Gale, MD
Assistant Professor
Department of Neurology
Harvard Medical School;
Associate Neurologist
Department of Neurology
Brigham and Women's Hospital
Boston, Massachusetts

Kathryn E. Hall, DNP, ANP-BC, NE-BC
Nurse Director
Translational and Clinical Research Centers
Massachusetts General Hospital
Medfield, Massachusetts;
Assistant Professor
Assistant Dean Master's Programs
Graduate School of Nursing
MGH Institute of Health Professions
Boston, Massachusetts

G. Kyle Harrold, MD
Clinical Instructor
Department of Neurology
Brigham and Women's Hospital;
Assistant in Neurology
Department of Neurology
Massachusetts General Hospital;
Instructor in Neurology
Harvard Medical School
Boston, Massachusetts

Michael T. Hayes, MD
Neurologist
Department of Neurology
Brigham and Women's Hospital;
Assistant Professor, Part Time
Department of Neurology
Harvard Medical School
Boston, Massachusetts

Manisha G. Holmes, MD
Section Chief of Epilepsy
Department of Neurology
Westchester Medical Health Network
Valhalla, New York

Danielle M. Howard, MD
General Neurologist
Department of Neurology
Tufts Medical Center
Boston, Massachusetts

Sultana Jahan, MD
Clinical Research Trainee
Department of Neurology, Autoimmune Neurology
Harvard Medical School, Brigham and Women's
    Hospital
Boston, Massachusetts

Alexandra Knief, PA-C
Physician Assistant
Department of Neurology
Brigham and Women's Hospital
Boston, Massachusetts

Eudocia Q. Lee, MD, MPH
Director of Clinical Research
Center for Neuro-Oncology
Dana-Farber Cancer Institute
Boston, Massachusetts

Thomas C. Lee, MD
Neuroradiologist
AdventHealth Orlando;
Associate Professor
University of Central Florida
Orlando, Florida

Giovanna S. Manzano, MD
Physician
Department of Neurology
Massachusetts General Hospital;
Physician
Department of Neurology
Brigham and Women's Hospital;
Instructor
Department of Neurology
Harvard Medical School
Boston, Massachusetts

Sadie P. Marciano, PA-C
Physician Assistant
Department of Neurology
Brigham and Women's Faulkner Hospital
Boston, Massachusetts

Tracey A. Milligan, MD, MS, FAAN, FAES, FANA
Director
Department of Neurology
Westchester Medical Center Health Network;
Professor and Chair
Department of Neurology
New York Medical College
Valhalla, New York

Orly Moshe-Lilie, MD
Faculty
Division of Neuromuscular Medicine
Department of Neurology
VA Boston Healthcare System;
Assistant Professor
Department of Neurology
Boston University
Boston, Massachusetts

William J. Mullally, MD
Associate Neurologist
Department of Neurology
Brigham and Women's Hospital;
Associate Chief of Clinical Neurology
Department of Neurology
Brigham and Women's Faulkner Hospital
Boston, Massachusetts

Peter Novak, MD, PhD
Physician
Department of Neurology
Brigham and Women's Hospital, Harvard Medical
    School
Boston, Massachusetts

Mary Angela O'Neal, MD
Assistant Professor
Department of Neurology
Brigham and Women's Hospital
Roslindale, Massachusetts;
Clinical Director of the Neurosciences,
Director of the Women's Neurology Program
Department of Neurology
Brigham and Women's Hospital
Boston, Massachusetts

Milena Pavlova, MD
Medical Director, Faulkner Sleep Testing Center
Department of Neurology
Brigham and Women's Hospital;
Associate Professor of Neurology
Department of Neurology
Harvard Medical School
Boston, Massachusetts

Sashank Prasad, MD
Professor
Clinical Neurology
University of Pennsylvania Perelman School of
    Medicine;
Chief
Department of Neurology
Penn Presbyterian Medical Center
Philadelphia, Pennsylvania

William Renthal, MD, PhD
Associate Professor of Neurology
Harvard Medical School, Brigham and Women's
    Hospital
Boston, Massachusetts

Gretchen Reynolds, PhD
Neuropsychologist
Department of Neurology
Brigham and Women's Hospital
Boston, Massachusetts

Paul B. Rizzoli, MD, FAAN, FAHS
Associate Professor, Director
John R. Graham Headache Center
Department of Neurology
Brigham and Women's Hospital, Harvard Medical
    School
Boston, Massachusetts

Daniel B. Rubin, MD, PhD
Assistant Professor
Department of Neurology
Massachusetts General Hospital, Harvard Medical
    School
Boston, Massachusetts

Reza Sadjadi, MD
Assistant Neurologist
Department of Neurology
Massachusetts General Hospital;
Assistant Professor in Neurology
Department of Medicine
Harvard Medical School
Boston, Massachusetts

Mohammad Kian Salajegheh, MD
Chief
Neuromuscular Division,
Deputy Chief
Department of Neurology
VA Boston Healthcare System;
Neuromuscular Staff
Department of Neurology
Brigham and Women's Hospital;
Associate Professor of Neurology
Harvard Medical School
Boston, Massachusetts

Ananya Ruth Samuel, MA
Doctoral Student
Clinical Psychology
William James College
Newton, Massachusetts

Andrew G. Schneider, MD, MPH
Resident Physician
Department of Radiology
Brigham and Women's Hospital
Boston, Massachusetts

Michael P.H. Stanley, MD
Fellow
Department of Neurology
Brigham and Women's Hospital
Boston, Massachusetts

Manisha Thakore-James, MD
Assistant Professor
Department of Neurology Neuromuscular Division
Boston VA Medical Center
Boston, Massachusetts

Angeliki Vgontzas, MD
Assistant Professor
Department of Neurology
Brigham and Women's Hospital, Harvard Medical
    School
Boston, Massachusetts

Victor C. Wang, MD, PhD, MBA
Physician
Department of Neurology
Boston Advanced Medicine
Waltham, Massachusetts

Gregory T. Whitman, MD
Neurologist
Department of Neurology
Cedars-Sinai Medical Center
Los Angeles, California

Kim C. Willment, PhD
Neuropsychologist
Department of Neurology
Brigham and Women's Hospital
Boston, Massachusetts

Gilbert Youssef, MD
Neuro-Oncologist
Center for Neuro-Oncology
Dana-Farber Cancer Institute;
Instructor
Department of Neurology
Harvard Medical School;
Neuro-Oncologist
Brigham and Women's Hospital
Boston, Massachusetts

Jonathan Zurawski, MD
Instructor
Department of Neurology
Brigham and Women's Hospital
Boston, Massachusetts

FOREWORD

It is not a surprise that neurology continues to mystify physicians in other specialties. People inside the field have been trying to figure out why this is so and how to rectify it for over half a century. The problem arose when neurology split off from internal medicine, and the gap between the two fields only expanded over time. The iconic chairman of internal medicine at the University of Washington and President of the Association of American Medical Colleges, Robert Petersdorf, warned at the time publicly and privately that this divorce was a mistake and that both neurology and medicine would pay the price in the future. They have. The limited number of neurologists has been required to deal with problems that only a few decades ago would have been considered mundane issues in general medicine and physicians in other fields have had to interminably consult neurologists and lose out on an appreciation of their patient's problems in their entirety.

The neurological exam, in contrast to conventional medical bedside examination, seems to have presented a challenge to both the patience and attention of nonneurologists. Part of this has been the squishy nature of interpreting neurological signs and the time it takes to conduct a thorough examination. I have felt there has also been a desire by all physicians to quantify everything and have a definitive test to supplant the classical approach to diagnosis and treatment, neither of which is entirely satisfied by the neurological examination and the synthetic mental process that follows. Finally, the now-old trope that nothing can be done to help neurological diseases is perpetuated as a counter-phobic reason for avoiding neurology. And yet, there is a modern thirst for knowledge about the brain and nervous system.

How can one practice medicine without a confident grasp of the most important organ system and one that is affected by so many diseases? It is true the field is vast. Raymond Adams pointed out that there are more nameable muscle diseases than there are all pulmonary diseases, and that is just one small corner of neurology. A fundamental problem remains of a lack of appreciation that neurology is a bedrock part of internal medicine and other fields such as psychiatry, anesthesia and pain medicine, rehabilitation medicine, emergency medicine, and pediatrics. All these have to be reversed by providing a practical approach to neurological problems that is accessible to all practitioners.

What Dr. Mullally and his colleagues have accomplished in this insightful book is to provide a practical framework for addressing prevalent neurological challenges faced by professionals across the entire spectrum of medical practice, including primary care physicians, medical specialists, nurse practitioners, physician's assistants, and medical students. In doing this, they begin to improve care provided by all practitioners to patients with a long list of problems ranging from headache to Parkinson disease. The writing is crisp and instructive. Virtually every important neurological disorder has been covered in a pleasing and uniform manner by seasoned senior practitioners. The authors of each chapter have distilled material that every well-educated physician should and can easily know.

Taken together, the chapters in this book are invaluable for anyone wishing to improve their neurological skills and thinking at a level that is applicable to our patients every day. As a primer, refresher, or resource for practice, this book hits the mark.

Allan H. Ropper, MD
Associate Neurologist, BWH
Professor of Neurology, Harvard Medical School
Deputy Editor, *New England Journal of Medicine*

Conquering Neurophobia

The evaluation of a patient with neurological disease remains one of the most daunting and anxiety-provoking tasks in clinical medicine. From the perspective of physicians who are not trained in neurology the performance and interpretation of the neurological examination is shrouded in mystery. The angst associated with the study of neuroscience begins in medical school and continues throughout residency, and the term "Neurophobia" was coined in 1994 to define this fear.

While clinicians usually acknowledge that neurology is the most interesting medical specialty, they also consider it the most complex and it is the only medical subspecialty that requires its own residency training program after internship. Both in the inpatient and outpatient setting, the neurologist is totally relied upon to diagnose and treat disorders of the brain and nervous system, as nonneurologists feel uncomfortable managing neurological disease. It is also the perception of patients that the treatment of their neurological disease rendered by a neurologist is superior to that of other physicians. With the impending shortage of neurologists, in conjunction with the explosion of new therapy and diagnostic techniques for neurological disorders, a crisis is looming that can only be assuaged by advancing the clinical skills and comfort level of the primary care physicians, medical specialists, nurse practitioners, and physician associates with regard to diseases of the nervous system. Medical schools and medical residency programs have started to initiate a curriculum that places more emphasis on clinical neuroscience training.

Neurology is a rapidly evolving field that has witnessed remarkable advancements in our understanding of the brain's structure, function, and the multitude of conditions that can affect it. From the complex neural networks responsible for our thoughts, emotions, and actions, to the intricate interplay between genetics, environment, and disease, the study of neurology provides an awe-inspiring window into the mysteries of human consciousness. In this book, we will be presenting a comprehensive review of principles and concepts that form the foundation of neurology, beginning with the neurological examination. We have carefully curated the content to cater to a wide range of readers. Each chapter is designed to explore a specific aspect of neurology with the goal of providing clinical medicine practitioners and students with a basic understanding of neurological disorders and a pragmatic approach to their diagnosis and treatment. The chapters are an update and expansion of the neurology series published in the *American Journal of Medicine*, and all the authors are experts in their field who have dedicated their lives to advancing the frontiers of neurology. The book can be used both as an easy reference in the office, clinic, or hospital and as a basic textbook of clinical neurology.

It is our hope that *Practical Approach to the Neurological Patient: A Clinician's Guide* will serve as a trusted companion on your path to becoming proficient in diagnosing and managing neurological disorders. Our goal is to unravel the mysteries of the nervous system and forever vanquish "Neurophobia."

CONTENTS

The Neurological Examination*

Michael P.H. Stanley, Kathryn E. Hall, and William J. Mullally

Today's neurological examination originates from those of Wilhelm Erb, Joseph Babinski, and William Gowers in the 1800s. Erb emphasized a systematic, comprehensive structure; Babinski uncovered signs distinguishing organic from hysterical paralysis; Gowers incorporated familiar tools like the ophthalmoscope and reflex hammer. Their legacy affords us a library of textbooks for clinicians to choose for their purposes, but whether it be antique Monrad-Krohn or modern Berkowitz, the key is to select neurological examination textbooks guiding functional-anatomical correlation through standardized, objective, and reproducible techniques.

The intimidation many feel toward the neurological examination derives from the observation that an impoverished examination betrays poor reasoning, whereas an image yields a result seemingly definitive. Obtaining an image does not guarantee an answer, however, and there has been little sense made and many dollars wasted imaging the head when the lesion was in the patient's hand (and the provider's thinking). All radiographic and electrophysiologic studies are at best secondary extensions of a primary physical examination. An orderly, objective examination focuses on the differential diagnosis, thereby narrowing the remaining workup. Oftentimes, the neurological examination is all the testing required.

Just as a history, no matter the order the patient relates it, should be reorganized with a beginning,

*Based on Stanley MPH, Hall KE, Mullally WJ. The neurologic exam. *Am J Med*. 2023;136(7):638–644. ISSN 0002-9343, https://doi.org/10.1016/j.amjmed.2023.03.016 (https://www.sciencedirect.com/science/article/pii/S0002934 32300219X).

middle, and end, with attention paid to the rate of rising or falling action, so too should your examination. There are acute, subacute, and chronic histories, and there are acute, subacute, and chronic examinations. In the emergency room a hyperacute screen to determine "stroke or not" and to what degree requires a National Institutes of Health Stroke Scale and nothing more, while weakness in the foot will require a broader assessment from head to toe and adjustments on one's area of focus as the examination progresses. But fast or slow, one's examination should screen sequentially at every step of the neuroaxis to establish location and gauge the degree of impairment. Test each neurological faculty for what normally should be the easiest thing that now the patient finds difficult to do, and what remains the most difficult thing that the patient still easily does. Combinatorial and complex maneuvers trade specificity for sensitivity, allowing clinicians to survey the nervous system at a glance to exonerate much of it. Then, a detailed diagnostic battery can be focused on a few potential sites of nervous injury for further targeted ancillary studies.

The examiner is like a detectorist trying to ascertain what lies beneath the surface of their patient, and what the examiner should keep in mind is that the structure-function relationship of the nervous system is what is being detected. The nervous system is ordered. In the words of Oliver Sacks, "it doesn't become disordered, but strangely ordered." The polyneuropathic patient's stance broadens not *because* of the lesion but to *accommodate* the function lost to the lesion. This may seem a trivial distinction but is even more important when problems of higher cortical function (disturbance in articulation vs. language) are at issue. The cooperation of multiple pathways forms modular functional units (perception or locomotion) that the patient and the examiner appreciate. Knowing what a component part does for the performance of a cognitive or behavioral operation will help you zero in on where along the chain of causation a symptom or sign arises. The examination is not a ritual but an exercise of the medical imagination made manifest by mapping historical points to parts of the body. While you should aim to know the examination by rote, it should not be performed as such, but tailored to the specific question you are trying to address.

As therapeutic as it is diagnostic, patients say a caring examiner's careful examination makes them feel not *inspected* but truly *seen*.

EXAMINATION

Inspection

Because one is speaking to the diseased organ, but addressing the ill patient, and doing so in a heightened environment of observation, it is important to assess function "by bush glasses and by opera glasses." Try to catch a few moments at least of the patient before they sense you are observing them and look for how the patient holds themselves, moves, talks, and engages with others or with objects. It may be quite different than with the clinician or provide a sense of ecological validity that standard examination maneuvers can never be extrapolated to reveal.

Follow the patient to the examination room to observe their gait and compare it to the demonstration they provide when you are standing in front of them asking to test their walk. There may be differences that indicate malingering or functional neurological conditions. Often the instructions given during examination maneuvers can be loaded with placebo and nocebo by clinicians; this can be of great advantage when psychiatric overlay is suspected in mixed conditions or there is an "effort-dependent" examination. Alternatively, there may be some gestalt sense that comes about when you see the person in the waiting room (how stiff they hold themselves) that you would miss during your busy history taking. Use the walk to and from the waiting room and some conversation as an opportunity to get a view of their form and function, which will help you estimate if the minute findings of your microscopic maneuvers on examination are insightful or incidental.

A Brief Note About Dominance

Ascertaining so-called "dominance" is a classical attribution of the neurological examination, because by it we orient our findings to a map of functional anatomy. We will not know our right hemisphere from our left hemisphere based on the deficits. There are scales for estimating dominance. The modern clinician should consider what is meant by this provocative and problematic term. Dominance of one hemisphere implies subordination of the other, but by what criteria? A clinician should try to identify the "eloquent" hemisphere (the one primarily responsible for language functions). Generally the handedness of the individual will be contralateral to the eloquent hemisphere, but even amongst "left-handers" a strong faction is believed to localize language to the left hemisphere, and it would seem other faculties arrange themselves accordingly. A safe bet is to assign eloquence to the left hemisphere unless other parts of the examination point otherwise.

Depth of Consciousness

First, determine the depth of consciousness (described as hypervigilant, alert, confused, drowsy, stupor, or coma), which is accomplished by establishing the threshold of response to environmental cues (Does the patient arouse or respond to voice, touch, or noxious stimulation?). The level of consciousness must be determined to the satisfaction of the examiner, because the level constricts the scope of subsequent properties of the mental status—and in many cases, the rest of the neurological examination.

For example, if a person is in a coma, the clinician cannot determine anything about the faculty of speech. It is no use to ask the patient to repeat, "No ifs, ands, or buts." A facetious and extreme example, it nevertheless emphasizes a point that in more nuanced cases—such as general confusional or inattentive states—becomes particularly important. If a patient has poor attention, can the examiner be sure the patient truly has lost certain faculties of speech, or are they merely too inattentive to follow the examiner's question.

MENTAL STATUS IN THE AWAKE AND ALERT PATIENT

MMSE, SLUMS, MoCA, BLESSED, ACE-R—there is an alphabet soup of acronymistic assessments principally for finding and following cognitive impairments, both in the general practitioner's office and in the research setting. They have their unique strengths and weaknesses but they all explore the major cognitive domains, and many have accompanying norms that offer some prognostic insight into presumed degree of functional impairment or support suggested at home. Try a few on colleagues to identify the one that seems to fit your needs for duration and completeness, and, generally speaking, they are organized above in increasing degree of granularity and time.

Orientation

After establishing that the patient is conscious and possesses enough attention and concentration to be coherent to the present circumstance, and communicates reliably, the clinician can then begin to explore other structures of mental life. Orientation is a sense of one's whereabouts and "whenabouts," for without knowing our place in the present moment, we cannot direct ourselves to purposeful ends. Orientation is mapped by asking the patient who they are, where are they, why are they here in this place, how did they get here, and what is going on currently in personal, local, and national news? There is a difference between the historical or remembered orientation (the map) versus the ability to orient when needed (the use of a compass). Traditionally, orientation refers to the historical or remembered sense, rather than the patient's ability to orient. There is a value judgment in the ecological validity of historical/remembered orientation. What is "Tuesday" to a retired person with no schedule but his meals and TV shows or a medical resident whose day begins Tuesday morning but ends Wednesday afternoon? Find out what the patient does with his days and then you can try to ascertain if his degree of orientation is sufficient for the schedule he offers. In some sense, we should be paying attention to the patient's ability to reorient to updated information or new circumstances, and so cues should be provided to see if the patient can guide themselves to the same lights you steer by.

Language

Although there is implicitly a rudimentary test of communication during the attentional and concentrative assessment, more is required to evaluate language's several features. The briefest assessment would be to determine if a person's speech is fluent or nonfluent (which assesses their ability to make themselves known to us) and if they can comprehend what is being told to them (which assesses our ability to make our wishes known to them). Language is the bridge of ideas and will play a substantial role in further assessment, and, more importantly, in management and recovery. Traditionally, in right-handers and many left-handers, the seat of language production is in the left frontal lobe and its reception in the left temporal lobe.

When listening to the patient, we naturally hear the thematic content of the message, but the language evaluation requires the examiner to tune into the compositional elements of the message (words *qua* syntax like in primary school sentence diagraming). Put another way, the patient can be talking nonsense because the content of the message is delusional or the composition of the message is denatured. Are their words vague, general terms (saying "animal" for "squirrel") and they seem to understand what the examiner is saying? This could be a semantic issue. Are their words mispronounced and a struggle to get out with their slurred, slowed speech? This could be a nonfluency issue. Do they speak slowly and have trouble putting together sentences because they cannot think of the words anymore? This could be a logopenic issue. Are they smoothly speaking but the lyric sounds like a foreign language? This could indicate a fluent aphasia.

After listening to the patient's fluency the first screening test is word finding and confrontational naming. In the former a definition is given and the patient is requested to provide the word (e.g., "What do soldiers wear on their backs when they jump out of a plane?" is answered with "parachute."), while the latter is tested by confronting patient with an object or an image. Impairments of either indicate an "anomia" (difficulty naming) and signify some insult to the faculty of language.

Next, a patient is asked to repeat phrases of increasing length and complexity, which indicate how robust conduction from the posterior temporal to the anterior opercular processes are intact. The power of repetition is not dependent on intelligibility and patients could be asked to repeat "no ifs, ands, or buts" versus "passoogmetunkapil" for short sensical and nonsensical phrases and longer ones like, "The clowns are in the circus ring" or "Twas brillig and the slithy toves did gyre and gimble in the wabe." Commending to memory a pangram containing all the phonemes (e.g., "With tenure, Suzie'd have all the more leisure for yachting, but her publications are no good.") will provide you with an opportunity to listen for articulation issues as well. The same is true for writing, and it may be useful to commend to memory a few sentences that use all the letters (e.g., "The quick brown fox jumped over the lazy dog."). In repetition, one is paying attention to how long and how complex a sentence can be repeated, and when the repetition fails, how is it being denatured. Is their elision and substitution of words but overall preservation of the sentence's theme signaling a working memory issue, or, are there impairments in the production of the word itself or tripping in the cadence of the phrases as they are being spoken to completion, which would indicate a language problem?

Comprehension is another element of language testing. An impression of comprehension will manifest during the give-and-take of a history in the precision of patient responses to the examiner's questions. Some questions can purposefully stress syntax to betray subtle deficits. Asking the patient, "If the lion is eaten by the lamb, which one died?" could by probability of the nouns be guessed the lamb, but one who comprehends the grammar will name the lion. Command following of increasing linguistic complexity is another way to assess language comprehension with single commands, then multistep commands, then out-of-sequence commands, then contralateral commands, and all this in composite. Asking the patient, "Before sticking out your tongue, but after pointing to the ceiling with your left hand, put your right hand over your eyes" should result in the raising of a left hand, the covering of eyes with the right hand, and the sticking out of their tongue in that order.

Fluency, naming, and repetition, and comprehension are the key components of characterizing traditional aphasia patterns. Language is a matter of linking ideas formulaically; impairments in speech are almost always present in writing. If the patient is literate, asking the patient to follow a written command, read a sentence aloud, or write a written response to a written prompt are ways of assessing how the apparatus of reading engages other language processes. Every patient with a communication problem should be asked to speak and to write to determine if it is an articulation problem (dysarthria) or a language problem (aphasia), because communication is impaired in both speech and written word in language disorders.

To demonstrate the above categorization, consider three classic aphasias: Broca, Wernicke, and conduction aphasia. Broca aphasia is nonfluent with a better preservation of comprehension. Wernicke aphasia is the converse of Broca, preserving fluency but losing comprehension of others. Wernicke predicted that there must be a band connecting the comprehending temporal lobe to the fluent frontal lobe for which repeating or dictating speech is carried through. Sure enough, a conduction aphasia localizes to the arcuate fasciculus that bridges Broca and Wernicke areas and is an aphasia marked by the inability to repeat (a loss of parroting) with relative sparing of other fluent or comprehensive elements.

There are additional properties of communication that can be evaluated. While the left frontal-temporal structures are involved in language as described above, the right frontal-temporal structures are involved in related processes like prosody (the musicality and rhythmicity of speech), with additional localizations to the cerebellum and the coarse scanning speech of a robocaller or the inebriated. Offering poetic lines of different meters will detect the ability to entrain prosodic rhythms (e.g., "Shall I compare thee to a summer's day?" vs. "Much of a which of a wind"). The difference between "lighthouse keeping" and "light housekeeping" is in its prosody. Some patients cannot produce this distinction, which is a more anterior or frontal lesion, while others cannot hear the difference, which is a more posterior and temporal lesion.

Attention and Concentration

Attention is a flashlight. It can be focused to accomplish a simple task among competing stimuli. It has an *object*. This can be tested by simple commands such as inviting the patient to open or close their eyes, stick out their tongue, or count the number of fingers shown to them. Concentration is a bucket. It holds vigilance across time and environmental disturbance. It has an *objective*. This can be tested by sustained or complex commands like inviting the patient to count backward by threes or spell WORLD or TRUCK backward. For standardized tests, Trails A (connecting a sequence of dots from 1 to 25) and Trails B (connecting a sequence of set-shifting numbers and letters 1–13 and A–L) have easily obtained norms by age and education and reflect attention and concentration, respectively.

Impulsivity and perseveration are the dark sides of attention and concentration. Contradictory commands like, "tap once when I tap twice; tap twice when I tap once," or "tap once when I tap once; don't tap when I tap twice," catch perseveration or impulsivity.

Deficits in attention, concentration, or excesses of impulsivity and perseveration implicate the frontal lobes and their attendant circuits.

Memory

The resilience of prior experience and knowledge's traces on the brain and the pathways for their recovery are traditionally tested by immediate registration of a few words, items, or a task; then short-term recall of items, words, or tasks at longer and longer intervals such as after 5 minutes, 10 minutes, or 15 minutes. There may be some lateralization with language-based memories processed through the left hippocampus and spatially based memories in the right hippocampus. Therefore one trick at the start of the interview is to show the patient an object and where you are hiding it, telling them as you do that it is the patient's task to remind you before you leave the room that there is a hidden object and where it is located. Episodic memory of recent autobiographical or current events can be inquired of but demands corroboration by another source. Semantic memory of common facts about their world is essentially a game of high-frequency *Jeopardy* (e.g., Who was the first president of the United States? On what continent can the country Slovenia be found?), but educational background impacts responses, so it becomes important to determine the baseline fund of world knowledge. Patients often know much about something that the clinician knows precious little. A brief biography of the person (e.g., Where did they grow up?, What is their occupation?, Do they have any hobbies?) is needed for assurances of semantic memory. A chronology of their disease is insufficient.

Spatial, Constructive, and Gestural Properties

The inner world tries to make sense of the outer world to perform many day-to-day functions, from tying one's shoes to getting around town. Space is divided into the personal (body), peripersonal (within our grasp), and extrapersonal (the environmental stage across which we move and navigate). Humans' midline symmetry makes questions of right-left discrimination easy enough to assess by asking the patient to indicate the side of a specific body part. Praxis is the ability to carry out overlearned sequence commands by miming or with the materials necessary to complete it set before them. Manual praxis should be tested on both sides for one-limb actions (e.g., swat a bug, brush off

a shoulder; hammer a nail, cut with scissors, use a key to unlock and open a door) as well as a few cooperative maneuvers (e.g., shuffle and deal a deck of cards or thread a needle and sew, tie your shoes or a necktie). Oral-buccal praxis is demonstrated by pretending to blow out a candle, lick an ice cream cone, suck on a straw, grin, or scowl. Emblematic gestures can be assessed by asking the patient to show you disagreement and agreement (thumbs-up, thumbs-down). Constructional abilities can be investigated by having the patient draw or copy shapes or build forms from blocks, navigate, or interpret directions of familiar places or locations.

Integrative Functions of Mental Status

Insight into a patient's own case and circumstance can be impaired (an anosognosia), and those patients who recognize their deficit can be impaired by judging the impairment with indifference (an anosodiaphoria). These are crucial components to assessing a person's capacity in making medical decisions. Reasoning can be assessed through presenting hypothetical scenarios in which a problem is to be solved or a moral dilemma is to be resolved. The patient's answers only tell us what they say they should do. It tells us with no assurance if, when actually in that situation themselves, they would act as they say they do.

Some basic thematic perception or consequential reasoning can be obtained by showing the patient an illustration depicting a dynamic interpersonal issue and asking the patient to surmise the consequences of it or the reasons for its outcome. In the classic "Cookie Thief" illustration used in stroke assessment a distracted mother is unaware of both an overflowing sink as well as her son about to fall off a stool in his pursuit of a top-shelf cookie jar. One could ask the patient why the sink is overflowing, or why the child might not have just asked his mother for the cookies, or what the mother will feel when she discovers her fallen child. Like physical strength, metaphysical strength testing is confrontational and is only reliably graded if the examiner is without deficiencies of their own.

While talking with the patient and observing their behavior, the patient's mood (how they feel) and affect (how they display how they feel) are not to be neglected, and if needed can be provoked by asking the patient to act out in voice and gesture a short script (e.g., I want you to say this line, "The snow will be melting soon," as if you are happy and then as if you are disappointed), or asking them to read your emotion as you act out a line.

Cranial Nerves

It is here deficits disclose a localization to the brainstem. There are 12 paired cranial nerves (CNs). Each pair should be compared to its fellow for relative deficits too subtle to apprehend if tested twinly.

For olfactory testing, ask the patient to close their eyes and depress first one nostril and then the other as various familiar scents such as chocolate or coffee are presented. Avoid a noxious substance like alcohol or ammonia, which tests the trigeminal nerve's afferent divisions.

Optic testing includes visual acuity with a Snellen chart or using a newspaper (headlines are about 20/400, subheadlines 20/200, column 20/60, and want ads 20/40). For visual field testing, divide the visual fields like a cartesian plot, and, checking each eye individually, briefly present one, two, or five fingers for their counting. Holding out your fingers too long and patients will throw a saccade in their direction, but just a flash of one, two, or five fingers briefly is all that is required for it to register in their vision for counting. Funduscopic assessment and pupillary reaction should be tested after vision screening so that the blinding light does not interfere with acuity.

Extraocular movements are innervated by the oculomotor, trochlear, and abducens nerves. A sweep of superior, inferior, and inward eye movements as well as presence of ptosis would identify oculomotor nerve problems and, if partial, could indicate partial nerve, individual nerve, or primary muscular problems. Failure of lateral eye movements abducting an eye from primary gaze would signify an abducens nerve or muscle injury. A head tilt to correct one's vision would indicate trochlear nerve weakness. When assessing a patient with double vision, it is important to test the movements with both eyes open and with one eye closed at a time. Double vision in one eye only is an eye or lens problem, not a neuro-ophtho problem. Double vision that resolves when one eye is covered suggests a neuro-ophtho problem.

Trigeminal nerve function is assessed gently by applying a bitter cold instrument (or pinprick, or the sharp end of a broken Q-tip) and by light touch of facial sensation on the forehead (V_1), the maxillary prominence (V_2), and between the lower corner of the mouth and the chin (V_3). The trigeminal nerve controls the muscles of mastication, so asking the patient to bite or clamp down and feeling these muscles can give a sense of atrophy or weakness.

The muscles of facial expression, tearing and salivation, sensation of external ear canal, and taste on the anterior two-thirds of the tongue are controlled by the facial nerve. A screening assessment includes how the patient can wrinkle their brow, smile, and puff out their cheeks, and slowed or reduced activation compared to the fuller and faster side would indicate a weakness.

Hearing is facilitated by the vestibulocochlear nerve. The cochlear apparatus's appreciation of a finger rub agitating the air near the ear assesses high-frequency hearing, whereas a finger tap near the ear assesses low-frequency hearing. An asymmetric impairment can then be defined with a low-frequency tuning fork under a modified Rinne test. Tell the patient they are going to listen to the tone of the tuning fork in one of two positions, off the mastoid process behind the ear or next to the ear itself. Those who hear the tone clearer through the mastoid have better bone than air conduction and this represents a conductive hearing loss; those who hear the tone better in the air have better air conduction and therefore have a sensorineural hearing loss. Further definition of whether the hearing loss is cochlear or retrocochlear (i.e., of the nerve as from schwannoma or cortical deafness from stroke or tumor) can be discerned by whispering 5 or 10 words in each ear clearly. Unless the cochlear-based sensorineural loss is quite severe, a close whisper will still be intelligible, but if the damage is retrocochlear in the nerve or cortex, then fewer words will be intelligible on the affected ear than the unaffected ear. The vestibular system is embarrassed when balance and torsional, latent, non–direction changing nystagmus is present.

Swallowing and the gag reflex are accomplished by the glossopharyngeal and vagus nerves, so observation of palatal asymmetry can indicate weakness. Asking the patient to stick their tongue out to look for atrophy or deviation can indicate ipsilateral hypoglossal weakness. If the patient knows they could previously roll their tongue lengthwise, asymmetry in the roll-up can indicate both side and severity of impairment. In cases of functional tongue weakness, recovery of weakness by tongue curling can be the essential and only positive feature to make the diagnosis.

Assessing shoulder shrug and rotation of the head for asymmetric weakness will expose a defect in spinal accessory nerves.

Movement and Power

Inspection of the muscle should begin with a simple differentiation of increased or decreased bulk. If there is reduced bulk, are fasciculations seen? If there is increased bulk, is it hard or spongy? In testing motor activity of a muscle, ensure good support and rest of all joints except the one about which the muscle attends.

Next, consider movements. Are they purposeful and voluntary or are there additional movements including tremor, dystonia, chorea, and dyskinesia, or are there reduced movements such as bradykinesia or breakdown in the smooth nature of the movements? Having the patient tap their fingers, or if arthritis is their excuse, rotate their hand at the wrist as if screwing in a light-bulb can betray these slower, ratcheting movements. These are considerations both while the person is distracted and when they are focusing on their movements. At times, an examiner may ask a patient to rest their hands in their lap, relax as best they can, and then tell the months of the year backward or count backward by fours. The goal is not their accuracy but that in distraction, sometimes hyperkinetic movements emerge. Examination of finer impairments in the fingers and hands can sometimes be exposed by having the patient hold a pen at the terminus and draw Archimedes spirals and a large "X's" across the page with both hands to look for oscillations or micrographia.

In passive range of motion about a joint, consider whether a muscle's tone is either increased or decreased. If tone is increased, define its character as spastic (velocity dependent), paratonic (force dependent), or lead pipe rigid (constant, independent of force or velocity).

Assessment and grading of power are better described as full to confrontation, partial resistance, maintains posture against gravity, facilitated with gravity removed, activation of muscle without movement across the joint, or no activity whatsoever. Numbers are really only helpful if kept to the strict Medical Research Council grading scale and are best when tested by the same clinician over time rather than with intra-clinician scoring. The limb should be positioned by the clinician so that the muscle's action is isolated across one joint in the face of gravity, and the remainder of the limb otherwise supported. Take, for example, a wrist-drop. It could

be a stroke at the hand-knob area of the frontal lobe contralateral to the injured hand, which would result in all the actions of the hands to be weakened. It could also be a radial nerve palsy at the spiral groove, which should spare muscles controlled by the median and ulnar nerves. If the hand's strength is assessed flailing about and flopped over the wrist, the leverage exerted by even well-working tendons controlled by median and ulnar nerves is limited, so all the fingers appear weak. But once the hand is aligned on a plane, strength of the flexor pollicis longus and the abductor digiti minimi seem to reappear, but wrist extension and finger extension (properties of the radial nerve) remain weakened. The patient is prescribed a tincture of time for a stunned nerve instead of tissue plasminogen activator for a presumed stroke, and all because of an examiner's punctilious technique in assessing power.

Once the patient is positioned for testing, the clinician then tells the patient to activate the muscle *before* providing you provide resistance. Avoid saying "don't let me pull you" which can be confusing. Rather instruct to "push," "pull," "lift," and "keep it strong" are straightforward. This gives you a chance to see and feel: no activation (0), a flicker (1), activation in the plane of rest (2), sustained activation against gravity (3), some engagement against the clinician's resistance (4), and full strength (5). Strength is graded by the maximum achieved, not what was maintained. A patient that almost beats you in an arm wrestling match had a 5, even if in the end you overpowered him.

Sensation

The sensory examination should consider both primary modalities, including pain and temperature, light touch, vibration, joint position, and, if these are sufficiently intact, integrative higher cortical sensory modalities such as texture, shape, forms, weights, stereognosis, and graphesthesia.

For the primary modalities, it is useful to have access to diagrams of the dermatomes (the arrangement of sensation of a given nerve root) as well as a chart of the individual territories of the peripheral nerve so you have something to compare your findings to. If the patient makes a specific complaint of sensory changes, ask them with one finger to trace as best they can the areas involved and you take note of it (sometimes even asking them to use a marker to outline it). Next, the examiner should start in the center of the involved area and work outward to inward with the stimulus (temperature, pinprick, vibration, proprioception, light touch) to see if they all track in a similar territory or if there is splitting or irregularities, as these have localizing value (presence of temperature and pinprick but absence of vibration or proprioception, e.g., indicate a large-fiber neuropathy, and even a dorsal column spinal cord disorder). The distribution of the impairment across a territory on the skin is important, but so is the dispersal of the degree of its impairment. Something equally impaired distally and proximally without a gradient may be more central, whereas something which is worse distally and improves proximally suggests a peripheral process.

The "degree" of impairment is tested differently for different stimuli. Sharp does not require you to carry pins. Snap off a Q-tip or a tongue depressor and hold it between your fingers loose enough that with a quick light jab into your hand, the sharp end makes contact with the palm but yields to it, rebounding gently backward through your fingers rather than pressing forward into your skin. A sense of sharp with minimal depression on the surface is what you are looking for. Some examiners assess a patient's response to cold, but one should ensure that the cool metal of a tuning fork is sufficient; if not it can be run under cold water. For vibration a low-frequency tuning fork should be placed firmly on a bony protuberance to resonate while the examiner waits until the vibration extinguishes. In the case of testing vibration on a finger or toe the examiner places their finger on the undersurface being tested. In this way if they still feel the vibration coursing through flesh and bone to the opposite side while the patient no longer does, the examiner can be sure confrontationally there is an impairment. Position sense (proprioception) is an alternate to vibration. The examiner passively moves a finger or toe across a joint and marks the degree of excursion from a neutral position that the patient first appreciates *when* it moved and *in what direction*.

Extinction of stimuli is an important parietal sign. It can be specific and affect personal space (does not dress/wash/shave one side of face/body, or when touching the patient's left and right hands simultaneously, they appreciate only one hand being touched). It can affect peripersonal space (in line bisection the division is displaced off the meridian, or in cancellation/word-finding tests targets are missed on one side of the visual field, or when presented with two stimuli, they ignore one side's stimulus). It can also affect extrapersonal space (does not appreciate a side of the room and/or sounds/sights/activity on a particular side of the room). A visually impaired patient moves their head to get the rest of their world into the remaining visual field. A neglectful patient sees no reason to; their world is a fragment viewed as complete.

These tests are usually performed on the appendages where sensitivity will be greatest, such as the fingertips or palm, but axial proprioceptive health should be examined by having the patient perform a Romberg test. The patient stands with feet together heel to heel and toe to toe with arms outstretched before them and then closes their eyes. If they broaden their stance or move to support themselves with a wall or offered arm, the test is positive.

Coordination

Appendicular coordination of movements can be assessed by finger to nose, heel to shin, or rapid alternating movements for signs of dysmetria, inconsistent in amplitude, and degree of impaired estimation of the target. Having the patient's index finger follow yours around but not make contact, as if your mirrored twin, can be very sensitive and reduces the excuse of arthritis at the shoulder inhibiting accuracy. Indeed, an arm cast to the hand, so long as the metacarpophalangeals are exposed, can mirror minute movements accurately. Incidentally, asterixis can be assessed with just a raised finger, too, not only with a hyperextended hand at the wrist. Some examiners are not able to *see* subtle irregular movements, but they can *hear* them. Have the patient tap a rhythm out with their finger on the table, an overturned cup, or the pendant of their wearable telemetry and listen for the wobble in the rhythm. Alternatively, making a small circle on a piece of paper and asking the patient to peck with their pen as accurately as they can in the circle with both hands will provide a measurable account of the accuracy and precision lost to dysmetrias. Axial coordination is judged from dysmetria of the trunk during changes in the patient's position from lying to sitting, sitting to standing, and maintaining

Gait and Stance

The patient's spontaneous gait should be examined for signs of broadening stance (a general sign of imbalance), reduced clearance (dropped foot), a reduction in stride length (shuffling), a scissoring gait, the number of steps to complete a turn, and an inefficient or uneconomical gait. The examiner can influence the gait to put stress on the nervous system by asking the patient to walk backward, run, or walk heel to toe.

Reflexes

A reflex is a short arc between afferent sensory and efferent motor components. Testing reflexes can quickly survey the general health of the nervous system because a careful balance must be maintained for normal reflexes. We describe the reflexes here, but generally, they should be incorporated into your examination when you are evaluating the relevant portion of the neuroaxis (those pertaining to the cortex when evaluating cortical function, cranial nerve reflexes when evaluating the cranial nerves, etc.). But for convenience, we present them here.

Cortical (or "frontal") release signs, the glabellar tap for parkinsonism, or the suck, snout, and grasp represent higher cortical inhibitions that govern certain behavioral reflexes. More localizable cortical reflexes are the antigravity reflexes of decortication posturing (flexed arms and legs extended) and decerebration posturing (extended and pronated arms and legs extended).

Pupillary constriction to direct and consensual light as well as near are important for evaluating CN II-III connectivity. The corneal reflex tests CN V and VII, the jaw jerk tests CN V and VII, and the gag reflex tests CN X actions.

There are superficial, nociceptive reflexes whose irritation results in motor response (e.g., abdominal, cremasteric, bulbocavernosus, anal wink, plantar). And there are the deeper proprioceptive reflexes elicited with a hammer on tendons. Reduced proprioceptive reflexes signify either weakened sensory inputs (from neuropathy) or weakened motor outputs (lower motor neuron injuries in the peripheral nervous system). In contrast, increased reflexes bespeak loss of governing inhibitor mechanisms and therefore signal aberrant upper motor neuron injuries of the central nervous system. To test a reflex, support the limb isolating the joint across which the muscle and tendon are to be tested. The muscle should be slightly loaded by this position so that the tendon is a little stretched. Then the tendon is lightly struck. If clonus is provoked, this is a grade of 4. If activation of the muscle is accompanied by an unrelated muscle across an additional joint, that is a grade of 3. If only the muscle in question is activated, that is a grade of 2. If the muscle does not activate unless a distracting maneuver is performed (e.g., clenched jaw, patient hooks fingers and pulls apart), that is a grade of 1. If despite such maneuvers there is no activation, that is a grade of 0.

The Functional Examination

Conversion disorders, today referred to as "functional neurological disorders," are disturbances in which the complaint is superficially mimicking a neurological symptom (weakness, ataxia, aphasia), and yet the fundamental integrity of the nervous system's anatomic structure is preserved. Hence the word "functional," indicating somehow an uncoupling between structural and functional impairments. This can sometimes be called a "hardware" versus "software" dichotomy in which functional syndromes are bugs in the "software" of planning and feedback in experience or execution of action. The core element on examination for functional phenomena is to demonstrate distractible recovery and/or entrainable distortions to the presentation. A person with an essential tremor in their left hand when outstretched will maintain the same frequency and amplitude regardless of if they start to waffle and waver their right hand fast or slow. However, in a functional disorder the speed or amplitude in the nonaffected hand will influence the affected hand, thus entraining it. The "astasia abasia" of functional gaits can often be distracted into normal function when the patient is asked to walk backward or slide across the floor as if ice skating, or waltz with the interviewer, or hop. A functionally blind person can be asked to read random words on cards, but inserting a card with profanity can often elicit a smile or blush or dilation of the pupils to indicate it was read and registered subconsciously. The Hoover test is a familiar test that has its application for functional neurological presentations. Functional examinations often require the clinician to consider the patient's problem and devise bespoke maneuvers to distract or entrain in such a way that it can definitely be shown that components of the nervous system seemingly lesioned are in fact working perfectly. In other words, the examiner demonstrates the person has preserved function that would be incompatible with the symptom in question if those structures responsible for that function were actually lesioned. Functional examinations can pose a challenge to the uninterested clinician, but their successful application yields a diagnosis and provides means of explaining afterward to patient how the test shows whatever they fear, like multiple sclerosis or stroke, cannot be. That physical reassurance can often be curative.

CONCLUSION

In all of medicine the neurologic examination represents the most elegant means of arriving at a clinical diagnosis without the complete reliance on technological tools. For well over a century, the examination has been expertly crafted and refined and always performed in a systematic sequential manner so that it is reproducible and easily understood when presented. The examination comprehensively describes the normal functioning nervous system and it slowly evolved over time to correlate every abnormality or deviation from the norm with a specific neuropathologic finding. Localization is the hallmark of the neurologic examination (Figs. 1.1–1.3). While the examination taken in toto can seem intimidating, if it is always performed in the same careful stepwise manner, it becomes relatively easy and routine, much like learning a new language. When performed properly, it directs us toward a focused differential diagnosis eliminating the need for unnecessary testing, which can be both expensive and, in some cases, pose significant risk.

The examination can be performed in any setting, ambulatory or emergency, and modified in critical care situations. In an emergency situation a rapid assessment can properly direct care leading to a reduction in disability and an improved survival rate. It is also useful in monitoring the progress of a patient over time. Once the examination has been mastered by the examiner, it can then be tailored depending on the specific disease presentation. A complaint of diplopia would be approached differently in an elderly patient with cognitive decline than a young female. While the main principle of the neurologic examination is to arrive at an accurate diagnosis with an understanding of the underlying pathology, it serves another important purpose that is often overlooked. The comprehensive examination creates a bond between the patient and the clinician. From the patient's perspective, their complaints are being taken seriously and the clinician is taking great pains to find clues to diagnose their problem, alleviate their fears, and help solve the problem. In conclusion, our goal is to make every primary care clinician and healthcare professional who is likely to see neurologic patients comfortable with performing and interpreting the neurologic examination.

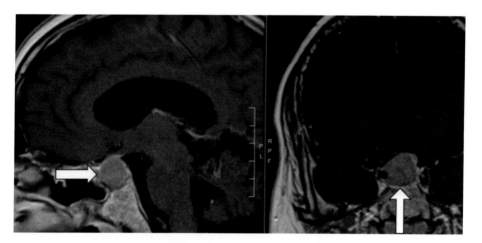

Fig. 1.1 Examination notable for positional headache worsened lying down. Fundoscopic examination shows right greater than left papilledema and optic nerve atrophy. There is blurred visual acuity and there is a reduced visual perception in the temporal fields, left greater than right. No other obvious signs. Axially we have no cortical signs but general cephalgia to indicate the lesion is in the skull, and there are no brainstem signs lower than II. Coronally we have a temporal predominant hemianopia, which localizes to central compression on the optic chiasma. Sagittally we have right greater than left papilledema and left greater than right temporal field deficits, which would indicate a right-sided predominant lesion. Below is the lesion's location.

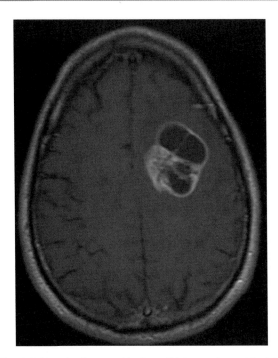

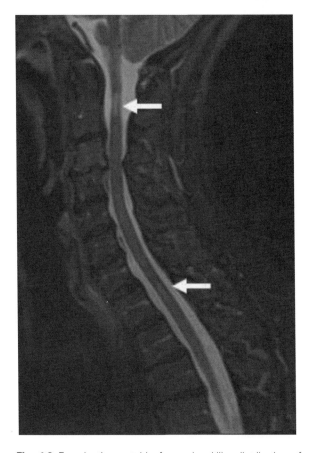

Fig. 1.2 Examination notable for mild inattention with right-sided gaze preference, nonfluent aphasia, some incoordination, clumsiness, and mild weakness in right hand for complex gestures. No other findings. A higher cortical function like nonfluent aphasia provides sagittal localization (language being of the left hemisphere) as well as coronally (frontal-temporal), and no other findings like cranial nerve findings or lower suggest the lesion is axially limited to the cortex and subcortex.

Fig. 1.3 Examination notable for a shawl-like distribution of reduced sensation to pinprick and temperature as well as an additional floating level of sensory loss above the navel. The reflexes are hyperreflexive throughout with sustained clonus bilaterally in the feet. The localization of a shawl-like distribution and a floating level suggests central cord involvement, and increased tone and reflexes indicate cortical tract involvement which as bilateral and sparing higher cortical function. This would place the lesion in the spinal cord. Of particular note, the shawl-like distribution indicates a high lesion in the cervical spine, whereas the additional floating level of denser anesthesia indicates a lesion a few vertebrae above T10 or so.

Basic Neurologic Examination

Mental Status Examination
a. Level of consciousness—alert, drowsy, stupor, coma
b. Orientation—person, place, time
c. Attention—name the days of the week and spell WORLD backward
d. Language—spontaneous speech, naming to confrontation, comprehension, repetition, prosody, reading out loud and for comprehension, writing
e. Memory—immediate recall, short and long term
f. Praxis, right-left discrimination, calculations, gnosis, constructional ability

Cranial Nerve Examination
1. Olfactory—smell check each nostril separately with a nonnoxious odor
2. Optic—visual acuity, visual fields, funduscopic examination, pupils (afferent pathways)
3. 4, and 6—Oculomotor, trochlear, abducens—extraocular movements, ptosis, pupils (efferent pathways)
5. Trigeminal—facial sensation in ophthalmic, maxillary and mandibular divisions, muscles of mastication, jaw jerk, sensory component of corneal reflex
7. Facial—muscles of facial expression, tearing and salivation, sensation of external ear canal, motor component of corneal reflex, taste on the anterior two-thirds of the tongue
8. Vestibulocochlear—hearing, vestibular function, balance
9. Glossopharyngeal—gag reflex sensory component, sensation on soft palate, taste on the posterior one-third of the tongue
10. Vagus—gag reflex motor component describing symmetric or asymmetric elevation of the palate
11. Spinal accessory—sternocleidomastoid and trapezius muscles
12. Hypoglossal—tongue strength and bulk, are fasciculations detected? Is protrusion midline or is there deviation to one side?

Motor Examination
a. Power—grade as 0–5
0. No muscle activation
1. Muscle contraction without movement
2. Movement with gravity eliminated
3. Movement against gravity only
4. Movement against gravity and some additional resistance
5. Movement against full resistance
b. Muscle tone—hypotonia, hypertonia, spasticity, paratonia, lead pipe rigidity
c. Muscle bulk—is atrophy present?
d. Observation for tremor, fasciculations, myokymia, myoclonus, asterixis

Sensory Examination
a. Primary modalities—pain and temperature, touch, vibration, joint position
b. Cortical modalities—graphesthesia, stereognosis, two-point discrimination, extinction to double simultaneous stimulation

Coordination
a. Finger to nose, heel to shin, rapid alternating movements

Gait
a. Stance, unassisted ambulation, tandem gait

Reflexes
a. Deep tendon reflexes—grade as 0–4
0. Absent
1. Diminished but present
2. Normal
3. Hyperactive
4. Clonus (unsustained or sustained)
b. Plantar, abdominal, cremasteric, bulbocavernosus, anal wink
c. Cortical release—suck, rooting, snout, grasp, palmomental, glabellar

"For the full bibliography list, please use the pincode on the inside front cover to access the electronic version of the text at ebooks.health.elsevier.com."

Introduction to Neuroimaging*

Thomas C. Lee and Andrew G. Schneider

INTRODUCTION

Neurologic symptoms such as headache and low back pain are common reasons for patients to present to their primary care physician. Imaging plays a crucial role in the diagnosis of a wide range of neurologic disorders. However, radiology training in medical school or non-radiology residencies is sparse, and clinicians often have limited knowledge of different imaging modalities, imaging study appropriateness, and interpretation of emergent findings. Moreover, neuroimaging routinely employs advanced modalities such as magnetic resonance imaging (MRI) and is rapidly evolving in both technological developments and the understanding of imaging manifestations of pathophysiology. A significant number of these advanced imaging studies are requested by primary care physicians. Furthermore, overutilization of imaging resources has come under much scrutiny. The American College of Physicians emphasizes the appropriate use of diagnostic tests and has identified 37 situations in which a test does not reflect high-value care; these include three neuroimaging scenarios: imaging for low back pain, recurrent classic migraine, and simple syncope.

An understanding of imaging as it pertains to the diagnosis and management of neurologic disorders will aid the primary care physician in ordering the most appropriate examination, interpreting the radiologists'

reports, determining the next steps in management, and making appropriate referrals to specialists. The purpose of this chapter is to review the basic concepts of neuroimaging that are relevant to the primary care physician, specifically the appropriateness of imaging tests, typical imaging techniques and terminologies, factors to consider prior to contrast agent administration, and the imaging findings of common pathologies.

APPROPRIATENESS OF IMAGING

While the care of the individual patient is paramount, imaging resources are limited in most clinical environments. Certain imaging modalities are better suited to evaluate specific patient presentations or neurologic conditions, and responsible stewardship of these limited resources allows for better care of the entire community. Unnecessary or unwarranted imaging increases the burden of care on the patient, can be psychologically or emotionally stressful for the patient, and incurs additional financial costs. There are also small health risks to the patient with some imaging studies, such as the exposure to ionizing radiation from x-ray and computed tomography (CT) studies.

To help clinicians make informed decisions about imaging studies, the American College of Radiology (ACR) maintains an online list of Appropriateness Criteria (https://acsearch.acr.org/list). This resource summarizes the current literature regarding the role of imaging in the evaluation of common neurologic presentations and serves as a guide for choosing an appropriate imaging test. These recommendations assess the utility and safety of different imaging studies and rank them from most to least appropriate for each clinical scenario.

*Based on George E, Guenette, JP, Lee TC. Introduction to neuroimaging. *Am J Med*. 2018;131(4):346–356. ISSN 0002-9343, https://doi.org/10.1016/j.amjmed.2017.11.014. (https://www.sciencedirect.com/science/article/pii/S0002934317312068)

Patient-friendly summaries of many Appropriateness Criteria recommendations are also available to download or print.

Multiple other organizations publish guidelines that include recommendations on diagnostic and interventional imaging studies specific to their field, such as the American Academy of Neurology (https://www.aan.com/practice/guidelines) and the American Heart Association (https://professional.heart.org/en/guidelines-and-statements). While the ACR Appropriateness Criteria attempts to synthesize the recommendations from other organizations, clinicians are encouraged to consider the recommendations that are best suited for their patient.

IMAGING TECHNIQUES AND TERMINOLOGY

Modern radiology offers multiple imaging modalities and techniques for the evaluation of neurologic conditions. In the primary care environment, CT is often the best modality for evaluating acute presentations. MRI is preferred for diagnosis or monitoring of chronic conditions, or in situations in which minimizing radiation exposure is important (e.g., pregnancy). Certain clinical presentations can also be well evaluated via ultrasound or nuclear medicine studies. Plain film radiographs (x-rays) have limited utility in neuroradiology outside of specific scenarios.

Computed Tomography

CT uses ionizing radiation (x-rays) to generate three-dimensional images of the body's internal structures, generally correlated with their relative densities. Materials with significant density differences are easier to distinguish between (e.g., bone and air), while tissues with more subtle variations in density can appear less differentiated (e.g., gray matter and white matter). Compared to other types of imaging, the speed, ubiquity, and cost often make CT imaging the most accessible modality.

CT scans of the head and spine are often performed without contrast. Administration of iodinated contrast can be considered for patients who cannot undergo MRI if there is suspicion of intracranial metastases or spinal surgery complication such as infection. Spine CT with intrathecal contrast (CT myelography) is useful to assess the patency of the spinal canal and neural foramen in patients with radicular symptoms when MRI is contraindicated or nondiagnostic.

On head CT, common causes of increased density/attenuation (bright areas) within the brain are calcifications, hemorrhage, or contrast. Decreased density/attenuation (dark areas) is a nonspecific finding in the brain that can be due to infarct, mass, or edema. While the density difference between gray matter and white matter is subtle, careful adjustment of the imaging window can allow for the parenchymal characteristics to be discerned. Normal cerebrospinal fluid (CSF) is low density (dark) and surrounds the brain, which makes it useful for assessing the cortical sulci, brain symmetry, and ventricular size.

Magnetic Resonance Imaging

MRI uses strong magnetic fields and nonionizing radio waves to measure variations in the magnetic properties of tissue. The chemical composition and conditions within a tissue impart particular magnetic signatures that allow for imaging characterization. While a straightforward head CT scan can often be completed in a matter of seconds, the subtlety of the magnetic fields within the human body means that a brain MRI usually takes several minutes to complete. A patient who is unable to lie supine and motionless within the MRI machine for this duration of time may require additional accommodations (e.g., anxiolytic medications) or a differing imaging modality.

Because the strong magnetic fields of MRI interact with metallic objects within the body, certain precautions are necessary to avoid catastrophic outcomes. Electronic devices (e.g., pacemakers, pumps, stimulators) can malfunction, and small metallic objects (e.g., aneurysm clips, shrapnel, orbital foreign bodies) can become dislodged. Since the MRI magnetic field is variable and dynamic, a previous MRI of a different body part does not guarantee safety. The presence of a metallic object or device is not necessarily an absolute contraindication for MRI, however, and clinicians are recommended to refer to their institution's guidelines or speak with a radiologist to clarify the risks and options.

By altering the magnetic fields and patterns of radio waves in an MRI, the characteristic signals from different tissues can be used to compose unique sequences or image types. Institutional protocols vary, but a brain MRI may include diffusion-weighted images (DWI), susceptibility-weighted images (SWI), gradient echo (GRE) images, T1- and T2-weighted images, and T2-weighted images with fluid suppression (T2-fluid attenuation inversion recovery [FLAIR]). MRI contrast agents have high T1 signal (bright), and additional post-contrast T1-weighted sequences are obtained in contrast-enhanced exams.

Areas of high signal (bright) on DWI with corresponding low signal (dark) on apparent diffusion coefficient (ADC) maps are referred to as areas of low or restricted diffusivity. These denote areas of infarction, pus, or high cellularity and are important for the evaluation of suspected stroke, infection, or malignancy. Given the high sensitivity of DWI for these critical pathologies, the DWI/ADC series will often be prioritized if the patient is unable to tolerate a complete MRI scan. In a similar vein, SWI/GRE images are particularly sensitive to metal such as iron or calcium and are useful for identifying areas of hemorrhage and calcification.

Spine MRI typically involves T1- and T2-weighted images, and a fat-suppressed T2-weighted sequence such as short tau inversion recovery (STIR). As in the brain, the postcontrast images will be T1-weighted sequences. Due to the geometric constraints of the strong magnetic field involved, MRI has an innate tradeoff between the size of the imaging field and the level of imaging detail. While this is not often an issue in the head, attempting to image the entire length of the spine all at once results in decreased image resolution and interpretability. The spine is therefore usually imaged in segments, and clinicians should provide guidance to the radiology team regarding the patient's symptoms or area of interest within the spine to ensure optimum image quality.

Angiography

Both CT angiography (CTA) and MR angiography (MRA) can be used to assess intracranial vasculature. CTA requires administration of iodinated contrast and has the advantage of superior spatial resolution at the cost of radiation exposure. MRA is often performed based on the phenomenon of flow-related enhancement (called "time-of-flight MRA") without the need for contrast administration. Importantly, a noncontrast MRA is only for assessment of vasculature and will not identify enhancing lesions.

Other

Although CT and MRI are the primary tools in neuroimaging and the most likely to be encountered by the clinician, ultrasound, nuclear medicine studies, and radiographs (x-rays) have certain specific and limited roles.

Beyond the neonatal period, ultrasound is not routinely employed to assess intracranial structures. Instead, ultrasound is primarily used in adult neuroimaging to evaluate carotid artery flow in the setting of transient cerebral ischemia or cerebral embolism.

Nuclear imaging studies also have specific functions in neurologic evaluation. The cortex avidly metabolizes glucose and so appears bright on 18F-fluorodeoxyglucose positron emission tomography (18FDG PET) studies. Some metastatic lesions, however, can display even greater avidity than normal brain tissue and therefore can be detected and followed on PET imaging. Gallium-68 radiotracers can be used to assess the patency of shunt catheters as well as for obstructive hydrocephalus. Nuclear medicine DaTscans are routinely used to assess basal ganglia function in the diagnosis of parkinsonism. PET imaging can also readily display malignant lesions in the head, neck, and vertebral bodies of the spine.

Finally, plain film radiographs (x-rays) have a limited role in modern neuroimaging. Their primary roles are ruling out metallic objects in the orbits before MRI; osseous assessment of subacute, posttraumatic, or postsurgical lumbar back pain; and assessing the integrity of VP shunt catheters and shunt valve settings.

CONTRAST CONSIDERATIONS

Intravenous contrast is primarily used to highlight vascular structures and to better detect and characterize lesions. Because of the increased time, higher costs, and small risk of contrast extravasation or reaction, contrast-enhanced studies should be requested only for specific indications. CT contrast is best indicated for detecting intracranial metastases, vascular assessment (CTA), and postsurgical spinal infections. MRI contrast is useful for assessing tumors, infections, demyelinating disease, vascular pathologies, and posttreatment changes. If there are any questions about the appropriateness of a contrast-enhanced study, clinicians are advised to speak with a radiologist.

Renal Function

In nondiabetic patients without acute kidney injury (AKI) and with an estimated glomerular filtration rate (eGFR) greater than $30\,\text{mL/min/1.73 m}^2$, there is little evidence that iodinated contrast media is an independent risk factor for AKI. There is, however, an increased risk of AKI in diabetic patients with eGFR less than 44 mL/min/1.73 m². Neither threshold is an absolute contraindication to contrast administration, and intravenous fluids can be given prophylactically if needed. Patients with anuric end-stage renal disease on dialysis can safely receive iodinated contrast media, as there is no risk of further renal damage. There is no need to adjust the patient's hemodialysis schedule following contrast administration. In patients on hemodialysis, patients with AKI, or patients with severe or end-stage renal disease (eGFR <30 mL/min/1.73 m²) who are not on hemodialysis, certain classes of gadolinium-based MRI contrast agents (GBCA) are contraindicated due to the risk of nephrogenic systemic fibrosis.

Contrast Reactions

Reactions to iodinated contrast are rare (0.6%) and usually mild. The most common reactions are self-limited and resolve without progression, including nausea, vomiting, vasovagal reaction, pruritis, and cutaneous edema. Some of these reactions are purely physiologic (e.g., vasovagal reaction) while others are allergic-like (e.g., pruritis). Importantly, these reactions are not true allergies, in that they are not IgE-mediated. This means that there is no need for sensitization, and a reaction can occur to a patient's first exposure.

The greatest risk factor for a contrast reaction is a previous reaction to the same class of contrast. In patients with a known allergic-like reaction to iodinated CT contrast media, steroid premedication should be strongly considered prior to administration. The ACR provides guidance on premedication regimens, though clinicians should refer to their institution's guidelines. While patients with unrelated allergies (including allergies to shellfish and other iodine products) or asthma may be at increased risk of contrast reaction, the risk does not warrant steroid premedication.

Allergic reactions to GBCA are very rare (<0.2%), though in patients with a prior contrast reaction it may be prudent to premedicate with steroids and administer a different GBCA. There is no cross-reactivity between GBCA and iodinated contrast agents.

Pregnancy and Other Considerations

In instances when CT imaging is performed during pregnancy, the effect of iodinated contrast on the fetus is minimal, and it should be used when clinically indicated. The effect of GBCA on a fetus is unclear, and MRI contrast should be administered in pregnancy only when there is a potential for significant clinical benefit that outweighs the possible risk of fetal exposure. In these situations there should be a discussion between the clinician and patient regarding the risks, and informed consent is needed.

During breastfeeding, only a minuscule amount of contrast is excreted into breast milk and absorbed by the infant, so no precautions are needed for lactating patients. If desired, however, a lactating patient can abstain from breastfeeding for 24 hours following contrast administration and dispose of any milk produced during that time.

Gadolinium has been found to be deposited in the brain in patients who have received multiple doses of GBCA, though the clinical consequences of this are unknown and investigations are ongoing. There is also an uncertain relationship between iodinated contrast and exacerbation of myasthenia gravis symptoms. The iodine in CT contrast has a minimal effect on a normal thyroid, but iodinated contrast risks potentiating thyrotoxicosis in cases of acute thyroid storm.

IMAGING FINDINGS

Brain Pathologies
Stroke

In cases of suspected stroke, imaging is used to help decide whether a patient is likely to benefit from therapy. Treatment for acute embolic stroke often consists of thrombolysis with tissue plasminogen activator (tPA, alteplase) or thrombectomy. Intracranial hemorrhage, however, is an absolute contraindication to thrombolysis, as it may worsen the bleeding.

Emergent noncontrast CT of the head is performed prior to initiation of tissue plasminogen activator to exclude intracranial hemorrhage. Although hyperacute (<6 hours) infarcts are not reliably detected on CT, several imaging signs may be present to suggest the diagnosis (Fig. 2.1). The insular ribbon sign is the loss of the gray-white differentiation along the insula and may be best appreciated lateral to the lentiform nucleus. Occasionally a dense vessel sign is identified at the site of vascular occlusion (often most apparent in the proximal middle cerebral artery [MCA]), in which a hyperattenuating (white) thrombus is seen within the vessel.

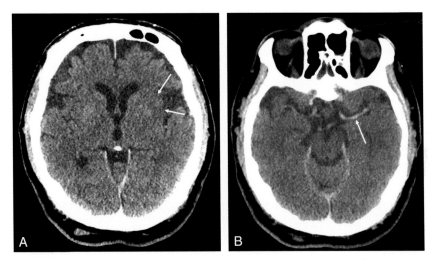

Fig. 2.1 Noncontrast computed tomography findings in a hyperacute infarction from a proximal left middle cerebral artery (MCA) thrombus. (A) The insular ribbon sign, with subtle loss of the gray-white differentiation in the left insula *(arrows)*. (B) The dense MCA sign, in which the hyperattenuating thrombus can be seen within the left MCA (arrow).

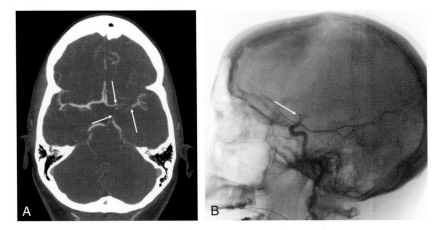

Fig. 2.2 (A) Maximum intensity projection reconstruction of a contrast-enhanced head CT demonstrating occlusion of the left internal carotid artery terminus, the M1 segment of the left middle cerebral artery, and the A1 segment of the left anterior cerebral artery (ACA) (with retrograde filling from the patent right ACA) *(arrows)*. (B) A selective left internal carotid artery diagnostic cerebral angiogram confirms the site of occlusion *(arrow)* distal to a large posterior communicating artery *(asterisk)*.

Acute hemorrhagic blood products appear hyperdense on CT imaging and are discussed in the section of this chapter titled "Trauma." After excluding intracranial hemorrhage on a noncontrast CT, emergent noninvasive vascular imaging (CTA or MRA) is recommended prior to endovascular intervention to identify the site of occlusion. Administration of tPA, however, should not be delayed for vascular imaging. An abrupt cutoff of a vessel at the site of embolism with diminished or absent contrast perfusion of the distal vasculature may be most readily appreciated on maximum intensity projection imaging reconstructions (Fig. 2.2).

Although MRI takes longer to perform than CT and is not suitable for all patients, DWI is the most sensitive imaging tool for detecting hyperacute infarcts (within minutes of ischemia). Areas of acute infarction display restricted diffusivity (DWI bright with matching ADC dark), without corresponding signal abnormalities on other sequences. As the ischemia progresses, other MRI findings can help to characterize chronicity. For example, T2/FLAIR hyperintensity is seen at >6 hours in the affected gray matter, and gyriform contrast enhancement is typically seen after 5 days.

Embolic occlusive infarcts most commonly affect the middle cerebral artery distribution. Small lacunar infarcts are due to occlusion of deep perforating arteries, most often within the basal ganglia, pons, internal and external capsule, and corona radiata (Fig. 2.3). The presence of multiple *bilateral* infarcts in an anterior and posterior circulation distribution raises concern for a cardiac source of emboli (Fig. 2.3D), especially in patients with known arrythmias, cardiac wall motion abnormalities, or endocarditis. A right-to-left shunt (e.g., patent foramen ovale) can also allow emboli from

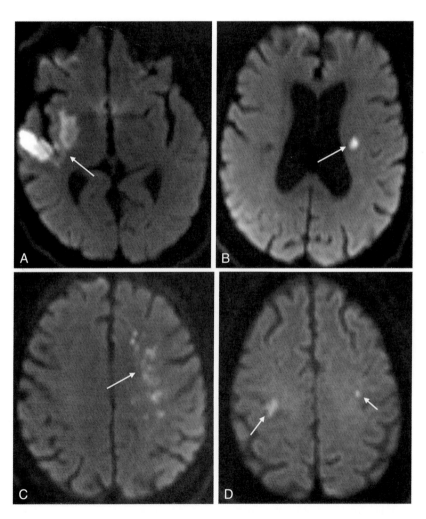

Fig. 2.3 Different distributions of infarcts, all characterized by hyperintensity on diffusion-weighted MRI imaging. (A) Right middle cerebral artery territory infarct involving the basal ganglia and right temporal lobe (*arrow*). (B) Lacunar infarct of the left corona radiata (*arrow*). (C) Watershed infarcts in the border zone between the anterior cerebral artery and middle cerebral artery circulation (*arrow*). circulation. (D) Infarcts in bilateral frontal lobes, suggesting cardioembolic phenomenon (*arrows*). (From George E, Guenette JP, Lee TC. Introduction to neuroimaging. *Am J Med.* 2018;131(4):346–356.)

venous thromboses to ascend into the cerebral circulation. Multiple *unilateral* anterior and posterior infarcts may be related to a fetal origin of the posterior cerebral artery, a common anatomic variant in which a large posterior communicating artery allows emboli to pass readily from the internal carotid artery into the posterior circulation (Fig. 2.2B).

Systemic hypotension in the presence of high-grade carotid stenosis/occlusion can result in "watershed" infarcts. These affect the border regions of the cerebral vascular territories, which are more susceptible to perfusional insufficiency. The most common areas are in the frontal cortex along the a nterior cerebral artery (ACA)/MCA border (Fig. 2.3C) and in the parieto-occipital region along the MCA/PCA border. Less commonly, a watershed infarction can occur at the triple border of the ACA, MCA, and PCA in the parieto-occipital region posterior to the lateral ventricles.

Perfusion imaging with CTA or MRA measures the affected ischemic core of nonsalvageable brain parenchyma and the surrounding penumbra of threatened tissue that may recover if it is reperfused (Fig. 2.4). This is most useful for patients who are beyond the window for tPA (>6 hours) but who still may benefit from mechanical thrombectomy (<24 hours). Although the specific technique differs by vendor, perfusion imaging measures the volume and timing of cerebral blood flow to provide a color-coded map of the parenchyma that can assist in clinical decision-making.

CTA/MRA of the neck is often performed along with vascular imaging of the brain to assess for atherosclerotic disease of the carotid vessels and to create a map of the cervical vessels for potential endovascular intervention. Stenosis is quantified by using the North American Symptomatic Carotid Endarterectomy Trial or Asymptomatic Carotid Atherosclerosis Study criteria. Patients with symptomatic high-grade stenosis (>70%) are likely to benefit from carotid endarterectomy.

Ultrasound evaluation of the carotids can be conducted at the bedside to assess for stenosis using Doppler imaging to measure peak systolic velocity. Normal carotid flow is considered to be <125 cm/sec, with >230 cm/sec indicating >70% stenosis. Luminal narrowing and calcified plaques may also be directly visualized in real time on ultrasound.

In cases of severe or widespread ischemia, the imaging characteristics of diffuse anoxic/hypoxic injuries are similar to those of focal ischemia except manifested globally. On CT, there is a diffuse loss of the gray-white junction that is often most apparent along the bilateral insula. These changes are often delayed (>12 hours) compared to focal ischemia, and so a normal head CT shortly after an anoxic/hypoxic episode may be misleading. Additionally, diffuse cerebral vasogenic edema will result in sulcal and ventricular effacement. MRI imaging is again more sensitive in the acute period, though extensive diffusion restriction may be more difficult to identify without normal brain parenchyma for comparison.

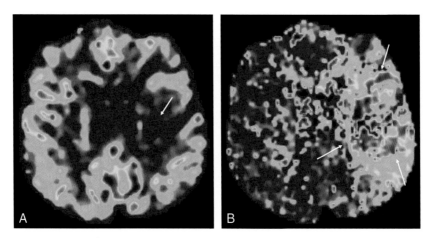

Fig. 2.4 Perfusion imaging in a patient with an acute left middle cerebral artery infarct. (A) Cerebral blood flow demonstrates an ischemic core in the left frontal white matter (dark blue) (*arrow*). (B) The time to maximum blood flow shows delayed perfusion (red) surrounding the infarct core, representing brain tissue with collateral blood flow that may be salvageable (*arrows*).

Transient Ischemic Attack

Transient ischemic attack (TIA) presents as an acute functional neurologic deficit limited to a discrete vascular territory, secondary to a temporarily inadequate blood supply. Although classically a TIA was defined retrospectively based on the duration of the symptoms (<24 hours), up to 67% patients had evidence of acute infarction on imaging. Hence, the definition has been updated to "a transient episode of neurologic dysfunction caused by focal brain, spinal cord, or retinal ischemia, without acute infarction," and brain imaging—preferably MRI—is recommended within 24 hours of symptom onset. Even if acute infarction is not present on initial imaging, there is an increased risk of progression to cerebral infarction within the acute to subacute period. Noninvasive imaging of the cervical and intracranial vessels (CTA, MRA, or carotid ultrasound/transcranial Doppler) should be routinely performed, as this has demonstrated ≥50% intracranial or extracranial stenosis in ~23% patients. Although TIAs have previously been associated with a high stroke risk of ~5% within 48 hours, aggressive management strategies have improved the prognosis. As many cases of TIA are likely missed due to their transitory nature, clinicians should have a low threshold for pursuing an MRI if there is clinical suspicion.

Trauma

Along with the physical and neurologic exam, imaging is one of the most critical components in evaluating patients following known or suspected head trauma. While some pathologies may manifest obviously on exam, imaging can identify conditions before they become critical. The clinical picture may also be complicated by multiple simultaneous traumatic injuries that can be identified and followed on imaging.

The CT and MRI appearance of blood products is related to their chronicity. On CT imaging, assessment of the evolution of blood products is based on density. In the hyperacute or actively bleeding stage, blood can appear isodense or hypodense (darker, gray) and may be difficult to identify compared to normal brain parenchyma and CSF. As the blood begins to clot over the next few minutes, however, it becomes denser (brighter, white) than the surrounding tissue. Two important corollaries are that (1) a thin rim of dense clot adjacent to bone may be challenging to identify, and (2) the blood of anemic patients will be less dense/bright. Continued

bleeding leads to heterogeneity in the collection (swirl sign), and over time the blood products will separate into layers of clotted blood and serum. Eventually, the body will begin to resorb the blood, with the collection slowly decreasing in density over the course of several weeks to months.

On MRI, the appearance of hemorrhagic blood products is more complex and depends on the chemical state and metabolism of the iron within the hemoglobin. Hyperacute blood in the form of intracellular oxyhemoglobin (<6 hours) is T1 isointense (gray) and T2 hyperintense (bright). As the hemoglobin deoxygenates (6–72 hours), the blood signal becomes T1 and T2 hypointense (dark). The MR signal of the blood continues to evolve as the iron is metabolized into methemoglobin in the subacute period and eventually into ferritin and hemosiderin. As with CT imaging, a heterogeneous signal usually indicates blood products in various stages.

Extra-axial Fluid Collections. Blunt or penetrating injury to the head can result in hemorrhage into several compartments, including the epidural, subdural, and subarachnoid spaces (Fig. 2.5).

An epidural hemorrhage/hematoma (EDH) is caused by bleeding into the potential space between the inner table of the skull and the dura mater (Fig. 2.5A). Because the dura adheres tightly to the cranium at the sutures, EDHs have a lens shape and do not cross the suture margins. The most common etiology (90%) is laceration of the middle meningeal artery secondary to temporal bone fracture (which itself will be best evaluated on CT). The classic presentation of a lucid interval followed by loss of consciousness is seen in up to 50% of patients with EDH. This delay occurs as blood gradually accumulates within the epidural space before causing rapid midline shift and brain herniation. Thus a suspected EDH warrants prompt recognition and close follow-up, as it may require surgical evacuation. Venous EDHs are much less common, and a small venous EDH in the anterior aspect of the middle cranial fossa is likely to be indolent.

A subdural hemorrhage/hematoma (SDH) is caused by bleeding into the potential space between the dura mater and the arachnoid mater (Fig. 2.5B). SDHs are crescentic, can cross suture lines, and may extend along an entire cerebral hemisphere. Although they can involve the falx, they will not cross the midline. SDHs are usually caused by tearing of the bridging veins. This is more common in elderly patients in whom parenchymal

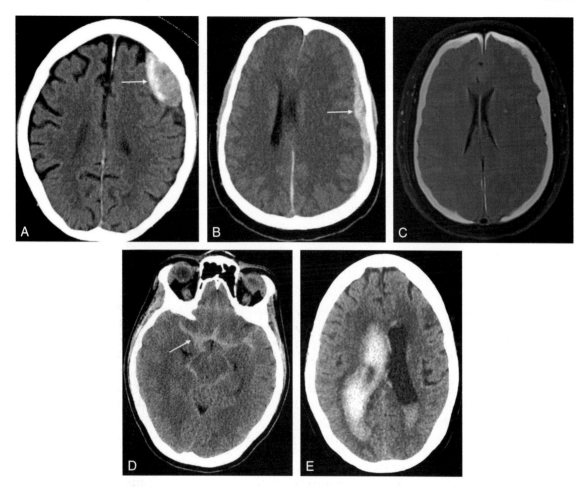

Fig. 2.5 Extra-axial fluid collections. The lenticular hyperdense appearance of an epidural hematoma (*arrow*) (A) compared to the crescentic appearance of a subdural hematoma (*arrow*) (B). (C) Bilateral fluid attenuation inversion recovery (FLAIR)-bright subdural hygromas (vs. the FLAIR-dark cerebrospinal fluid [CSF] in the lateral ventricles) (*arrow*). (D) Hyperdense appearance of the basal cisterns representing subarachnoid hemorrhage (*arrow*). (E) Dense blood products filling the right lateral ventricle and a blood-CSF level in the left occipital horn (*arrow*). (A and B) (From George E, Guenette JP, Lee TC. Introduction to neuroimaging. *Am J Med.* 2018;131(4):346–356.)

volume loss has stretched the veins, and it may be exacerbated by systemic anticoagulation. Unfortunately, that same parenchymal volume loss may also lead to delayed diagnosis, as the SDH has greater room to expand before becoming symptomatic from mass effect. Isodense or bilateral symmetric SDHs can be challenging to identify, since they can appear similar to brain parenchyma and may not cause midline shift. In elderly patients with normally prominent sulci, the effacement (compression or absence) of the sulci should warrant extra attention.

A subdural hygroma is a collection of (nonblood) fluid within the potential space between the dura mater and the arachnoid mater. Subdural hygromas may be due to a tear in the arachnoid mater that allows CSF to accumulate in the subdural space, or they can represent the fluid remnants of a degenerated chronic SDH. They are often difficult to differentiate from normal CSF on CT imaging with their similar densities, though are more apparent on MRI because of the higher protein content in the hygroma (FLAIR bright) (Fig. 2.5C). While most subdural hygromas are asymptomatic, intervention may be warranted if there is evidence of mass effect.

A subarachnoid hemorrhage (SAH) is caused by bleeding into the space between the arachnoid mater and the pia mater (Fig. 2.5D). Trauma and ruptured aneurysm are the most common causes of SAH, with nontraumatic SAHs classically presenting as a "thunderclap" headache. Blood in a SAH will infiltrate along the sulci, with larger hemorrhages extending into the cisterns and fissures. The pattern of the SAH can indicate the site of aneurysm, such as hemorrhage in the anterior interhemispheric fissure (anterior communicating artery) or in the suprasellar cistern (posterior communicating artery), though blood may redistribute with time and patient positioning. There are multiple complications of SAH that are well assessed on imaging, including hydrocephalus and vasospasm. Hydrocephalus occurs when clotted blood obstructs arachnoid granulations and impairs CSF resorption. It can result in brain herniation and may warrant ventricular shunt placement. Vasospasm occurs around 7 to 10 days following SAH and can result in cerebral ischemia. Although monitoring of vasospasm is best done via interventional angiography, CTA of the head is often a more practical method.

Intraventricular hemorrhage (IVH) can occur from a number of injuries and is most often secondary to direct extension of a SAH or intraparenchymal hemorrhage. Primary IVH may occur from the tearing of subependymal veins, vascular malformations, or intraventricular tumors. Although IVHs are often secondary to other trauma (Fig. 2.5E), they are particularly important to note because of the risk of a clot causing obstructive hydrocephalus.

Traumatic Brain Injury. Primary traumatic brain injuries include cortical contusion, intraparenchymal hematoma, and diffuse axonal injury. The coup-contrecoup injury pattern most commonly manifests with cerebral contusions and traumatic subarachnoid hemorrhages. In the coup-contrecoup pattern, soft tissue and fracture injuries occur at the site of initial impact and brain contusion/hemorrhage occurs at the opposite side of the head (e.g., left frontal and right parietal) (Fig. 2.6). Any visible brain injury at the site of the initial impact is often less severe than that on the opposite side. Therefore identification of the site of trauma is important, and an injury anywhere in the brain should prompt a close examination of the opposing site where the brain impacts the inner skull.

Cortical contusions are the most common primary traumatic brain injury. They occur from blunt head trauma resulting in the collision of the brain against the inner table of the skull. Because of their etiology and the irregular shape of the skull base, they are most common in the frontal lobes along the anterior cranial fossa and the anterior temporal poles along the middle fossa. In the hyperacute setting, these injuries can be difficult to see on CT and may manifest only as small hypodense or hyperdense subcortical irregularities. As the contusions

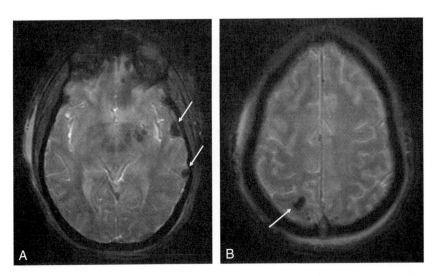

Fig. 2.6 Coup-contrecoup injury pattern. Susceptibility-weighted magnetic resonance imaging imaging demonstrates hemorrhagic contusions in the left temporal lobe and basal ganglia (*arrows*) (A) and in the opposing right parietal lobe (*arrows*) (B).

slowly bleed over the course of hours to days, however, the intraparenchymal hematomas (IPH) may become more apparent on CT. Focal areas of high density (white) surrounded by low density represent the clotted blood products with adjacent parenchymal edema (Fig. 2.7A). Although MRI is not often used for assessing acute injuries, it can be more sensitive within the first 24 hours and will demonstrate hypointense (dark) foci on SWI/GRE sequences at the sites of microhemorrhages. Diffuse axonal injury (DAI) results from shearing due to differential motion of the gray and white matter during acceleration and deceleration and typically results in loss of consciousness at the time of impact. Initial head CT is often negative, so DAI should be suspected in a patient with discrepant clinical and imaging findings with a reported mechanism of severe trauma. MRI dark foci on SWI/GRE often identify sites of DAI at the gray-white junction, splenium and posterior body of corpus callosum, brain stem, basal ganglia, internal capsule, and superior cerebellar peduncle (Fig. 2.7B).

Additional Trauma Considerations. Brain herniation is a life-threatening condition that occurs when the parenchyma is forced past a rigid barrier and into an adjacent space. These changes in brain position and volume can compress or stretch vascular structures and nerves. Some of the more common causes include increased parenchymal volume (e.g., edema, tumor, IPH) or increased extraparenchymal volume (e.g., obstructive hydrocephalus, SDH, meningioma). Subfalcine herniation is the most common type and occurs when the cingulate gyrus is forced under the falx and into the contralateral side, with risk to the anterior cerebral artery and internal cerebral veins (Fig. 2.8). Inferior transtentorial herniation involves herniation of the temporal lobe uncus into the posterior fossa, possibly compressing the oculomotor nerve (cranial nerve III), posterior cerebral arteries, and midbrain. Mass effect in the posterior fossa can result in ascending transtentorial herniation or inferior tonsillar herniation through the foramen magnum. CT imaging is a fast and effective way to identify herniation, and CTA and MRI can identify vasculature that is at risk or signal abnormalities in adjacent nerves and brain parenchyma. As herniations can progress rapidly with catastrophic results, however, additional imaging should not delay emergent interventions.

Any history of significant head trauma should also prompt an evaluation for skull fractures. CT imaging using a bone reconstruction is most sensitive, and 3D rendering may help to visualize complex fracture structures (Fig. 2.9A). Normal suture lines are generally

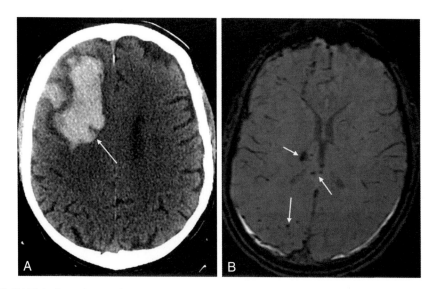

Fig. 2.7 (A) Right frontal parenchymal hemorrhage (*arrow*). (B) Susceptibility-weighted magnetic resonance imaging imaging demonstrates multiple foci of microhemorrhages (hypointense foci) at the gray-white junction, corpus callosum, and right thalamus, consistent with diffuse axonal injury (DAI) (*arrows*). (From George E, Guenette JP, Lee TC. Introduction to neuroimaging. *Am J Med.* 2018;131(4):346–356.)

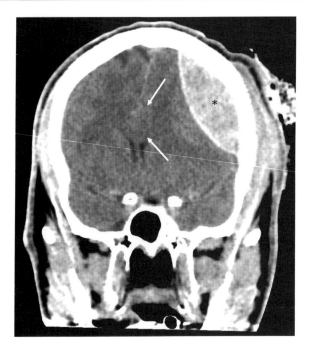

Fig. 2.8 Rightward subfalcine herniation (*arrows*) in a patient with a large left epidural hematoma (*asterisk*).

symmetric and should not be mistaken for fractures. Overlying soft tissue swelling or hematomas may indicate an underlying fracture, and an EDH should prompt a thorough evaluation of the underlying bone. Because of the complex structure of the skull, skull base fractures can be more challenging to identify; hemorrhage within the paranasal sinuses should prompt close evaluation. Any fracture involving the carotid canals, jugular foramen, or major venous sinuses should warrant a CTA/CTV to evaluate the vascular structures. Temporal bone fractures can be also difficult to identify and may be suggested by blood in the external or middle ear (including the mastoid air spaces) (Fig. 2.9B). Fractures involving the sinuses, face, temporal bones, or cervical spine deserve dedicated CT imaging with thin-slice bone reconstructions.

Finally, in any case of trauma, the clinical team must consider the possibility of a nonaccidental cause. In children, complex and/or depressed skull fractures, bilateral chronic SDHs, and multiple intracranial bleeds of different ages raise concern for nonaccidental trauma. In elderly patients and adults with limited capabilities or who require caregivers, these types of injuries should also prompt consideration of neglect or intentional harm. Nonaccidental trauma is a complex medical, social, and legal issue, and if there is any question about the nature of a patient's injuries, the clinician should consult directly with a radiologist.

Other Vascular

One of the most common pathologies seen on brain imaging is the manifestation of chronic microvascular disease in the bilateral white matter. These changes appear primarily in the periventricular and subcortical white matter as hypoattenuating (dark) foci on CT and as hyperintense (bright) spots on T2/FLAIR sequences. Unlike acute infarctions, there is no associated diffusion restriction or enhancement. These foci are common in older adults and represent areas of chronic microischemia that may coalesce over time. Although most often incidental and asymptomatic, they can be associated with cognitive decline and vascular dementia.

Nontraumatic parenchymal hemorrhage is most often due to chronic hypertension and classically involves the basal ganglia, thalamus, brain stem, and cerebellum. Like other parenchymal hemorrhages, they manifest on CT as expansive, hyperdense (white) foci. There is often only mild mass effect in the hyperacute phase, though over the following 24 to 48 hours patients usually develop worsening symptoms as the surrounding edema increases. Smaller hemorrhages can be relatively asymptomatic and go ignored or unnoticed by the patient. These small bleeds are commonly seen incidentally as dark foci on SWI.

Another cerebrovascular disorder that appears as dark foci on SWI is cerebral amyloid angiopathy (CAA). CAA is caused by the accumulation of cerebral amyloid-β in the walls of the cortical vessels, resulting in vascular fragility and multiple hemorrhagic events. While most of these hemorrhages are tiny and self-limited, a lobar IPH in a normotensive elderly patient should raise concern for CAA. Chronic CAA, like chronic white matter microvascular disease, can lead to cognitive decline. Although there is a rare familial form of CAA, the vast majority of cases are sporadic, and there is no known treatment.

The most common nontraumatic cause of SAH is a ruptured aneurysm, and the imaging manifestations of SAH are discussed in the section of this chapter titled "Trauma." Widespread use of neuroimaging has resulted in increased detection of incidental intracranial aneurysms, with an estimated prevalence of ~3% (Fig. 2.10).

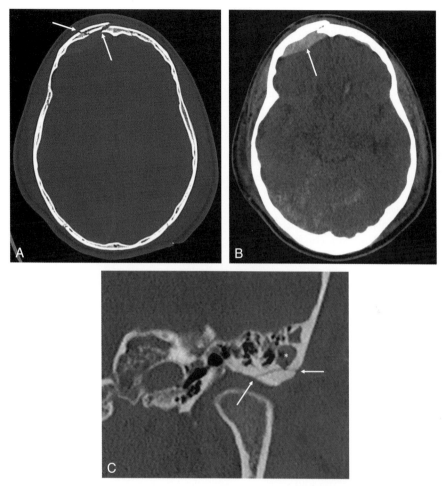

Fig. 2.9 Skull fractures. (A) A right frontal cranial fracture overlies an epidural hematoma (*arrows*) (B). (C) Coronal imaging of a left temporal bone fracture (*arrows*) with blood in the mastoid air spaces (*asterisk*).

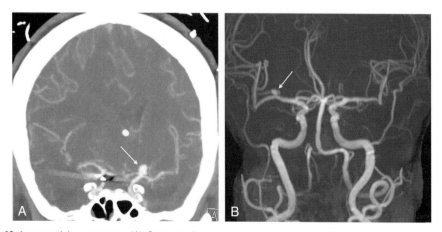

Fig. 2.10 Intracranial aneurysms. (A) Computed tomography angiography (CTA) coronal maximum intensity projection image demonstrates an aneurysm of the left internal carotid artery terminus (*arrow*). (B) Magnetic resonance angiography (MRA) demonstrates an aneurysm of the right middle cerebral artery bifurcation (*arrow*). (From George E, Guenette JP, Lee TC. Introduction to neuroimaging. *Am J Med.* 2018;131(4):346–356.)

The American Heart Association recommends offering aneurysm screening with CTA or MRA for patients with polycystic kidney disease or with two or more family members with intracranial aneurysm or subarachnoid hemorrhage. The decision to intervene is based on the presentation, aneurysm size, and patient risk. Patients who are medically managed are typically followed with CTA or MRA within 6 to 12 months of initial discovery and then yearly or every other year. Follow-up imaging is also indicated in patients who have undergone surgical or endovascular repair, particularly those with high-risk features.

Nontraumatic SAH or IPH in a young person should raise concern for a vascular malformation. An arteriovenous malformation (AVM) is a congenital, high-flow, arterial-venous connection, with a 2% to 4% risk of rupture per year. Most AVMs will appear on CT as a hypodense (dark) area within the brain parenchyma without mass effect. CTA is best to assess the complex vascular nidus and feeding/draining vessels. MRI shows "dark" vascular flow voids and changes to the surrounding parenchyma on T2 sequences (Fig. 2.11). Dural arteriovenous fistulas (dAVF) are high-flow shunts between meningeal arterioles and dural venules, which can present with hemorrhage or venous hypertension. CTA will demonstrate an enlarged and tortuous vessel in the subarachnoid space and may show early contrast flow into the dural venous sinuses. A carotid-cavernous fistula (CCF) is a subtype of dAVF caused by posttraumatic fistulation between the cavernous carotid artery and cavernous sinus, often presenting with pulsatile exophthalmos or visual changes. CCF is characterized on imaging by dilatation of the superior ophthalmic vein and early contrast filling of the cavernous sinus.

Venous thrombosis is a challenging diagnosis that can present with nonspecific symptoms and varying appearances on imaging depending on the chronicity and location. It is a common cause of stroke in younger patients, however, and should be considered in patients who are pregnant, who are on oral contraceptives, or who have thrombophilia, malignancy, or signs of infection. The thrombus usually begins in the superior sagittal or transverse sinuses, though it may extend into other veins (Fig. 2.12). On unenhanced CT, an acute thrombus may appear as a linear density (white) within the vessel (cord sign). A contrast-enhanced CT venogram is more sensitive and will demonstrate a dark filling defect within the vessel (e.g., the empty delta sign in the superior sagittal sinus). Similarly, an MR venogram will show an absence of flow in the affected vessel. Blood products within the clot evolve over time, however, and its appearance will vary. A secondary sign of chronic

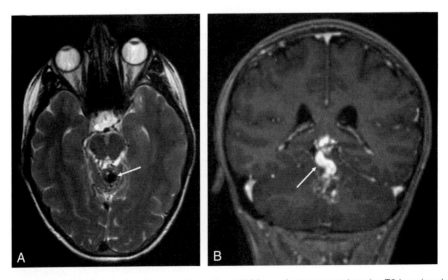

Fig. 2.11 Cerebellar vermis arteriovenous malformation. (A) Magnetic resonance imaging T2 imaging demonstrates an abnormal dark vascular flow void in the superior vermis (*arrow*). (B) Coronal T1 postcontrast imaging demonstrates a large serpentine vessel in the vermis (*arrow*).

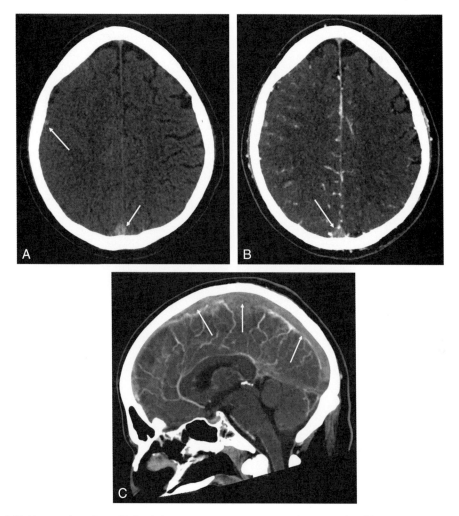

Fig. 2.12 Venous thrombus. (A) Cord sign on noncontrast computed tomography (CT) imaging with a dense clot within the superior sagittal sinus and right vein of Trolard (*arrows*). (B) Empty delta sign, with absent flow within the superior sagittal sinus on a venous-phase contrast-enhanced head CT (*arrow*). (C) A midline sagittal view in the same patient demonstrates a large filling defect within the superior sagittal sinus (*arrows*).

venous obstruction is the development of collateral draining vessels. Obstructed venous drainage can lead to hypoperfusion and infarction, though unlike embolic arterial strokes they will not be confined to a normal arterial vascular territory.

Infection

Meningitis, the inflammation of the pia and arachnoid mater, is a clinical diagnosis based on CSF analysis. Imaging is often not indicated and may be negative in early or treated meningitis. Prior to a lumbar puncture,

however, CT imaging may be used to rule out space-occupying intracranial lesions, particularly in the posterior fossa. MRI in acute meningitis can demonstrate FLAIR hyperintensity of the subarachnoid fluid, hydrocephalus, and parenchymal swelling leading to herniation.

Pyogenic brain abscesses are due to hematogenous spread, direct extension from the paranasal sinuses, or as a complication of meningitis. They are often seen in patients with congenital heart disease, intravenous drug use, or HIV/AIDS. Abscesses frequently occur at the gray-white junction and evolve over the course of

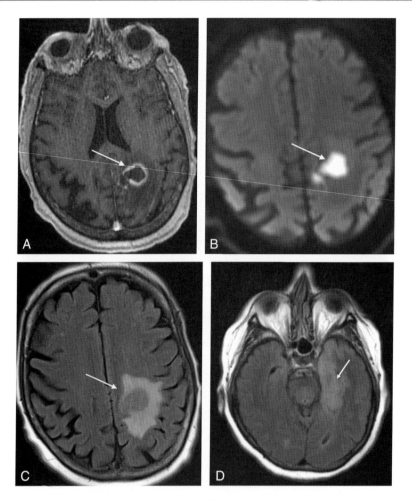

Fig. 2.13 Intracranial infections. Cerebral abscess (A–C) characterized by a rim-enhancing mass (*arrow*) (A) with central low diffusivity (*arrow*) (B) and surrounding vasogenic edema (*arrow*) (C). (D) Herpes simplex virus encephalitis with T2/fluid attenuation inversion recovery hyperintensity in the medial left temporal lobe (*arrow*). (From George E, Guenette JP, Lee TC. Introduction to neuroimaging. *Am J Med.* 2018;131(4):346–356.).

about 2 weeks from a focus of inflammation to a mature abscess. These are best evaluated with MRI. They have a thin, smooth, enhancing rim with central low diffusivity, surrounding vasogenic edema (Fig. 2.13), and occasionally a thin T2-hypointense (dark) rim. If the abscess is periventricular, the thin abscess wall adjacent to the ventricle can be easily ruptured. This will spill the infectious contents into the ventricle resulting in ventriculitis, which has high mortality.

Herpes simplex virus-1 (HSV-1) is another common culprit of encephalitis. While CT imaging is often nonspecific with ill-defined hypoattenuation in the temporal lobe, MRI will show T2/FLAIR hyperintensity of the medial temporal lobe, insula, and cingulum, with possible associated gyriform low diffusivity, enhancement, or hemorrhage (Fig. 2.13D). The clinical symptoms in herpes encephalitis are often nonspecific, and since early diagnosis and treatment greatly improve clinical outcomes, radiologists are often aggressive in querying HSV encephalitis on imaging.

A number of CNS fungal infections can present with nonspecific imaging findings, such as abscesses, cerebritis, meningitis, vasculitis, and mycotic aneurysms. The distribution of the findings and the patient's immune status can help to differentiate between different fungal organisms. *Cryptococcus*, *Aspergillus*, and *Rhizopus/Mucor* all commonly affect immunocompromised patients. Cryptococcosis results in gelatinous pseudocysts in the basal ganglia perivascular space that appear T2 hyperintense (bright) on MRI and can produce ring-enhancing granulomas in the choroid plexus. Aspergillosis has a predilection for vascular invasion, mycotic aneurysms along the distal arteries, and abscesses with a T2/GRE-dark rim corresponding with hemorrhagic blood products. Mucormycosis displays aggressive osseous destruction of the affected sinuses, and parenchymal infarctions with hemorrhagic necrosis secondary to angioinvasion.

Intracranial parasitic infections are unfortunately common in some parts of the world. Four stages of parenchymal neurocysticercosis have been described on imaging, progressing from CSF-intensity cysts (T2 bright, FLAIR dark), to ring-enhancing lesions, to shrinking cysts with thickened walls, and finally small parenchymal calcifications. The entire sequence takes approximately 5 years on average, and the resulting calcifications of the final stage appear as scattered bright spots on CT and dark spots on T2/SWI MRI sequences. Intraventricular neurocysticercosis is a common complication, with a FLAIR hyperintense (bright) cyst in the Sylvian aqueduct or fourth ventricle resulting in obstructive hydrocephalus. Toxoplasmosis is most common in immunocompromised patients and often appears as a ring-enhancing lesion in the basal ganglia with significant surrounding edema (CT dark, FLAIR bright).

While Creutzfeld-Jakob disease is thankfully rare, early recognition is important for correct patient care and protection of involved healthcare workers, given its resistance to standard sterilization techniques including autoclave. MRI will display FLAIR hyperintensity and restricted diffusion along the cerebral cortex (cortical ribboning), often with sparing of the motor cortex. Similar signal intensity may be seen in the thalamus.

Neoplasm

The World Health Organization (WHO) 2021 classification system has an exhaustive list of intracranial neoplasms classified based on histology and molecular markers. This also includes a grading system, with Grades 1 and 2 representing low-grade and Grades 3 and 4 representing high-grade tumors. In previous editions, this grading system was applied equivalently across all CNS tumor types, allowing for a rough comparison of tumor aggressiveness between different types. With the most recent update, however, the grading system is shifting toward being specific to each tumor type, so two tumors of different types but of similar grade may now display different levels of aggressiveness. This is coupled with a move away from relying on tumor grade as a marker of prognosis, since treatment outcomes continue to improve with new and emerging therapies.

Although imaging alone is not always able to determine the exact type or subtype of a tumor, CT and MRI are often used for primary tumor detection, assessing the extent of the tumor, and determining the involvement of adjacent vessels or structures. Intracranial tumors are broadly divided into extra-axial (outside the brain parenchyma) and intra-axial (within the brain parenchyma), with extra-axial tumors accounting for the majority. Extra-axial lesions can be identified by the presence of a rim of CSF interposed between the lesion and the brain, as well as a thin rim of gray matter separating the lesion from the white matter. Conversely, intra-axial lesions directly abut the white matter.

The most common extra-axial tumor is meningioma, a dural-based mass that is prevalent in middle-aged women and is WHO Grade 1 in ~85% of cases (Fig. 2.14A). Meningiomas can be found anywhere along the dura (including the spine), though they are most frequently found along the parasagittal dura and convexities. Although usually asymptomatic and incidental, larger meningiomas can result in a mass effect causing brain herniation or obstructive hydrocephalus. On CT they may appear slightly hyperdense (brighter) than the adjacent brain tissue, and up to 25% will have calcifications. Contrast-enhanced MRI is excellent for assessing meningiomas, which can be heterogeneous on T1 and T2 sequences but will strongly enhance and display an elongated "tail" along the adjacent dura.

The most common (~35%) intra-axial neoplasms in adults are metastases, seen as well-defined, enhancing masses, typically at the gray-white junction (Fig. 2.14B). In a patient with any history of malignancy, an enhancing intraparenchymal mass should raise concern for metastasis. Because of their highly vascular nature, metastatic lesions are prone to hemorrhage.

Glioblastoma, the most common primary intra-axial neoplasm (~25%), is a WHO Grade 4 tumor with a peak incidence in the fifth and sixth decades of

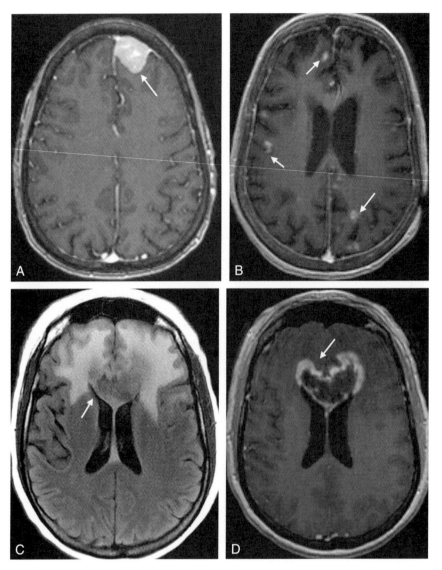

Fig. 2.14 Intracranial neoplasms. (A) Extra-axial dural-based mass consistent with a meningioma (*arrow*). (B) Multiple enhancing foci, predominantly at the gray-white junction, representing metastases (*arrows*). (C, D) Peripherally enhancing centrally necrotic mass of the corpus callosum with marked surrounding T2 hyperintensity representing glioblastoma (*arrow*). (From George E, Guenette JP, Lee TC. Introduction to neuroimaging. *Am J Med.* 2018;131(4):346–356.)

life and a median survival of 15 months. The typical appearance is of a heterogenous, necrotic mass with peripheral enhancement and surrounding T2 hyperintensity, representing a combination of infiltrating non-enhancing tumor, edema, and gliosis (Fig. 2.14C and D). Glioblastomas are able to spread through white matter tracts, CSF, and the meninges. When they cross the midline via the corpus callosum they are termed "butterfly"

lesions. Because of their ability to metastasize through CSF, MRI imaging of the spine is recommended to look for "drop metastases."

Diffuse astrocytoma, another common primary intra-axial neoplasm (~10%), can range from WHO Grade 2 to Grade 4. As the name suggests, they appear as somewhat ill-defined white matter lesions that are T2/FLAIR hyperintense (bright). Lower-grade tumors

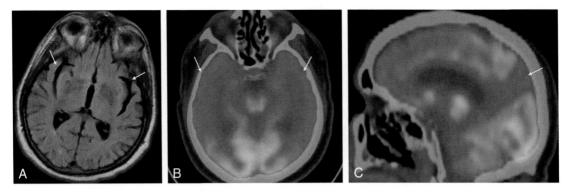

Fig. 2.15 Alzheimer disease. (A) Magnetic resonance imaging demonstrates bilateral temporal lobe atrophy (*arrows*). 18F-fluorodeoxyglucose positron emission tomography (PET) demonstrates marked hypometabolism of the temporal lobes (*arrow*) (B), and posterior cingulate cortex and precuneus (*arrow*) (C). (From George E, Guenette JP, Lee TC. Introduction to neuroimaging. *Am J Med.* 2018;131(4):346–356.)

do not enhance, and areas of enhancement or necrosis indicate higher grade. Similarly, increased restricted diffusion and blood perfusion are associated with higher grade. Because they expand the white matter, there is often bulging or displacement of the overlying cortex.

Neurodegenerative Diseases

Along with clinical assessment, structural imaging can play a role in diagnosing neurodegenerative causes of dementia and excluding alternative etiologies such as hydrocephalus, intracranial hemorrhage, or mass. There is normal atrophy of the brain parenchyma with age, most apparent on imaging with diffuse widening of the sulci and the proportional and symmetric dilation of the ventricles. These normal changes must be distinguished from hydrocephalus, in which the ventricles are dilated but the sulci are effaced. CT is effective at differentiating between atrophy and hydrocephalus, though for more detailed anatomical assessment of neurodegenerative changes, MRI is better suited. MR spectroscopy and nuclear medicine studies also have a role in differentiating between the underlying causes.

Multiple neurodegenerative diseases also result in parenchymal atrophy, though the early imaging findings may be nonspecific and should be correlated with clinical findings.

Alzheimer disease (AD) is the most common cause of neurodegenerative dementia, accounting for ~60 of cases, and is characterized by diffuse cortical atrophy that is most pronounced in the hippocampi and medial temporal lobes. On 18FDG PET, the earliest abnormality is

hypometabolism in the posterior cingulate cortex, with later involvement of the hippocampi, medial temporal lobes, precuneus, and lateral temporoparietal lobes. The frontal lobes eventually become involved in advanced Alzheimer disease (Fig. 2.15).

Focal cortical atrophy and hypometabolism of the frontal and/or temporal lobes are the hallmarks of frontotemporal dementia. Vascular or multiinfarct dementia is characterized by multiple areas of chronic white matter infarcts and deep gray matter lacunar infarcts (FLAIR bright). Dementia with Lewy bodies can have an imaging pattern similar to that of AD but with more pronounced cortical atrophy in the occipital lobes. Dementia symptoms occur later in Parkinson disease, and there are rarely anatomic findings on imaging that allow it to be differentiated from other pathologies. PET scans using I-123 ioflupane (DaTscan) or 18F-DOPA can differentiate early Parkinson disease from other causes of tremor (e.g., essential tremor) by identifying decreased dopamine transporter density in the striatum.

Demyelinating Disorders

Multiple sclerosis (MS) is the most common demyelinating disorder in the United States, with a female predominance and a peak in early adulthood. Diagnosis is based on the McDonald criteria, which require evidence of lesions disseminated in both time (appearance of a new lesion or simultaneous presence of both enhancing and nonenhancing lesions) and space (juxtacortical, periventricular, infratentorial, or spinal cord lesions). These lesions appear on MRI as flame-shaped areas of

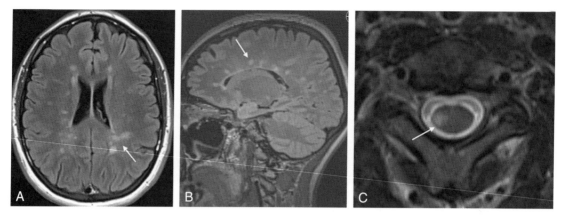

Fig. 2.16 Multiple sclerosis. Numerous flame-shaped areas of T2/fluid attenuation innversion recovery hyperintensity in the periventricular white matter (*arrow*) (A), callososeptal interface (Dawson fingers) (*arrow*) (B), and peripheral T2 hyperintense lesion in the cervical spinal cord (*arrow*) (C). (From George E, Guenette JP, Lee TC. Introduction to neuroimaging. *Am J Med*. 2018;131(4):346–356.)

T2 hyperintensity (bright) that enhance during active demyelination and often appear at the callososeptal interface oriented perpendicular to the long axis of the ventricles (Dawson fingers) (Fig. 2.16). In the most common form of MS (relapsing-remitting), these lesions will not enhance during the quiescent phase. MS often also involves the spinal cord, in which the lesions appear as short segments of T2 hyperintensity.

Acute disseminated encephalomyelitis (ADEM) is an immune-mediated demyelinating process, commonly affecting children, that can mimic the appearance of MS or tumors. Monophasic ADEM lesions typically resolve by 3 months with full recovery. Posterior reversible encephalopathy syndrome (PRES) is associated with a failure of autoregulation that leads to hypertension and vasogenic edema within the posterior circulation, though multiple other causes, such as sepsis and chemotherapy, have been identified. PRES appears as symmetric subcortical edema in the posterior parietal and occipital lobes on CT (hypodense, dark) and MRI (T2/FLAIR hyperintensity, bright) (Fig. 2.17).

Demyelinating disorders secondary to HIV and immunosuppression include progressive multifocal leukoencephalopathy (PML) and HIV encephalitis. PML is caused by the JC virus, manifesting as *asymmetric*, confluent white matter lesions *involving* the arcuate (subcortical U) fibers. HIV encephalitis represents the direct infection of CNS lymphocytes and microglial cells by HIV and is the most common CNS infection in AIDS

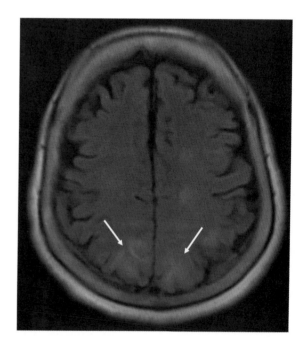

Fig. 2.17 Posterior reversible encephalopathy syndrome. Cortical/subcortical edema of the posterior parietal and occipital lobes (*arrows*).

patients. It appears similar to PML except that there is *symmetric* white matter involvement that *spares* the subcortical U fibers. Diffuse cerebral atrophy is also more common in HIV encephalitis.

Several metabolic disorders result in demyelinating conditions. Osmotic demyelination (central pontine myelinolysis) is seen in the setting of rapid changes in extracellular osmolality, often with the rapid correction of hyponatremia in patients with poor nutritional status. On MRI, this is seen as bilateral T2 hyperintensity in the thalami, basal ganglia, white matter, and pons. Thiamine (vitamin B1) deficiency can also be seen in nutritionally poor patients and manifests as symmetric T2/FLAIR hyperintensity and restricted diffusion in the medial thalami, mammillary bodies, and inferior hypothalamus.

Spine Pathologies

The majority of patients presenting with low back pain do not require imaging. Imaging should be considered if there is concern for cauda equina syndrome, malignancy, fracture, or infection, or if there is little or no improvement after 6 weeks of physical therapy. MRI is superior to CT in patients who have persistent radiculopathy, who are candidates for intervention, or who have a prior history of surgery. CT is beneficial in the postoperative setting to assess for hardware complications. For chronic neck pain, an x-ray study of the cervical spine is the recommended initial diagnostic examination, with MRI reserved for cases with neurologic symptoms, persistent pain despite conservative management, or concern for infection or malignancy.

Degenerative disease

The spine degenerates over time in response to chronic stress, with gradual formation of bone spurs at the vertebral body endplates. This is different from disc herniation, which can result in acute spinal canal stenosis and nerve impingement. Although there can be a fair amount of interobserver variability, MRI best demonstrates the extent of disc degeneration, facet arthropathy, and spinal canal and neural foraminal stenosis (Fig. 2.18). Contrast administration is generally reserved for concerns of malignancy or infection, or to distinguish postsurgical granulation tissue from recurrent disc herniation.

Infection

Unlike metastases of the spine, which usually are within the vertebral bodies, infections of the spine are predominantly centered in the relatively avascular discs. These patients typically present with back pain, fever, and elevated inflammatory markers. On MRI, there is T1 hypointensity (dark) and T2/STIR hyperintensity (bright) involving discs and endplates. Enhancement of the bone marrow, discs, and prevertebral and paraspinal soft tissues is often seen (Fig. 2.19). And while concurrent inflammatory degenerative disease can confound the picture, the presence of a paravertebral psoas or epidural abscess is definitive. MRI is the best method for detecting complications such as abscess or phlegmon, leptomeningeal

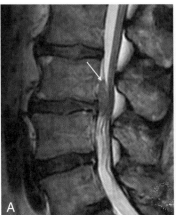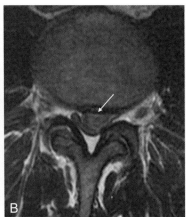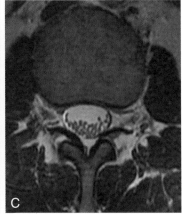

Fig. 2.18 Lumbar disc degenerative disease. Lumbar spine MRI demonstrates an extruded disc fragment (A, B) causing severe spinal canal stenosis. (C) Normal appearance of a widely patent spinal canal at an adjacent level for comparison. (From George E, Guenette JP, Lee TC. Introduction to neuroimaging. *Am J Med.* 2018;131(4):346–356.)

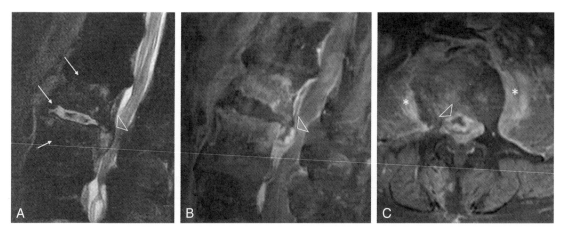

Fig. 2.19 Discitis/osteomyelitis. Lumbar spine magnetic resonance imaging with fat-suppressed T2 sequence demonstrates (A) hyperintensity of the disc and the adjacent vertebral bodies (*arrows*) with epidural soft tissue (*arrowhead*). The soft tissue demonstrates peripheral enhancement consistent with abscess (B, C, *arrowhead*). Note paraspinal soft tissue enhancement (C, *asterisk*). (From George E, Guenette JP, Lee TC. Introduction to neuroimaging. *Am J Med*. 2018;131(4):346–356.)

involvement, or compression of the thecal sac. Contrast enhancement is beneficial in differentiating diffusely enhancing phlegmon from centrally nonenhancing abscess, which is essential in determining medical versus surgical management. In the setting of florid MR changes without definitive clinical or imaging evidence of infection, CT can be helpful in distinguishing between chronic degenerative endplate changes versus rapidly developing infective bony erosions of the endplates. On follow-up, MRI findings can lag behind clinical improvement.

Trauma

Although CT is the preferred imaging modality in the setting of trauma, MRI can be complementary if there are neurologic deficits or concerns for ligamentous injury or to assess for bone marrow edema when differentiating between acute versus chronic compression fractures. Evaluation of stability of spinal fractures includes a combination of clinical and radiologic assessments. The spinal column is divided into anterior, middle, and posterior columns, and involvement of more than one column is generally considered an unstable injury. The thoracolumbar injury classification and severity score guides treatment decisions and is based on the morphology of fracture, neurologic involvement, and involvement of the posterior ligamentous complex.

Neoplasm

Tumors of the spinal canal are often classified based on their location into intramedullary (within the spinal cord), intradural extramedullary, and extradural lesions. The most common intramedullary spinal tumors are astrocytomas, ependymomas, and hemangioblastomas. Multiple simultaneous intramedullary lesions should raise concern for a demyelinating or inflammatory disease. Extramedullary intradural lesions include meningiomas and nerve sheath tumors such as neurofibroma or schwannoma. In the cauda equina, myxopapillary ependymomas are the most common intradural extramedullary tumors. Metastatic disease can also infiltrate the arachnoid and pia mater (leptomeninges) focally or diffusely (Fig. 2.20). The most common extradural/epidural neoplastic lesion is a metastasis, which often extends into the anterior epidural space from an adjacent vertebral body metastasis and can cause narrowing of the thecal sac with resultant neurologic symptoms. These metastases are characterized by T1 hypointensity (dark), T2/STIR hyperintensity (bright), and heterogenous enhancement. Other common extradural neoplasms that affect the spinal canal also usually arise from the adjacent bone and include lymphoma, plasmacytoma, chordoma, and chondrosarcoma.

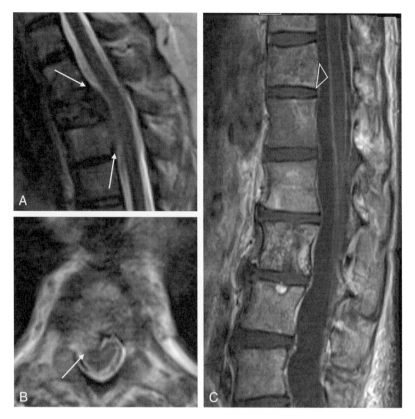

Fig. 2.20 Spinal metastases. (A) T2 hyperintensity of multiple thoracic vertebral bodies representing vertebral metastases with epidural extension (*arrow*) causing spinal canal stenosis and deformation of the cord (B). (C) Diffuse leptomeningeal enhancement (*arrowhead*) in this patient represents leptomeningeal carcinomatosis. (From George E, Guenette JP, Lee TC. Introduction to neuroimaging. *Am J Med.* 2018;131(4):346–356.)

Inflammatory Lesions

Guillain-Barré syndrome is an immune-mediated polyneuropathy, often preceded by an infection. MRI can support this diagnosis by demonstrating enlarged, enhancing nerve roots, usually at the cauda equina, and can exclude alternative etiologies such as myelopathy or an infiltrative or compressive radiculopathy. Transverse myelitis manifests as rapidly progressive neurologic dysfunction with edematous expansion of the cord and possible patchy enhancement, typically extending over multiple vertebral body levels and involving the entire cross section of the cord. Multiple sclerosis lesions commonly affect the cervical spinal cord. These also demonstrate T2/STIR hyperintensity (bright) but are often located peripherally (Fig. 2.16C), are less than two vertebral body segments in length, and rarely cause cord enlargement or enhancement.

Head and Neck Pathologies

Head and neck imaging falls within the realm of neuroradiology and includes CT and MRI with contrast, often performed for evaluation of neck masses. The most common cause of a neck mass in adults is lymphadenopathy, either inflammatory or metastatic. Other less frequent etiologies for neck masses include congenital, neoplastic, traumatic, and infectious/inflammatory (Fig. 2.21).

Branchial cleft cysts and thyroglossal duct cysts are usually incidental findings in younger patients. They are generally benign, but when they become infected the patient may present with a painful and/or swollen neck mass. Second branchial cleft cysts are the most common type of branchial cleft cyst and are typically located near the angle of the mandible. Thyroglossal duct cysts occur in the midline neck, anywhere between the tongue base

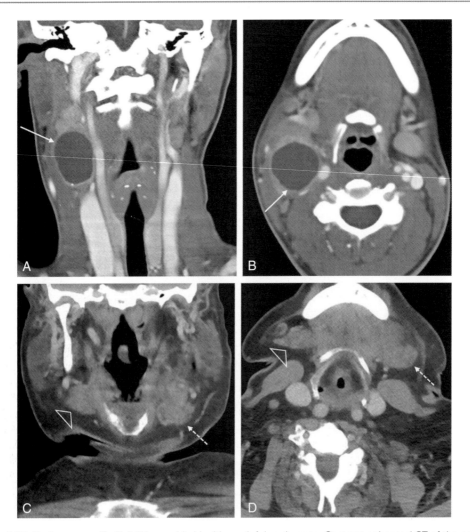

Fig. 2.21 Neck masses. (A, B) A 15-year-old girl with a painful neck mass. Contrast-enhanced CT of the neck demonstrates an abscess (*arrow*) in a right cervical lymph node, corresponding to the neck swelling. (C, D) A 67-year-old male with sudden-onset left neck swelling and pain. Contrast-enhanced CT of the neck demonstrates asymmetric enlargement of the left submandibular gland (*dashed arrow*) with surrounding fat stranding, representing sialadenitis. The right submandibular gland is normal (*arrowhead*). (From George E, Guenette JP, Lee TC. Introduction to neuroimaging. *Am J Med*. 2018;131(4):346–356.)

and the thyroid gland, and will elevate with tongue protrusion.

Thyroid cancer is the most common primary malignancy within the neck, and ultrasound is the best modality for the initial assessment of thyroid findings. In cases of malignancy, CT and MRI may be used to assess for local invasion and metastases. Although there are no definitive characteristics of thyroid cancer on ultrasound, nodules with microcalcifications, irregular margins, and a taller-than-wide shape are highly suspicious and may warrant biopsy. Per ACR guidelines, incidental thyroid nodules without suspicious features on CT/MRI that measure <1 cm in patients <35 years old or <1.5 cm in patients >35 years old do not require further evaluation.

Infections within the neck are of particular clinical concern due to the limited space, multiple critical blood vessels, and risk of rapid spread to critical structures.

The neck is divided anatomically into multiple longitudinal spaces that allow infections to quickly expand both superiorly and inferiorly. One of the most important compartments is the retropharyngeal space, which is located between the posterior pharynx and the anterior spine. Infections and fluid collections in this space can compress the airway and have the potential to spread inferiorly into the mediastinum.

Image-Guided Intervention

There are many image-guided head, neck, and spine interventions performed for diagnosis and therapy, including facet injections, nerve root blocks, and epidural steroid injections. In all of these cases, it is important to first establish a clinical correlation between the patient's symptoms and imaging findings so as not to miss an unexpected pathology. These procedures are conducted under fluoroscopic (x-ray), CT, or MRI guidance. Short-term symptom relief is often possible with injections, but the underlying disease will remain, and symptoms usually recur. When injections have worked but temporarily, ablation of the associated nerve can lead to more durable relief, though this may be nonpermanent. Ablation of neoplasms can be curative but may be temporizing in metastatic situations. Patients should be made aware of limitations prior to the intervention.

Vertebral augmentation procedures are often performed for osteoporotic vertebral compression fractures.

The two primary percutaneous vertebral augmentation procedures are vertebroplasty and kyphoplasty. In both cases, a needle is inserted through the skin and used to inject surgical cement into the fracture space to stabilize it and manage the patient's symptoms. The difference between the two is that in a kyphoplasty, a small balloon is inflated within the fracture space to expand the compressed vertebra before the cement is injected. The goal is to reduce the risk of extravasation, and may be more beneficial in cases of tumor infiltration of the marrow. Although these procedures often help with pain control, there are mixed data on the long-term benefits.

The more recently developed interventional procedures include CT- and MRI-guided ablation of head, neck, and spine tumors. These procedures often use cryoablation or heat-based modalities such as radiofrequency ablation to target lesions in real time under direct imaging guidance, allowing for precise tumor treatment while reducing risks to critical adjacent structures such as the cord and cervical arteries. Although this is still a developing field, clinicians should keep in mind these emerging treatment options.

"For the full bibliography list, please use the pincode on the inside front cover to access the electronic version of the text at ebooks.health.elsevier.com."

3

Introduction to Neurogenetics*

Angeliki Vgontzas and William Renthal

INTRODUCTION

Neurogenetics has evolved considerably over the last 25 years. Advancements in human genome sequencing have led to the identification of mutations that cause neurologic disease and to fundamentally new insights into disease pathophysiology. These advances, along with technological breakthroughs in gene therapy, have already translated genetic insight into disease treatments for previously incurable diseases, a process that will continue to accelerate. Given the increasing role genetic diagnosis and treatment are playing in neurological care, we aim to summarize basic genetic concepts and provide a framework for approaching both rare and common neurogenetic diseases.

BASIC CONCEPTS

The human genome is composed of over 3 billion DNA nucleotides organized into 23 pairs of chromosomes. Genes are sequences of DNA that are transcribed into RNA and translated into proteins. Although all cells contain the same DNA, gene expression is customized to the specific cell type and physiological stimulus. These complex gene expression patterns are controlled by gene enhancers, which are short, noncoding regions of DNA that recruit transcription factors required for gene activation of nearby protein-coding genes.

*Based on the article—Vgontzas A, Renthal W. Introduction to neurogenetics. *Am J Med.* 2019;132(2):142–152, ISSN 0002-9343, https://doi.org/10.1016/j.amjmed.2018.07.041 (https://www.sciencedirect.com/science/article/pii/S0002934318307708).

Humans inherit two copies of each gene, one from each parent. Rare genetic diseases often follow Mendelian inheritance patterns, in which the disease is the direct result of a single-gene mutation. Diseases that follow an autosomal dominant inheritance pattern require only one mutant allele and typically affect every generation of a family (e.g., neurofibromatosis, Huntington disease, and myotonic dystrophy). Autosomal recessive diseases require the inheritance of two mutant alleles, which often results in asymptomatic or mildly symptomatic carriers (e.g., Friedrich ataxia, Tay-Sachs disease). X-linked diseases are more commonly observed in males because they only have a single X chromosome, while females can be asymptomatic or mildly symptomatic carriers (e.g., Duchenne and Becker muscular dystrophy). Spontaneous mutations are not inherited but occur during development because of DNA replication errors. Somatic and germline mosaicism can occur when mutations occur in later stages of development, such that only certain cell lineages are affected by the mutation, while other cell and tissue types remain normal. Mosaicism may result in diverse phenotypes depending on where in the developmental process the mutation occurs. Mosaicism can also be observed in heterozygous females with X-linked mutations because X-inactivation randomly silences either the wild-type or mutant X chromosomes in each cell. Rare and phenotypically severe neurologic diseases can also be caused by mutations in the maternally inherited mitochondrial DNA.

The phenotypic severity of a genetic mutation depends on how the DNA sequence is altered. Point mutations occur when a single nucleotide is changed and can result in silent, missense, or nonsense mutations. Silent mutations, which are asymptomatic, do not affect the encoded protein because the mutated DNA sequence still codes for the wild-type amino acid. Missense mutations change a specific amino acid within a protein, and the phenotypic severity of this largely depends on how the amino acid change alters the protein's function. A nonsense mutation results in a stop codon that terminates the translation of messenger RNA into protein. The severity of nonsense mutations depends on where in the protein the stop codon occurs, but they often result in severely truncated proteins. If more than a single nucleotide is mutated (e.g., insertions or deletions), a frameshift mutation can occur that disrupts the entire reading frame of the gene and usually results in severely dysfunctional protein. Several neurologic diseases, such as Huntington disease, are also caused by repeat expansions. Trinucleotide repeats often increase with each generation and are thought to result in progressively toxic RNA or protein products that correlate with disease severity. Lastly, noncoding DNA mutations may be significant if they prevent a transcription factor from binding to a gene regulatory element (gene promotor or enhancer) that is needed to activate the expression of a nearby gene. Distal enhancers can be at great distances from their target genes and form long chromatin loops to make contact with and regulate their expression.

The majority of common neurologic diseases are polygenic, caused by the summation of small effects from mutations in many genomic loci (e.g., Alzheimer disease, Parkinson disease, migraine). Genome-wide association studies (GWASs) have revolutionized the study of polygenic diseases. GWAS may identify genetic variation that is statistically more common in the disease of interest. Because multiple statistical comparisons are needed to study every genomic locus, large numbers of cases and controls are required to sufficiently power these studies. Initial GWASs were met with criticism because of insufficient sample sizes to detect susceptibility loci, but the ongoing development of collaborative international consortia has led to more recent high-quality studies.

RARE GENETIC DISEASES

Advances in DNA sequencing have resulted in the identification of numerous rare single-gene mutations in a wide spectrum of neurological diseases. Although these diseases are rare and may not be encountered in the primary care setting, collectively, they are not uncommon. Given recent improvements in gene therapy, it is important to recognize and refer these patients to specialists. The tables at the end of the manuscript serve as a reference and contain a detailed listing of rare monogenic neurologic diseases, organized by cellular function affected (see Tables 3.1–3.5). Below, we will review the key cellular processes that are disrupted in neurogenetic disorders to provide a framework for understanding their pathophysiology and clinical presentation.

Metabolic diseases affect energy homeostasis within the cell via mitochondrial dysfunction, toxic metabolite buildup secondary to lysosome dysfunction, urea cycle dysfunction, or deficiencies in the processing of vitamins, minerals, and lipids. These diverse diseases may have severe phenotypes that present during infancy, although milder subtypes can present during adolescence and early adulthood (see Table 3.1). Clinical identification has traditionally been important for symptomatic management and surveillance. However, the identification of causative genes in some cases has led to significant changes in clinical management. One example of this was the identification of the gene responsible for GLUT1 deficiency, in which a defective transporter results in poor ability to transport glucose across the blood-brain barrier, manifesting with expected severe neurological symptoms within the first 6 months of life (epileptic encephalopathy, global developmental delay, complex movement disorders, and paroxysmal events triggered by exercise, exertion, or fasting). Identification of the gene that encodes this glucose transporter, *SLC2A1*, created more accurate and less invasive diagnostic testing and identified the need to place patients on a strict ketogenic diet, which increases ketones in the blood and can be used as an alternative energy source in the brain.

Genetic disorders of axon guidance are a small group of rare disorders caused by mutations in genes involved in normal axonal growth, axon signaling, transport molecules, and structural proteins. They include several anatomical abnormalities, including corpus callosum agenesis, Joubert syndrome, and albinism. They have been traditionally difficult to diagnose and phenotypically characterize without the assistance of imaging. Genome sequencing has led to better characterization and diagnosis of some of these disorders, as well as creation of mouse models to better understand these disorders.

TABLE 3.1   Major Neurometabolic Diseases With Causative Genes, Pathophysiology, and Phenotypic Features

| Type | Disease | GENETICS | | | Pathophysiology | Phenotypic Features |
		Gene(s)	Location	Inherit		
Mitochondrial	MELAS	*MTTL1*	Mit.	M	Dysfunctional tRNA results in improper translation.	Seizures, ataxia, ischemic events, short stature, hearing loss, exercise intolerance, migraine.
	MERFF	*MTTK*	Mit.	M	Dysfunctional tRNA results in improper translation.	Seizures, ataxia, myoclonus, weakness, ptosis (may overlap with MELAS).
	LHON	*MTND4* *MTND1* *MTND6*	Mit.	M	Malfunctioning proteins involved in oxidative phosphorylation.	Subacute loss of central vision. 50%–85% of people with the mutation are asymptomatic.
Lysosomal	Gaucher disease (types 2 and 3)	*GBA*	1q22	AR	Glucocerebroside toxicity within cells secondary to abnormal β-glucocerebrosidase.	Type 2 may include brainstem dysfunction, apnea, hepatosplenomegaly, anemia, failure to thrive, thrombocytopenia, high mortality rate < age 2.
	Niemann-Pick disease	*SMPD1*	11p15.4	AR	Sphingomyelin excess due to abnormal sphingomyelinase.	Hepatosplenomegaly, cherry-red spot, and profound psychomotor regression; rare survival after age 2. Type B: without CNS involvement.
		NPC1 *NPC2*	18q11.2 14q24.3	AR	Lipid accumulation due to dysfunctional lipid movement within cells.	Ataxia, supranuclear gaze palsy, dystonia, hepatosplenomegaly, interstitial lung disease.
	Fabry disease	*GLA*	Xq22.1	XR	Glycosphingolipid excess in lysosomes due to α-galactosidase deficiency.	Classic: paresthesias, pain crises, GI manifestation, angiokeratoma, hypohidrosis, corneal/lenticular opacities, early death from renal or vascular disease. Later onset: no vascular endothelial involvement, but develop cardiac and renal disease in maturity.

Category	Disease	Gene	Locus	Inheritance	Mechanism	Presentation
Metal metabolism disorders	Wilson disease	*ATP7B*	13q14.3	AR	Excess copper accumulation secondary to dysfunctional copper transporter ATPase 2.	Cirrhosis and neuropsychiatric symptoms (tremors, gait difficulty, mood disturbance), Kayser-Fleischer ring.
	Menkes disease	*ATP7A*	Xq21.1	XR	Maldistribution of copper (deficiency) in mitochondria, collagen, vascular tissue, and neuronal degeneration.	Presentation in neonate with hypothermia, feeding difficulties, seizures, palor, and kinky hair.
	PKAN	*PANK2*	20p13	AR	Lack of functional pantothenate kinase 2 disrupts the production of coenzyme A and results in iron deposition in the basal ganglia.	Neurodegeneration with brain iron accumulation, childhood-onset dystonia and pigmentary retinopathy, dementia, parkinsonism, and neuropsychiatric features.
Vitamin disorders	Holocarboxylase synthetase deficiency	*HLCS*	21q22.13	AR	Accumulation of abnormal urea cycle metabolites secondary to inability to utilize biotin.	Severe metabolic acidosis, feeding and breathing difficulties, hypotonia, lethargy in neonatal period.
	Pyridoxine-dependent epilepsy	*ALDH7A1*	5q23.2	AR	Accumulation of pyridoxine (B6).	Encephalopathy and seizures, intractable to antiepileptic drugs, treated with pyridoxine supplementation.
Lipid metabolism	Cerebrotendinous xanthomatosis	*CYP27A1*	2q35	AR	Lipid accumulation in brain parenchyma and myelin results in its destruction.	Defective bile acid synthesis—tendon/tuberous xanthomas, juvenile cataracts, nervous system dysfunction (epilepsy, movement disorders, peripheral neuropathy, dementia).

(continued)

TABLE 3.1   Major Neurometabolic Diseases With Causative Genes, Pathophysiology, and Phenotypic Features—cont'd

| Type | Disease | GENETICS | | | Pathophysiology | Phenotypic Features |
		Gene(s)	Location	Inherit		
Urea cycle	Carbamoyl phosphate synthetase I deficiency	CPS1	2q35	AR	The enzyme is responsible for catalyzing entry of ammonia into the urea cycle.	Neonatal presentation starts secondary to hyperammonemia and includes poor feeding, vomiting, lethargy, seizures, coma, tachypnea, cerebral edema, and death if untreated. Treatments are sodium phenylacetate/benzoate and arginine. Partial deficiencies may present in adulthood in the setting of stress (e.g., surgery) and may present as encephalopathy, behavioral and psychiatric disorders, vomiting, alterations in consciousness.
	Ornithine transcarbamylase deficiency	OTC	Xp11.4	XR	The enzyme catalyzes production of citrulline from ornithine and carbamylphosphate in the liver and small intestine.	
	Argininosuccinate synthase deficiency	ASS1	9q34.11	AR	The enzyme catalyzes conversion of citrulline and aspartate to arginosuccinic acid.	
	Argininosuccinate lyase deficiency	ASL	7q11.21	AR	Catalyzes conversion of arginosuccinate to arginine and fumarate.	
	Arginase deficiency	ARG1	6q23.2	AR	Catalyzes conversion of L-arginine into L-ornithine and urea.	
	HHH	SLC25A15	13q14.11	AR	Ornithine translocase is a mitochondrial transporter.	

AR, Autosomal recessive; CNS, central nervous system; GI, gastrointestinal; HHH, hyperornithinemia-hyperammonemia-homocitrullinuria; LHON, Leber hereditary optic neuropathy; mit., mitochondria; M, maternal; MELAS, mitochondrial encephalomyopathy, lactic acidosis, and stroke-like episodes; MERRF, myoclonus epilepsy and ragged-red fibers; PKAN: pantothenate kinase–associated neurodegeneration; tRNA, transfer RNA; XR, X-linked recessive.

TABLE 3.2 Genetic Channelopathies With Principal Causative Genes and Key Phenotypic Features

Channel Affected	Disorder	Gene	Loc.	Inherit	Key Phenotypic Features
Sodium	Simple febrile seizures (part of GEFS+ syndrome)	SCN1A	2q24.3	AD	Seizures associated with fever in childhood. There is an overall benign course, although the risk of future epilepsy syndromes is increased.
	Dravet syndrome (or SMEI—severe myoclonic epilepsy of infancy) (part of GEFS+ syndrome)	SCN1A (in 80% of cases)	2q24.3	AD	Infantile-onset encephalopathy with epilepsy (tonic, tonic-clonic, or clonic seizures), typically presenting in the context of fever, continues to involve multiple seizure types and significant cognitive dysfunction. May have normal development in the first year of life, followed by regression.
	FHM3	SCN1A	2q24.3	AD	Attacks of migraine with fully reversible motor weakness and visual, sensory, or language problems.
Potassium	KCNQ2-related disorders (BFNE; NEE)	KCNQ2	20q13.33	AD	These are a continuum of disorders. BFNE—seizures starting within the first week of birth, normal interictal periods, and spontaneously disappearing by 1 year of age. NEE—In addition, patients have encephalopathy from birth and persist after seizures end (age 1–4 years) with moderate-severe developmental impairment.
	Episodic ataxia, type 1	KCNA1	12pq13.32	AD	Brief episodes of ataxia (minutes), provoked by exercise, with facial and hand myokymia. Treated with phenytoin.
Calcium	FHM 1	CACNA1A	19p13.3	AD	Attacks of migraine with hemiplegia that may be accompanied by vertigo or mild ataxia.
	Episodic ataxia, type 2	CACNA1A	19p13.3	AD	Episodes of ataxia for days and vertigo provoked by stress. Treated with acetazolamide.

(continued)

TABLE 3.2   Genetic Channelopathies With Principal Causative Genes and Key Phenotypic Features—cont'd

Channel Affected	Disorder	Gene	Loc.	Inherit	Key Phenotypic Features
AChR	AD familial nocturnal frontal lobe epilepsy	CHRNA4, CHRNB2	20q13.33 1q21.3	AD	Nocturnal seizures during NREM sleep with tonic, clonic, and hyperkinetic movements, normal cognition, and development. Ictal EEG with bifrontal spike wave discharges.
GABA	Juvenile myoclonic epilepsy	GABRA1	5q34	AD	Myoclonic seizures, usually in the morning on awakening. Presentation starts in adolescence. Comorbid with absence seizures and generalized tonic-clonic seizures. EEG with 4–6Hz polyspike wave complexes.
	Childhood absence epilepsy	GABRG2, GABRA1, GABRB3	5q34 5q34 15q12	AD	Multiple daily absence seizures in developmentally normal children 4–10 years old; 3-Hz spike and wave pattern.

[a]Spinocerebellar ataxia 6 (SCA6) is also a notable channelopathy affecting P/Q type calcium channels; however, in this review, it has been classified along with the other SCAs as a repeat expansion disorder (see Table 3.4).

GEFS+ is a spectrum of seizure disorders that may be associated with fevers (simple febrile seizures are considered the mildest form, and Dravet syndrome is the most severe form). *AChR*, Acetylcholine receptor; *AD*, Alzheimer disease; *BFNE*, benign familial neonatal epilepsy; *EEG*, electroencephalogram; *EIEE*, early infantile epileptic encephalopathy; *FHM3*, familial hemiplegic migraine type 3; *GABA*, gamma aminobutyric acid; *GEFS+*, generalized epilepsy with febrile seizures plus; *NEE*, neonatal epileptic encephalopathy; *NREM*, non–rapid eye movement.

TABLE 3.3 Disorders of Gene Regulation With Major Causative Genes, Pathophysiology, and Phenotypic Features

Disease	GENETICS			Pathophysiology	Phenotypic Features
	Gene(s)	Location	Inherit		
Facioscapulohumeral muscular dystrophy—type 2	SMCHD1 DUX4	18p11.32 4q35.2	Digenic[a]	SMCHD1 protein affects DNA methylation in the D4Z4 region—preventing the normal silencing of the DUX4 gene.	Progressive muscle weakness and atrophy starting in face, scapula, and upper arms starting in adolescence may progress to lower extremity weakness and hearing loss.
Angelman syndrome[b]	UBE3A	15q11.2	Sporadic	Altered ubiquitin protein ligase results in altered proteostasis (rate of protein synthesis and degradation) at synapses.	Developmental delay, ataxia, epilepsy, microcephaly, happy demeanor, frequent smiling, laughter and hand-flapping movements, hyperactivity, coarse facial features, fair skin, light-colored hair, scoliosis.
Rett syndrome	MECP2	Xq28	XD	MeCP2 protein has various roles in transcription regulation.	Primarily in girls. Classic phenotype involves regression of normal development 6-18 months, with progressive dementia, motor loss, and stereotypies.
Rubinstein-Taybi syndrome	CREBBP	16p13.3	AD	CREB-binding protein important in gene regulation in many tissues (cell growth, division, and normal fetal development).	Short stature, moderate to severe intellectual disability, distinctive facial features, broad thumbs, increased risk of malignancies.
X-linked intellectual disability, Siderius type	PHF8	XP11.22	XR	Altered PHF8 protein (part of zinc finger proteins) is not able to bind chromatin, affecting chromatin remodeling, altering normal gene expression.	Only males are affected. Intellectual disability, cleft lip/palate, and developmental delay may have characteristic facial features (long face, sloping forehead, broad nasal bridge, prominent supraorbital ridge, upslanting palpebral fissures).
Early infantile epileptic encephalopathy 1	ARX	Xp21.3-XP22.1	XR	Altered transcriptional factor that is part of homeobox genes that act during early embryonic development to control cell differentiation.	Infantile spasms, developmental delay, and EEG with hypsarrhythmia pattern. Cases may evolve to LGS.

AD, Alzheimer disease; *EEG*, electroencephalogram; *LGS*, Lenox-Gastaut syndrome; *XR*, X-linked recessive.

[a]Digenic—two independent genetic changes are necessary to cause the disorder. Individuals typically inherit the *SMCHD1* gene mutation from one parent and the "permissive" chromosome 4 from the other parent.

[b]In Angelman disease, the maternal copy of the gene is the only one that is active in the brain. The parent-specific gene activation results from genomic imprinting.

TABLE 3.4 Neurologic Disorders Caused by Sequence Repeats—Including Select Ataxias, such as Spinocerebellar Ataxias (SCA), Friedrich Ataxia, and Myotonic Dystrophies

Disease	GENETICS			Pathophysiology	Phenotypic Features
	Gene(s)	Location	Inherit		
SCA1	ATXN1	6p22.3	AD	CAG repeats in the ataxin protein form cytotoxic intranuclear aggregates.	Ataxia with ophthalmoparesis and nystagmus, speech and swallowing difficulties, spasticity, and cognitive impairment. May develop peripheral neuropathy, atrophy, dystonia, chorea.
SCA2	ATXN2	12q24.12	AD	CAG repeats in the ataxin-2 protein are cytotoxic.	Ataxia, ophthalmoparesis, saccadic slowing. May develop peripheral neuropathy, atrophy, dystonia, chorea, and dementia; comorbid RLS or REM sleep behavior disorder.
SCA3	ATXN3	14q32.2	AD	CAG repeats, codes for ubiquitin protease (waste clearing system), which becomes inactivated with polyglutamine aggregates, MJD-ataxin 3.	Ataxia with ophthalmoparesis, variable pyramidal, extrapyramidal, and amyotrophic signs, mild dementia.
SCA6[a]	CACNA1A	19p13.2	AD	CAG repeats in the calcium channel gene result in its inactivation.	Ataxia dysarthria, nystagmus.
SCA36	NOP56	20p13	AD	GGCCTG repeat.	Ataxia, motor neuron disease, muscular atrophy, fasciculations.
Friedrich ataxia	FXN	9q21.1	AD	GAA repeats result in abnormal frataxin, resulting in abnormal regulation of mitochondrial iron metabolism and iron accumulation.	Ataxia, cardiomyopathy, diabetes mellitus, foot deformities, optic atrophy.
Dentatorubropallidoluysian atrophy	ATN1	12p13.31	AD	CAG repeats resulted in abnormal atropine.	Ataxia, chorea, dystonia, seizures, myoclonus, dementia.

Disease	Gene	Locus	Inheritance	Mechanism	Clinical features
Fragile X syndrome	FMR1	Xq27.3	XD	CGG repeat (>200x) is expanded within the FMR1 gene, silencing it. This affects FMRP protein, which shuttles mRNA molecules involved in synapse development.	>200 repeats: delayed language, intellectual development, anxiety, hyperactivity, autism spectrum disorder, seizures, physical features (narrow face, large ears, prominent jaw/forehead) 55–200 repeats: intellectually normal, may have mild physical features and autism-like behaviors.
DM1	DMPK	19q13.3	AD	CTG repeat expansion in myotonic dystrophy protein kinase, important in myocytes, also found in brain and heart.	Progressive muscle weakness and atrophy (most prominent in lower legs, hands, neck, and face), myotonia (prolonged muscle contractions), cataracts, cardiac conduction defects, endocrine abnormalities.
DM2	CNBP	3q21.3	AD	CCTG repeat expansion in a regulatory gene found in heart and skeletal muscles.	Similar, but less severe presentation than DM1, but with greater proximal than distal muscle weakness pattern.

For a more complete listing of SCAs, *Rosenberg's Molecular Basis of Neurologic and Psychiatric Disease* is recommended. SCA3 is also known as Machado-Joseph disease. *AD*, Alzheimer disease; *CAG*, Cytosine-adenine-guanine; *DM1*, myotonic dystrophy type 1; *DM2*, myotonic dystrophy type 2; *XD*, X-linked dominant.

[a]SCA6 may also be classified as a channelopathy, but it was included in this table with the other SCAs.

TABLE 3.5 Peripheral Inherited Neuropathies (Charcot-Marie-Tooth [CMT] or Hereditary Motor and Sensory Neuropathies)

Syndrome	Phenotypic Features	Subtype	GENETICS			
			Gene(s)	Location	Inherit	Protein
CMT1 (autosomal dominant)	Distal muscle weakness and atrophy, sensory loss, slow nerve conduction velocity. Slowly progressive, associated with pes cavus foot deformity and bilateral foot drop. Age of onset is 5–25 years of age. Life span preserved.	CMT1A (70%–80% of all CMT1)	PMP22	17p12	AD	Peripheral myelin protein 22
		CMT1B (6%–10%)	MPZ	1q23.3	AD	Myelin protein P0
		CMT1C (1%–2%)	LITAF	16p13.13	AD	Lipopolysaccharide-induced TNF-α
		CMT1D (<2%)	EGR	10q21.3	AD	E3 SUMO-protein ligase EGR2
		CMT1E (<5%)	PMP22	17p12	AD	Peripheral myelin protein 22
		CMT1F (<5%)	NEFL	8p21.2	AD	Neurofilament light polypeptide
CMT2	Distal muscle weakness, mild sensory loss, normal/near-normal nerve conduction velocities. Usually less severe than CMT1. CMT2A1 can have MS-like white matter lesions on brain MRI.[a]	CMT2A1 (rare)	KIF1B	1p36.22	AD	Kinesin-like protein
		CMT2A2 (10%–30% of CMT2)	MFN2	1p36.2	AD, AR	Kinesin-like protein
		CMT2B (rare)	RAB7A	3q21.3	AD	Ras-related protein
		CMT2B1 (rare)	LMNA	1q22	AR	Prelamin-A/C
		CMT2C (rare)	TRPV4	12q24.11	AD	Transient receptor potential cation channel
		CMT2D (rare)	GARS	7p14.3	AD	Glycine-tRNA ligase
		CMT2E/1F (rare)	NEFL	8p21.2	AD	Neurofilament light polypeptide
		CMT2F (4% of CMT2)	HSPB1	7q11.23	AD	Heat shock protein beta-1
		CMT2I/J (1%–8% of CMT2)	MPZ	1q23.3	AD	Myelin protein P0
		CMT2H/K (rare)	GDAP1	8q21.11	AR, AD	Ganglioside-induced differentiation-associated protein

			Gene	Locus		Protein
CMT4	Distal muscle weakness and atrophy associated with sensory loss and pes cavus foot deformity.	CMT4A (1%–5%)	GDAP1		AR	
		CMT4B1 (1%)	MTMR2	11q21	AR	Myotubularin-related protein 2
		CMT4B2 (4%)	SBF2	11p15.4	AR	Myotubularin-related protein 13
		CMT4C (1%–12%)	SH3TC2	5q32	AR	SH3 domain and tetratricopeptide repeat containing protein 2
		CMT4D (rare)	NDRG1	8q24.22	AR	Protein NDRG1
		CMT4E (1%)	EGR2	10q21.3	AR	E3 SUMO-protein ligase EGR2
		CMT4F (5%)	PRX	19q.32	AR	Periaxin
		CMT4H (3%)	FGD4	12p11.21	AR	FYVE, RhoGEF, and PH domain containing protein 4
CMTX	Males with distal weakness, foot drop, sensory loss. Females may be minimally affected. Sensorineural hearing loss and optic neuropathy (more common in type 5).	CMTX1	GJB1	Xq13.1	XD, XR	Connexin-32 (gap junction beta-1)
		CMTX5	PRPS1	Xq22.3	XR	Phosphoribosyl pyrophosphate synthetase 1

AD, Alzheimer disease; *AR*, Autosomal recessive; *MRI*, magnetic resonance imaging; *TNF-α*, tumor necrosis factor alpha; *tRNA*, transfer RNA; *XD*, X-linked dominant; *XR*, X-linked recessive.

aMany more CMT2 subtypes have been discovered and are frequently unique to a single family; please see the reference for a complete listing.

Channelopathies can be associated with diverse clinical presentations, such as epilepsy, encephalopathy, periodic paralysis, or pain disorders (see Table 3.2). Ion channels are vital for initiating and propagating action potentials in neurons as well as establishing their resting membrane potential. The specific neurological symptoms can often be predicted by the electrophysiological consequences of the ion channel mutation and the cell types in which it is expressed. The sodium channel Nav 1.7, which is expressed in primary sensory neurons, exemplifies the close link between channel physiology and neurologic symptoms. Mutations in Nav 1.7 that block sodium conductance in primary sensory neurons result in congenital insensitivity to pain, while mutations in the same channel that increase sodium conductance result in severe pain disorders.

Disorders of gene regulation have been implicated in multiple neurologic diseases (see Table 3.3). Coordinated gene expression programs are critical for normal neuronal development, synapse formation, and plasticity. The translational potential of basic research on gene regulation in the nervous system is exemplified by the survival motor neuron 1 gene (*SMN1*) in infantile-onset spinal muscular atrophy. *SMN1* gene mutations affect how messenger RNA is processed in the cell, such that it is not translated into the correct amino acid sequences needed for spinal motor neuron survival. Clinically, this manifests as a profound, progressive weakness in feeding and respiratory functions. The severity of this condition partly depends on the expression of the related survival motor neuron 2 gene (*SMN2*), which can compensate for the *SMN1* mutation and lead to motor neuron survival. This observation resulted in the development of Nusinersen, a novel drug administered intrathecally that selectively increases expression of the *SMN2* gene product to ensure motor neuron survival. Nusinersen clinical trials resulted in dramatic improvements in motor outcomes, and the drug is US Food and Drug Administration (FDA) approved for treating infantile-onset spinal muscular atrophy. Two other drugs have been FDA-approved for SMA: Risdiplam, a daily pill that enhances the splicing of *SMN2* to the full-length SMN protein and onasemnogene abeparvovec-xioi, a one-time intravenous (IV) gene therapy utilizing a nonpathogenic viral vector called adenovirus-associated virus (AAV) that replaces the *SMN1* gene in vivo with a functional SMN transgene.

Several novel gene therapies are approved for the treatment of Duchenne muscular dystrophy (DMD), an X-linked recessive disorder presenting in young boys characterized by muscle atrophy and progressive loss of ambulation, cardiac dysfunction, and death due to mutations in the largest known human gene, dystrophin. Eteplirsen, an exon skipping weekly IV gene therapy, was the first to gain accelerated FDA approval in 2016. Eteplirsen has been shown to increase dystrophin and prevent loss of ambulation in patients with a mutation in the dystrophin gene amenable to exon 51 skipping (15% of patients with DMD). By excising the problematic exon segment and linking the two remaining functional ends together, the drug was shown to increase dystrophin protein in patients, albeit the gene is less functional and a smaller version compared to normal type. Three other weekly IV exon-skipping gene therapies were subsequently approved for DMD—golodirsen and vitolarsen, which target exon 53 (a mutation found in 8% of those with DMD), and casimersen, which targets exon 45 (affecting 9% of patients with DMD), and ongoing trials for these and several other new exon-skipping drugs are currently underway. Ataluren is an oral drug that bypasses a nonsense mutation in the dystrophin gene (present in 10% of patients with DMD) that results in a stop codon and early termination of dystrophin translation; it is approved by the European Medicines Agency but not the FDA. Individual phase 2 and 3 trials did not meet their primary endpoints (mean change in 6-min walk test in all participants), but subsequent post hoc analyses and meta-analyses showed significant improvement in a prespecified group (those in the ambulatory transition phase, with more severe disease burden). Multiple DMD clinical trials of AAV gene therapies are currently underway. AAV aims to deliver mini/micro-dystrophin genes in vivo with the goal to increase dystrophin expression, with early clinical trials showing promising results. A major advantage of these AAV therapies is that they can be used in all patients with DMD, regardless of individual genetic mutations. While there remain challenges to the broader application of gene therapies in neurology (e.g., toxicity, cost), the early successes described above have led to great excitement and investment in this area and will likely lead to improved treatment options for many patients with neurological disease in the near future.

Disorders of repeat expansion can cause neurological diseases such as Huntington disease, spinocerebellar ataxia, and myotonic dystrophy (see Table 3.5). These short nucleotide repeats may expand in subsequent generations through a process termed anticipation, in which subsequent generations develop symptoms at an earlier age. Therefore family history of milder symptoms becomes incredibly important when these diseases are suspected. The mechanisms by which short nucleotide repeats cause disease is an area of active research, but recent evidence suggests that pathogenic numbers of nucleotide repeats cause RNA or protein to form large macromolecular aggregates within cells that could disrupt normal cell functions. Indeed, this has been observed in amyotrophic lateral sclerosis, another disorder in which a repeat expansion of C9ORF72 results in intracellular aggregates that directly damage intracellular processes.

Perhaps the most well-known repeat nucleotide disorder is Huntington disease, an autosomal dominant disorder caused by cytosine-adenine-guanine (CAG) repeats in the huntingtin gene (*HTT*). Phenotypic expression of disease occurs at >37 CAG repeats, with the classic disease presentation (chorea, dystonia, cognitive decline, and depression) manifesting once there are >41 CAG repeats. The CAG repeats within *HTT* encode an abnormal protein, which results in cytotoxic neuronal inclusions. In rodent models of Huntington disease, decreasing the levels of mutant *HTT* reversed disease symptoms and suggests a potential avenue for drug development. Early-stage clinical trials with an antisense oligonucleotide that targets *HTT* mRNA show promising results in reductions of mutant *HTT* in CSF in patients, giving hope for ongoing clinical trials in patients with this progressive neurodegenerative disease.

COMMON GENETIC DISEASES

The majority of neurologic diseases that are encountered in clinical practice are polygenic and result from the combined effects of multiple DNA variants. The development of GWAS was integral for the identification of common variants that increase the likelihood of disease transmission.

Alzheimer Disease

Alzheimer disease is the most common neurodegenerative disorder, affecting 4.5 million Americans, with the prevalence expected to increase to over 13 million by 2050. Genetic studies in both the rare early-onset subtype and more common late-onset disease presentation have provided significant insights into AD pathophysiology.

The earliest genetic studies of Alzheimer disease focused on the rare familial early-onset subtype. Familial Alzheimer disease occurs before age 65, affects <1% of those with Alzheimer disease, and is inherited in an autosomal dominant pattern. Linkage analysis of the familial subtype in the 1990s identified three fully penetrant mutations in amyloid beta (A4) precursor protein (*APP*), presenilin 1 (*PSEN1*), and presenilin 2 (*PSEN2*). Molecular characterization of genes converged on the common pathway of amyloid beta processing, a known pathologic marker of Alzheimer disease. These insights resulted in a better understanding of the mechanisms involved in amyloid plaque formation and in the development of animal models. These molecular genetic insights observed from single-gene mutations in the familial subtype likely have relevance to the more common form of Alzheimer disease (sporadic) because the clinical presentation and neuropathological changes (neuronal loss, neurofibrillary tangles, amyloid plaques, and cerebral amyloid angiopathy) are very similar between the two conditions.

Alzheimer disease has also been associated with a common polymorphism in the *APOE* gene termed *APOE-ε4*. The *APOE* gene encodes a protein that functions as a major cholesterol carrier in both the periphery and the brain. In contrast to the three autosomal dominant mutations that cause disease in all carriers, *APOE-ε4* confers an increased *risk* of disease development with an effect size that varies widely in different populations. It thus follows that *APOE-ε4* alleles are not observed in all patients with Alzheimer disease, and all individuals with *APOE-ε4* alleles do not develop Alzheimer disease. *APOE-ε4* is also a risk factor for cardiovascular disease, which raised the possibility that there may be an interaction between vascular and dementia pathophysiology, as observed in diabetics.

While much insight into pathophysiology has been obtained from mutations with very strong effects, GWASs have identified over 75 common loci associated with small effects on the risk of developing Alzheimer disease. It is thought that the aggregation of risk alleles (large, medium, and small effects) in an individual determines their ultimate likelihood of developing the disease.

Migraine

Migraine is a prevalent and debilitating neurologic disorder characterized by episodic, prolonged severe headaches with nausea, photophobia, and phonophobia, causing significant disability. Attack pathophysiology involves cortical spreading depression (in at least those with aura) followed by activation of trigeminal afferents surrounding meningeal and dural vessels. Activation of trigeminal afferents results in the release of nociceptive and inflammatory substances, causing vasodilation, pain sensitization, and activation of brainstem and thalamic nuclei that are likely involved in migraine-associated features such as photophobia and nausea.

Family studies have revealed an approximate two- to threefold increased risk of migraine among first-degree relatives of those with migraine. Rare subtypes, such as familial hemiplegic migraine (FHM), presented an opportunity to gain insight into rare migraine genes with strong effect sizes. FHM is characterized by multiple attacks of migraine with aura, including motor weakness, typically in those with a first-degree relative with the same condition. Linkage studies have identified autosomal dominant mutations in three ion channels—*CACNA1A* (calcium channel), *ATP1A2* (sodium-potassium ATP pump), and *SCN1A* (sodium channel). Of note, there has also been the more recent identification of mutations in *PRRT2*, the exact function of which remains unknown. Although each of these disorders shares some similarities with common migraine, they also tend to be associated with more severe focal neurologic deficits and are not observed in patients with common migraine. The genetics of other migraine-related conditions have provided insight into migraine pathophysiology. One such disorder is cerebral autosomal dominant arteriopathy with subcortical infarcts and leukoencephalopathy, which is caused by a mutation in the *NOTCH3* gene that results in alterations in vascular smooth muscle cell function and manifests as migraine with aura and subcortical infarcts and vascular dementia. The *NOTCH3* gene polymorphism has been found to be associated with migraine susceptibility for common migraine with aura in a modest sample, and further studies may help elucidate if this contributes to increased stroke risk in migraine.

GWASs have recently identified over 100 susceptibility loci for migraine. The familial aggregation of these loci was examined, and the common variant burden (the polygenic accumulation of common variants) was found to be significantly higher in familial cases compared to population cases. Furthermore, the greatest contribution of common variants was in cases of hemiplegic migraine, suggesting that common variants are not only needed for the expression of known FHM genes but may perhaps be contributing even more than the FHM gene mutation. While these studies identified key genetic mechanisms associated with migraine, it was unclear precisely how these genetic variants contribute to pathophysiology. Analysis of gene expression from specific human brain cell types identified enrichment of migraine-associated genes in neurons, glia, and neurovascular cells. Several migraine-associated genes also show preferential cell-type expression in the peripheral nervous system and neurovasculature. Once the gene variants that contribute to migraine susceptibility have been localized to the correct cell types, their role in migraine pathophysiology can be studied directly. It may also be possible to stratify migraine patients by their risk alleles to predict which groups of patients are most likely to respond or have significant side effects to specific treatments.

FUTURE DIRECTIONS

The field of neurogenetics is growing exponentially. Genetic testing is becoming common in monogenic disorders and in cancer, where genotypes can determine treatment regimens. We will continue to see widely available treatment developments for monogenic diseases, such as infantile-onset spinal muscular atrophy and Duchenne muscular dystrophy. The clinical implications for polygenic neurologic diseases are less predictable. However, larger GWAS studies combined with new gene therapy technologies, such as CRISPR, are already contributing to our knowledge of common diseases. We are optimistic that continued advances in neurogenetics will lead to better treatments and help predict individualized treatment response with current therapies.

"For the full bibliography list, please use the pincode on the inside front cover to access the electronic version of the text at eBooks.health.elsevier.com."

4

Neuro-ophthalmology*

Sashank Prasad

INTRODUCTION

Visual symptoms can be the presenting feature of a wide range of important neurological diseases. It is important for primary care clinicians to be familiar with the approach to these clinical scenarios to be able to triage care and direct appropriate initial diagnostic assessment, treatment, and referral for further evaluation. This chapter encompasses a practical, up-to-date overview of important considerations in the management of acute monocular visual loss, papilledema, visual field deficits, anisocoria, limitations of eye movements, and nystagmus.

ACUTE MONOCULAR VISUAL LOSS

Acute visual loss of one eye is a common symptom that requires urgent evaluation and management, usually requiring ophthalmologic consultation. As a first step, it is critical to identify whether visual loss is due to a lesion in the eye (especially retinal disease) or the optic nerve. A retinal lesion may be suggested by reported symptoms of metamorphopsia (wavy, warped images), positive phenomena (flashing or colored lights), or a sudden increase in "floaters" in one eye. In contrast, optic nerve lesions tend to present with visual loss (often with significant color desaturation), without prominent metamorphopsia, positive phenomena, or floaters.

*Based on Article—Prasad S. A window to the brain: neuro-ophthalmology for the primary care practitioner. *Am J Med*. 2018;131(2):120–128. ISSN 0002-9343 (https://doi.org/10.1016/j.amjmed.2017.10.008. (https://www.sciencedirect.com/science/article/pii/S0002934317310458).

The tempo of visual loss is key to making an accurate diagnosis; for example, with optic neuritis visual loss evolves quickly and then subsequently improves; with ischemic optic neuropathy, it is sudden and fairly static; with compressive lesions, its discovery may be sudden, but its occurrence is more likely to be insidious and slowly progressive. The presence or absence of pain is also important to establishing the correct diagnosis; for example, pain is typically present in disorders such as optic neuritis or giant cell arteritis (GCA) but absent in nonarteritic ischemic optic neuropathy (NAION).

A dilated fundus examination typically must be performed to diagnose conditions such as retinal or vitreous detachment, arterial or venous occlusion, or other retinal pathology. Occlusion of the central retinal artery is characterized by diffuse retinal whitening with a macular cherry-red spot (Fig. 4.1). This occurs because the inner layers of the retina, which are normally transparent, become swollen due to acute ischemia and obscure the normal color observed in the pigment epithelial layer in the outer retina. The cherry-red spot is seen in the macula because the normal retina is thinnest in this location, so there is less swelling of the inner layers. With branch retinal artery occlusion the areas of retinal ischemia are more circumscribed. Diabetic macular ischemia often produces macular edema in association with retinal microhemorrhages and cotton wool spots (cotton wool spots also represent areas of ischemia where the inner retinal layers are no longer transparent to light). A retinal vein occlusion produces profuse intraretinal hemorrhages (Fig. 4.2).

The hallmark of unilateral optic neuropathy is the relative afferent pupillary defect (RAPD) (Fig. 4.3). The RAPD is identified by the swinging flashlight test,

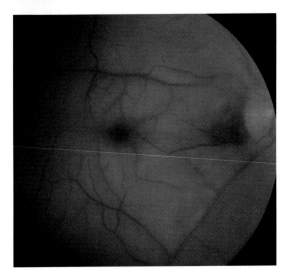

Fig. 4.1 Central retinal artery occlusion, with whitening of the retina and a cherry-red spot in the region of the macula. (Reprinted with permission from Prasad and Galetta 2012. Prasad S, Galetta SL. Approach to the patient with acute monocular visual loss. *Neurol Clin Pract.* 2012;2:14–23.)

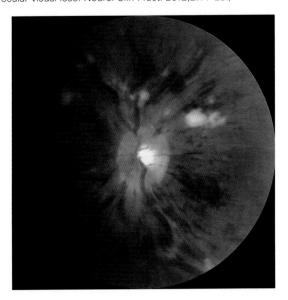

Fig. 4.2 Central retinal vein occlusion, with extensive intraretinal hemorrhages and scattered cotton wool spots. (Reprinted with permission from Prasad and Galetta 2012. Prasad S, Galetta SL. Approach to the patient with acute monocular visual loss. *Neurol Clin Pract.* 2012;2:14–23.)

during which light is alternately directed toward each pupil. When light is shined into the unaffected eye, both pupils constrict normally. When light is swung to the affected eye, both pupils should stay constricted.

However, dilation of both pupils when the light is swung to the affected eye indicates an RAPD and strongly suggests an optic neuropathy on that side.

A slit-lamp examination provides detailed inspection of the anterior structures of the eye, allowing the diagnosis of conditions such as uveitis. In some circumstances, the ophthalmologic evaluation will include additional imaging and electrophysiologic studies such as optical coherence tomography (which provides high-resolution cross-sectional images of the retina), fluorescein angiography, or electroretinography.

Magnetic resonance imaging (MRI) of the orbit is often the most helpful diagnostic test in patients with a suspected optic nerve disorder and can help distinguish inflammatory, ischemic, and neoplastic causes. As opposed to standard MRI of the brain, MRI of the orbit includes coronal views with suppression of the orbital fat, thus permitting better visualization of the optic nerve.

Optic Neuritis

Optic neuritis most often occurs between the ages of 20 and 50 and is three times more frequent in females. Visual loss usually reaches its nadir within 7 to 10 days and begins to recover within 1 month. Retro-orbital pain, particularly with eye movements, occurs in almost all cases.

The likelihood of optic neuritis progressing to multiple sclerosis (MS) is best predicted by brain MRI at the time of diagnosis. Patients with other white matter lesions are at very high risk of a subsequent clinical relapse; consultation with a neurologist or MS specialist is needed to assess the benefit and risk of a growing number of available disease-modifying treatments.

Treatment with intravenous corticosteroids may hasten the recovery of visual deficits from optic neuritis, although it does not significantly affect long-term visual outcomes. Treatment with oral corticosteroids, on the other hand, may be associated with an increased risk of recurrence of optic neuritis, and this therapy should be avoided.

Neuromyelitis optica spectrum disorder (NMOSD) is a rare autoimmune condition that causes severe optic neuritis and myelitis, but many patients will not have both. Aggressive treatment in the form of plasma exchange may be warranted in suspected cases, because spontaneous recovery can be poor. The aquaporin

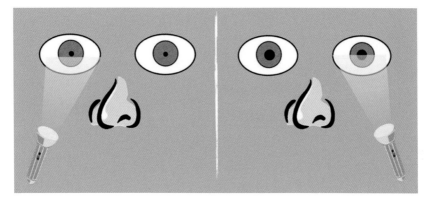

Fig. 4.3 Left relative afferent pupillary defect. A light source is swung back and forth. The pupils both constrict when the light is shined into the right eye. The pupils both dilate when the light source is shined into the left eye. (From Prasad S. A window to the brain: neuro-ophthalmology for the primary care practitioner. *Am J Med.* 2018;131(2):120–128.)

4-IgG (anti-AQP4) and anti–myelin oligodendrocyte glycoprotein serum tests are highly specific for NMOSD. The identification of these antibodies has implications for prognosis and optimal long-term immunosuppressive treatment, compared to patients with typical optic neuritis.

Ischemic Optic Neuropathy

Ischemic injury to the optic nerve can be either arteritic or nonarteritic. NAION most commonly affects adults over the age of 50 and causes acute, painless visual loss. Nocturnal hypotension (possibly precipitated by antihypertensive therapy) may provoke the ischemic event. The affected optic disk is swollen and often has surrounding hemorrhages in the acute phase. Recovery tends to be poor.

Ischemic optic neuropathy can also occur in the setting of GCA. The prevalence of GCA increases with age and is rare under the age of 60. Systemic symptoms may include myalgia, jaw claudication, fever, malaise, and scalp tenderness. The diagnosis is suggested by an elevated erythrocyte sedimentation rate and C-reactive protein and confirmed by evidence of inflammation on a temporal artery biopsy. Depending on the level of clinical suspicion, temporal artery ultrasound can provide useful information to determine whether additional diagnostic testing or empiric treatment should be pursued. Given the potentially high risk of progressive, irreversible visual loss, empiric treatment with corticosteroids should be initiated promptly in suspected cases, without delaying for a biopsy to be performed.

PAPILLEDEMA

Papilledema refers to optic disk swelling specifically caused by elevated intracranial pressure (ICP) (Fig. 4.4). Papilledema may be one manifestation of a neurologic emergency, and its presence therefore requires immediate diagnostic evaluation. The more generic term "optic disk edema" is used to describe other causes of intrinsic optic nerve swelling (e.g., optic neuritis, NAION) in which the ICP is not elevated. True papilledema must also be differentiated from other optic nerve anomalies, such as optic disk drusen (Fig. 4.5). One key feature that helps distinguish papilledema from so-called "pseudo-papilledema" is the obscuration of vasculature across the optic disk margins. The observation of spontaneous venous pulsations is not considered highly reliable for the distinction of various causes of optic disk edema.

Symptoms of elevated ICP that accompany papilledema include headache, pulsatile tinnitus, nausea, vomiting, and diplopia. Transient visual obscurations are common, consisting of fleeting, painless blackouts of vision that occur on changing posture.

It is important to recognize that visual acuity is often normal in the presence of papilledema, as opposed to other causes of optic disk edema, in which the acuity is commonly reduced. Acuity becomes compromised from papilledema when optic nerve damage is severe or peripapillary retinal swelling has extended to the macula itself.

Automated visual field assessment is essential to the evaluation and management of patients with papilledema. Enlargement of the blind spots and constriction

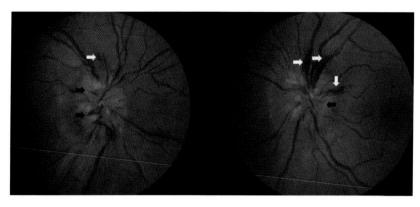

Fig. 4.4 Acute papilledema. Swelling of the peripapillary nerve fiber layer obscures the view of retinal vessels (*black arrows*). Splinter hemorrhages are present around the optic disk (*white arrows*). (From Prasad S, Volpe NJ, Balcer LJ. Share approach to opticneuropathies: clinical update. *Neurologist.* 2010;16(1):23–34.)

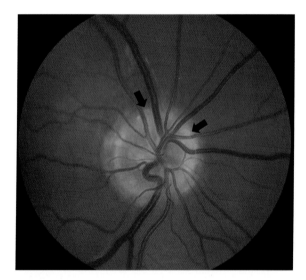

Fig. 4.5 Optic disk drusen. Refractile excrescences visible on the optic disk (*arrows*). (From Prasad S. A window to the brain: neuro-ophthalmology for the primary care practitioner. *Am J Med.* 2018;131(2):120–128.)

of peripheral vision are typical. Progression of visual field abnormalities is a critical parameter that affects treatment decisions.

The differential diagnosis for elevated ICP includes an intracranial or intraspinal mass lesion, cerebral venous thrombosis, meningitis, subarachnoid hemorrhage, and intracranial hypertension secondary to medication or systemic medical conditions. Appropriate imaging studies include either a computed tomography (CT) or MRI study of the brain, with CT- or MR venography to evaluate the possibility of venous thrombosis.

Lumbar puncture provides critical diagnostic information in a patient with papilledema and can generally be performed safely (unless there is a space-occupying lesion that poses increased risk of herniation). Basic cerebrospinal fluid (CSF) studies help identify infectious, inflammatory, and neoplastic conditions affecting CSF circulation and provide a measure of the ICP.

The diagnosis of idiopathic intracranial hypertension (IIH, pseudotumor cerebri) is established when neuroimaging and spinal fluid examination yield no other explanation for elevated ICP. IIH shows a female predominance and is highly associated with obesity or recent weight gain. Weight loss is a critical component of effective treatment for IIH. Medical therapy often includes acetazolamide, a carbonic anhydrase inhibitor that decreases CSF production. Topiramate may be considered as an alternative. When visual loss progresses despite medical treatments for papilledema, surgical treatments, including cerebrospinal shunting procedures, are considered. Patients with IIH often have narrowing of cerebral venous sinuses, visible on MRI or CT venography. In some cases of medically refractory IIH, catheter venography may demonstrate a venous stenosis that is hemodynamically significant and amenable to stenting, which can reduce the ICP.

PROGRESSIVE VISUAL LOSS FROM OPTIC NEUROPATHIES

Glaucomatous optic neuropathy is among the most common causes of progressive visual loss. Open angle glaucoma typically produces fairly symmetric progressive visual field loss with optic disk cupping and elevated intraocular pressure (Fig. 4.6). A variety of mass lesions (including meningioma and pituitary adenoma) can also cause progressive vision loss from compression of the optic nerve. Therefore while imaging studies are not necessary for a typical case of glaucoma, they are necessary in any case that the presentation is atypical.

Toxic or nutritional optic neuropathy causes painless, symmetrical visual loss affecting central vision. Vitamin B_{12} deficiency, as may occur with pernicious anemia or following gastric bypass surgery, is an important and reversible cause. Ethambutol toxicity is an important cause in regions where tuberculosis is endemic.

VISUAL FIELD DEFICITS

Axons in each optic nerve represent the temporal field of that eye decussate in the optic chiasm. A lesion affecting the optic chiasm therefore causes temporal field loss in each eye. Posterior to the optic chiasm, in the optic tract, the decussating axons from the contralateral eye join the axons representing the nasal field of the ipsilateral eye. Lesions affecting any part of the visual pathway

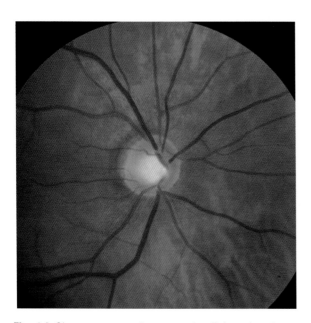

Fig. 4.6 Glaucomatous optic neuropathy. Enlarged optic cup (approximately 0.6 cup:disk diameter ratio). (From Prasad S. A window to the brain: neuro-ophthalmology for the primary care practitioner. *Am J Med.* 2018;131(2):120–128.)

posterior to the optic chiasm, therefore, cause a contralateral visual field deficit, respecting the vertical meridian of each eye.

Confrontation visual field testing has value as a screening test to identify substantial visual field deficits, but more sensitive techniques such as automated perimetry are required to identify more subtle abnormalities. Once a visual field deficit is identified, a neuroimaging study is typically necessary to establish the underlying cause.

The most common cause of a bitemporal field deficit is pituitary macroadenoma (Fig. 4.7). A lesion of the inferior optic radiation produces a contralateral superior quadrantanopia (Fig. 4.8), while a lesion affecting the parietal radiations produces a contralateral inferior quadrantanopia. Homonymous hemianopia that spares the macula has high localizing value, suggesting a contralateral posterior cerebral artery (PCA) infarction (Fig. 4.9). This occurs because representation of the macula in the occipital cortex is at the occipital pole, which often receives dual collateral blood supply from the PCA and branches of the middle cerebral artery. Other lesions in the occipital lobes typically do not cause macular sparing.

ANISOCORIA

Examination of the pupils can often provide a meaningful clue about an underlying neurological disease. The normal pupillary light reflex is consensual, meaning that light directed into either eye drives constriction of both pupils. The optic nerve fibers that mediate the pupillary light reflex exit the optic tract to synapse in the dorsal midbrain, connecting bilaterally with the Edinger-Westphal nuclei, which give rise to the parasympathetic fibers that travel with the third nerve to innervate the iris sphincter muscle and cause pupillary constriction.

Pupillary dilation is mediated by sympathetic input to the eye via a three-neuron pathway that begins in the hypothalamus. From the hypothalamus the first neuron projects through the brainstem to the lower cervical spinal cord. After synapsing, the second neuron exits the spinal cord into the sympathetic chain and synapses in the superior cervical ganglion. The third neuron ascends along the internal carotid artery, enters the cavernous sinus, and then follows the ophthalmic branch of the trigeminal nerve (V1) to innervate the pupillary dilator muscles.

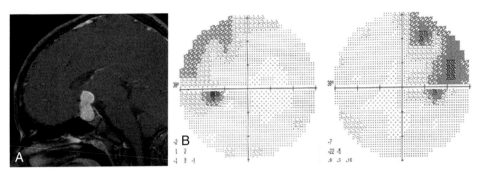

Fig. 4.7 (A) Sagittal postcontrast magnetic resonance imaging demonstrating a pituitary macroadenoma compressing the optic chiasm. (B) Superior bitemporal hemianopia. (From Prasad S. A window to the brain: neuro-ophthalmology for the primary care practitioner. *Am J Med.* 2018;131(2):120–128.)

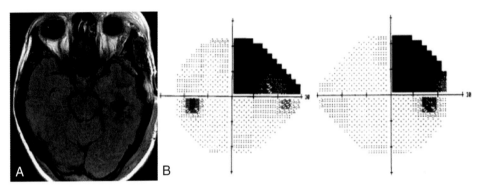

Fig. 4.8 (A) Magnetic resonance imaging following resection of a right temporal cavernoma. (B) Contralateral superior quadrantanopia resulting from injury to the inferior optic radiations. (From Prasad S. A window to the brain: neuro-ophthalmology for the primary care practitioner. *Am J Med.* 2018;131(2):120–128.)

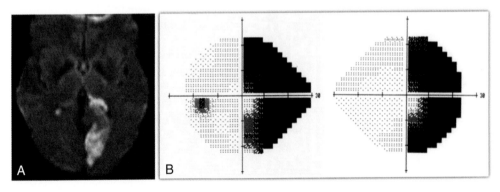

Fig. 4.9 (A) Diffusion-weighted imaging showing infarction of left occipital lobe from a posterior cerebral artery stroke, sparing the occipital pole. (B) Right homonymous hemianopia with macular sparing. (From Prasad S. A window to the brain: neuro-ophthalmology for the primary care practitioner. *Am J Med.* 2018;131(2):120–128.)

Anisocoria refers to a difference in the size of the two pupils and can either be physiologic or pathologic. With physiologic anisocoria the difference in the size of the pupils is fairly consistent in both light and dark. In contrast, anisocoria that is more pronounced in darkness (with normal pupillary reactivity to light but slow dilation of one pupil) suggests sympathetic dysfunction on the side of the smaller pupil (i.e., Horner syndrome). Accompanying clinical signs often provide the best way to localize the causative lesion to either the brainstem, spinal cord, lung apex, carotid artery, or cavernous sinus. Horner syndrome with ipsilateral neck pain is concerning for carotid dissection (Fig. 4.10). Targeted imaging studies of the head, neck, and upper chest can then help disclose the underlying lesion.

Pupillary asymmetry that is greater in light (with a larger pupil that shows a sluggish reaction to light) indicates parasympathetic dysfunction of the larger pupil and can be a sign of a third nerve palsy when eye movement abnormalities and ptosis are also present. Patients with pupil-involving third nerve palsy must undergo imaging studies to evaluate for a compressive lesion; aneurysm of the posterior communicating artery is the most worrisome condition in the differential diagnosis (Fig. 4.11). An isolated dilated pupil, with normal eye movement and eyelid function, may occur with inflammation of the ciliary ganglion (i.e., tonic pupil) or pharmacologic blockade.

LIMITED EYE MOVEMENTS

Normal eye movements ultimately depend on the ocular motor nerves (cranial nerves three, four, and six), which innervate the six extraocular muscles of each eye. The oculomotor (third) nerve innervates the medial rectus, inferior rectus, superior rectus, inferior oblique, levator palpebrae (the main eyelid muscle), and the pupillary constrictor. The trochlear (fourth) nerve innervates only the superior oblique muscle, and the abducens (sixth) nerve innervates only the lateral rectus muscle.

Binocular diplopia is the symptom caused by misalignment of the eyes; it is present only when both eyes are open and resolves when either eye is closed. Diplopia that persists when one eye is closed is termed monocular diplopia; it is not caused by ocular misalignment and usually arises from an abnormality within the eye itself (affecting the cornea, lens, or retina).

The first step in determining the cause of binocular diplopia is to examine the eye movements directly. Weakness in a particular direction of gaze may be partial or complete and may result from dysfunction at the level of the cranial nerve, eye muscle, neuromuscular junction, or from mechanical restriction of an extraocular muscle. Other methods, such as alternate cover testing of the eyes, provide a more sensitive method to detect ocular misalignment. While the patient fixates on a target, the examiner alternately covers each eye. If there is ocular misalignment, each time an eye is uncovered there will be a corrective saccade to refixate on the target.

Complete, isolated third nerve palsy causes weakness of elevation, depression, and adduction of the eye, in combination with ptosis and pupillary dilation. In some cases, a lesion in the brainstem can affect the third nerve before it has exited the midbrain. These syndromes are characterized by crossed neurological findings, with deficits such as contralateral hemiparesis or ataxia accompanying the ipsilateral third nerve palsy.

In cases of isolated third nerve palsy, it is critical to distinguish microvascular third nerve palsy, which is relatively benign, from compressive lesions such as aneurysm

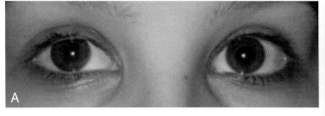
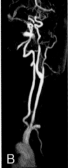

Fig. 4.10 Horner syndrome. (**A**) Left miosis and ptosis associated with neck pain after a motor vehicle accident. (**B**) Magnetic resonance angiogram of the neck demonstrating tapering of the left internal carotid artery consistent with dissection (*arrow*). (From Prasad S. A window to the brain: neuro-ophthalmology for the primary care practitioner. *Am J Med.* 2018;131(2):120–128.)

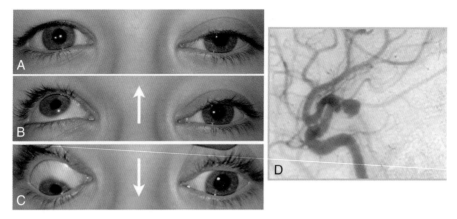

Fig. 4.11 Pupil-involving third nerve palsy. (**A**) Left pupillary enlargement, ptosis, and hypotropia. (**B**) Impaired left upgaze. (**C**) Impaired left downgaze. (**D**) Angiography revealed a posterior communicating artery aneurysm compressing the third nerve. (From Prasad S. A window to the brain: neuro-ophthalmology for the primary care practitioner. *Am J Med.* 2018;131(2):120–128.)

of the posterior communicating artery. Microvascular third nerve palsy is commonly associated with vascular risk factors including hypertension, diabetes, and hyperlipidemia. There is an excellent prognosis for recovery, typically over 8 to 12 weeks. If the isolated third nerve palsy is partial or involves the pupil, urgent imaging with CT/CT angiography or MRI/MR angiography is necessary to exclude compression from an aneurysm or other mass. However, a growing number of reports of lesions are diagnosed by MRI in patients who mimicked microvasculopathic third nerve palsy. Therefore in clinical practice, it may be prudent to obtain imaging studies for these patients as well.

The pattern of diplopia caused by isolated fourth nerve palsy is vertical diplopia that increases with contralateral gaze and with ipsilateral head tilt. Patients often manifest a compensatory contralateral head tilt. The most common cause of acquired fourth nerve palsy is trauma, because the trochlear nerve is the longest and thinnest of all the cranial nerves and is particularly vulnerable to crush or shearing injury. Decompensated congenital fourth nerve palsy is also relatively common and may present with the insidious onset of intermittent vertical diplopia in adulthood.

Sixth nerve palsy causes weakness of the lateral rectus, presenting with horizontal diplopia worse when looking to the affected side (Fig. 4.12). Often, the limitation of abduction is easily observed, but in more subtle cases, the misalignment must be demonstrated by alternate cover testing to assess binocular alignment.

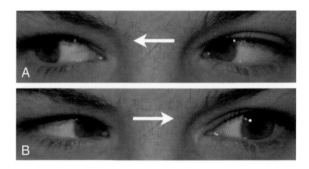

Fig. 4.12 Left sixth nerve palsy. (**A**) Normal right gaze. (**B**) Limited abduction of the left eye. (Reprinted with permission from Prasad S, Volpe NJ. Paralytic strabismus: third, fourth, and sixth nerve palsy. *Neurol Clin.* 2010;28(3):803–833.)

Lesions in the cavernous sinus are an important cause of combined third, fourth, and/or sixth nerve palsy. Diagnostic considerations include meningioma, pituitary adenoma, lymphoma, infection, or inflammatory conditions.

Internuclear ophthalmoplegia refers to impaired adduction of one eye during an attempted rapid horizontal movement of both eyes (Fig. 4.13). It occurs with a lesion affecting the medial longitudinal fasciculus, which connects the sixth nucleus in the pons to the third nucleus in the midbrain. Demyelination from MS is the most common cause.

Disorders of the neuromuscular junction or ocular muscles are also often on the differential diagnosis for binocular diplopia. Approximately one-half of patients with myasthenia gravis initially present with visual symptoms. The examination may demonstrate weakness

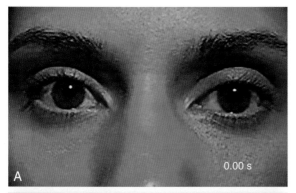

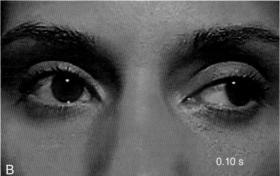

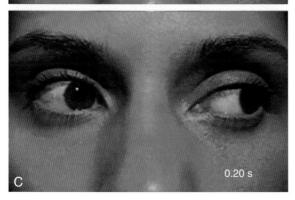

Fig. 4.13 Right internuclear ophthalmoplegia. (**A**) Primary gaze. (**B**) Adduction lag of the right eye at the onset of a leftward saccade. (**C**) Completion of the leftward saccade. (Reprinted with permission from Prasad S, Galetta SL. Eye movement abnormalities in multiple sclerosis. *Neurol Clin.* 2010;28(3):641–655.)

of a variety of eye muscles and variable ptosis. The deficits often worsen with fatigue and improve after rest. Serological testing for the acetylcholine receptor antibody has good specificity but poor sensitivity, particularly in patients with isolated ocular manifestations.

Thyroid eye disease is the most common disorder of the ocular muscles. The abnormal autoimmune response in this condition causes enlargement and fibrosis of the eye muscles. Patients commonly present with eyelid retraction, proptosis, and ocular misalignment (Fig. 4.14). Although many patients are hyperthyroid, this is not a prerequisite, and some patients are euthyroid or hypothyroid.

One way to eliminate the symptom of binocular diplopia is by patching one eye. If the ocular misalignment remains stable, prisms may be placed in glasses to alleviate the double vision. Once ocular misalignment from an ocular motor palsy has been stable for 6 to 12 months, strabismus surgery may be considered.

NYSTAGMUS

Nystagmus refers to involuntary, rhythmic oscillations of the eyes and can be either physiologic or pathologic. Physiologic end-gaze nystagmus is typically at the extremes of horizontal gaze and extinguishes after several beats. Pathologic nystagmus results from either central or peripheral vestibular lesions. Features suggesting a central etiology include pure vertical or pure torsional nystagmus, nystagmus that changes direction depending on the position of gaze, nystagmus that does not suppress with visual fixation, and nystagmus that does not easily fatigue. In contrast, nystagmus from a peripheral lesion (such as vestibular neuritis) causes unidirectional nystagmus that can vary in amplitude in different positions of gaze but does not change its direction.

In some cases, provocative maneuvers are used to try to elicit nystagmus. Transient vertical/torsional nystagmus that is elicited when the patient is recumbent with the head turned so that one ear is down (i.e., the Dix-Hallpike maneuver) is diagnostic of benign positional peripheral vertigo (BPPV). BPPV is a common condition that occurs because of displaced otoconia lodged most commonly in the posterior semicircular canal. It is treated with the Epley maneuver, which is a series of positions intended to reposition the dislodged canalith.

An important examination technique in patients with acute vertigo is direct testing of the vestibulo-ocular reflex (VOR) (by performing horizontal head thrusts while the patient maintains visual fixation). Catch-up saccades that occur when the VOR is deficient are indicative of peripheral vestibular dysfunction. In contrast, horizontal head thrusts are normal (without catch-up saccades) in patients with central forms of nystagmus.

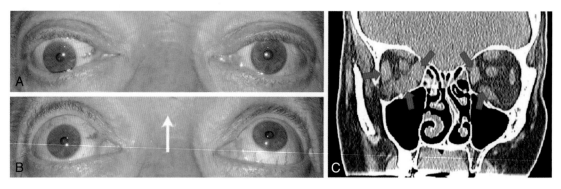

Fig. 4.14 Thyroid eye disease. (**A**) Eyelid retraction and left hypertropia. (**B**) Impaired upgaze bilaterally, worse on the right. (**C**) Coronal computed tomography of the orbits demonstrating marked thickening of the right lateral, inferior, and medial rectus muscles as well as the left medial and inferior rectus muscles. (From Prasad S. A window to the brain: neuro-ophthalmology for the primary care practitioner. *Am J Med*. 2018;131(2):120–128.)

Central, gaze-evoked pathologic nystagmus results from lesions of the vestibulocerebellum and its brainstem connections. It results from failure of the "neural integrators" that normally maintain visual fixation in an eccentric position. This type of nystagmus has a fast-phase direction that changes according to the direction of gaze (i.e., the nystagmus will be right beating in right gaze, left beating in left gaze, and upbeating in upgaze). In addition to structural lesions of the cerebellar pathways, metabolic derangements, thiamine deficiency (Wernicke encephalopathy), and some medications (e.g., antiepileptics, lithium) are other important causes.

In general, medical treatments for nystagmus are not very effective, but certain drugs may provide symptomatic benefit for some patients. Clonazepam, baclofen, gabapentin, memantine, and aminopyridines are reasonably well tolerated and may be effective. Vestibular rehabilitation therapy can be effective for improving gaze and gait stabilization. Many patients take meclizine to reduce the symptoms of vertigo that can be associated with a variety of vestibular disorders. They should be advised that meclizine can help with symptoms in the short term, but it should not be used chronically because it dampens function in the vestibular system and could perpetuate chronic dizziness.

SUMMARY

The diagnosis and management of neuro-ophthalmologic disorders begin with the accurate localization of pathology in the visual system through careful analysis of a patient's history and examination. Primary care clinicians play a pivotal role in framing the initial differential diagnosis and identifying situations when visual symptoms should trigger targeted evaluation for potential neurological disease.

"For the full bibliography list, please use the pincode on the inside front cover to access the electronic version of the text at eBooks.health.elsevier.com."

5

Cerebrovascular Disease

Steven Feske

INTRODUCTION

Cerebrovascular diseases commonly confront primary care providers. Stroke, the most common serious manifestation of cerebrovascular disease, is the fifth leading cause of death in the United States and a major cause of severe disability. It is the leading cause of hospitalization for neurologic disease. This review addresses many issues in the prevention, diagnosis, and management of cerebrovascular diseases, causing both ischemic and hemorrhagic stroke, that commonly confront primary care physicians.

EPIDEMIOLOGY

The 2022 update of the American Heart Association report "Heart Disease and Stroke Statistics" estimates that the prevalence of stroke in the United States in 2018 was approximately 2.7%, which translates into 7.6 million Americans 20 years of age or greater who had suffered a stroke, nearly 800,000 new or recurrent stroke events yearly and over 160,000 deaths. Age is the most important demographic risk factor, and although the incidence of stroke has fallen in recent years, the lifetime risk of stroke has increased due to the aging of the population. Female sex and African American race confer added risk. The estimated annual direct and indirect cost of stroke in 2017–18 was $52.8 billion.

The falling incidence of stroke since 1999 correlates with improvements in control of cardiovascular risk factors—improved control of hypertension, diabetes mellitus, and hyperlipidemia and lower rates of smoking—and in better stroke preventive treatment of cardiac arrhythmias. This means that primary care physicians are in the most important position to minimize the burden of stroke in the population.

ISCHEMIC STROKE

Ischemic Stroke: Pathology, Pathophysiology, and Stroke Types

Pathophysiology and Classification of Ischemic Stroke

The primary lesion of ischemic stroke is cerebral infarction. With an inadequate supply of blood to cerebral tissue, there is first a reversible loss of tissue function and, given enough time, infarction of tissue with loss of neurons and supportive structures. Ischemia sets off a cascade of events that begins with loss of electrical function and passes through disturbance of membrane channel function with calcium influx, leading to calcium-dependent excitotoxicity, generation of reactive oxygen species, and ultimately completes destruction of cell membranes and lysis of cells at its extreme, leaving a cavitation at the site of infarction.

There are several different mechanisms of vascular occlusion and many diseases that may underlie them (Boxes 5.1 and 5.2).

Embolism is the commonest mechanism of stroke (Fig. 5.1). The great majority of emboli are blood clots generated from the heart (*cardioembolism*) due to cardiac disease. Common cardiac disorders leading to stroke include atrial fibrillation, valvular heart disease, and cardiomyopathy from coronary artery disease with myocardial infarction or hypertension. Less common causes of cardiomyopathy (e.g., viral, drug-induced, infiltrative, hereditary, or idiopathic) leading to low

---

BOX 5.1   Mechanisms of Ischemic Stroke[a]

Embolism
   Cardioembolism
   Artery-to-artery embolism
   Paradoxical embolism
Large vessel disease
   Atherosclerotic stenosis of occlusion
   Arterial dissection
Small vessel disease
Other identifiable underlying causes
   Hypercoagulability etc.
No identified cause despite extensive evaluation

[a]Based on the TOAST classification.

BOX 5.2   Some Uncommon Causes of Ischemic Stroke

Embolism
   Infective endocarditis
   Nonbacterial thrombotic (marantic) endocarditis
   Embolism of other materials: calcium, fat, air, amniotic
     fluid, medical devices
   Hypercoagulability (see below)
Large vessel disease
   Moyamoya disease and moyamoya syndrome
   Large vessel vasculitis
Small vessel disease
   Small vessel vasculitis
   CADASIL[a] and other inherited vasculopathies
   Cerebral amyloid angiopathy (more commonly causes
     hemorrhage)
Hypercoagulability
   Hypercoagulability of malignancy
   Antiphospholipid antibody syndrome
   Inherited and acquired clotting disorders (most
     commonly cause venous thrombosis)
   Hypercoagulability of pregnancy
Sickle cell disease (with or without secondary moyamoya
   syndrome)
Infections
   Infective endocarditis (see above)
   Zoster ophthalmicus (an infectious form of vasculitis)
   Syphilis
   Tuberculosis and angioinvasive fungi (e.g., *Aspergillus*)
Cerebral venous thrombosis

[a]Cerebral autosomal-dominant arteriopathy with subcortical infarcts and leukoencephalopathy.

---

left ventricular ejection fraction, arrhythmia, and intracardiac thrombus formation may also cause embolic strokes. Right-to-left shunting, most commonly from patent foramen ovale or from congenital heart disease, may lead to *paradoxical embolism* from the venous circulation. *Artery-to-artery embolism* occurs when a thrombus, usually in association with atherosclerotic plaques or at sites of arterial dissection, is dislodged from a large vessel wall and flows distally to lodge in smaller downstream vessels. Much less common, but important to consider in the right circumstances, material other than thrombus may embolize to cause strokes. Calcium may embolize from calcified atherosclerotic lesions. Fat may embolize after fracture of or surgery on long bones and in the setting of sickle cell crisis. Air may embolize during the placement or removal of intravenous catheters or during open heart and intravascular surgery. Amniotic fluid may embolize in the course of labor and delivery. Finally, intravascular medical devices may embolize when fractured or dislodged.

Large vessel disease is another common underlying cause of stroke (Fig. 5.2). *Large vessel atherosclerotic disease*, most commonly in the proximal cervical internal carotid arteries, but also at times in the more distal internal carotid arteries, in the aorta, the vertebral and basilar arteries, or intracranially, may cause strokes. Arterial dissection affecting any of these vessels is the next most common cause of large vessel disease. Arterial dissection is a common cause of stroke in young patients without alternative risk factors and in patients with certain predisposing conditions. The most common cause of arterial dissection is major trauma or minor trauma from vigorous coughing, vomiting, or chiropractic manipulation. Diseases that compromise the integrity of connective tissues may predispose patients to arterial dissection, including fibromuscular dysplasia, Marfan syndrome, vascular Ehlers-Danlos syndrome, and Loeys-Dietz syndrome. Many arterial dissections occur without any apparent provocation and without any of these disorders. Many such patients likely harbor genetic polymorphisms that render them vulnerable to minor traumas of everyday life. The commonest mechanism by which large vessel disease leads to stroke is artery-to-artery embolism so large vessel disease and embolism are overlapping categories defining stroke mechanisms. Large vessel stenosis or occlusion may alternatively lead to low flow in distal branches, typically causing infarction in the border zones of converging perfusion fields (Fig. 5.3).

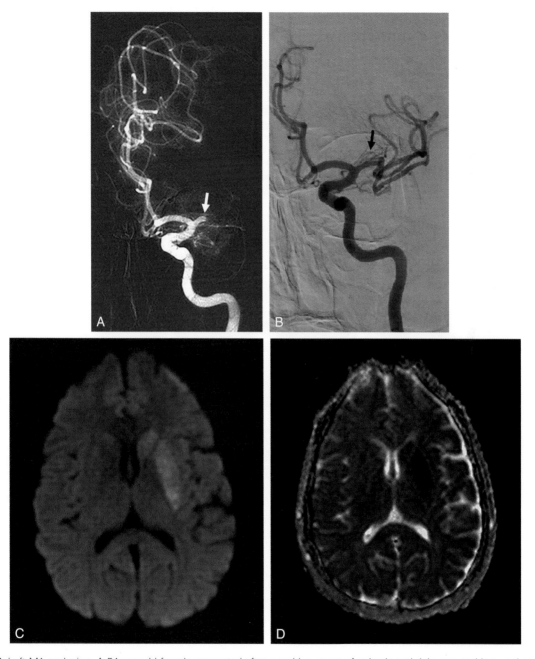

Fig. 5.1 Left M1 occlusion. A 54-year-old female presented after a sudden onset of aphasia and right arm and leg weakness. On examination she had global aphasia, right hemianopsia, impaired rightward gaze, and severe weakness and sensory loss of the left arm and leg. Computed tomography angiography showed occlusion of the left middle cerebral artery (MCA) stem (not shown). The patient was transferred to a comprehensive stroke center for urgent endovascular thrombectomy. Digital subtraction angiogram confirms the left M1 occlusion (A, *arrow*). Stent retriever thrombectomy achieved early full (TICI 2c) reperfusion. The postthrombectomy digital subtraction angiogram shows the left MCA stem to be open and filling the distal branches (B, *arrow*). MRI the next day shows an acute ischemic stroke limited to the left basal ganglia and adjacent white matter of the corona radiata with sparing of the cortex (C, diffusion-weighted imaging, and D, apparent diffusion coefficient). Follow-up echocardiogram showed hypokinesis of the left ventricle (LV) apex and LV mural thrombus as the embolic source.

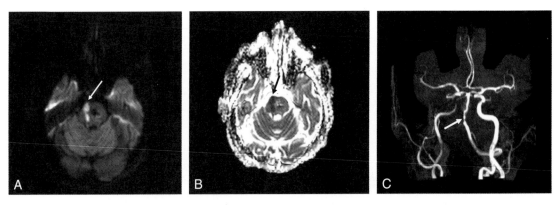

Fig. 5.2 Basilar artery stenosis and pontine infarct. A 75-year-old female with type II diabetes and hypertension with a history of a recent prior pontine ischemic stroke presented with worsened dysarthria and left hemiparesis. Magnetic resonance imaging shows diffusion restriction with a linear hyperintensity in the right side of the basis pontis on the diffusion-weighted imaging sequence (A, *arrow*) and corresponding hypointensity on the apparent diffusion coefficient sequence (B, *arrow*). Magnetic resonance angiography showed irregularity and stenosis of the proximal and mid basilar artery at the level of the stroke (C, *arrow*).

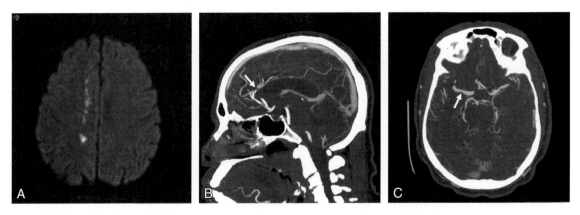

Fig. 5.3 Borderzone infarct. A 65-year-old male with uncontrolled hypertension presented with several hours of left arm and leg weakness. On examination he had mild dysarthria and mild left arm weakness. Magnetic resonance imaging showed a watershed "string of pearls" pattern of acute infarction in the right middle cerebral artery (MCA)-ACA border zone (A). CT angiography multiple areas of intracranial arterial stenosis including severe stenosis of the right ACA (B, *arrow*) and mild stenosis of the right MCA stem (C, *arrow*) suggesting low flow as the mechanism of infarction. There is more severe stenosis of the asymptomatic left MCA consistent with intracranial cerebral atherosclerotic disease. *ACA,* anterior cerebral artery.

Small vessel disease typically causes small, deep strokes. Ischemia extends around occluded distal arteries to create oval "little lakes" of infarction, so-called lacunar strokes. Small penetrating arteries, which are most vulnerable to the effects of chronic hypertension and other risk factors, are most commonly affected. Common sites for lacunar infarction that may cause recognizable clinical presentations include the posterior limb (*pure motor hemiplegia* and *ataxic hemiparesis*) and genu (*clumsy hand-dysarthria*) of the internal capsule, the basis pontis (*pure motor hemiplegia* and *clumsy hand-dysarthria*), the thalamus (*pure hemisensory and contralateral cerebellar syndrome*) (Fig. 5.4), and the cerebellum. Other sites of deep white matter infarction may cause symptoms that are referable to their locations.

Many other uncommon vascular and hematologic lesions may cause vascular disease with occlusion or embolism leading to strokes. Many of these less common causes of stroke are listed in Box 5.2.

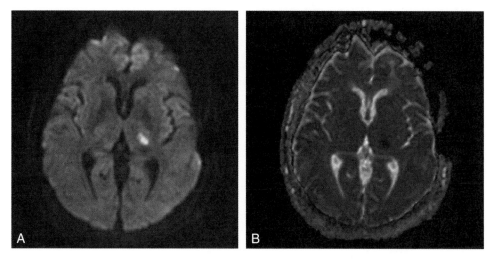

Fig. 5.4 Lacunar infarct. A 54-year-old male with type II diabetes, hypertension, and hypercholesterolemia presented after the sudden onset of right arm numbness. On examination he had mild right arm weakness found as orbiting and pronator drift, decreased sensation throughout the right arm, and right arm ataxia. Magnetic resonance imaging shows an acute lacunar stroke with diffusion-weighted imaging showing hyperintensity (A) and the apparent diffusion coefficient sequence showing corresponding hypointensity (B) in the lateral portion of the left thalamus. Computed tomography angiography showed no vascular occlusion or stenosis (not shown).

Pathophysiology: Time Course of Blood Flow Deficit

The progression of cerebral tissue to irreversible infarction depends on the magnitude of the drop in cerebral blood flow and the duration of this drop. With a fall in cerebral blood flow by approximately 50%, the oxygen extraction from perfusing blood is increased to compensate for the drop in flow, and the patient remains asymptomatic. With a further fall in cerebral blood flow, reversible neuronal dysfunction occurs, leading to ischemic symptoms, typically deficits of function corresponding to the location of the ischemia and the topographic representation of function. If flow is restored rapidly enough, neuronal function returns without infarction, and the patient is said to have had a *transient ischemic attack.* If, on the other hand, flow-causing ischemia lasts long enough, irreversible tissue injury occurs, leading to the pathophysiologic events described above for *cerebral infarction* or *ischemic stroke.* The time from the onset of symptoms until the onset of irreversible tissue injury depends, in each area of the brain, on the magnitude and duration of the drop in cerebral blood flow (Fig. 5.5). Infarction occurs earlier, sometimes within minutes, in the core of the lesion, where flow is lowest, and it may occur much later in the periphery of the lesion, where flow is nearer the threshold of reversibility. This understanding of the time course of cerebral

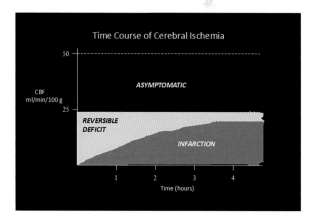

Fig. 5.5 Cerebral infarction depends on the magnitude and duration of reduced perfusion.

infarction leads to the concept of the infarct core surrounded by a periphery of tissue at risk and the penumbra surrounded by a periphery of oligemic tissue that is not at risk of infarction (Fig. 5.6). The delay in the development of infarction depends in large part on the adequacy of collateral circulation, the supply of blood to the peripheral zone of ischemia by alternative vessels that normally perfused adjacent areas. The duration of delay until the completion of infarction varies from minutes

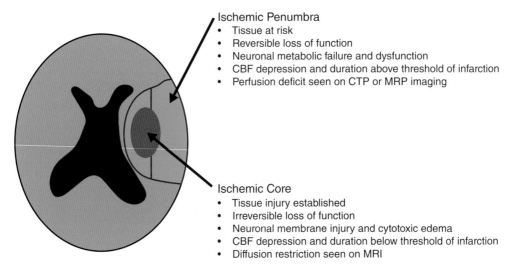

Ischemic Penumbra
- Tissue at risk
- Reversible loss of function
- Neuronal metabolic failure and dysfunction
- CBF depression and duration above threshold of infarction
- Perfusion deficit seen on CTP or MRP imaging

Ischemic Core
- Tissue injury established
- Irreversible loss of function
- Neuronal membrane injury and cytotoxic edema
- CBF depression and duration below threshold of infarction
- Diffusion restriction seen on MRI

Fig. 5.6 Infarct core and penumbra.

to many hours. This provides both an opportunity for urgent therapy to restore blood flow and an imperative to act rapidly before the window of opportunity to minimize the stroke volume closes.

Ischemic Stroke: Diagnostic Imaging

After initial evaluation to establish airway and circulatory stability, a patient presenting with acute onset of a focal neurologic deficit should undergo a rapid, focused history and examination. The history should elicit, as nearly as can be determined, the time the patient was last seen well, relevant details of onset risk factors, medications, and clues of possible relevant illness. A rapid focused examination should record the vital signs, including the heart rate and rhythm, blood pressure (BP), and the presence or absence of fever, and signs of possible endocarditis or other immediately relevant illness. The patient should then proceed immediately to the scanner for urgent brain imaging.

A noncontrast head computed tomography (CT) is, in most institutions, the first study of choice. CT is widely available and can be completed rapidly. The CT is reviewed with special attention to the following: (1) hemorrhage or other alternative nonstroke diagnoses that might explain the presentation, (2) signs of infarction, and (3) evidence of the site of vascular occlusion. Hemorrhage appears as hyperdensity on the head CT. Acute hemorrhage represents an absolute contraindication for intravenous thrombolytic therapy, so it

is important to review the images carefully to rule it out. Early in the evolution of an ischemic stroke in the middle cerebral artery territory, the earliest signs of infarction are most commonly in the insula and the deep basal ganglia, especially the putamen. Early signs of infarction include loss of gray-white differentiation due to decreased density in gray matter structures such as the insular cortex (*insular ribbon sign*) or the deep gray matter (loss of putaminal definition). Loss of gray-white differentiation might be seen elsewhere as well. With more time, sulcal effacement due to tissue swelling, other signs of mass effect, and frank hypodensity are seen. The ASPECTS score is a grading scale that is commonly used to standardize communication about the extent of early infarction (Fig. 5.7). Head CT may be normal early after onset of acute ischemic stroke, so the lack of hemorrhage or of an alternative cause for the focal deficit and the lack of a large completed stroke on CT provide adequate imaging to support urgent intravenous thrombolysis with alteplase or tenecteplase.

To plan for possible urgent endovascular thrombectomy, many centers typically add vascular imaging with CT angiography (CTA) to the initial CT study. This adds only a few minutes and offers much needed information. However, care must be taken that this does not delay initiation of treatment with IV thrombolysis.

CTA from the aortic arch to the crown allows the identification of large vessel occlusions that might be amenable to endovascular therapy and allows the

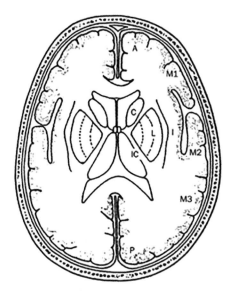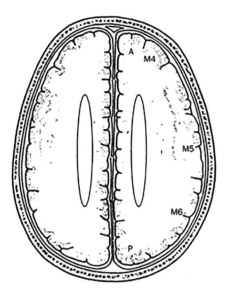

Fig. 5.7 ASPECTS score. A = anterior circulation; P = posterior circulation; C = caudate; L = lentiform nucleus; IC = internal capsule; I = insular ribbon; M1 = anterior middle cerebral artery (MCA) cortex; M2 = MCA cortex lateral to the insular ribbon; M3 = posterior MCA cortex; M4, M5, and M6 = anterior, lateral, and posterior MCA territories immediately superior to M1, M2, and M3 rostral to the basal ganglia. One point is subtracted from 10 for each affected area to give a score from 10 (no ischemic change) to 0 (all areas affected). (Reprinted with permission from Elsevier., Barber PA, et al. Validity and reliability of a quantitative computed tomography score in predicting outcome of hyperacute stroke before thrombolytic therapy. *Lancet.* 2000;355:1670–1674.)

endovascular team to plan their approach to therapy. It is important to review the entire study, including the chest, neck, and intracranial arteries, and the arteries outside of the area of the suspected stroke, to avoid errors in diagnosis.

Magnetic resonance imaging (MRI) is more sensitive for the early identification of acute ischemic stroke, yet it is not commonly used as the initial study because it takes longer to complete. However, when there is doubt about the diagnosis of stroke or when the timing of presentation or other aspects of the case demand a clearer early definition of the infarcted core or when iodinated contrast is contraindicated and urgent vascular imaging is needed, MRI may be useful. Diffusion-weighted (DWI) and apparent diffusion coefficient (ADC) sequences are nearly 100% sensitive in identifying acute infarction (Figs. 5.2 and 5.4). MRI lesions that are bright on DWI and dark on ADC without early changes on the fluid attenuated inversion and recovery (FLAIR) are typical of acute strokes imaged less than approximately 6 hours after onset.

Magnetic resonance angiography (MRA) can demonstrate flow or stenosis or occlusion in the arteries of the chest, neck, and head. MRA is more likely than CTA to overestimate loss of flow.

Perfusion imaging to define the core and penumbra can be done with CT or MRI, and these studies are recommended in many cases presenting late and being considered for endovascular thrombectomy.

Diagnostic digital subtraction angiogram (DSA) remains the gold standard for vascular imaging, and DSA will be done urgently before proceeding to endovascular thrombectomy (see Fig. 5.1).

Ischemic Stroke: Acute Treatment

Acute treatment of stroke is directed at early reperfusion of tissue at risk with intravenous thrombolysis and/or endovascular thrombectomy and with optimization of hemodynamic status through management of fluid volume, BP, and cardiovascular status.

A revolution in acute stroke care began with the publication in 1995 of the NINDS trial of IV tissue-plasminogen activator (tPA alteplase) for acute ischemic stroke. This trial showed a benefit of urgent treatment for selected patients when IV tPA was started within 3 hours of onset, which was defined as the time the patient had last been seen well. A subsequent trial and meta-analyses extended the window for treatment with IV tPA to 4.5 hours in selected patients (Box 5.3). Although beneficial overall many patients, especially those with proximal large vessel occlusions middle cerebral artery, stem, and internal carotid artery), do not respond to IV tPA with early recanalization. Fine-tuning of techniques of urgent endovascular thrombectomy has led to a second revolution in reperfusion therapy for patients with these common large vessel occlusions. All patients presenting within 6 hours of onset with significant functional deficits with a large vessel occlusion, without a large established stroke on CT or MRI, and without contraindications and selected patients up to 24 hours should be considered for endovascular thrombectomy. Selection for late-window (>6 hours) intervention is defined by imaging to confirm the likelihood of recoverable tissue at risk and a small established core infarct. Recent data suggest that many patients with significant areas of established infarction, and hence low ASPECTS scores, may still benefit from urgent endovascular thrombectomy.

Prevention of Ischemic Stroke

While work in the last 25 years has greatly extended our capability to minimize the volume of acute strokes and preserve neurologic function in many cases, we can make our greatest contribution to stroke care and patient health by preventing strokes. The great majority of this care falls ultimately to primary care physicians. Stroke has fallen from the third to the fifth leading cause of death in the United States with a decreasing incidence in the last 25 years. However, the lifetime risk of stroke has increased, due to aging of the population, so the need for vigilance in preventive care has only increased. Success depends on the proper application of the various modalities of therapy, optimizing our choices of antiplatelet and anticoagulant therapies, optimal control of treatable risk factors, and selective referral for surgical therapies, when indicated.

Antiplatelet agents

Except when displaced by anticoagulants or when contraindicated due to bleeding risks, antiplatelet agents should be given for secondary stroke prevention in almost all patients after TIA or ischemic stroke. Low-dose aspirin is the mainstay of such therapy. Doses as low as 30 mg daily have shown success in clinical trials with endpoints including MI and cardiovascular death

BOX 5.3   Protocol for IV tPA for Acute Ischemic Stroke

Indications for IV thrombolysis
1. Acute ischemic stroke with disabling deficit
2. Onset time within 3–4.5 hours with these added exclusions:
   a. Age > 80 years
   b. NIHSS > 25
   c. Taking oral anticoagulants
   d. History of both diabetes mellitus and prior stroke
3. Head CT without well-established infarct, hemorrhage, or alternative explanation for the focal neurologic deficit

Absolute contraindications
1. Head CT showing hemorrhage, or well-established infarct, or other diagnosis that contraindicates treatment, such as tumor, abscess
2. Known CNS vascular malformation or tumor (except certain benign tumors, such as small meningiomas)
3. Mild deficit
4. Added exclusions for 3–4.5 hours, use (see above)

Relative contraindications[a]
   1. Bacterial endocarditis
   2. Significant trauma within 3 months
   3. Stroke within 3 months
   4. History of intracranial hemorrahge or symptoms suspicious for SAH
   5. Major surgery within 14 days; minor surgery within 10 days, including liver or kidney biopsy, thoracocentesis, lumbar puncture
   6. Arterial puncture at noncompressible site within 7 days
   7. Gastrointestinal, urologic, or pulmonary hemorrhage within 21 days
   8. Known bleeding, diathesis, or hemodialysis
   9. aPTT > 40 seconds; INR >1.5; platelet count <100,000/mm³
   10. SBP >185 or DBP >110, despite therapy to lower BP acutely
   11. Seizure at onset of stroke[b]
   12. Glucose <50 or >400 mg/dL[b]

[a]In clinical practice where the risk of permanent disability due to stroke is felt to be great, judgments may favor therapy.
[b]This relative contraindication is intended to prevent the treatment of patients with focal deficits due to a cause other than stroke. If the deficit persists after correction of the glucose abnormality or if the rapid diagnosis of a vascular occlusion can be made by CT or MR angiography, then treatment may be indicated.
DBP, Diastolic blood pressure; NIHSS, National Institutes of Health Stroke Scale; SAH, subarachnoid hemorrhage; SBP, systolic blood pressure.

in addition to stroke. However, some patients with aspirin resistance will respond best to doses from 81 to 325 mg daily. This dose lowers the relative risk of recurrent stroke by approximately 20% per year. Clopidogrel and aspirin combined with dipyridamole confer risk reduction similar to that of aspirin. Clopidogrel may be chosen in patients with sensitivity to aspirin. Ticagrelor, like clopidogrel, blocks platelet P2Y12 receptors; however, it does not require metabolic activation and therefore may offer advantages over clopidogrel, especially in patients who carry the CYP2C19 trait, which limits the activation of the prodrug clopidogrel. Prasugrel is another prodrug that inhibits the platelet P2Y12 receptor. It has some potential pharmacologic advantages over clopidogel. Clinical trials so far suggest a clinical benefit for stroke prevention comparable to that of clopidogrel. Any of these alternatives may be chosen for patients who have events despite proper aspirin use.

Dual antiplatelet therapy for long-term use was tested in three trials and found to confer no long-term advantage over single-agent therapy. However, after TIA and nondisabling stroke, the greatest risk of recurrent stroke occurs in the first couple of weeks after the event. Dual antiplatelet therapy with combined aspirin and clopidogrel has been found in two large trials to confer lasting benefit if given for the first 3 weeks after TIA or a small stroke. The second of these trials gave aspirin for 3 months with no benefit over the 3-week regimen and a higher rate of adverse hemorrhagic effects.

Anticoagulants

Many clinical situations call for anticoagulation rather than antiplatelet therapy (Box 5.4). The mainstay of oral anticoagulation was for many years warfarin. Since 2009 several new oral anticoagulants have been shown to be equivalent to warfarin, and in some cases safer, and they are more convenient, since they do not require INR monitoring.

For nonvalvular atrial fibrillation (AF), stroke risk depends on the presence of other risk factors. This risk is commonly estimated based on the $CHADS_2VA_2Sc$ score (Box 5.5). Patients with a true lone AF $CHADS_2$ score 0–1 may not benefit from anticoagulation; those with scores ≥ 2 do benefit. Age is not a contraindication to anticoagulation. Although age does confer greater risk of hemorrhage from anticoagulant use, the proportional increase of stroke risk with age is yet greater, so the relative benefit of anticoagulation increases with age.

The three factor Xa inhibitors, apixaban, rivaroxaban, and edoxaban, and the direct thrombin inhibitor dabigatran have all been shown to be roughly equivalent (noninferior) to warfarin for stroke prevention in AF. All may serve as appropriate substitutes. We typically choose apixaban based on the low risk of adverse effects and the favorable pharmacokinetics for twice daily dosing. Several studies suggest that rivaroxaban and apixaban may substitute for cancer-associated hypercoagulability. So far, studies comparing warfarin to the newer agents have not been promising in patients with antiphospholipid antibody syndrome; therefore we continue to recommend warfarin for that indication. Warfarin also remains the recommended anticoagulant for protection in patients with mechanical heart valve prostheses.

The 2017 COMPASS trial of low-dose rivaroxaban plus rivaroxaban versus aspirin alone is the first trial to

---

BOX 5.4 Indication for Anticoagulation for Stroke Prevention

Mechanical heart valve prosthesis
Atrial fibrillation (see also Box 5.5)
Intracardiac thrombus
Hypercoagulable states
Cerebral venous sinus thrombosis

BOX 5.5 $CHADS_2VA_2Sc$ Score

CONDITION	POINTS
C—Congestive heart failure	1
H—Hypertension	1
A_2—Age $\geq$75 years	2
DDiabetes mellitus	1
S_2—Prior stroke or TIA or other thromboembolism	2
V—Vascular disease CAD, PAD, aortic plaque)	1
A—Age 65–74 years	1
Sc—Sex category (female)[a]	1

[a]A point is given for female sex only if at least one other point is given.
CAD, Coronary artery disease; PAD, peripheral artery disease.

show a benefit of anticoagulation in patients outside of the indications discussed previously. In this study, rivaroxaban 2.5 mg twice daily plus aspirin 100 mg daily was superior to rivaroxaban alone 5 mg twice daily and to aspirin alone 100 mg daily for primary prevention of stroke in patients with coronary or peripheral atherosclerotic vascular disease. This benefit came with a small increased risk of major bleeding.

Risk Factor Management

The major decline in the incidence of stroke in recent decades correlates with major improvements in the management of vascular risk factors, including smoking cessation and control of hypertension, hypercholesterolemia, and diabetes mellitus. Therefore it is most important to address all of these conditions for both primary and secondary stroke prevention. High-intensity statins with a goal LDL <70 are recommended for secondary stroke prevention in patients with atherosclerotic risk factors. It is also very important to encourage and support healthy lifestyles, including weight reduction, healthy diet, and regular exercise. We also recommend screening for obstructive sleep apnea and treatment of affected patients.

Surgical Therapies for Ischemic Stroke Prevention

Carotid endarterectomy. Patients with symptomatic stenosis of the cervical internal carotid artery of ≥50% benefit from carotid endarterectomy (CEA) if surgeons maintain low surgical risk. Endovascular placement of carotid artery stents (CAS) may be an alternative to CEA in selected patients. Studies from approximately 20 years ago found benefit of CEA in patients with asymptomatic carotid stenosis. However, a fall in the risk of stroke since these studies were done has raised doubt concerning the benefit of CEA or CAS in asymptomatic patients. This issue is currently under investigation in a large clinical trial. Until this issue is settled we recommend consultation with a vascular neurologist to help with optimal patient selection for CEA or CAS.

PFO closure. Patent foramen ovale (PFO) is a very common and usually benign condition with estimates of approximately 25% in the general population, depending on the mode of assessment. When patients with no or few vascular risk factors have embolic strokes and are found to have PFO the questions arise: Is the PFO related to the stroke? As a conduit for paradoxical embolism or

by another mechanism? Will closure of the PFO lower the risk of recurrent stroke? And is it safe? There is good evidence that paradoxical embolism is a cause of stroke in many otherwise low-risk patients. The RoPE score is a useful tool to estimate the attributable risk in a particular patient. Initial trials of device closure for presumed symptomatic PFO suggested that the procedure can be done safely; however, they failed to establish clear benefit. More recent trials have shown benefit. Consultation with a vascular neurologist and interventional cardiologist with experience in this procedure is now recommended in patients with embolic stroke or TIA without apparent alternative cause and PFO.

External carotid-internal carotid (EC-IC) bypass and indirect surgical revascvariztion procedures. Controlled trials of EC-IC bypass for carotid occlusion have not shown benefit. However, in expert surgical hands, and in patients with cervical or intracranial vascular stenoses with high risk of stroke, especially in moyamoya syndrome, such procedures may be beneficial. This therapy remains unvalidated, and we recommend that symptomatic patients with such vascular occlusions be evaluated by neurologists and surgeons with expertise in this area.

Intracranial stenting. Studies of the placement of intracranial arterial stents in patients with symptomatic intracranial stenoses have not shown benefit. In fact, these studies have shown an excess of events in surgically treated patients. We currently treat such patients according to the protocol used in the medical arm of the SAMMPRIS trail, saving the option of intervention for exceptional patients with demonstrated higher risk.

Future Directions

Advances in recent decades in medical and surgical therapy have had a major impact on stroke care. The most important interventions continue to be the optimal application of available medical therapies for primary and secondary stroke prevention, that is, those interventions introduced and maintained by primary care physicians. Expertise is available to properly select patients for surgical therapies. Since 1995 there has been a revolution in the management of acute stroke which has led to the development of effective thrombolytic and endovascular therapies that can in many cases minimize the disability from strokes. The availability of these therapies has prompted the development of enhanced systems of stroke care to maximize patients' access to advanced care.

Future refinements of stroke care will fine-tune the development of revascularization therapies and the systems of care to make them as accessible as possible. Further advances in vascular imaging will add to our understanding of cerebrovascular disease and to the most precise diagnosis and best management of patients. Neuroprotection, the use of drugs that protect neurons from ischemia and minimize stroke size or allow greater time for the application of reperfusion therapies, remains an unmet goal, and efforts to find such agents should continue. Genetic studies and studies of basic pathophysiology will help us to understand the basic mechanisms of cerebrovascular disorders and will, we anticipate, lead to improved therapies to allow us to further reduce the burden of ischemic stroke.

HEMORRHAGIC STROKE

Hemorrhagic Stroke: Pathology, Pathophysiology, and Types of Hemorrhage (Differential Diagnosis)

Pathophysiology and Classification of Hemorrhagic Stroke

The primary lesion of hemorrhagic stroke is extravascular blood that has escaped from the intravascular compartment to the brain or surrounding compartments. With escape of blood into these tissues, there may be displacement of normal structures, mass effect with elevation of intracranial pressure (ICP), and resultant compromise of cerebral perfusion, inflammation, release of bioactive substances with toxic effects, such as iron and endothelin, tissue edema, and swelling and herniation of cerebral contents outside of their normal containing boundaries, and vasospasm. Elevation of ICP, local edema, herniation, and vasospasm may compromise cerebral perfusion and lead to secondary infarction. These processes may ultimately lead to destruction of cerebral tissue and cavitation however if mitigated may result in reversible injury to tissues.

It is clinically useful to classify hemorrhagic strokes into the tissue compartments into which the bleeding occurs. Hemorrhage may occur in the parenchyma of the brain or spinal cord, within the brain's ventricles, or in the subarachnoid space. (Hemorrhage may also occur within the subdural or epidural spaces; however, we do not classify such hemorrhages as strokes.) Many different vascular lesions and disorders may underlie hemorrhage into each of these locations (Boxes 5.6 and 5.7).

BOX 5.6 Types of Hemorrhagic Stroke Based on Location

Intraparenchymal (IPH)
  Deep
  Lobar
Intraventricular (IVH)
  Primary IVH
  Intraventricular extension from IPH or subarachnoid (SAH)
SAH
  Basal cisterns
  Convexal
Multicompartmental

BOX 5.7 Some Causes of Hemorrhagic Stroke

Intraparencymal (IPH)
Deep
  Hypertensive hemorrhage
Lobar
  Cerebral amyloid angiopathy (CAA)
Either or Both
  Hypertensive hemorrhage
  Vascular malformations
  Pseudoaneurysms
  Mycotic aneurysms and septic embolism
  Hemorrhagic transformation of an infarct
  Hemorrhagic tumor
  Vasculitis and vasculopathy
  Clotting disorders
  Trauma
  Cerebral venous sinus thrombosis
Intraventricular (IVH)
  Primary IVH
  Intraventricular extension from IPH or subarachnoid (SAH)
  Vascular malformation
Subarachnoid
  Basal cisterns
    Aneurysmal SAH
    Perimesencephalic SAH
  Convexal
    Trauma
    CAA
    Reversible cerebral vasoconstriction syndrome

Multicompartmental
Trauma
Cerebral venous sinus thrombosis

Hemorrhagic Stroke: Causes

It is important to establish, as accurately as possible, the underlying cause of cerebral hemorrhage. The determination of the cause will govern further evaluation and therapies for prevention of recurrence.

Hemorrhage due to trauma. We typically exclude traumatic hemorrhage from discussions of hemorrhagic stroke so we will dispense with trauma quickly. However, it merits mention here, because especially when trauma is not apparent, it remains in the differential diagnosis of hemorrhage seen on brain imaging. Traumatic hemorrhage may occur in any compartment, parenchyma, ventricles, subarachnoid space, subdural space, or epidural space, and it is a common cause of multicompartmental hemorrhage. When in the subarachnoid space, it is a common cause of convexal hemorrhages at the site of trauma or at points of contact of the brain with the rigid fold of dura, the falx cerebri or tentorium. When in the brain substance, it is typically a manifestation of a contusion. These most commonly occur at sites of collision of the brain contents against the hard cranium (*coup*) or at the opposite pole (*contracoup*) as the brain accelerates and decelerates with blows to the head. The most common sites are the frontal and temporal poles. The history and external injuries are often decisive in making the diagnosis of traumatic hemorrhage. When considering possible hemorrhagic strokes, it is important to keep occult trauma in the initial differential diagnosis.

Hypertensive hemorrhage is the commonest type of nontraumatic hemorrhage (Figs. 5.8 and 5.9). Hypertensive hemorrhage results from spontaneous rupture of small arteries that feed the deep structures of the brain. With every beat of the heart the vessels expand and contract leading to wear and tear over the years. This wear and tear leads to degenerative hyalinosis and thickening of vessel walls. This vascular degeneration causes a loss of compliance of the vessel wall, often gradual compromise of the lumen as the walls thicken and encroach on the luminal space but also sometimes expansion of the lumen, causing enlarged, dolichoectasia arteries and sometimes small, so-called Charcot-Bouchard aneurysms of the microscopic small vessels. The loss of integrity of the vessel wall may culminate in rupture. Because hypertension greatly accelerates this process of age-related small vessel disease, such hemorrhages are considered hypertensive hemorrhages, although they may occur in elderly patients, without a

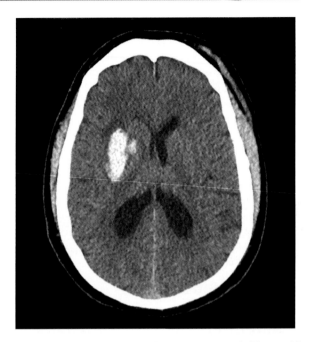

Fig. 5.8 Hypertensive hemorrhage, putamen. A 52-year-old male was found down with left hemiparesis. Noncontrast shows an acute right putaminal hemorrhage typical of hypertensive hemorrhage. Computed tomography angiography (not shown) was normal.

history of hypertension. Because this underlying pathology may also lead to ischemic strokes of the lacunar type (see above), as one might expect, hypertensive hemorrhages are most commonly located in the same deep locations as lacunes, most typically in the putamen, caudate, thalamus, pons, and cerebellum. For this reason, it is useful to classify hemorrhages into deep, suggesting hypertension, or lobar, often suggesting cerebral amyloid angiopathy, as the underlying cause (see below).

Cerebral amyloid angiopathy (CAA) refers to the vascular deposition of A-ß amyloid in the small vessel walls. This is the same amyloid that is implicated in the pathogenesis of Alzheimer's disease. The vascular amyloidosis renders the small vessel walls friable and subject to spontaneous rupture. This may occur as the result of a familial disorder of amyloid processing, and many family pedigrees have been described; however, like Alzheimer disease, it is most commonly sporadic. The prevalence of CAA is not certain but estimated to be 5%–7% in elderly patient who are cognitively normal and 50%–57% in elderly patients with lobrar hemorrhage. In contradistinction to hypertensive hemorrhage, bleeding typically occurs spontaneously more superficially in the lobar regions (Figs. 5.10 and 5.11). Spontaneous focal convexal subarachnoid hemorrhage may also occur, presenting with acute symptoms or found upon imaging asymptomatic patients. Such convexal subarachnoid hemorrhage is seen as superficial siderosis on MRI (see Fig. 5.11). Commonly, asymptomatic microhemorrhages in the same lobar locations, and visible on MRI sequences sensitive to hemosiderin, occur before larger symptomatic hemorrhage. Though definite diagnosis depends on pathologic examination of a specimen taken during brain biopsy or autopsy, for practical reasons, biopsy is seldom done, and so diagnosis of CAA is established based on clinical criteria. The modified Boston criteria offer widely used, validated guidelines for clinical diagnosis (Box 5.8).

Vascular malformations may underlie hemorrhages in any compartment. *Developmental cerebral aneurysms* are expansions of the cerebral arterial walls typically causing a localized, thin-walled outpouching of the vessel. All three layers of the arterial wall make up the aneurysm, but with weakened areas that render the aneurysm liable to spontaneous rupture. Rupture of such *saccular aneurysms* usually leads to subarachnoid hemorrhage (SAH), though rupture of an aneurysm adherent to the adjacent cortex may cause isolated intracerebral hemorrhage (for example rupture of a anterior communicating artery aneurysm directly into the interior frontal lobe) (Figs. 5.12 and 5.13). Risk factors for cerebral aneurysm rupture include (1) fixed risk factors: age, family history of aneurysmal rupture, Japanese or Finnish ancestry; (2) modifiable risk factors: hypertension, smoking, heavy alcohol consumption, cocaine use; and (3) various anatomic features of the aneurysm (size, location, and irregularity of the dome contour). Large studies allow us to

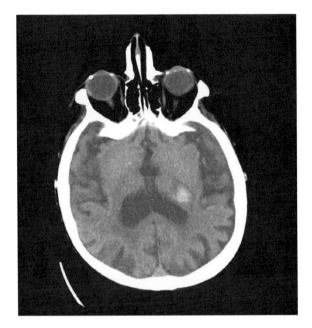

Fig. 5.9 Hypertensive hemorrhage, thalamus. A 98-year-old male with hypertension on apixaban for atrial fibrillation presented with right hemiparesis and sensory loss affecting the right face, arm, leg, and torso. Noncontrast shows an acute left thalamic hemorrhage typical of hypertensive hemorrhage. Computed tomography angiography (not shown) was normal.

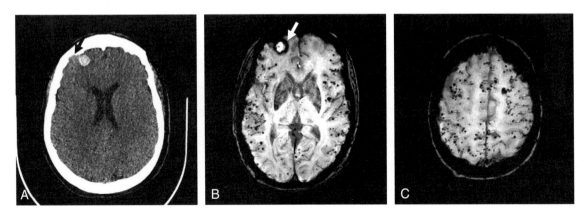

Fig. 5.10 Cerebral amyloid angiopathy. A 65-year-old female with new-onset confusion was found to have multiple acute cerebral hemorrhages (A, noncontrast head computed tomography [CT] shows an acute right frontal hemorrhage). CT angiography (not shown) showed no vascular lesions. Magnetic resonance imaging, susceptibility-weighted sequence shows the right frontal hemorrhage (B) and innumerable chronic microhemorrhages throughout the lobar regions of the hemispheres (B and C), strongly suggesting cerebral amyloid angiopathy.

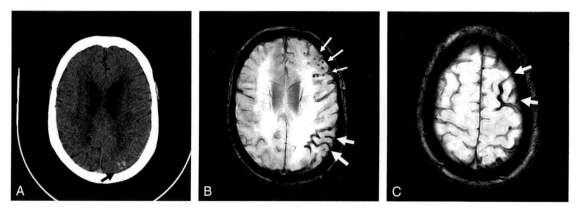

Fig. 5.11 Cerebral amyloid angiopathy with superficial siderosis. A 67-year-old female with a history of past left temporal lobar hemorrhage and sudden onset of fluent aphasia. Computed tomography (CT) shows small subarachnoid hemorrhage in the left parietal convexity (A, *arrow*). CT angiography (not shown) showed no vascular lesions. Magnetic resonance imaging (MRI), susceptibility-weighted sequence shows lobar microbleeds (A, *small arrows*) and the parietal SAH (A, *large arrows* and B, *arrows*) strongly suggesting cerebral amyloid angiopathy. The areas of subarachnoid hemorrhage persist as chronic superficial siderosis on subsequent MRIs.

BOX 5.8   The Modified Boston Criteria for Diagnosis of Cerebral Amyloid Angiopathy[a]

Definite CAA

Full postmortem examination demonstrating:

    Lobar, cortical, or cortical-subcortical hemorrhages

    Severe CAA with vasculopathy

    Absence of other diagnostic lesion

Probable CAA with supporting pathology

Clinical data and pathologic tissue (evacuated hematoma or cortical biopsy) demonstrating:

    Lobar, cortical, or cortical-subcortical hemorrhage (including ICH, CMB, or cSS)

    Some degree of CAA in specimen

    Absence of other diagnostic lesion

Probable CAA

Clinical data and MRI or CT demonstrating:

Multiple hemorrhages (ICH, CMB) restricted to lobar, cortical, or cortical-subcortical regions (cerebellar hemorrhage allowed), or single lobar, cortical, or cortical-subcortical hemorrhage and cSS (focal or disseminated)

    Age ≥ 55 years

    Absence of other cause of hemorrhage

Possible CAA

Clinical data and MRI or CT demonstrating:

Single lobar, cortical, or cortical-subcortical ICH, CMB, or cSS (focal or disseminated)

Age ≥ 55 years

Absence of other causes of hemorrhage

[a]From Greenberg (2018).

CAA, Cerebral amyloid angiopathy; *CMB,* cortical microbleed; *cSS,* cortical superficial siderosis; *CT,* computed tomography; *ICH,* intracerebral hemorrhage; *MRI,* magnetic resonance imaging.

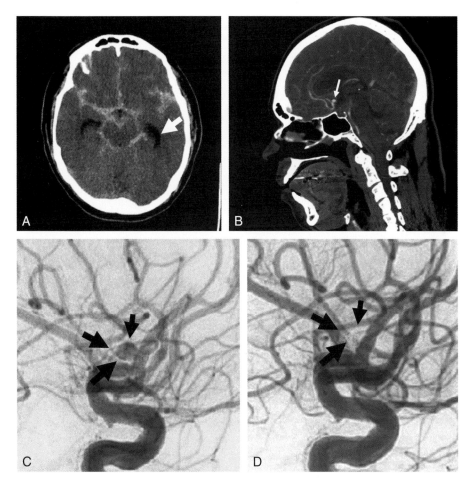

Fig. 5.12 Subarachnoid hemorrhage (SAH), anterior communicating artery aneuyrysm. A 49-year-old male presented with a thunderclap headache. Noncontrast head CT shows acute SAH with hyperdensites corresponding to blood in the basal cisterns, Sylvian fissure, and sulci and early hydrocephalus with expansion of the temporal horns of the lateral ventricle (A, *arrow*). CT angiogram shows an aneurysm of the anterior communicating artery (B, *arrow*). Digital subtraction angiogram confirms the anterior communicating artery aneurysm (C, *arrows*). After coil occlusion of the aneurysm, it no longer fills with contrast and only a faint shadow of the coils is seen (D, *arrows*).

estimate risk of hemorrhage based on these risk factors; however, such estimates are complex and uncertain, and many SAHs occur in patients who might be deemed low risk in population-based studies. Large SAH may cause elevated ICP, hydrocephalus (Figs. 5.12 and 5.13), recurrent hemorrhage, arterial vasospasm, and delayed cerebral ischemia, all of which place patients at high risk of major neurologic injury and death. *Cerebal arteriovenous malformations* (AVM) are vascular malformations characterized by abnormal development of a focal area of circulation in which arteries bypass normal cerebral (or spinal) tissues and flow directly into veins via

a tangle of vessels, the *nidus*. AVMs may occur as part of a syndrome, such as Olser-Weber-Rendu, Sturge-Webert, or von Hippel Lindau syndrome, or they may occur in isolation. They typically become symptomatic when they cause headaches, seizures, intraparencymal or subarachnoid hemorrhage, or mass effect with focal neurologic deficits. Treatment decisions concerning cerebral AVMs are complex, depending on the size and location of the AVM and the neurologic function it threatens, the nature of the symptoms, the risks for further neurologic symptoms, such as seizures or recurrent hemorrhage, and other features that influence surgical

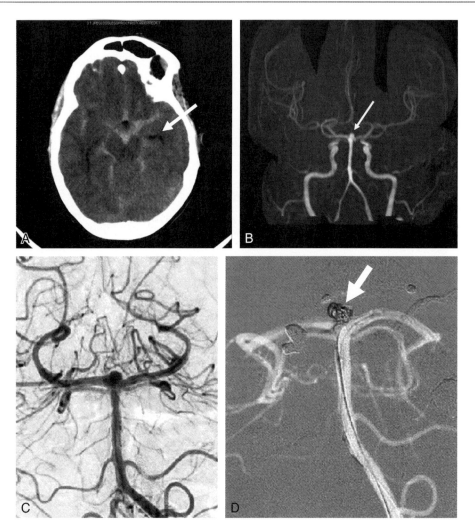

Fig. 5.13 Subarachnoid hemorrhage (SAH) basilar tip aneuyrysm. A 52-year-old female presented with sudden onset of severe headache and vomiting followed by loss of consciousness. Noncontrast head computed tomography shows acute SAH with hyperdensites corresponding to blood in the basal cisterns, Sylvian fissure, and sulci and early hydrocephalus with expansion of the temporal horns of the lateral ventricle (A, *arrow*). Magnetic resonance angiogram shows the basilar tip aneurysm (B, *arrow*). Digital subtraction angiogram confirms the basilar tip aneurysm (C, *arrow*). "Roadmap" (silhouette) of the digital subtraction angiogram shows a catheter in place deploying coils to fill the aneurysm (D, *arrow*).

risk, such as the anatomy of the drainage of the AVM and patient age and comorbidities. *Dural arteriovenous fistulas* (DAVF), like AVMs, are vascular malformations in which an artery bypasses capillary channels to flow directly into draining veins (Fig. 5.14). DAVFs are distinguished from AMMs because they arise from feeding arteries of the pachymeninges (dura) rather than the brain parenchyma, and they have no nidus. These lesions are thought to be acquired in most cases, probably from normal microscopic arteriovenous channels that expand as a result of aging or injury. Like AVMs they may cause headache, hemorrhage, or focal neurologic deficits due to cerebral (or spinal cord) edema. Spinal DAVFs represent a significant and treatable cause of myelopathy. *Cerebral cavernous malformations (CCM)* are foci of expanded thin-walled channels. They have only small, low-flow connections to their arterial supply so that they are typically not seen with CTA or digital

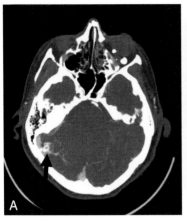 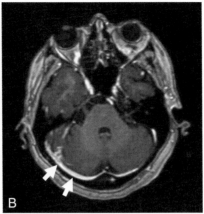 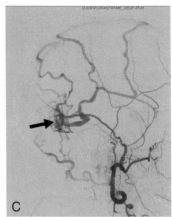

Fig. 5.14 Dural AV fistula. A 59-year-old female presented with 2 weeks of persistent right occipital headache. Head computed tomography (CT) (not shown) showed no hemorrhage. CT angiography shows dilated, irregular vessels just above and adjacent to the right transverse sinus with enlarged draining veins (A, *arrow*). MRV shows a patent right transverse sinus with no venous sinus thrombosis (B, *arrow*). Digital subtraction angiogram shows a dural arteriovenous fistula (DAVF) with middle meningeal artery supply and drainage into the transverse sinus (C, *arrow*). The DAVF was occluded by endovascular embolizaton.

subtraction angiography. They most commonly occur sporadically, although pedigrees with familial CCM have been identified. They often cause small hemorrhages in any part of the CNS, although they can cause large hemorrhages. They typically become symptomatic when they bleed or cause seizures or focal neurologic deficits. *Developmental venous anomalies (DVA)* are developmental varicose venous channels. They are typically small low-flow lesions that are found incidentally by neuroimaging. Rarely, they may cause symptoms by bleeding or causing edema. They are usually asymptomatic, but they may be associated with adjacent CCMs. *Cerebral capillary telangiectasias* are foci of dilated capillaries that can be seen on brain MRI. Like DVAs they are typically asymptomatic and of no clinical significance.

Distinct from vascular malformations, *pseudoaneurysms* occur when an artery is injured, either by trauma or due to underlying vulnerabilities that lead to arterial dissections. Such vulnerabilities may be due to systemic disorders of connective tissue, such as Marfan syndrome, Ehlers-Danlos syndrome, or Loeys-Dietz syndrome; however, they are more commonly due to fibromuscular dysplasia or occur in patients with no known predisposing condition, likely from minor connective tissue variations due to common polymorphisms. Unlike developmental aneurysms, they result from an injury to the artery so that the wall of the expanded aneurysm does not contain all three

vascular layers. Pseudoaneurysms in the cerebral circulation occur most often extracranial in the cervical carotid and vertebral arteries so they usually cause neurologic symptoms when they cause ischemic stroke as a result of artery-to-artery embolism on low flow, but they may cause subarachnoid hemorrhage when dissections extend to the incranial arteries. *Cerebral mycotic aneurysms* are focal expansions of intracranial arteries due to septic embolism from infective endocarditis. Septic emboli, either luminal or via the *vasa vasorum*, cause focal sites of vascular inflammation that weaken the arterial wall leading to aneurysmal expansion and sometime rupture and parenchymal or subarachnoid hemorrhage. Vessel rupture and hemorrhage may also occur after septic embolism without prior visible expansion of the vessel. Neurologic injury from cerebral hemorrhage (and infarction) is a major cause of death and long-term disability from infective endocarditis.

Cerebral hemorrhage may occur within CNS tumors. Though they do not typically present with hemorrhage, lung and breast metastases to the brain may hemorrhage, and, because they are common, they represent the most common hemorrhagic tumors. Some less common tumors are more prone to hemorrhage, which may be the initial finding that leads to diagnosis, such as melanoma, renal cell carcinoma, thyroid carcinoma, and choriocarcinoma.

Hemorrhagic transformation of an infarction most commonly occurs after large embolic strokes, presumably from reperfusion into damaged distal vessels. When hemorrhage is present on the initial presentation, it may be hard to distinguish from primary hemorrhage.

Vasculitis and noninflammatory vasculopathies most commonly cause cerebral infarction; however, they may also cause hemorrhage. As noted earlier, septic embolism causes focal areas of infective vasculitis which may lead to cerebral hemorrhage in patients with infective endocarditis. Fungal infections with angioinvasive organisms, such as *Aspergillus*, may cause cerebral hemorrhage and infarction.

Disorders of clotting such as thrombocytopenia from any cause (TTP, ITP, DIC, HIT, TMA, hypersplenism, and chemotherapy and other drug toxicities) may lead to cerebral hemorrhage in any compartment. Clotting disorders from hepatic failure and, more commonly, from the use of therapeutic anticoagulants may cause spontaneous hemorrhage, and these disorders render patients more vulnerable to traumatic hemorrhage and hemorrhage from other causes such as HTN and CAA.

Cerebral venous thrombosis may cause increased venous pressure leading to edema, venous infarction, and, in some cases, hemorrhage into any compartment.

Reversible cerebral vasoconstriction syndrome (RCVS) can also cause cerebral hemorrhage. This syndrome of disrupted cerebral vasomotor control classically presents with thunderclap headache, transient focal neurologic symptoms and signs, and angiography evidence of cerebral vasospasm. In addition to focal ischemic manifestations, patients with RCVS may present with intraparenchyal or subarachnoid hemorrhage. Along with CAA, RCVS is one of the common causes of small atraumatic convexal subarachnoid hemorrhages. CAA most commonly affects those >60 and RCVS in those ≤60 years of age.

Hemorrhagic Stroke: Diagnostic Imaging

The pattern of hemorrhage seen on head CT and brain MRI along with the clinical context often strongly suggests the cause of the hemorrhage. A healthy person with a thunderclap headache and subarachnoid hemorrhage in the basal cisterns probably has suffered rupture of a saccular cerebral aneurysm (Figs. 5.12 and 5.13). However, a restricted perimesencephalic (or perpontine, permedullary, or supracellar) pattern of SAH suggests that venous bleeding may be the cause and that no aneurysm will be found (Fig. 5.15). A patient without coagulopathy who is found to have a small subarachnoid hemorrhage isolated to a convexal surface of the brain likely has had trauma, or, if not, likely has CAA, if older (Fig. 5.11), or RCVS, if younger, although many other causes are possible. A patient with a history of HTN and

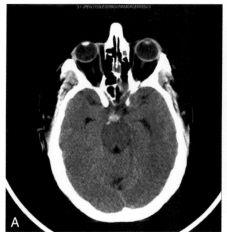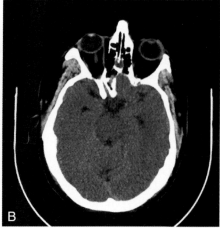

Fig. 5.15 SAH prepontine. A 62-year-old male presented with a severe sudden-onset headache followed by neck stiffness. He had suffered no trauma. His neurologic examination was normal. Noncontrast head computed tomography (CT) shows a focal subarachnoid hemorrhage restricted to the suprasellar and prepontine cisterns (A). CT angiography showed no aneurysm or vascular malformation (not shown). Two digital subtraction angiograms showed no aneurysm or other vascular malformation. A follow-up head CT a week later showed resolution of the SAH (B).

a hemorrhage in the putamen, thalamus, basis pontis, or cerebellum has probably had a hypertensive hemorrhage, due to rupture of a small penetrating artery (Figs. 5.8 and 5.9). An elderly patient with a lobar hemorrhage with no other apparent cause likely has CAA. Further imaging with an MRI sequence sensitive to iron remnants (susceptibility-weighted imaging [SWI], gradient-echo imaging, and T2* imaging, depending on the scanner) that shows one or many lobar microbleeds or superficial siderosis greatly increases the likelihood of CAA (Box 5.8 and Figs. 5.10 and 5.11). The diagnosis of isolated intraventricular hemorrhage (IVH) requires careful scrutiny of the image looking for a small parenchymal component, often in the thalamus or caudate head. When this is present, the lesion is often a hypertensive hemorrhage at a typical site with intraventricular extension. When there is true isolated IVH, it is important to look for AVM or other vascular malformation, though such hemorrhages are often cryptogenic. A patient with multiple round hemorrhages may have a hemorrhagic tumor, such as a melanoma; however, there are many other possible causes. In the case of tumor, further scanning with MRI and contrast will usually show the enhancing mass. Simultaneous hemorrhage into multiple compartments (intraparenchymal, subarachnoid, subdural) may occur from many causes, but trauma, cerebral venous sinus thrombosis (CVT), and coagulopathy, including from anticoagulant therapy, should be considered. Coagulopathy is most commonly due to anticoagulant therapy, thrombocytopenia from many possible causes, or deficits of clotting factors, most often acquired from alcohol toxicity. Patients with coagulopathies may present with many different patterns of hemorrhage. It is prudent practice to take a moment to consider, in addition to coagulopathy, CVT and infective endocarditis early in the consideration of every hemorrhage, since these disorders may present in many different ways, and their diagnosis is often delayed.

The initial diagnostic image for suspected cerebral hemorrhage should usually be noncontrast head CT. Hemorrhage is almost always apparent as hyperdensity on the CT, and this study can be done quickly to allow the early identification of threatening instability, such as from mass effect or hydrocephalus, and initial clues about the cause. This should be followed by vascular imaging. CT angiogram (CTA) offers quick and sensitive information about the presence of vascular lesions, such

as aneurysm, or AVMs, vascular stenoses that might suggest other diagnoses, including vasospasm or vasculitis. CT or MRI with contrast can look for evidence of tumor or inflammatory lesions. Brain MRI adds detail to CT, and it is especially useful when, done with contrast, looking for tumor, when trying to define anatomic precision, for example, the extent of involvement of brainstem structures, when timing the onset of hemorrhage, and when looking for old microhemorrhages (SWI GRE or T2* sequence). MRA is an alternative modality for cerebrovascular imaging. MRA imaging is less sensitive or specific than CTA for visualization of the more distal vessels; however, it offers a high level of accuracy for proximal arteries and the advantage of vascular imaging without contrast using the time-of-flight technique. Digital subtraction angiography (DSA) remains the gold standard for imaging of the cerebral vasculature. All patients with possible cerebral aneurysm, AVM, or AVDF should undergo DSA for the most sensitive diagnostic look and, in many cases, for endovascular treatment (Fig. 5.13). For many other conditions, such as RCVS, cerebral angiitis, DSA adds invaluable diagnostic information when CTA is not definitive. Vessel wall imaging (VWI) relies on the enhancement of vessels walls highlighted against a suppressed, black lumen. Though this technique is new, and its specificity remains too low for reliable differentiation of inflammatory from noninflammatory disorders, it holds promise to support such significant clinical distinctions as those between arteritis and noninflammatory arteropathies or between active, recently ruptured, and quiescent aneurysms.

Hemorrhagic Stroke: Acute Treatment

The acute management of patients with cerebral hemorrhage should be approached hierarchically proceeding in order through early stabilization, precise diagnosis, definitive treatment, and prevention of recurrence. Initial assessment includes a rapid physical and neurologic examination to establish cardiorespiratory and neurologic stability. This should include a history of the onset and subsequent events and a history of relevant medications, most importantly anticoagulants, and other conditions that might allow the direction of therapies to the cause of hemorrhage. The examination includes assessment of vital signs and cardiopulmonary function and screening for trauma and evidence of coagulopathy or septic embolism. Neurologic assessment includes level of consciousness, cranial nerve (including

BOX 5.9   The Modified Hunt & Hess Scale

Grade 0—Unruptured aneurysm

Grade I—Asymptomatic, or minimal headache and slight nuchal rigidity

Grade Ia—No acute meningeal or brain reaction, but with fixed neurologic deficit

Grade II—Moderate to severe headache, nuchal rigidity, no neurologic deficit other than cranial nerve palsy

Grade III—Drowsiness, confusion, or mild focal deficit

Grade IV—Stupor, moderate to severe hemiparesis, possibly early decerebrate rigidity and vegetative disturbances

Grade V—Deep coma, decerebrate rigidity, moribund appearance

vision, pupillary size and reactivity, and eye movements) and motor function, especially laterality. The findings of these critical examinations are commonly communicated among physicians using the Glasgow Coma Score (GCS) and for SAH, the modified Hunt & Hess scale and World Federation of Neurosurgical Societies scale (WFNS), which provide a common structure and terminology for early assessment (Box 5.9). After having addressed any issues of cardiopulmonary stability, patients should have immediate head CT to look for hemorrhage and for potential complications which might demand rapid neurosurgical intervention, such as hydrocephalus with impaired level of consciousness or impending or established hernation. Such patient will need urgent neurosurgical consultation for placement of intraventricular drains or urgent decompressive surgery, as indicated. In addition, interventions should be made to minimize continued and recurrent hemorrhage. The BP should be controlled rapidly, and patients should have urgent laboratory testing for platelets and INR. Rapid BP control should be achieved with nicardipine or other intravenous agents. Patients on warfarin should be given prothrombin complex concentrate (PCC) (preferable a 4-factor agent) or fresh frozen plasma, if PCC is not available, and intravenous vitamin K. Patients on dabigatran, apixaban, rivaroxaban, or other oral anticoagulants should receive PCC or specific reversal agents (idarucizumab for dabigatran or andexanet alpha for direct anti-Xa agents, such as apixaban and rivaroxaban). Patients with thrombocytopenia should receive platelet transfusions. Although benefits have not been confirmed in clinical trials, it is common practice in urgent situations to give platelet transfusions and/or DDAVP for patient with disorders expected to cause platelet dysfunction, such as alcoholism and renal insufficiency. After stabilization has been accomplished, neurologic, neurosurgical, and intensive care consultants should collaborate to plan for further testing as needed to establish a precise diagnosis and to provide early critical care and surgical therapy, as indicated. Vascular imaging with CTA and, when indicated, DSA should be done.

Patients with SAH should be evaluated for aneurysms, and ruptured aneurysms should be surgically secured as soon as medically feasible. The choice of therapies for surgical control of aneurysms requires the expertise of vascular neurosurgeons and interventionists. These decisions depend on neurologic factors, such as the Hunt & Hess grade, medical factors, such as cardiopulmonary stability, and neurosurgical factors, such as the size, configuration, and location of the implicated aneurysm. Possible interventions include open craniotomy and aneurysm clipping and endovascular control procedures, including coiling (Figs. 5.12 and 5.13), stenting, and flow diversion. Patients with aneurysmal SAH are at risk for delayed hydrocephalus, if not present on presentation, and cerebral vasospasm and delayed cerebral injury, and these patients should be monitored closely in a critical care unit for diagnosis and treatment of these potential complications. Patients with intraparenchymal hemorrhage should be evaluated for urgent neurosurgical complications, and the potential benefits of early hematoma evacuation and/or craniectomy should be considered. Indications and the methods for early hematoma evacuation are evolving under active clinical study. Early trials of early hematoma evacuation did not show benefit. However, recent clinical trials of minimally invasive techniques have shown promise so it is expected that the early decompression surgery will be undertaken more frequently in coming years. Patients with large intraparenchymal hemorrhages are at risk for brain swelling and secondary neurologic injury from hydrocephalus, elevated ICP and hernation. Patients with hydrocephalus and depressed level of consciousness should be treated with external ventricular drainage. Patients with severely elevated ICP and impending herniation may benefit from craniectomy, hemicraniectomy or suboccipital craniectomy, for decompression to add to the early medical management of edema and brain swelling.

Patients with hemorrhage from any cause will benefit from therapies directed at the cause. Therefore, after immediate stabilization, a full diagnostic evaluation should be undertaken to establish the cause and to treat endocarditis, other infections, malignancy, or inflammatory disorders appropriately.

Patients with infective endocarditis (IE) and cerebral hemorrhage usually have hemorrhage due to septic embolism and vascular rupture with or without mycotic aneurysms. Appropriate intravenous antibiotics are the mainstay for therapy in all such patients. Although uncommon, mycotic aneurysms pose a great risk for poor neurologic outcome, and they should be sought in all patients with IE who have headache, focal neurologic deficits, CSF pleocytosis, or brain imaging showing ischemic stroke, hemorrhage, or brain abscess. If found, small mycotic aneurysms may respond to antibiotic therapy. If not secured surgically these small aneurysms must be followed with frequent serial imaging for potential expansion and heightened risk of hemorrhage. Large or expanding mycotic aneurysms should be treated surgically when possible to avoid rupture. Because most mycotic aneurysms are distally located in the arterial tree, are circumferential rather than arising from a narrow neck, and occur in tissue with poor structural integrity due to infection, surgical clipping is rarely an option. Current endovascular techniques allow canalization of the artery and embolization to isolate the aneurysm from the circulation. Because the aneurysms are typically distal, this can usually be accomplished with low risk of significant ischemic stroke due to vessel occlusion. Mycotic aneurysms may evolve very rapidly and so they should be addressed early to avoid cerebral hemorrhage and to allow safe cardiac surgery when this is needed. The diagnosis and management of IE is complex, and it is optimally accomplished with an interdisciplinary team, including experts in cardiology, infectious disease, cardiovascular surgery, neurology, interventional neurosurgery/radiology, diagnostic radiology, and addiction medicine.

Prevention of Hemorrhagic Stroke

Primary and secondary prevention of cerebral hemorrhage is critical to sound medical care. Many of its aspects are in the hands of primary care physicians, and preventive measures will have the greatest population-level impact on outcomes. Because brain imaging is commonly done for many conditions, including headaches, it is now common for asymptomatic, unruptured cerebral aneurysms to be found. Large cohort studies have provided data to help define the risk of subsequent rupture, based on aneurysm size, location, and morphologic features, and on age, and other risk factors, both fixed and treatable. The International Study of Unruptured Intracranial Aneurysms (ISUIA) found a low rate of rupture of unruptured aneurysms <10 mm in diameter in patients with no prior history of SAH. However, most ruptured aneurysms are <10 mm in diameter. These facts and the other features complicating the question of optimal surgical risk:benefit balance, including patient and aneurysm features and evolving surgical techniques, make decisions about if and when and how to operate complex. As a result of this complexity, there is not full consensus about which aneurysms to treat and how best to treat them. Therefore it is important to have such patients evaluated and monitored in collaboration with a vascular neurosurgeon and/or neurointerventionalist. When the decision is made to monitor patients with unruptured aneurysms without immediate surgical intervention, it is important to follow such patients with periodic cerebrovascular imaging to look for aneurysm growth and morphologic change.

Asymptomatic AVMs may also be found by imaging screening for other conditions. A large unblinded, randomized trial of patients with unruptured cerebral AVMs (ARUBA) found that patients fared better overall with medical rather that interventional therapy. However, the interpretation of these results has led to much controversy. Given the complexity of these patients and the evolution of surgical techniques, all such patients should be referred to a vascular neurosurgeon and/or neurointerventionalist to guide decision-making concerning when and how to intervene.

A family history of cerebral aneurysm and SAH confers risk, therefore after an aneurysm has been identified, we must also consider screening of family members at risk. Data on which to base selection of those who should benefit from screening imaging are limited; therefore decision analysis methods have been applied to the question of screening. The current practice among many experts is to screen all patients with two or more first-degree relatives with an aneurysm or SAH. The current guideline from the American Heart Association/American Stroke Association is to consider screening of patients with a first-degree relative with a history of aneurysmal SAH.

Management of treatable risk factors for subarachnoid hemorrhage is a critical component of optimal preventive care. Major predictors of SAH include fixed (age, history of SAH, aneurysm size, aneurysm location, and Finnish or Japanese heritage) and treatable risk factors (HTN, smoking, excessive alcohol intake). These treatable risk factors each increase risk by over twofold (relative risk: HTN 2.5, smoking 2.2, excessive alcohol intake 2.1); therefore, as for ischemic stroke, optimal control of these conditions and behaviors will have the greatest impact on outcomes of SAH. HTN is the most common cause of intraparenchymal hemorrhage, and therapeutic anticoagulant use with or without HTN is another major cause. Therefore both optimal treatment of HTN and therapies for the prevention of cardiovascular disease that leads to AF and ischemic stroke, thus diminishing the need for therapeutic anticoagulation, will have the greatest impact on the outcome of intraparenchmal hemorrhage.

Future Directions

In recent years, we have seen major advances in the understanding and care for patients with hemorrhagic stroke. Our understanding of hemorrhagic stroke has been advanced by the elucidation of the role of amyloid angiopathy in common senile lobar hemorrhage. With insight into the pathology of CAA and the pathophysiologically-related Alzheimer disease, we might hope for the emergence of novel therapies to prevent amyloid-related hemorrhage. We have also seen the development of refined surgical techniques that are now leading to new successes for surgical evacuation of hemorrhages, and we might expect a continuation of this trend. Prevention of all types of stroke has been more effective with better agents for the treatment of HTN, hypercholesterolemia, diabetes, a trend that has not yet run its course. Finally, we have seen the introduction of safer and more convenient anticoagulants which will, we hope, reduce this iatrogenic contribution to hemorrhagic stroke risk.

CONCLUSION

We have seen great advances in the prevention and treatment of stroke, both ischemic and hemorrhagic in recent decades. Yet, stroke remains the most common disabling neurologic condition and a major cause of long-term disability and death. New therapies for both ischemic and hemorrhagic stroke have been developed, and others are on the horizon. It is our task as clinical scientists to contribute to the development of stroke therapies and as clinicians to develop the protocols and coordinated systems of care that will promote the widespread applications of these advances, making them as widely available as possible.

"For the full bibliography list, please use the pincode on the inside front cover to access the electronic version of the text at ebooks.health.elsevier.com."

6

Traumatic Brain Injury*

William J. Mullally and Kathryn E. Hall

INTRODUCTION

Traumatic brain injury (TBI) is a major cause of death and disability in the United States. Each year approximately 2.5 million people are evaluated in a hospital emergency room for a TBI. In 2019, 223,135 individuals were hospitalized indicating that they had suffered a moderate or severe TBI. There were 64,362 TBI-related deaths in 2020. Falls are one of the main causes of TBI-related hospitalizations, especially among older adults. The highest rates and numbers of TBI-related hospitalizations and deaths occur in patients 75 and older. Children aged 0 to 4, adolescents aged 15 to 19, and adults 65 and older are most likely to sustain a TBI. Falls are the leading cause among children, and motor vehicle accidents for adolescents and persons aged 15 to 44. Motor vehicle accidents are the principal cause of TBI-related death. From 2010 to 2016 there were on average 283,000 TBI-related emergency room visits each year in persons under the age of 17 for sports and recreation-related TBIs and approximately 45% of the injuries were due to contact sports. The direct and indirect lifetime cost of TBIs is estimated at $76.5 billion/year and 90% is attributed to the moderate and severe TBIs that require hospitalization.

In this chapter we will review moderate and severe TBI, but the emphasis will be placed on concussion, including sports concussion, as concussion is a common problem encountered in primary care practice.

*Based on Mullally WJ. Concussion. *Am J Med.* 2017;130(8): 885–892. ISSN 0002-9343. https://doi.org/10.1016/j.amjmed. 2017.04.016.

MODERATE AND SEVERE TRAUMATIC BRAIN INJURY

Definition

When a patient suffers a head injury the initial concern is whether the traumatic insult has resulted in a severe traumatic brain injury (TBI). If, based on the clinical presentation of the injured person, a severe TBI is suspected then the patient should be immediately transported to the hospital emergency room. Indications for performing imaging of the brain using the New Orleans and Canadian criteria are listed in Box 6.1.

Severe injuries include cerebral contusion, subarachnoid hemorrhage, subdural and epidural hemorrhage, intraparenchymal hemorrhage, cerebral edema, skull fracture, and diffuse axonal injury. These injuries may result in death or major disability and must be diagnosed and treated without delay. While brain magnetic resonance imaging (MRI) will detect more intraparenchymal lesions it may miss skull fractures and a computed tomography (CT) scan is the modality of choice. CT can be performed expeditiously and will accurately detect acute structural abnormalities. The Glasgow Coma Scale (GCS) (Table 6.1) provides diagnostic guidance in the acute setting with scoring using eye, motor, and verbal scales. Moderate TBIs have a GCS score of 9 to 12 and severe, 8 or less. Moderate TBIs, as defined by the World Health Organization (WHO) and the Center for Disease Control (CDC) classifications, have abnormal or normal structural imaging, loss of consciousness of 30 minutes to 24 hours, altered mental state of >24 hours and post-traumatic amnesia >1 day and <7 days. Severe TBIs usually have abnormal structural imaging but occasionally imaging will be normal. Loss of consciousness and

BOX 6.1   Neuroimaging Guidelines

Abnormal neurologic exam including testing of gait
Progressive headache
Recurrent vomiting >2 episodes
loss of consciousness
Anterograde amnesia longer than 30 minutes
Age >60
Seizure
GCS score <15 2 hours post injury
Skull fracture
Signs of basilar skull fracture including hemotympanum,
   raccoon eyes, Battle's sign with ecchymosis around
   the mastoid, CSF rhinorrhea or otorrhea
Alcohol or drug intoxication
Coagulopathy
Dangerous mechanism including fall from >5 feet,
   ejection from a motor vehicle, pedestrian struck by
   a vehicle

TABLE 6.1   Glasgow Coma Scale

Best eye response (E)	Spontaneous—open with blinking at baseline	4
	Opens to verbal command, speech, or shout	3
	Opens to pain, not applied to face	2
	None	1
Best verbal response (V)	Oriented	5
	Confused conversation, but able to answer questions	4
	Inappropriate responses, words discernible	3
	Incomprehensible speech	2
	None	1
Best motor response (M)	Obeys commands for movement	6
	Purposeful movement to painful stimulus	5
	Withdraws from pain	4
	Abnormal (spastic) flexion, decorticate posture	3
	Extensor (rigid) response, decerebrate posture	2
	None	1

alteration of mental status are >24 hours, and posttraumatic amnesia is >7 days.

Pathogenesis

Both moderate and severe TBIs are serious injuries and require management in a specialized neurocritical care unit. Patients have often suffered multiple bodily injuries requiring multidisciplinary treatment. The mechanism of TBI, including closed head injury, penetrating head injury, blast injury, or crash injury, may provide valuable information regarding treatment and prognosis. The traumatic insult causes an injury to the skull or intracranial structures through direct, rotational, and shearing forces leading to focal contusions, intracranial hemorrhage, subarachnoid hemorrhage, cerebral edema, skull fracture, or diffuse axonal injury. Secondarily, damage occurs from oxidative stress, free radical formation, apoptosis, calcium-related axonal injury, and inflammation. Increased intracranial pressure, cerebral hypoxemia, and edema potentiate the damage.

A traumatic subarachnoid hemorrhage occurs when blood flows into the subarachnoid space from a tear of small capillaries. Unlike a subarachnoid aneurysmal bleed, the blood enters the space at low pressure (Fig. 6.1). An intraventricular hemorrhage may occur leading to hydrocephalus.

Contusions are the result of a direct injury to the brain and are described as a coup injury at the site of impact and contrecoup on the contralateral side (Fig. 6.2). Clinical signs and symptoms can be quite variable ranging from mild to severe.

An epidural hematoma (Fig. 6.3) is usually the result of direct trauma to the temporal region causing disruption of the middle meningeal artery and at times a skull fracture. The bleeding is outside of the dura and characteristically does not cross suture lines. The injury usually results in loss of consciousness followed by a "lucid" period where the patient is essentially asymptomatic, followed by a rapid decline due to increased intracranial pressure. Herniation leading to death may occur.

Subdural hematomas (Fig. 6.4) are the result of direct trauma causing a tear of a bridging vein and can cross suture lines. The acute form is usually associated with a significant brain injury due to mass effect on the underlying brain and cerebral edema and is dependent on the size of the hematoma. Subacute, chronic, and mixed forms of subdural hematomas may occur. A chronic subdural hematoma usually occurs in patients over the age of 60 who have brain atrophy. The most common

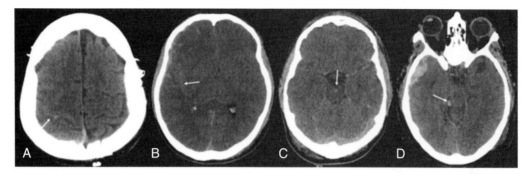

Fig. 6.1 Subarachnoid hemorrhage. Computed tomography demonstrating localized acute subarachnoid hemorrhage (*arrows*) in (A) cerebra sulci at the vertex, (B) the right Sylvian fissure, (C) the interpeduncular fossa, and (D) the ambient cistern. (From Adams A, Dixon AK, Gillard JH, Schaefer-Prokop C. *Grainger and Allison's Diagnostic Radiology.* 7th ed. 2020.)

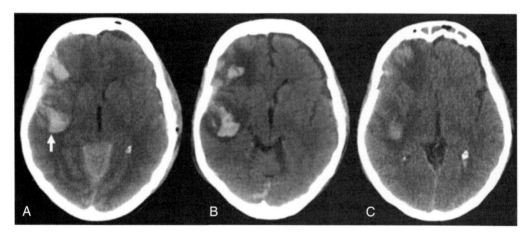

Fig. 6.2 Cerebral contusion axial unenhanced computed tomographic images showing a reduction in the density of acute hemorrhage within cerebral contusions. (A) Day 1; (B) day 5; (C) day 10. (From Adams A, Dixon AK, Gillard JH, Schaefer-Prokop C. *Grainger and Allison's Diagnostic Radiology.* 7th ed. 2020.)

initial complaint is headache, but the patient may then slowly develop cognitive difficulty and a hemiparesis and occasionally seizures. Small subdural hematomas may have very few symptoms.

Traumatic intraparenchymal hemorrhage (Fig. 6.5), due to vascular injury and disruption, portends a poor prognosis. Hematomas with associated brain edema tend to expand over time and a volume of more than 50 mL is associated with a very high mortality. Coagulopathies contribute to hematoma formation and expansion.

Vascular stretching may lead to arterial dissection with disruption in the intimal layer resulting in an intra-mural hematoma that can cause stenosis, limiting blood flow and increasing the risks of embolic infarcts. The cervical internal carotid artery just below the skull base is most often affected.

Diffuse axonal injury is the result of significant rotational acceleration-deceleration forces causing extensive axonal shearing. Hemorrhagic foci are seen in the thalamus, brainstem, internal capsule, corpus callosum, and corona radiata. The diffuse injury is associated with disorders of consciousness, and prognosis for recovery is poor. MRI scan is more sensitive than CT in detecting diffuse axonal injury (Fig. 6.6).

Acute Management

Patients who have suffered a moderate to severe acute TBI may require intubation and mechanical ventilation

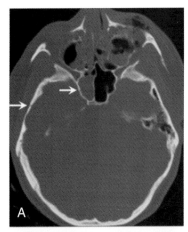

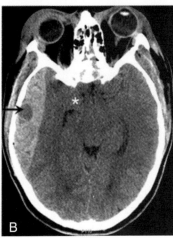

Fig. 6.3 Axial bone window computed tomography indicates a comminuted fracture through the squamosal portion of the right temporal bone. Also, note the extension of the fracture through the lateral wall of the right sphenoid sinus (*arrows*). (B) Corresponding brain window image reveals a large lentiform hyperdense epidural hematoma. Note the central rounded hypodensity, or "swirl sign" (*arrow*) that represents unclotted blood and indicates active extravasation. Also, note the ipsilateral uncal herniation. (From Aiken AH, Gean AD. Imaging of head trauma. *Semin Roentgenol.* 2010;45(2):63–79.)

moderate to severe TBIs should receive an antiepileptic medication for 7 days. There are no data to support treatment for a longer period. Expedited surgical intervention is warranted for epidural and subdural hematomas when there is significant mass effect, and for intraparenchymal hematomas and contusions with a large volume of blood.

Medical interventions to lower intracranial pressure (ICP) should be instituted. Elevation of the head of the bed and hyperosmolar fluids, such as mannitol or hypertonic saline, may be used acutely to reduce intracranial pressure. The use of prophylactic hyperventilation is not recommended as it will cause vasoconstriction and decrease in cerebral blood flow. Studies evaluating therapeutic hypothermia to decrease oxidative stress have revealed mixed results as it effectively reduces intracranial pressure but does not improve outcomes. Glucocorticoids are not recommended and a large study comparing the use of steroids within 8 hours of presentation to placebo revealed that mortality was higher in the group that received the steroid. Patients may be placed in a medically induced coma to reduce the metabolic demand in the brain. Prophylactic use of phenobarbital is not recommended as it has not been shown to influence functional outcome or mortality and will induce systemic hypotension and lead to a more prolonged stay in the intensive care unit. There are some data that support the use of the antifibrinolytic agent, tranexamic acid, in reducing mortality and death when administered within 3 hours after the severe traumatic brain injury but a systematic review and meta-analysis on the efficacy and safety of the drug found no statistically significant difference between patients treated with tranexamic and placebo for mortality, long-term outcome, or risk of adverse events.

An intracranial pressure monitoring device may be placed after the patient is stabilized to reduce early mortality as both cytotoxic and vasogenic edema causing cerebral hypoperfusion may result in death. The intracranial compartment comprises brain parenchyma (83%), cerebrospinal fluid (CSF) (11%), and arterial and venous blood (6%). The structures create a transcortical pressure gradient referred to as intracranial pressure. The homeostatic environment is dependent on each of these contents. An increase in intracranial volume in the traumatized brain due to blood, edema, and venous congestion may result in pathological compression of the brain. ICP may be effectively lowered by CSF drainage.

to protect airways. Cardiac arrest may occur. A head CT must be performed as soon as possible to define the intracranial pathology and neurosurgery should be consulted. The cervical spine must be immobilized, and a cervical CT performed to evaluate for fracture or subluxation. The occurrence of early posttraumatic seizures significantly increases the risk of developing posttraumatic epilepsy and to reduce the risk all patients with

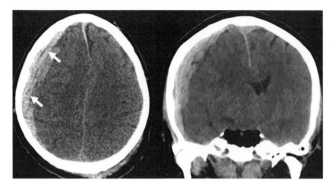

Fig. 6.4 Computed tomographic axial and coronal images of an acute subdural hematoma (*arrows*) overlying the right cerebral convexity. The classical crescentic appearance of a subdural hemorrhage is shown with the hemorrhage extending over the cerebrum limited medially by the falx. There is subfalcine herniation. (From Adams A, Dixon AK, Gillard JH, Schaefer-Prokop C. *Grainger and Allison's Diagnostic Radiology*. 7th ed. 2020.)

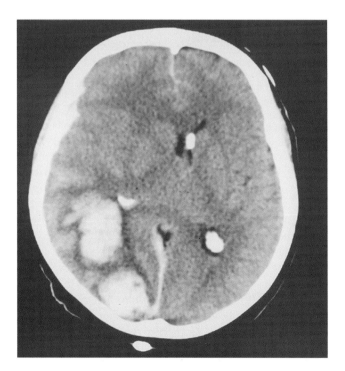

Fig. 6.5 Non–contrast-enhanced computed tomographic scan of right occipital and temporal intracerebral hematomas, surrounded by mild edema and hemorrhagic contusion. A small, interhemispheric, subdural hematoma is visible in the posterior interhemispheric fissure. Midline shift is obvious. A ventriculostomy has been placed and is visible as a high-density image within the ventricles. (From Walls R, Hockberger R, Gausche-Hill M, Erickson TB, Wilcox SR. *Rosen's Emergency Medicine: Concepts and Clinical Practice*. 10th ed. 2022.)

Intracranial monitoring for ICP is indicated if the head CT is abnormal and the GCS score after resuscitation is between 3 and 8. If the CT is normal and the GCS score is 3 to 8 it is still indicated with two of the following: the systolic blood pressure is less than 90, motor posturing is observed, and the patient is over 40 years of age. CSF

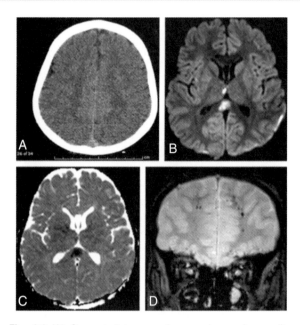

Fig. 6.6 (A) Computed tomography reveals no abnormality. Magnetic resonance imaging images (B) DWI and (C) ADC reveal restricted diffusion in the splenium of the corpus callosum. (D) Coronal T2 GRE depicts multiple hemorrhagic foci at the gray-white junction of the corpus callosum. *ADC*, Apparent diffusion coefficient; *DWI*, diffusion-weighted image; *GRE*, gradient echo. (From Altmeyer W, Steven A, Gutierrez J. Use of magnetic resonance in the evaluation of cranial trauma. *Magn Reson Imaging Clin N Am.* 2016;24(2):305–323.)

drainage using the external ventricular drain will effectively reduce pressure but carries the risks of infection and hemorrhage. Refractory elevation of the intracranial pressure may require a decompressive craniectomy.

Immediate and Delayed Complications

There are several complications that may occur in the acute setting including a coagulopathy, most significantly in patients who are on an anticoagulant. Immediate reversal must be administered with either fresh frozen plasma or prothrombin complex concentrates. No mortality benefit has been shown with the use of platelet transfusions for patients on antiplatelet therapy.

Thrombosis of venous sinuses along fracture lines is a common complication and increases the risk of in-hospital mortality. Treatment is difficult as full anticoagulation is contraindicated and there are no data to support the use of antiplatelet therapy or venous thrombosis

prophylaxis. Decompressive craniectomy can be considered if there is rapid clinical deterioration.

Cerebral vasospasm is common following a traumatic subarachnoid hemorrhage resulting in cerebral hypoperfusion and ischemia. The vasospasm begins in the first three days and usually persists for 5 to 10 days. Transcranial doppler may detect vasospasm before the onset of ischemic complications and if suspected then a CT or MR angiogram should be performed. Digital subtraction angiography, however, remains the gold standard. The 1,4-dihydropyridine calcium channel blocker, nimodipine, administered orally or intravenously is the treatment of choice.

In the weeks after the patient has regained consciousness neurobehavioral symptoms may be observed including delusions, agitation, impulsiveness, aggression, and cognitive disturbance. Treatment with propranolol, clonidine, and sertraline has been shown to be efficacious. Amantadine, an N-methyl-D-aspartate receptor antagonist which may protect neurons against glutamate excitotoxicity, has been demonstrated to accelerate functional recovery, improve cognition and reduce aggression. Disruption of the sleep-wake cycle is a common sequela of TBI. Insomnia or hypersomnia may occur due to involvement of the reticular activating system, posterior hypothalamus, and cortical projections. Insomnia is treated with cognitive behavioral therapy and benzodiazepines. Hypersomnia responds to stimulants such as modafinil and methylphenidate.

Approximately 10% of patients who sustain a head injury will suffer a seizure during the first week with 50% occurring in the first 24 hours. The incidence is higher in children and correlates with the severity of the injury. Seizures during the first week are referred to as early seizures. Late seizures are those that occur after 1 week and as the risk of recurrence following a late seizure is 70% one episode is sufficient to make a diagnosis of posttraumatic epilepsy. Eighty percent of initial late seizures occur within 2 years of the injury. Ten percent of patients who are hospitalized with a head injury will suffer a seizure. The cumulative incidence of posttraumatic epilepsy (PTE) in patients who have suffered a severe TBI is 25% at 5 years and 32% at 15 years. Three percent of patients who do not suffer an early seizure will develop PTE, however PTE will develop in 25% who experienced an early seizure. Patients who have suffered a concussion may exhibit convulsive activity characterized by tonic posturing followed by myoclonic jerks of the extremities. These episodes, however, may not be epileptic but rather similar to what is observed in convulsive syncope. The incidence of epilepsy is not increased in patients who have suffered a concussion. Risk factors that increase the risk of posttraumatic epilepsy include subdural hematoma, brain contusion, penetrating head injury, depressed skull fracture, focal neurologic deficits, early posttraumatic seizures, premorbid alcohol use disorder, and severity of the injury. Eighty percent of posttraumatic seizures are generalized and 20% are focal. Treatment is with antiepileptic medication.

Clinical deterioration with ataxia, worsening cognitive function, urinary incontinence, lethargy, and lack of progress with rehabilitation may be observed in patients who develop posttraumatic communicating hydrocephalus. Placement of a ventriculoperitoneal shunt is required.

Neuroendocrine disorders occur commonly in patients who have suffered a severe TBI. Problems include diabetes insipidus, syndrome of inappropriate adrenocorticotropic hormone (SIADH), human growth hormone, and adrenocorticotropic hormone deficiencies. The disorders may impede emerging consciousness and should be promptly treated. Patients who suffer a severe TBI have increased caloric needs and there is evidence to suggest that early enteral feeding can decrease neuroendocrine complications.

Spasticity with impaired motor function may occur with moderate to severe TBI and may be painful and interfere with rehabilitation. Management includes physical therapy, medication including baclofen or tizanidine and Onabotulinum Toxin A injections.

Paroxysms of sympathetic hyperactivity, usually beginning 1 to 2 weeks after the TBI, may occur with symptoms including hypertension, diaphoresis, tachycardia, tachypnea, and hyperthermia. Pharmacologic treatment may include propranolol, clonidine, and bromocriptine.

Posttraumatic agitation and neuropsychiatric disorders including depression, anxiety, psychosis, aggression, and posttraumatic stress disorder should be managed with the assistance of Psychiatry. Some patients will exhibit a pseudobulbar affect with inappropriate outbursts of laughing or crying which may respond to a combination of dextromethorphan and quinidine sulfate.

Long-term rehabilitation of patients who have suffered a severe TBI consists of a multimodal interdisciplinary approach with intensive care provided by physical, occupational, and speech therapy, Psychiatry and Rehabilitation Medicine. A brain MRI is helpful in defining the extent of brain damage. Behavioral and environmental strategies are extremely important. Patients who receive intensive inpatient rehabilitation demonstrate earlier gains in independence.

CONCUSSION

Concussion has been recognized as a clinical entity for more than 1000 years. Throughout the 20th century it was studied extensively in boxers but did not pique the interest of the general population, as it is the ultimate goal of a boxer to inflict a concussion on their opponent. In 2005 Dr. Bennet Omalu, a neuropathologist, published a report of a postmortem examination which he had performed on a former football player. Mike Webster played the position of center for the Pittsburgh Steelers and competed in 245 games from 1974 until his retirement in 1991. He died from a myocardial infarction in 2002 at the age of 50 and his family reported that he had exhibited behavioral issues and cognitive difficulty in the 10 years prior to his death. The autopsy revealed amyloid plaques, neurofibrillary tangles, and tau deposits in the neocortical areas interpreted as consistent with chronic traumatic encephalopathy. The documented presence of a neurodegenerative disorder, presumably due to multiple concussions sustained over a long career, raised the level of appreciation of the gravity of the cumulative effect of repetitive mild head injuries that had previously been minimized and often been described as "getting your bell rung." Since that time concussion has been a frequent topic of conversation and has become a major focus of sports programs in communities and schools at all levels. All 50 states and the District of Columbia, and the NCAA have enacted laws and rules to protect the athlete. The National Football League has made significant changes to prevent the occurrence of concussion, immediately recognize athletes who may have suffered a concussion, and properly treat and manage the injured player. It is the responsibility of medical practitioners who care for patients who have suffered a concussion to have a thorough understanding of the disorder, and know how to recognize, manage, and treat the postconcussion symptoms. Additionally, if the injured patient is an athlete, determine when and if they may resume participation in their sport.

It has been estimated that up to 3.8 million sports-related concussions occur in athletes annually, but the exact number is unknown. Despite the NCAA mandatory concussion education program for student athletes, an anonymous survey of a cohort of college athletes from the University of Pennsylvania revealed that 43% had deliberately concealed their symptoms. In another survey of NCAA women's ice hockey athletes, 34.2% of players reported concussion-like symptoms after a head impact and 82.8% continued to play. An astounding 66.8% of the players did not disclose their symptoms. The studies give us an indication of the extent to which underreporting may take place. Given the magnitude of the problem, which has reached epidemic proportions, and the possibility of long-term neurologic sequelae, it is essential that we are able to diagnose concussion, provide effective treatment, and prevent recurrent episodes.

DEFINITION OF CONCUSSION

The term "concussion" comes from Latin *concussus* which means "to shake violently." While the first recorded description of concussion has been attributed to Hippocrates approximately 2400 years ago, it was not until the 10th century AD that the great Persian physician, Rhazes, made the distinction between concussion as an abnormal physiologic state as opposed to a brain injury. A European physician, Lanfrancus, in the 13th century described a transient paralysis of cerebral function secondary to head trauma from which patients would completely recover and referred to it as "commotio cerebri" in contrast to "contusio cerebri" which implied structural brain damage.

Concussion is often used interchangeably with mild traumatic brain injury (mTBI); however, it is a descriptive term for the mildest form of mTBI. The WHO and CDC consider a nonpenetrating head injury to be mild if structural imaging is normal, loss of consciousness is less than 30 minutes, posttraumatic amnesia is less than 24 hours, the GCS score is 13 to 15, and altered awareness is less than 24 hours. Most clinicians would argue that if their patient was rendered unconsciousness, for the sake of argument, for 29 minutes the injury would be considered far from mild. With a concussion, more than 90% of patients do not lose consciousness and if it does occur it is for only a short period of time. The anterograde amnesia is less than 30 minutes, and the GCS score is 14 or 15. Some patients may experience a slight sense of confusion for several hours. In 2013 the American

Academy of Neurology (AAN) defined concussion as a "clinical syndrome of biomechanically induced alteration of brain function typically affecting memory and orientation, which may involve loss of consciousness." While this description is accurate it is not particularly helpful for the clinician who is evaluating a patient, attempting to determine if a concussion has occurred. The Zurich Symposium on Concussion in Sport in 2016 placed emphasis on the presence of physical signs and symptoms following the head injury when diagnosing a concussion. From a clinician's standpoint the AAN, in 1997, provided the most useful definition describing concussion as a "trauma induced alteration in mental status that may or may not result in loss of consciousness."

Concussion occurs as a result of direct trauma, rapid acceleration-deceleration of the head such as a "whiplash" injury, or a blast injury commonly seen in military personnel serving in a war zone. In its mildest form, the patient is dazed or "star struck" and may be momentarily confused. Depending on the severity of the injury, loss of consciousness may occur followed by a brief period of amnesia, but loss of consciousness is seen in less than 10% of patients who suffer a concussion. The loss of consciousness is a result of the rotational forces exerted at the junction of the midbrain and thalamus causing a transient disruption of the reticular activating system.

While loss of consciousness does not always correlate with the outcome of a TBI, it does provide incontrovertible evidence that a significant injury has occurred and prolonged loss of consciousness is indicative of a more severe traumatic brain injury rather than a concussion or mTBI. There are some data that suggests that loss of consciousness may accentuate postconcussive cognitive dysfunction. The duration of posttraumatic amnesia, both anterograde (an inability to assimilate new memory) and retrograde (memory of events preceding the injury) may be an indication of the severity of the injury, however, it is often difficult to assess as the patient may recall what was related to them after the event by witnesses, family, friends, teammates, and coaches.

Research has been conducted to determine if blood biomarkers, including astroglial (glial fibrillary acidic protein- GFAP and S-100 calcium-binding protein B) and axonal (tau and ubiquitin *C*-terminal hydrolase-UCH-L1), would provide objective evidence of a concussion. To date they have shown promise in determining the severity of an injury and may predict outcomes but not specifically in identifying who has suffered a concussion.

Due to the confusion regarding the definition of concussion it is even more difficult to arrive at a consensus at to what represents a subconcussive injury. Clinicians who strictly adhere to the WHO definition of mild traumatic brain injury would likely consider a concussion without loss of consciousness or amnesia to be a subconcussive injury. What is commonly identified as a subconcussive injury may represent a concussion with axonal injury and disruption of neuronal integrity but without loss of consciousness or significant postconcussive symptoms. This type of injury can potentially be quite dangerous, especially if it occurs repeatedly in an athlete, as it is usually unrecognized and untreated and may potentially have long-term ramifications.

PATHOPHYSIOLOGY OF CONCUSSION

When trauma induces an alteration in neurologic function, a cascade of neurochemical changes develops over hours, as observed in animal studies. There is a sudden release of excitatory neurotransmitters, particularly glutamate, binding to NMDA receptors, causing the sudden release of potassium into the extracellular space followed by an influx of calcium into cell. This results in a transient hypermetabolic glycolytic state as ATP pumps become hyperactive to restore homeostasis causing depletion of energy stores and hyperglycolysis. The prolonged presence of intracellular calcium disrupts mitochondrial function. Lactate is produced impairing neuronal function and there is a reduction in cerebral blood flow. A diffuse spreading depression occurs and the state of impaired metabolism typically lasts 7 to 10 days in adult animals and during that time behavioral impairments in spatial learning are observed. During the time period of the altered metabolic state neural tissue is more vulnerable to repeated injury. Diminished blood flow to the brain may persist for days to weeks. Axonal injury occurs but there is generally little cell death, however chronic structural changes may evolve over time (Fig. 6.7). MRI spectroscopy and functional MRI studies in humans following a concussive injury reveal neurometabolic changes that correlate with the animal model, but recovery may occur over a longer period of time in humans.

EVALUATION OF CONCUSSION

Most traumatic brain injuries are mild, and concussion is the mildest form. More than 90% of patients who have suffered a concussion do not lose consciousness and when it occurs it is brief, lasting usually no more than 30 seconds, and posttraumatic amnesia is less than 30 minutes. The neurologic exam does not reveal focal abnormalities and the GCS score is 14 to 15. Guidelines for performing an imaging study of the brain are discussed in the previous section. Conventional neuroimaging of the brain with CT and MRI scans usually contributes little to the evaluation of concussion as routine imaging does not detect microscopic axonal injury. Diffusion tensor imaging, however, is an MRI technique that assesses white matter microstructural integrity and has been shown to detect white matter injuries in mTBI but whether the findings are clinically useful remains controversial.

When a patient is evaluated in a hospital emergency room and diagnosed with a mild traumatic brain injury they are usually observed for a few hours. If their exam is normal, and there are no worrisome symptoms, they are discharged to home to the care of a responsible party with a written list of instructions including symptoms that would warrant a reevaluation at the hospital. After a thorough evaluation has been performed there are no data to support waking the patient up at regular intervals during the night.

POSTCONCUSSION SYNDROME

Postconcussion syndrome describes a constellation of symptoms that occur after suffering a concussion (Box 6.2). Headache is the most common postconcussive symptom followed by dizziness which is more a sense of disequilibrium and imbalance than objective vertigo. Patients may also report orthostatic lightheadedness indicating mild autonomic dysfunction. A sense of mental "fogginess" is usually noted with word finding difficulty and mild problems with short-term memory and concentration. Reaction time is often slow. Nausea may be present in the first few days but usually quickly disappears. Emotional lability is not uncommon and other symptoms include photophobia, phonophobia, tinnitus, fatigue, and irritability. Initially patients experience hypersomnia but if symptoms persist, they usually develop insomnia. Patients report difficulty focusing with their vision and specifically problems with visual tracking. If symptoms persist, anxiety and depression may develop and patients with a history of an underlying mood disorder may experience a worsening of symptoms.

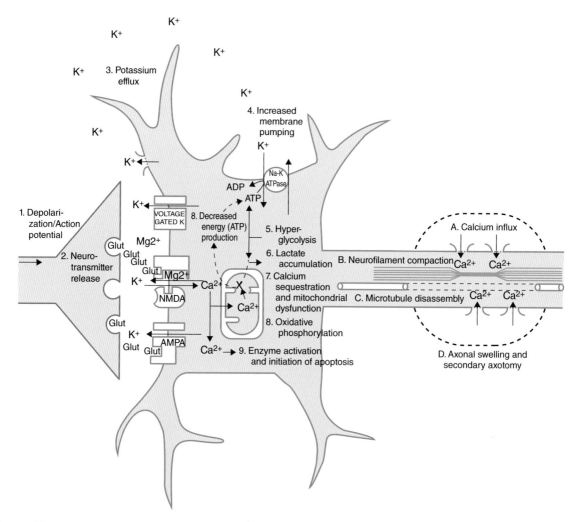

Fig. 6.7 Metabolic cascade in nerve cells following traumatic injury. (1) Changes in ion fluxes. (2) Release of glutamate. (3) Considerable efflux of potassium. (4) Increase activity of membrane pumps to restore homeostasis of ions. (5) Increase in glycolysis to generate energy in the form of ATP. (6) Lactate accumulation as a result of glycolysis. (7) Increased Ca2þ in mitochondria leading to impaired oxidative metabolism. (8) Decreased energy (ATP). (9) Activation of the enzyme calpain and initiation of programed cell death. (A) Damage of neuron cell. (B) Neurofilament damage. (C) Impaired neuronal transport. (D) Axon swelling. *Kþ*, potassium, *Naþ*, sodium, *Mg2þ*, magnesium, *Ca2þ*, calcium, NMDA, *N*-methyl-ᴅ-aspartate. (From Giza CC, Hovda DA. The new neurometabolic cascade of concussion. *Neurosurgery.* 2014;75 Suppl 4(0 4):S24–33.)

Most research suggests that the incidence of concussion is higher in females than males possibly due to anatomical differences, or the fact that migraine which is a risk factor for concussion is more common in females. A patient who has suffered a concussion has a significantly greater chance of suffering a subsequent concussion. Almost every patient who has sustained a concussion will experience transient postconcussion symptoms and it is the duration that is quite variable. Headaches have been reported to occur in 25% to 90% of patients and in 15% to 78% they are still present at 3 months. Twenty percent of patients continue to report headaches at 3 years. In the pediatric population, the prevalence of chronic posttraumatic headache is much lower at 7.6%. It is interesting that chronic headaches are more commonly seen following a mTBI as opposed

BOX 6.2 Postconcussion Syndrome

Somatic
Headache
Dizziness with a sense of disequilibrium and imbalance
Nausea
Photophobia
Phonophobia
Tinnitus
Difficulty with visual focusing and tracking
Anosmia
Postural lightheadedness
Fatigue

Cognitive
Mental "fogginess" with memory and word finding difficulty, and problems concentrating

Behavioral
Mood lability
Irritability
Hypersomnia/insomnia
Anxiety
Depression
Personality changes

to a severe brain injury. In 20% of patients who have suffered a concussion, the symptoms of postconcussion syndrome persist for years and do not respond to treatment. In addition, there are patients who despite resolution of most of their symptoms continue to experience photophobia or tinnitus.

In athletes the statistics are very different and postconcussion symptoms resolve in 2 to 3 weeks in 80 to 90%, although athletes 14 and younger may have a more prolonged course. Patients who have a high symptom burden immediately after suffering a head injury are more likely to experience persistent symptoms. It is not uncommon for patients who have recovered from a concussion to experience recurrent postconcussive symptoms without sustaining an actual concussion after suffering a very mild blow to the head. The symptoms usually last from a few days to 1 to 2 weeks.

The reason for the variable statistics regarding the persistence of postconcussive symptoms is that the populations studied are not uniform and we must consider the effects of psychosocial problems, psychiatric disorders, and pending litigation. Symptoms of postconcussion syndrome are also not unique to that disorder and may be seen in conditions such as chronic migraine. In a study of a cohort of patients in Lithuania where significant monetary compensation for injuries does not exist, Harald Schrader sent questionnaires about symptoms of PCS to subjects who had suffered a concussion with loss of consciousness and to a sex- and age-matched control group who had suffered a mild nonhead injury. At 3 and 12 months the prevalence of headache in both groups was no different. In a cross-sectional study by Philip Dean comparing subjects with an mTBI to those without a head injury, symptoms of persistent postconcussion syndrome were present in 31% of those who had suffered an mTBI and 34% of those who did not suffer a head injury. Chronic PCS has been a controversial topic since a financial compensation system was established for accident-related injuries on the Prussian railway system in the second half of the 19th century. Factors that may contribute to the chronicity of the symptoms include comorbid psychiatric disorders, a history of prior TBI, a history of migraine, litigation, and compensation. Attention deficit hyperactivity and learning disorders are risk factors for a more prolonged and more symptomatic recovery from concussion.

Military personnel deployed in war zones are at risk for mTBI, predominantly due to blast injuries, and approximately 20% of soldiers will suffer a mTBI during their tour of duty. Headache is the most common symptom and prevents more than 80% from returning to the combat theater.

While the phenotype of posttraumatic headache may resemble many of the primary headache disorders, most of the headaches meet the ICHD-3 criteria for migraine. Cervicogenic headache may occur when there is also an injury to the neck, and trauma to the skull may directly injure the occipital, supraorbital, or infraorbital nerves resulting in a neuralgic pain syndrome.

By ICHD-3 criteria, an acute headache attributed to traumatic injury to the head must present within 7 days of the injury as this will result in a higher specificity regarding the diagnosis. Updating criteria to recognize a more delayed onset in the weeks following the injury is being considered and in one study of military personnel only 37% of soldiers who had suffered a concussion reported a headache in the 7-day window. Headaches that continue for more than 3 months following the injury are officially referred to as persistent headache attributed to traumatic injury to the head rather than chronic posttraumatic headache. (Box 6.3)

BOX 6.3   ICHD-3 Headache Attributed to Head and/or Neck Trauma

1. Acute headache attributed to traumatic injury to the head (moderate or severe; mild)
   Persistent headache attributed to traumatic brain injury (moderate or severe; mild)
2. Acute headache attributed to whiplash
   Persistent headache attributed to whiplash
3. Acute headache attributed to craniotomy
   Persistent headache attributed to craniotomy

BOX 6.4   24-Hour Step: Return to Play Protocol

1. Light aerobic exercise
2. Sports specific exercise
3. Noncontact training drills
4. Full contact practice
5. Return to play

Posttraumatic headaches represent 4% of all headaches. Medication overuse with rebound must always be considered as a potential cause of chronic headaches.

CONCUSSION IN SPORTS

Forty-four million children and 170 million adults in the United States participate in sports-related activities. There are approximately 1.7 to 3.8 million sports-related concussions each year. In males the injury rate in student athletes is highest in football followed by hockey, lacrosse, wrestling, and soccer. In females the injury rate is highest in soccer followed by lacrosse, field hockey, and basketball. Five percent of student athletes will suffer a concussion and 20% of those who participate in contact sports. Fifteen percent of all sports injuries are concussions. Most participants in boxing and the martial arts will suffer a concussion at some point while participating in these sports.

Player to player contact is the most common cause of concussion and as many as 25% are the result of a prohibited activity. Soccer is the most popular sport worldwide and there is increasing concern about the cumulative effects of intentional heading. The ball is kicked at high velocity and players frequently report headache and a sense of imbalance after heading, suggesting a mild concussion, and may be the best example of a subconcussive injury. Consensus is building that athletes under the age of 13 should not head the ball. In football, the risk of concussion is higher on kickoffs when compared to plays from the line of scrimmage. As a result the NFL continues to make changes in the kickoff to reduce the risk of injury. Contrary to earlier reports, a recent systematic review and meta-analysis demonstrated a decrease incidence of head injury and concussion when contact sports are played on artificial turf. Athletes who have a history of a prior concussion are more likely to suffer another concussion and should be managed more conservatively. Research suggests that female athletes may be at more a risk for suffering a concussion. Young athletes are also more susceptible to concussion and have a more prolonged period of recovery. To reduce the number of concussions athletes are being taught new techniques to reduce the risk of direct head trauma. Contact drills in practice are being limited and many youth football programs are trending away from full contact in the younger athletes.

When a concussion is suspected the athlete must be immediately removed from play and evaluated by a licensed medical professional. A neurologic examination, including cognitive and balance testing, should be performed. Standardized tests, such as the Sports Concussion Assessment Tool 5 (SCAT 5) and Balance Error Scoring System (BESS), may be useful, but the reliability, validity, specificity, and sensitivity remain undefined without an individual baseline. If the athlete is diagnosed with a concussion, they cannot return to play on the same day and should be managed by a health care practitioner with expertise in the treatment of concussion. Athletes should be free of symptoms or back to their baseline before they are cleared to begin the five-step return to play (RTP) protocol (Box 6.4). Data suggest that the neurometabolic abnormalities of a concussion persist for at least 7 to 10 days and possibly longer, in younger athletes. While the asymptomatic athlete may begin the RTP protocol they should not be subjected to contact until they are 10 to 14 days post injury at the minimum, and for the athletes 14 and younger it may be as long as 4 weeks. Each step of the RTP protocol is 24 hours and athletes may only advance if they remain asymptomatic through each step. If they develop symptoms, they must return to the previous step. Case studies of catastrophic brain swelling, and death have been reported in, usually young, athletes who have suffered a second brain injury while still symptomatic from the first injury. This is referred to as second impact syndrome.

Neurocognitive testing, such as the computerized Immediate Post Concussion Assessment and Cognitive Testing (ImPACT), can be useful in assessing cognitive function in an athlete who has suffered a concussion. ImPACT tests verbal memory, visual memory, reaction time, processing speed, and impulse control. The testing is only helpful when it can be compared to a baseline test completed by the athlete before the injury occurred and it is not as reliable in athletes 14 and under. The testing is only another parameter to assist in the clinical management of the injured athlete. A diagnosis and recommendations cannot be made based solely on the results.

There are several grading systems that were developed to assist in the RTP decision process. The American Academy of Neurology recommends that each athlete who has suffered a concussion be assessed and managed individually without relying on a grading system with immutable RTP guidelines. Except for severe brain injuries, grading systems are arbitrary as there are no good prospective randomized controlled trials regarding the assessment and management of different grades of brain injury in sports. Clinical decisions are made based on consensus statements, retrospective data, limited prospective data, experimental models, and personal experience. Clinical guidelines should not preempt the judgment of the medical professional and should be only used as an adjunct when determining whether to release an athlete to full participation in their sport. The type of sport and the risk of recurrent head injury should factor into that decision.

The use of protective equipment does not reduce the risk of concussion. Helmets, headgear, and mouth guards may prevent lacerations, soft tissue trauma, and serious head, face, and oral injuries but do not protect against concussion.

The decision to retire from a sport because of repeated concussions is difficult and requires input from the athlete, health care providers, and family. The risk and benefits of continued participation in the sport must be considered and there is no clear evidence regarding the number of concussions to guide the decision. A discussion should begin after 3 to 4 concussions and the time interval between the episodes must be considered. With the more serious injuries the decision is much easier. Athletes who have suffered trauma-related structural brain injuries, have an abnormal neurologic examination, or persistent deficits on neuropsychological testing should not return to contact sports.

MANAGEMENT OF POSTCONCUSSION SYNDROME

The traditional management of concussion mandated complete physical and cognitive rest. Television, telephone, reading, texting, and video games were to be assiduously avoided and patients were told that all exercise including exertion with activities of daily living could be potentially harmful and delay recovery. Studies, however, have shown that early physical activity is beneficial and is associated with lower rates of persistent postconcussive symptoms. Patients should be encouraged to begin light exercise 1 to 2 days following the injury then gradually increase their level of exercise as tolerated. In athletes, more time spent in moderate and vigorous exercise early in recovery may bring about a more rapid resolution of symptoms. Exercise should be introduced below the threshold of symptoms then increased as tolerated. Controlled aerobic exercise may help restore cerebral blood flow regulation to normal. Regarding cognitive rest, the data indicate that maintaining full cognitive activity after a concussion will more than double the time to recovery. What is interesting is that continuing with moderate cognitive activity is equivalent to complete cognitive rest in reducing the postconcussive symptoms. In a study that looked at early return to school following a concussion, students aged 8 to 18 who returned to school in 2 days or fewer had a lower symptom burden at 14 days suggesting that prolonged absences from school may be detrimental to recovery.

For 3 to 5 days following a concussion patients should scale down their cognitive activity then increase as tolerated. Students should be encouraged to return to school within 2 days. Special accommodations should be made for the students including more time to complete assignments, prepare for tests, and take tests. Standardized tests must be avoided during the recovery period. When reading or working on a computer the patient should take scheduled breaks every 45 to 60 minutes and eyeglasses that filter blue light may help with the photophobia.

Unfortunately, there is a paucity of evidence from randomized controlled trials to assist the clinician in the treatment of the symptoms of postconcussion syndrome. For posttraumatic headaches, simple analgesics including nonsteroidal antiinflammatory drugs (NSAIDS) and acetaminophen are the first-line treatment, although the

NSAIDS should not be used in the first 24 hours because of the risk of bleeding. If they are not effective then the triptans or oral calcitonin gene-related peptide (CGRP) antagonists can be used for headaches with the phenotype of migraine. Metoclopramide and prochlorperazine are options both for the headaches and nausea. Narcotic analgesic agents and butalbital compound should be avoided. Care should be taken to avoid rebound and the development of medication overuse headache. For headaches that occur frequently more than 2 weeks following the concussion, a preventative medication should be considered. A tricyclic antidepressant medication (TCA), such as nortriptyline or amitriptyline, in low doses prior to bed may be effective both for the headaches and insomnia. If the headaches do not respond to the TCA alone, then a low dose of propranolol can be added but the beta blocker can potentially aggravate underlying depression and cannot be used if there is a history of asthma. Topiramate can be considered if the TCA does not help and there are data that indicate that it may be more effective than amitriptyline. Topiramate, however, may aggravate the feeling of mental fogginess. For persistent posttraumatic headaches with the phenotype of migraine that do not respond to a TCA, beta blocker or topiramate, or if the medicines are contraindicated or not tolerated, the oral CGRP antagonists, gepants, or the monoclonal CGRP antagonists that are administered monthly by subcutaneous injection, could be considered. Onabotulinum Toxin A injections are an option for refractory headaches that have the phenotype of chronic migraine, and there are data suggesting that the injections are effective in the treatment of persistent posttraumatic headaches. A randomized placebo-controlled trial did not find Onabotulinum Toxin A injections to be effective in the treatment of cervicogenic headache, however.

Spinal manipulative therapy for cervicogenic headaches may provide short-term benefits for pain intensity, frequency, and disability. The long-term impact is not significant, however. There are data that suggest that it may be somewhat effective in the treatment of migraine by reducing pain intensity and frequency. Cervical physical therapy may be of benefit for cervicogenic headache, posttraumatic headaches with the phenotype of tension-type headache and possibly migraine as well, but consistent evidence supporting benefit in migraine is lacking. Acupuncture has proved to be effective in the treatment of migraine and tension-type headache and is a viable nonpharmacologic option in the treatment of persistent posttraumatic headaches. Anesthetic nerve blocks can be administered for the neuralgic pain syndromes and there is some evidence suggesting efficacy in the treatment of cluster, migraine, tension-type, and cervicogenic headaches in both adult and pediatric patients. Medication options for neuralgic pain include TCAs, gabapentin, pregabalin, and duloxetine.

There are conflicting data regarding the use of cognitive behavioral therapy for the treatment of posttraumatic headaches and postconcussion syndrome. It was demonstrated to be effective for posttraumatic headache in an open-label study of 20 patients, but not effective in a randomized, controlled trial of 90 patients. A systematic review and meta-analysis of randomized controlled trials for the treatment of postconcussion syndrome did not find it to be effective in reducing the severity of symptoms but it appeared to promote improvement in depression, anxiety, and social integration.

There are some reports suggesting that the use of hyperbaric oxygen therapy for persistent postconcussion syndrome may improve cognitive function, depression, and anxiety. A systematic review, however, revealed it to be no better than sham treatment.

The constant sense of imbalance and disequilibrium that occurs following a concussion is a result of injury to vestibular structures, and the presence of dizziness may portend a longer recovery time. Patients often experience problems tracking with their vision and impaired convergence. If the symptoms persist for more than 2 weeks vestibular ocular rehabilitation therapy should be initiated. Meclizine is only mildly effective for the dizziness as a vestibular depressant and will cause a sense of lethargy.

For cognitive symptoms that persist for more than 1 month, cognitive rehabilitation therapy with a speech therapist may be helpful. If symptoms do not improve patients will require a neuropsychological evaluation. Persistent symptoms that are the result of underlying anxiety and depression should be managed by a behavioral medicine practitioner.

Research has been conducted to determine if nutritional supplements and vitamins, including omega-3 fatty acids, vitamins, melatonin, creatine, curcumin, and resveratrol, are effective in the prevention and treatment of concussion. To date, however, there is no convincing evidence in human studies that prove that they are of benefit.

CHRONIC TRAUMATIC ENCEPHALOPATHY

In 1928 Harrison Martland, a forensic pathologist in New Jersey, published the paper "Punch Drunk" which described a progressive neurologic syndrome characterized by ataxia, cognitive difficulty, dysarthria, tremor, and physical slowing in boxers. Postmortem examination of the brain of one afflicted boxer revealed perivascular microhemorrhages, gliosis, atrophy, and enlarged ventricles. In 1937 Millspaugh used the term dementia pugilistica to describe the syndrome. In 1949 MacDonald Critchley published the paper, Punch Drunk Syndromes: The Chronic Traumatic Encephalopathy in Boxers. In 2005 Bennet Omalu reported a tauopathy in the brain of a football player, Mike Webster, which he diagnosed as chronic traumatic encephalopathy (CTE). Until that time most studies focused on boxers. After Omalu's paper, Ann McKee et al. published multiple papers demonstrating pathologic changes on the postmortem examination of football players, boxers, and military veterans with a history of repetitive concussions consistent with a progressive tauopathy. The abnormalities were ascribed to CTE but in their 2013 analysis of 85 subjects (including athletes and military veterans), 65 with evidence of CTE, 37% had comorbid pathology consistent with Alzheimer's disease, frontotemporal dementia, motor neuron disease, or Lewy Body disease. In their 2017 paper CTE was diagnosed in 87% of 202 football players across all levels, and in 110 of 111 (99%) former National Football League players. A comorbid neurodegenerative disease was detected in 47% of the cases with severe CTE. In these case studies the vast majority of patient were symptomatic with behavioral or cognitive symptoms. While the findings revealed important clinical implications, they in no way reveal the incidence or prevalence of the disorder.

The pathologic findings of CTE have been divided into four stages based on a consensus of a panel of neuropathologists. The abnormalities become more pronounced with each stage and are characterized histologically by hyperphosphorylated tau in neurofibrillary tangles and astrocytic tangles deposited around small blood vessels in sulcal depths of the cerebral cortex. Unlike Alzheimer disease where there is extensive beta-amyloid deposition, amyloid is present in only 52% of CTE case. Macroscopically there is diffuse atrophy, enlarged ventricles, fenestrated cavum septum pellucidum, and pallor of the substantia nigra and locus coeruleus. The findings are directly attributed to repetitive mild head trauma.

CTE is a pathologic diagnosis and the clinical disorder that is now associated with the neuropathologic changes is referred to as traumatic encephalopathy syndrome (TES). TES begins years after repetitive concussions, is progressive for more than 2 years, and is characterized by behavioral changes (change in personality, violence, suicide), emotional dysregulation (depression, anxiety, paranoid ideation), cognitive impairment (short-term memory, executive function), and motor disturbance (ataxia, bradykinesia, tremor, dysarthria, rigidity).

The incidence of CTE in the at-risk population and the general population is unknown. There are data regarding the risk of developing a neurodegenerative disease in patients who have suffered a TBI. A study published by the National Institute for Occupational Safety revealed that NFL players may be at higher risk for developing a neurodegenerative disorder. Data from the studies on aging (Religious Orders, Memory and Aging Project, Adult Changes in Thought) revealed that a single TBI with loss of consciousness did not increase the risk of developing dementia although it slightly increased the risk of Parkinson's disease. A meta-analysis assessing the risk of dementia in military personnel who had suffered a TBI revealed an increased risk of dementia by a factor of 2 to 1. In a study of the records of 7676 former male professional soccer players in Scotland between 1900 and 1977 a neurodegenerative disorder was diagnosed in 5% of the soccer athletes compared to 1.6% in a matched population control group. The risk was highest among players with a career longer than 15 years and with those in defense positions where there is a higher frequency of heading. The lowest frequency was among goalkeepers. A 1969 book by Anthony Roberts examined the prevalence of traumatic encephalopathy in retired boxers. Eleven percent suffered from mild traumatic encephalopathy and 6% had severe disease. In a neuropathological study of deceased military personnel who had suffered a blast injury, 3 of 45 had evidence of CTE compared to 7 of 180 brains from those without a history of blast exposure. All ten who were diagnosed with CTE had participated in contact sports. Notably, 50% of those determined to have CTE had only a single pathognomic lesion. The risk of neurodegenerative disease in elite male soccer players in Sweden was assessed and compared to ten controls from the general population. Nearly 9% of soccer players and 6.2% of controls were diagnosed with a neurodegenerative disorder. The incidence of Alzheimer's disease and other dementias was higher in the soccer players, while the incidence of Parkinson's disease was lower. Group differences were not observed for motor neuron disease.

While studies have revealed an increased risk of developing a neurodegenerative disorder from one or multiple mild TBIs the numbers do not approach what has been implied by the published case studies that focused on retired NFL players.

Epidemiologic studies are currently being conducted to ascertain the frequency of CTE in professional NFL players and to determine the contributing factors that place the athletes at higher risk. Is it the number of concussions that potentially causes CTE or is it the fact that athletes are not given sufficient time to recover? In a study that looked at repeated concussive injuries in adult mice, worsening neurocognitive function and traumatic axonal injury was observed when injuries were spaced out by 3 to 5 days but not when the injuries were separated by 7 days. If a second injury occurred during the period of impaired glucose metabolism from the initial injury, the severity of hypometabolism and memory impairment was greater. If a second injury occurred after there was full metabolic recovery from the first injury, the mice behaved like they had sustained a single injury without the accentuated impairment. Perhaps we should allow athletes more time to recover and not be cleared to return to play for several weeks or longer. There is the possibility that some individuals may be more susceptible. Recent data suggest that individuals who carry the APOE4 gene have a higher risk of developing CTE. Depressive symptoms in younger retired NFL players are slightly higher than in the general population of men of the same age and race, and depression in young people is a risk factor for developing dementia later in life. Suicide has been widely cited as being associated with CTE but the risk of suicide in former NFL players is lower than in men in the general population. Former NFL athletes often suffer from chronic pain and substance abuse is not uncommon. There is a definite link between both chronic pain and substance abuse and depression but there is no evidence that would support the premise that opioid use is a risk factor for dementia.

Multiple concussions have been implicated as a potential cause of amyotrophic lateral sclerosis (ALS) as a TDP 43 proteinopathy is common to both CTE and ALS with deposition in the brain and spinal cord in both disorders. The incidence of ALS has been found to be higher in former NFL players but there is no compelling evidence linking it to multiple concussions. A higher risk of ALS has also been noted in long-distance cross-country skiers where there is no history of head injuries. The incidence of ALS is increased in physically active people in general. The tau pathology and TDP 43 proteinopathy seen in CTE is evident in ALS cases regardless of whether they have suffered a head injury and patients with ALS who suffer a head injury do not experience a more rapid decline in function.

CONCLUSION

Concussion has become a major health care concern and the number of people who suffer this type of injury has steadily risen. More than 50% of our population participates in sports or recreational activities and there are many unanswered questions. Hopefully prospective studies will furnish us with answers in the future not only to improve our clinical management of our patients but also help us to provide proper advice about how to avoid further injury and when to safely resume participation in their sport or recreational activity. The possibility of developing a progressive neurodegenerative disorder from repetitive concussions must be respected and will factor into the recommendations that we make to our patients.

"For the full bibliography list, please use the pincode on the inside front cover to access the electronic version of the text at ebooks.health.elsevier.com."

7

Encephalopathy*

Michael Erkkinen, William J. Mullally, and Aaron L. Berkowitz

INTRODUCTION

Encephalopathy is commonly encountered in inpatients and outpatients and has a broad and complex differential diagnosis including both primary neurologic and systemic causes. The term derived from the Greek *en-cephalo* (in the brain) and *pathos* (suffering) refers to a set of dysfunctional brain states associated with varying degrees of arousal/wakefulness, attention (and other aspects of other cognition and perception), and emotional/limbic processing. The presentation varies considerably in symptomatology and severity, and it has myriad underlying causes. Precise clinical characterization via a careful history, examination, laboratory testing, imaging, and other ancillary studies can narrow the differential diagnosis.

There are several related terms. Delirium is a type of encephalopathy characterized by fluctuating attention and arousal and is often associated with systemic conditions (i.e., toxic, metabolic, and infectious) rather than primary structural neurologic causes. An acute confusional state overlaps with encephalopathy and is preferred when describing cognitive-behavioral syndromes that spare arousal, attention, and limbic functioning, such as transient global amnesia (TGA), receptive aphasia, cortical blindness, or abulia.

Encephalopathy can present with a wide range of symptoms and severity, from subtle, intermittent confusion, fatigue, and irritability to lethargy, florid multimodal hallucinations, paranoid delusions, aggression, and others. It emerges with disruption, disorganization, and/or dyscoordination within and across functional neural networks supporting attention, arousal, awareness, and emotion. An encephalopathic patient manifests an altered mental status characterized by inattentiveness, disorientation, short-term memory impairment, and often an abnormal state of arousal. Neurologic dysfunction, as occurs in systemic conditions, is the most common precipitant, although focal or multifocal primary central nervous system (CNS) injury can also manifest as encephalopathy. The underlying mechanisms are complex and likely multifactorial.

A diagnosis of the syndrome of encephalopathy is made entirely from the history and neurologic exam; the history often requires input from a reliable informant given the compromised cognitive functioning. Encephalopathy must be distinguished from psychosis which may include delusions, paranoia, hallucinations, and abnormalities of arousal but with orientation and memory function intact. Determining the underlying cause of encephalopathy usually requires additional clinical data, including laboratory studies, neuroimaging (e.g., computed tomography [CT] and magnetic resonance imaging [MRI]), and in some instances additional testing such as electroencephalography and/or spinal fluid analysis.

Encephalopathy has many underlying causes. Categorizing these causes by the pace of onset of symptoms provides a useful clinical framework for narrowing this complex set of underlying etiologies. We present the differential diagnosis of encephalopathy at four different timescales: *hyperacute/sudden* (i.e., seconds to minutes), *acute* (i.e., hours to days), *subacute* (i.e., weeks to months),

*Based on article—Erkkinen MG, Berkowitz AL. A clinical approach to diagnosing encephalopathy. *Am J Med.* 2019; 132(10):1142–1147. ISSN 0002-9343. https://doi.org/10.1016/j.amjmed.2019.07.001.

and *chronic* (i.e., months to years). This chapter emphasizes primary neurologic causes, although systemic medical conditions may be more common, including infection, metabolic disturbances, inflammatory disease, anemia, end-organ dysfunction (e.g., renal, hepatic, cardiac, and respiratory), medication (and other drug) toxicity, and others. Encephalopathy is often multifactorial in origin, with both precipitating factors (e.g., infection, metabolic derangement, and stroke) and predisposing vulnerabilities (e.g., prior neurologic conditions and advanced age).

Categories of primary neurologic disease to consider for each time course are summarized in Table 7.1: hyperacute-onset encephalopathy should lead to consideration of cerebrovascular disease, seizure, trauma, or migraine; acute-onset encephalopathy should lead to consideration of neurologic infection (bacterial or viral meningitis or encephalitis) or acute demyelination (e.g., acute disseminated encephalomyelitis [ADEM] or flare of multiple sclerosis [MS]); subacute-onset encephalopathy should lead to consideration of neoplasia (primary brain neoplasm or metastasis), autoimmune conditions (such as antibody-mediated limbic encephalitis) and infections (fungal or tuberculous meningitis); chronic-onset encephalopathy should lead to consideration of neurodegenerative conditions (i.e. dementia). Toxic and metabolic insults can cause encephalopathy over any time course, depending on the toxin/metabolite and time course of its aberration.

HYPERACUTE CAUSES OF ENCEPHALOPATHY—ONSET WITHIN SECONDS TO MINUTES

Primary Neurologic Conditions

Intracranial Hemorrhage

Intracranial hemorrhage is categorized by the compartment where the bleeding occurs, including the brain parenchyma (e.g., intraparenchymal or intracerebral) and the subarachnoid, subdural, or epidural spaces. Encephalopathy can accompany acute hemorrhage into any of the intracranial compartments and is often associated with headache and/or focal neurologic deficits. This diagnosis is suspected clinically but made definitively by CT. An acute intracranial hemorrhage is a neurologic emergency given the potential for rapid elevations in intracranial pressure and cerebral herniation due to expansion of the blood, especially those under arterial pressure (e.g., aneurysmal subarachnoid hemorrhage and epidural hematoma).

Subarachnoid hemorrhage, particularly when caused by rupture of a cerebral artery aneurysm, is often

TABLE 7.1   Selected Causes of Encephalopathy by Time Course

	Hyperacute	Acute	Subacute	Chronic
Primary neurologic	• Vascular (IS, ICH) • Seizure • Migraine • Trauma	• Vascular (SDH) • Inflammatory (acute demyelination) • Infectious (bacterial/viral meningitis encephalitis)	• Vascular (SDH) • Neoplasm related (brain tumors, paraneoplastic syndromes) • Inflammatory • Infectious (fungal, TB, parasitic, complications of HIV)	• Vascular (SDH) • Degenerative • NPH • Infectious (syphilis, HIV associated neurocognitive disease)
Systemic	• Toxic/metabolic/drug related • Psychiatric			

	• Hypertensive encephalopathy	• Systemic infection	• Chronic systemic conditions:
			  • Heart failure
			  • Endocrinopathy
			  • Malignancy
			  • Autoimmune
			• OSA	

HIV, Human immunodeficiency virus; *ICH*, intracranial hemorrhage, including subarachnoid, subdural, epidural, intraparenchymal; *IS*, ischemic stroke; *NPH*, normal pressure hydrocephalus; *OSA*, obstructive sleep apnea; *SDH*, subdural hematoma; *TB*, tuberculosis.

associated with a sudden, severe headache and can be accompanied by signs of meningeal irritation (e.g., meningismus, photophobia, nausea), seizures, and encephalopathy characterized by a reduced level of arousal. Subarachnoid hemorrhages have many underlying causes, including cerebral aneurysm (e.g., idiopathic and mycotic), head trauma/traumatic brain injury (TBI), vascular malformation, reversible cerebral vasoconstriction syndrome, venous sinus thrombosis, cerebral amyloid angiopathy, and others.

Intraparenchymal hemorrhage typically presents with focal neurologic deficits that correspond to the location of hemorrhage and is often accompanied by headache, nausea, seizures, and hypertension. Encephalopathy can have different characteristics depending on the location and size of the hemorrhage. Wakefulness may be affected by large lesions causing elevations in intracranial pressure and/or smaller focal injuries to arousal centers (e.g., brainstem and thalamus). Cognitive, emotional, and motivational symptoms can develop with focal injury to the networks supporting these functions. The common causes of intraparenchymal hemorrhage include hypertension, cerebral amyloid angiopathy, head trauma, vascular malformation, coagulopathy, brain metastases, venous sinus thrombosis, and ischemic stroke with hemorrhagic transformation.

Epidural and subdural hematoma are almost always associated with head trauma. Epidural hematomas often cause encephalopathy with a depressed level of consciousness, although there may be a "lucid interval" prior to this change. Epidural hematoma usually occurs with damage to the middle meningeal artery, which allows arterial blood to collect in the epidural space, leading to rapidly increased intracranial pressure and the risk of herniation. Subdural hematomas are less apt to occur on hyperacute timescales, although they can cause seizures, which in turn can be hyperacute.

Ischemic Stroke

Ischemic stroke is caused by lack of blood flow to one or more regions of the brain leading to infarction. Most patients present with focal deficits, and the precise clinical syndrome depends on the functions supported by the ischemic tissue. Encephalopathic states with changes in arousal, cognition, and emotion can occur with lesions of the bilateral thalami (e.g., "top of the basilar" syndrome, artery of Percheron stroke), mesencephalic-diencephalic junction, and diffuse bilateral cortical-subcortical microemboli. A much broader set of focal cognitive, neuropsychiatric, and behavioral syndromes can also occur secondary to ischemic stroke depending on infarct location(s). Acute confusional states characterized by impaired orientation, inattention, and aberrant perception may occur as a result of right middle cerebral artery infarctions disrupting networks that subserve attention. Patients are alert but concentration is impaired, and memories are poorly formed. They may become agitated with awareness of irrelevant stimuli. The disorder may occur as a result of right parietal or right temporal lesions. The right temporal lesions may be more likely to produce a confusional state due to the proximity to the limbic system disrupting modulation of affective responses. Elderly patients with preexisting cognitive decline are more prone to develop a confusional state following a stroke.

Seizure

Seizures are caused by abnormal, excessive, rhythmic electrical discharges in the brain and usually occur as discrete events with a rapid onset. The clinical presentation of seizure (e.g., semiology) is highly variable and depends on where in the brain the aberrant electrical activity originates and whether it remains in one location (i.e., partial) or becomes more widespread (i.e., generalized). Generalized seizures lead to a loss of consciousness and are followed by a variable-length postictal period of encephalopathy with a return to baseline. Partial seizures often produce focal symptoms that reflect the function of the area where the aberrant electrical activity occurs (e.g., motor, sensory, and autonomic). Sudden changes in arousal, attention (e.g., absence), memory (e.g., focal dyscognitive), language (e.g., speech arrest), and/or emotion (e.g., ictal panic, gelastic) can occur and are important causes of encephalopathy. Nonconvulsive seizures (i.e., those without obvious motor manifestations) should also be considered in patients with sudden onset and/or fluctuating encephalopathy symptoms.

Migraine

Typical migraine is characterized by unilateral and throbbing headaches lasting several hours that are often accompanied by nausea, photophobia, and phonophobia. These headaches tend to build over the course of several minutes and may be preceded by an aura that is often visual (e.g., "scintillating scotoma") or somatosensory (e.g., spreading paresthesias). Migraine can occasionally produce symptoms of confusion ("confusional migraine"), which can rarely occur in the absence of headache ("acephalgic migraine"). Acute confusional migraine manifests with acute confusion, agitation, disorientation, altered mental status, and speech and memory difficulty and may be the first presentation of migraine in children or adolescents. Most patients develop a headache prior to the onset of the confusional state. The confusion may be a manifestation of cortical spreading depression and some patients may experience, visual, somatosensory, and/or speech difficulty prior to or during the period of confusion. The confusion resolves within 24 hours and acute confusional migraine is a diagnosis of exclusion. Infection, seizures, inflammatory, neoplastic, and vascular disorders, and metabolic abnormalities must be ruled out. In one adult study, acute confusional migraine was noted to be the initial presentation of cerebral autosomal dominant arteriopathy with subcortical infarcts and leukoencephalopathy (CADASIL).

Traumatic Brain Injury

Acute TBI is a common cause of hyperacute encephalopathy. Changes in both the level of arousal (e.g., lethargy and coma) as well as contents of consciousness (e.g., amnesia and disorientation) can occur, depending on the severity of injury.

The term *concussion* is used to describe the mildest form of traumatic brain injury associated with altered mental status and only occasionally loss of consciousness. Patients with concussion can experience a posttraumatic encephalopathy as part of a broader postconcussive syndrome (e.g., headaches, dizziness, mental fogginess, intolerance of loud noises or bright lights), and the onset of symptoms may be delayed by hours or days following impact. Neuropsychiatric symptoms may accompany the syndrome, including fatigue, excessive sleeping or insomnia, personality changes (e.g., irritability, labile affect), memory loss, poor concentration, and slow processing speed. Symptoms usually resolve within a few weeks but can persist for months or years.

Systemic Conditions

Sudden-onset encephalopathy can occur with hypertensive emergency (e.g., hypertensive encephalopathy), metabolic derangements (e.g., hyper- or hypoglycemia), medications/drugs/drug withdrawal, and other toxic exposures.

Psychiatric conditions such as panic attacks, nonepileptic seizures, fugue states, and psychosis can also present as sudden-onset encephalopathy.

ACUTE CAUSES OF ENCEPHALOPATHY— ONSET WITHIN HOURS TO DAYS

Primary Neurologic Conditions
Subdural Hematoma

Subdural hematoma is hemorrhage into the subdural space, often due to the injury of the bridging veins that connect the surface of the brain with the dura. Since the cause is generally venous bleeding, the slow accumulation of blood can take days or even weeks to cause a clinically significant mass effect. Common symptoms include headache, seizure, and encephalopathy with reduced arousal and cognitive impairment, sometimes with focal elemental deficits. Subdural hematoma may be caused by head trauma, coagulopathy, anticoagulant medications, and intracranial hypotension (often due to the lumbar puncture or shunt). In older adults, perhaps due to stretching of bridging veins due to aging-associated brain atrophy (i.e., larger space between the brain parenchyma and dura), subdural hematoma can develop after only mild TBI. Acute-to-subacute encephalopathy in this age group should prompt head CT to assess for subdural bleeding.

Posterior Reversible Encephalopathy Syndrome

Posterior reversible encephalopathy syndrome is caused by breakdown of the neurovascular autoregulation of blood pressure, which leads to vasogenic edema in the brain parenchyma, which has a predilection for posterior regions (e.g., occipitoparietal areas). Common symptoms include headache, seizures (occipital > others), and encephalopathy characterized by reduced arousal, confusion, and occasionally cortical blindness. It is associated with conditions that predispose to endothelial dysfunction, including hypertension, preeclampsia, and drug toxicity (e.g., cyclosporine, tacrolimus, and bevacizumab).

Demyelinating Conditions (e.g., Multiple Sclerosis and Acute Disseminated Encephalomyelitis)

Demyelinating diseases of the central nervous system include MS and ADEM. Although MS is a chronic disease, the most common form has a relapsing-remitting course that is often punctuated by acute flares that cause focal elemental neurologic deficits (e.g., optic neuritis and transverse myelitis). Encephalopathy can occur with focal or multifocal demyelination, leading to fatigue, cognitive slowing, and apathy, when focal cognitive/behavioral networks are involved. ADEM is an acute, multifocal demyelinating disorder of the CNS that usually occurs after an infection, most commonly in children.

Primary Central Nervous System Infections (Meningitis/Encephalitis/Abscess)

Central nervous system infections such as meningitis and encephalitis can present with acute encephalopathy, usually accompanied by headache and fever (as well as neck stiffness in the former). Acute bacterial, fungal, and parasitic meningitis may be fatal if untreated. Infectious encephalitis can cause encephalopathy via the disruption of arousal, cognitive, and limbic-affective networks. Herpes simplex virus can cause an acute change in personality, emotion, and cognition that rapidly progresses to coma if untreated.

Transient Global Amnesia

The syndrome of TGA is characterized by a temporary inability to form new episodic memories and presents with disorientation, repeated questioning, and a subsequent amnesia for the symptomatic period. Arousal and other aspects of cognitive and emotional functioning are typically normal. The condition always resolves within 24 hours and typically lasts only a few hours. TGA may be triggered by intense physiological or emotional stimuli (e.g., sexual intercourse, argument) or exposure to extreme environmental conditions (e.g., cold water). Although the condition is typically idiopathic, the syndrome may rarely be caused by posterior cerebral artery infarction or temporal lobe seizure.

Systemic Conditions

Systemic medical conditions associated with acute encephalopathy include systemic infections (e.g., septic encephalopathy), systemic autoimmune diseases (e.g., lupus, Sjögren syndrome, Behçet disease), metabolic disturbances including acute renal or hepatic failure, acute hypo- or hypernatremia, hyperammonemia, hypo- and hyperthyroidism, thiamine deficiency (e.g., Wernicke encephalopathy), drugs or drug withdrawal, medications (e.g., benzodiazepines, narcotics, anticholinergics, antihistaminics, sympathomimetics, dopamine blockers), toxin ingestions, and others.

Psychiatric illness can present with acute encephalopathy. Acute symptoms of mania, psychosis, panic, anxiety, and depression can produce symptoms of cognitive impairment, psychomotor agitation, or slowing.

Catatonia, which is associated with both psychiatric and general medical causes, can occur with characteristic motor dysfunction (e.g., inability to move, "waxy" flexibility, repetitive movements), reduced responsiveness, and other behavioral changes (e.g., agitation, mutism, negativism, echoing behaviors).

Intensive Care Unit Delirium

Delirium is the most common clinical manifestation of acute brain dysfunction in the intensive care unit (ICU) and always warrants a full evaluation. ICU delirium is characterized by the sudden onset of confusion, inattention, and altered consciousness. Certain factors increase the risk including older age, preexisting cognitive impairment, prolonged mechanical ventilation, severe illness, use of sedative medication, and history of alcohol or substance abuse. There is a broad differential, and the leading causes include infection, metabolic abnormalities, medications, Wernicke disease due to thiamine deficiency, seizures, stroke, hypoxia, vitamin deficiencies, trauma, endocrinopathies, and alcohol/substance withdrawal or intoxication. Patients with ICU delirium will require a longer stay in the ICU and often a longer duration of mechanical ventilation. There is also an increased risk of mortality and patients may continue to have cognitive impairment with a decline in their ability to perform activities of daily living after discharge from the hospital. Many patients, however, who experience ICU delirium will fully recover and the underlying medical illness and quality of care in the ICU play a role in determining the outcome. Treating ICU delirium involves treating the underlying causes and providing optimal supportive care. Maintaining a normal sleep-wake cycle, minimizing the use of sedative medication, involving family members in the care, and early mobilization with physical therapy are essential in preventing and managing ICU delirium.

SUBACUTE CAUSES OF ENCEPHALOPATHY—ONSET WITHIN WEEKS TO MONTHS

Primary Neurologic Conditions
Subdural Hematoma

Subdural hematoma (discussed earlier) can produce cognitive symptoms that emerge slowly, sometimes weeks after onset.

Brain Tumors and Complications of Chemotherapy/ Radiation

Primary brain tumors (e.g., glioblastoma, meningioma, primary CNS lymphoma) can cause encephalopathy. Symptoms may result from direct infiltrative damage to local tissue, edema, mass effect and intracranial shifts, effects on intracranial pressure, seizures, or hemorrhages. Headache is common during the course of the disease but rarely the sole presenting symptom.

Solitary parenchymal brain metastases commonly present with focal deficits that can affect arousal, cognition, emotion, and behavior depending on the involved brain region(s) affected. Widespread metastatic disease can mimic diffuse, systemic symptoms of encephalopathy. Headaches, seizures, and hemorrhages are common.

Subacute to chronic changes in cognition can occur as a side effect of treatments used for intracranial tumors, including tissue resection, radiation, and chemotherapy. Radiation is associated with tissue necrosis and vasculopathy. Leukoencephalopathy is reported with some chemotherapy agents (e.g., methotrexate). Episodic headaches, seizures, and other focal deficits, including those affecting cognition, can occur as part of the syndrome of stroke-like migraine attacks after radiation therapy (SMART syndrome).

Antibody-Mediated Autoimmune/Paraneoplastic Conditions

A growing number of recently described antibody-mediated autoimmune conditions can affect the central nervous system, causing subacute changes in cognition, emotion, and behavior due to the antibodies' affinity for limbic brain regions (i.e., autoimmune limbic encephalitis). Additional focal neurologic deficits are common and depend on the antibody's tropism for different parts of the neuraxis. These antibody-mediated encephalopathies can be isolated or occur as a paraneoplastic phenomenon. A well-described entity is the limbic encephalitis associated with autoantibodies against the glutamate N-methyl-D-aspartate receptor. Initial presentation with memory loss and personality/mood changes may be mistaken for primary psychiatric disease, though seizures and/or movement disorders often develop, revealing a neurologic rather than a primary psychiatric cause of the alterations in mental status.

Hashimoto Encephalopathy

Hashimoto encephalopathy (HE), also known as steroid-responsive encephalopathy associated with autoimmune thyroiditis, occurs in association with autoantibodies against thyroglobulin or thyroid peroxidase, although neither the antibodies nor the thyroid state itself have been clearly established to mechanistically underlie the symptomatology. HE can present with global or focal symptomatology, at times as a rapidly progressive dementia syndrome. Patients typically experience a robust improvement with intravenous corticosteroids.

Infectious Meningitis/Encephalitis

Subacute infectious meningoencephalitis can occur with fungal, tuberculous, viral (human immunodeficiency virus [HIV]), or syphilis infection. Typical meningeal symptoms may be present but often emerge more subacutely than in bacterial or viral meningitis. Seizures and strokes can occur. Immunocompromised patients are at higher risk for developing fungal meningitis.

Prion Disease/Jakob-Creutzfeldt Disease

Prion disease (e.g., Jakob-Creutzfeldt disease [CJD]) is a rare but important cause of rapidly progressive dementia in adults. Patients may present initially with cognitive impairment and behavioral changes (e.g., psychosis, paranoia, personality change), and movement disorders (e.g., myoclonus, parkinsonism), sensory changes, and altered sleep-wake cycles are common with disease progression. The Heidenhain variant of CJD is characterized by visual disturbances at onset due to prions targeting the occipital lobes early in the disease and may persist for weeks before there is cognitive involvement.

Central Nervous System Vasculitis

CNS vasculitis can present with subacute progressive cognitive decline. Nearly all patients have headaches, and neuroimaging generally shows subcortical infarctions of different ages. CNS vasculitis may be isolated to the CNS (i.e., primary) or secondary to systemic vasculitis (e.g., granulomatosis with polyangiitis or infection [e.g., varicella zoster]).

Neurosarcoidosis

Sarcoidosis is a granulomatous inflammatory condition that can affect multiple organ systems, including the brain. Neurosarcoidosis most commonly causes cranial nerve palsies, although subacute meningitis and/or direct parenchymal involvement may also occur, leading to cognitive and behavioral changes with encephalopathy. The observed neurologic deficits can be widespread or focal, depending on the location and extent of the pathology. Seizures may also occur.

Systemic Conditions

A number of systemic conditions can present with subacute encephalopathy. There can be overlapping causes, including toxic-metabolic causes (e.g., electrolyte disturbances, renal failure/uremia, liver failure, and cardiac failure), endocrinopathies (e.g., thyroid and adrenal disease), vitamin deficiencies (e.g., thiamine (B_1), vitamin B_{12}, and niacin), porphyrias, and toxins (e.g., heavy metals). The effects of systemic inflammation, as occurs in autoimmune disease (e.g., systemic lupus erythematosus [SLE], Sjögren syndrome, and peripheral vasculitides), malignancy, chronic infections (e.g., osteomyelitis), and other chronic conditions (e.g., diabetes and celiac disease), can produce cognitive slowing and neuropsychiatric symptoms. Primary psychiatric disorders (e.g., major depressive episode and postpartum psychosis) can cause altered cognition.

CHRONIC CAUSES OF ENCEPHALOPATHY—ONSET WITHIN MONTHS TO YEARS

Primary Neurologic Conditions

Degenerative Disease

In older adults, the most common causes of chronic symptoms with features of encephalopathy are the neurodegenerative diseases associated with cognitive decline. There is considerable syndromic variability across the spectrum of degenerative disease, and it can impact aspects of cognitive, perceptual, limbic-emotional, motor, sensory, autonomic, and arousal/sleep functions. Precise characterization of deficits can help predict the underlying pathology, prognosis, and treatment options. By their nature, all degenerative diseases tend to progress gradually over the course of years. Many degenerative diseases are associated with the accumulation and network-based spread of toxic proteins within the brain. Patients with neurodegenerative cognitive impairment are more susceptible to acute and subacute encephalopathy in the setting of systemic and/or other neurologic conditions, perhaps reflecting vulnerabilities (i.e., reduced resiliency) of the neuroanatomical networks supporting these disrupted functions.

Alzheimer disease is the most common degenerative disease and is associated with the excessive deposition of amyloid plaques and tau neurofibrillary tangles in brain tissues. Typical presentations of Alzheimer disease include early and disproportionate episodic memory loss, often accompanied to a lesser extent by deficits in visuospatial skills, aspects of language (e.g., lexical retrieval), and executive functions. Less common presentations of Alzheimer disease include those with relative sparing of episodic memory with disproportionate involvement of other domains, including language (e.g., logopenic variant of primary progressive aphasia), visuospatial functioning (e.g., posterior cortical atrophy), and a frontal-behavioral or dysexecutive variant. These "atypical" variants are more common in patients with an early age of onset. "Sundowning," a type of encephalopathy characterized by changes in cognition, arousal, limbic-emotional functioning at the end of the day, is common in later stages of AD even in the absence of a superimposed condition.

New disease-modifying antiamyloid therapies (e.g., lecanemab, donanemab) can slow cognitive and functional decline in patients with mild cognitive impairment or early dementia due to biomarker-positive Alzheimer disease (e.g., cerebrospinal fluid, amyloid-positron emission tomography). The benefits of this therapy need to be balanced against the risk of cerebral edema and brain hemorrhage. Diagnosing Alzheimer disease at an early stage is more urgent than previously, given the limited window for accessing this novel therapy.

Dementia with Lewy bodies, a synucleinopathy, often presents with fluctuations in arousal, cognitive impairment (especially executive and visuospatial impairment), parkinsonism (usually minimally responsive to dopamine replacement), dysautonomia, REM sleep behavior disorder, and psychosis with visual hallucinations.

Frontotemporal lobar degeneration (FTLD) is a set of neuropathological proteinopathies (e.g., Pick disease, corticobasal degeneration, progressive supranuclear palsy, and TDP-43) that are often associated with frontotemporal dementia syndromes. The most common syndromic presentation is the behavioral variant of frontotemporal dementia, which is characterized by early behavioral, personality, and social changes including apathy, disinhibition, loss of empathy, repetitive or stereotyped movements, hyperorality (e.g., increased appetite, new food preferences, putting things in one's mouth), and changes in executive functioning. FTLD pathologies also cause primary progressive aphasia syndromes (e.g., nonfluent/agrammatic and semantic variants), corticobasal syndrome, Richardson syndrome, and others, each reflecting tropism for other parts of the brain.

Cerebrovascular Disease

Vascular cognitive impairment is a common cause of chronic encephalopathy among older adults. Cerebrovascular disease can produce cognitive decline in several ways, including progressive accumulation of precisely located symptomatic strokes that leads to a stepwise reduction in function with each episode (e.g., multiinfarct dementia), or a slowly progressive accumulation of silent microinfarcts (often within the white matter), microhemorrhages, and other damage. When chronic and slowly progressive, vascular dementia often presents with deficits in executive functioning and visuospatial skill.

A rare but important cause of vascular cognitive impairment is CADASIL arising from Notch3 gene mutations and characterized by recurrent ischemic strokes accompanied by diffuse white matter lesions and subcortical infarcts. Patients with CADASIL often present with dementia at a younger age than those with atherosclerotic disease and may experience neuropsychiatric symptoms such as depression.

Normal Pressure Hydrocephalus

Normal pressure hydrocephalus is characterized by the excessive accumulation of cerebrospinal fluid without an accompanying elevation in intracranial pressure. The typical triad of symptoms includes gait unsteadiness with falls, urinary incontinence, and cognitive impairment. Cognitive involvement usually develops after the onset and progression of gait dysfunction. Cognitive and behavioral deficits reflect frontal-subcortical dysfunction and may include inattention, executive dysfunction (e.g., processing speed), apathy/abulia, impulsivity, and a tendency to perseverate.

Multiple Sclerosis

MS (as discussed earlier) is associated with chronic symptoms of cognitive impairment and fatigue. The cognitive syndrome typically affects attention, processing speed, executive functions, and episodic memory.

Infection

Chronic, smoldering infections can present with cognitive symptoms. Longstanding HIV infection is associated with progressive cognitive decline with motor slowing (i.e., HIV-associated neurocognitive disorder). Syphilis is a well-known cause of chronic cognitive impairment and behavioral changes. The neurologic phenotypes of syphilis are diverse, which may be due to the spirochete's tropism for several CNS compartments, including the meninges, cerebral vessels, and parenchyma.

Progressive multifocal leukoencephalopathy is an infectious disease associated with JC virus infections that is seen in patients with chronic immunosuppression, often due to HIV infection or immunomodulatory medication (e.g., natalizumab).

Chronic Traumatic Encephalopathy

Recent evidence suggests that repetitive head trauma, as occurs with contact sports such as football, boxing, and soccer, is associated with a delayed-onset neurodegenerative disease. The symptoms include cognitive impairment, neurobehavioral changes (e.g., personality changes, impulsivity, depression, suicide), and parkinsonism.

Adult-Onset Leukodystrophies

Leukodystrophies are diseases that affect metabolic pathways important for myelin development, maintenance, and destruction. The clinical manifestations are diverse and often include cognitive and behavioral changes, motor dysfunction (e.g., spasticity), and seizures.

Mitochondrial Disorders

Mitochondrial diseases often affect multiple neurologic (and systemic) systems and are associated with leukoencephalopathy. MELAS syndrome (mitochondrial encephalomyopathy, lactic acidosis, and stroke-like episodes) is a multiorgan disease with broad manifestations including stroke-like episodes, lactic acidemia, epilepsy, dementia, and myopathy. Most patients suffer migrainous headaches and peripheral neuropathy is common. The encephalopathy manifests as a wide range of neurologic symptoms including seizures, headaches, muscle weakness, and cognitive decline. These symptoms can occur episodically, hence the term "stroke-like episodes." Patients may develop cardiomyopathy, diabetes, gastrointestinal, renal, and pulmonary disease.

Systemic Conditions

There are many systemic conditions that cause a chronic, persistent encephalopathy syndrome, including several that are potentially reversible. Systemic conditions with potentially reversible cognitive symptoms include vitamin deficiencies (e.g., vitamin B_{12}, thiamine, and niacin), obstructive sleep apnea, endocrinopathies (e.g., adrenal and thyroid), metabolic disease (e.g., renal/liver failure), systemic autoimmune disease (e.g., Sjögren and Behçet), and porphyrias. Other important diagnoses include chronic alcohol exposure (e.g., Korsakoff syndrome, Marchiafava-Bignami disease, cerebellar atrophy), heavy metal exposure, celiac disease, Wilson disease, and fragile X-associated tremor/ataxia syndrome.

Chronic psychiatric conditions such as bipolar disorder and schizophrenia can be associated with cognitive impairment.

CONCLUSION

Encephalopathy is a broad term that encompasses dysfunction affecting the level of consciousness (e.g., wakefulness, arousal), cognition (especially attention), awareness, emotion, and behavior. It can occur in isolation or as part of a broader neurologic or systemic syndrome, and the precise phenotype depends on the affected regions of pathology within the CNS. The differential diagnosis depends on the time course of onset and evolution of symptoms and includes both primary neurologic and systemic conditions.

"For the full bibliography list, please use the pincode on the inside front cover to access the electronic version of the text at eBooks.health.elsevier.com."

8

Brain and Spine Tumors*

Gilbert Youssef and Eudocia Q. Lee

INTRODUCTION

The incidence of brain tumors, particularly brain metastases, has been increasing in certain patient groups, and the average annual adjusted incidence rate has been estimated to be 24.71 per 100,000 population between 2015 and 2019. This is mainly due to advances in the diagnosis of primary central nervous system (CNS) tumors (Table 8.1), and improved outcomes and survival from systemic malignancies. Malignant brain tumors are associated with poor survival outcomes and often lead to a decline in patients' functional and performance status. Hence, timely diagnosis, management, and coordination of care are crucial, and it is important for physicians, particularly primary care providers and internists, to be familiar with their basic approach and management. This chapter will review brain metastases, which are the most common malignant brain tumors in adults, along with meningiomas and gliomas, with an emphasis on their clinical presentation, diagnosis, and basic oncological management. It will also review some of the most common medical and neurologic complications of brain tumors and their management.

CENTRAL NERVOUS SYSTEM METASTASES

CNS metastases are the most common malignant CNS tumors, and are common among patients with advanced solid malignancies, leading to significant morbidity and mortality. The brain parenchyma is the most commonly involved site in the CNS. Leptomeningeal metastases (LM) refer to the tumor cell infiltration of the cerebrospinal fluid (CSF), and leptomeninges of the brain and spinal cord (i.e., the pia and arachnoid mater, the inner membranes of the meninges), whereas dural metastases refer to the infiltration of the dura mater, the outer membrane of the meninges, by tumor cells. Cancer may also metastasize to the spinal cord as intramedullary tumors, to the epidural spaces causing spinal cord compression, as well as to the nerve plexuses and even individual nerves.

The true incidence of brain metastases (BM) is challenging to determine due to lack of mandated reporting to local and federal registries and comprehensive epidemiology data. Also, screening for BM is only recommended by consensus guidelines for specific malignancies or stages of disease, including patients with small and non–small cell lung carcinoma, melanoma, testicular cancer, alveolar sarcoma, angiosarcoma, and left-sided cardiac sarcoma. The incidence ranges from 10% to 40% of patients with solid tumors, and the annual incidence is estimated to be 70,000 to 400,000 cases per year in the United States and has been increasing with better systemic therapies, improved survival, expanded use of surveillance imaging, and greater awareness among oncologists. The most common systemic malignancies to metastasize to the brain are lung cancer, breast cancer, and melanoma, which account for 67% to 80% of BM, whereas prostate cancer, head and neck cancer, non–melanoma skin cancer, esophageal cancer, and Hodgkin lymphoma rarely metastasize to the brain. Population data is limited, though recent studies shed light on the

*Based on Ricardo McFaline-Figueroa J, Lee EQ. Brain tumors. *Am J Med*. 2018;131(8):874–882. ISSN 0002-9343. https://doi.org/10.1016/j.amjmed.2017.12.039.

TABLE 8.1 Primary Central Nervous System Tumors	
Gliomas	Embryonal tumors
Astrocytoma, IDH-mutant	Medulloblastoma, WNT activated
WHO Grade 2, 3 and 4	Medulloblastoma, SHH activated and TP53 wild type
Oligodendroglioma, IDH-mutant, 1p/19 codeleted	Medulloblastoma, SHH activated and TP53-mutant
WHO Grade 2 and 3	Medulloblastoma, non-WNT/non-SHH
Glioblastoma	Other embryonal tumors
Diffuse midline glioma, H3K27-altered	Atypical teratoid/rhabdoid tumor
Diffuse hemispheric glioma, H3G34-mutant	Cranial and paraspinal nerve tumors
Other astrocytic tumors	Schwannoma
Pilocytic astrocytoma	Neurofibroma
High-grade astrocytoma with piloid features	Malignant peripheral nerve sheath tumor
Glioneuronal and neuronal tumors	Paraganglioma
Ganglioglioma	Tumors of the sellar region
Neurocytoma	Adamantinomatous craniopharyngioma
Ependymal tumors	Papillary craniopharyngioma
Ependymoma	Pituitary adenoma
Meningiomas	Germ cell tumors
Meningioma	Mature teratoma
Mesenchymal, nonmeningothelial tumors	Germinoma
Solitary fibrous tumor	Yolk sac tumor
Hemangioblastoma	Choriocarcinoma
Rhabdomyosarcoma	Mixed germ cell tumor
Choroid plexus tumors	Melanocytic tumors
Pineal tumors	Hematolymphoid tumors
Pineocytoma	Primary diffuse large B cell lymphoma of the CNS
Pineoblastoma	Immunodeficiency-associated CNS lymphoma
Histiocytic tumors	Intravascular large B cell lymphoma
	Other rare lymphomas of the CNS
	Histiocytic tumors
	Metastases to the CNS
	Metastases to the brain and spinal cord parenchyma
	Metastases to the meninges

CNS, Central nervous system; *IDH*, isocitrate dehydrogenase; *H3G34*, glycine codon of the H3 histone gene; *H3K27*, lysine codon of the H3 histone gene; *SHH*, sonic hedgehog gene; *TP53*, tumor protein p53; *WNT*, Wnt signaling pathway; *1p/19q codeleted*, codeletion of the short arm of chromosome 1 and the long arm of chromosome 19.

epidemiology of BM at the time of systemic cancer diagnosis (i.e., synchronous BM) using the National Cancer Institute (NCI) Surveillance, Epidemiology, and End Results (SEER) database. Cagney et al. estimate the overall annual incidence of synchronous brain metastasis at 23,598 patients per year in the United States, based on SEER data from 2010 to 2013. The incidence per tumor type for all stages of disease was highest in patients with small cell lung cancer, lung adenocarcinoma, and non–small cell lung cancer (NSCLC) not-otherwise specified, with a prevalence of synchronous brain metastasis of over 10%. Considering only patients with metastatic disease at the time of diagnosis, metastatic melanoma was the most likely to present with synchronous BM (28.2%), followed by lung adenocarcinoma, NSCLC not-otherwise specified, small cell lung cancer, squamous cell carcinoma of the lung, bronchioalveolar carcinoma, and renal cancer, all with a prevalence of over 10%. Analysis of SEER data by Kromer et al. revealed similar results.

As for LM, they are diagnosed in about 5% of patients with solid tumors and often identified concurrently with parenchymal and dural metastases. However, the incidence of undiagnosed or asymptomatic LM has been reported to be greater than 20% in autopsy series. Breast cancer, particularly of negative hormonal receptor and Her2 expression status, is the most common solid malignancy that causes LM, followed by lung cancer and melanoma.

Pathophysiology

Tumor cells often acquire epigenetic and proliferative changes, including the expansion of preexisting or development of new blood vessel networks, leading to vascular invasion and subsequent hematogenous spread to the brain. Other routes of tumor cell spread to the CNS include perineural invasion and anterograde or retrograde dissemination through the Schwann cells, which is often observed in head and neck squamous cell carcinoma, and intracranial retrograde dissemination from spinal tumors such as ependymoma. Once inside the brain, tumor cells interact with brain endothelia and adhere to the brain parenchyma via upregulation of particular cell surface proteins and growth factors, then secrete inflammatory cytokines, through interaction with the surrounding astrocytes, promoting cell motility, invasion, and survival. LM also develop through hematogenous spread to the arachnoid via the arterial circulation, particularly in hematological tumors, through endoneural or perineural and perivascular lymphatic spread from vertebral metastases or head and neck cancers, or direct spread from BM in close proximity to CSF spaces.

Clinical Presentation and Diagnosis

The clinical presentation of BM is quite variable. Headache is a common complaint, occurring in up to 50% of patients, though it is neither sensitive nor specific for the diagnosis. The classic headache is diffuse, mild at onset, occurring mainly in the recumbent position due to peritumoral edema and increased intracranial pressure (ICP). It begins when the patient awakens in the morning, disappears shortly after arising, and returns the following morning. The question of when to image those without the classic "brain tumor headache" or those with chronic headache is a difficult one for primary care providers, neurologists, and oncologists alike. The US Headache Consortium recommends consideration of neuroimaging to rule out a secondary cause of headaches for those patients with an abnormal neurological examination, those who develop consistent and progressive headaches at an older age, those with

atypical headache features, or headaches that do not fit the strict definition of migraine or other primary headache disorder. Atypical features include rapidly increasing headache frequency, history of lack of coordination, history of localized neurological signs, such as localized sensory or motor symptoms, and history of headache causing awakening from sleep.

Seizures are another common symptom in patients with BM and can occur at any time of the disease course. Neuroimaging should be considered for all adults presenting with a first unprovoked seizure. Patients may also present with focal neurological symptoms (i.e., aphasia, weakness, sensory loss, visual disturbances, ataxia), which often have a subacute onset, secondary to direct invasion or compression of eloquent brain structures. Cognitive or behavioral impairment is likewise common and often develops with multifocal BM (i.e., involving multiple areas of the brain responsible of memory encoding, registration, and recall, as well as personality changes) or secondary to increased intracranial pressure (ICP) or delayed brain tissue injury from radiation.

Classically, LM present with signs and symptoms of increased intracranial ICP due to decreased CSF reabsorption at the arachnoid villi and poor CSF ventricular outflow leading to hydrocephalus, and/or focal neurologic deficits involving multiple sites within the neuroaxis. Clinical manifestations include headache that is also worse in the recumbent position, dizziness, cognitive changes, speech problems, signs of focal cortical or cerebellar dysfunction, incontinence, and gait disorders. Malignant invasion of the arachnoid mater can lead to multiple cranial neuropathies and radiculopathies. Cranial nerves VI, VII, and VIII are most affected, leading to binocular diplopia, facial weakness, and/or hearing impairment. Nonspecific symptoms like hiccups and bilateral tinnitus can also be observed and should raise the suspicion of LM, particularly if they occur concurrently with the former symptoms. Involvement or compression of the small vessels in the subarachnoid space can occasionally lead to ischemic infarcts. Seizures from meningeal and cortical irritation are rare.

The National Comprehensive Cancer Network (NCCN) guidelines for CNS cancers provide an algorithm for establishing the diagnosis of BM. Magnetic resonance imaging (MRI) of the brain with and without contrast is the gold standard for brain tumor imaging, though computerized tomography (CT) with and

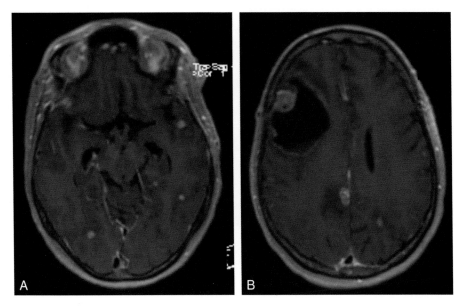

Fig. 8.1 A 65-year-old female, with a history of melanoma, BRAF V600E-mutant, presented with progressive headaches and confusion. She was found to have multiple enhancing, hemorrhagic lesions (A), the dominant of which was cystic and centered in the right frontal lobe (B). The right frontal lesion was resected, with pathology confirming metastatic melanoma. She was treated with a combination of the BRAF inhibitor dabrafenib and the MEK inhibitor trametinib to achieve a quick response, then was switched to the combination of PD-1 inhibitor nivolumab and CTLA-4 inhibitor ipilimumab. Her brain disease stabilized initially but then progressed 4 months later.

without contrast is a reasonable alternative for those that cannot undergo MRI. Imaging of the neuroaxis should be considered in all cancer patients who develop new neurologic symptoms, while screening for asymptomatic BM is only recommended in patients with cancers associated with high risk of BM, including small cell lung cancer, advanced NSCLC, and advanced melanoma. BM typically appear as well-demarcated, solid or ring-enhancing lesions located in the gray-white matter junction (Fig. 8.1). They involve the cerebral hemispheres in 80%, whereas the cerebellum and the brainstem are affected in about 15% and 5%, respectively. BM from melanoma, choriocarcinoma, germ cell tumors, thyroid carcinoma, and renal cell carcinoma are more likely to be hemorrhagic. In patients with a known history of cancer and little concern for alternative diagnoses, neuroimaging alone may be sufficient to make the diagnosis of BM. In those without a prior diagnosis, CT imaging of the chest/abdomen/pelvis or whole-body positron emission tomography (PET-CT) may reveal other sites of involvement outside the CNS that may be biopsied or resected for tissue confirmation. In

those without evidence of systemic malignancy (almost a third of patients), or those with concern for an alternative diagnosis based on neuroimaging, a stereotactic or open biopsy, or surgical resection of the brain mass is recommended to direct further care.

LM may manifest as diffuse opacification and thickening of the leptomeninges and enhancement along the cerebral surface, cranial nerves, and nerve roots, or as minute enhancing nodules particularly in the posterior fossa, basal cisterns of the brain, and cauda equina (Fig. 8.2). However, brain and spine MRI can be normal despite symptoms, as it has a sensitivity of only 70%. CSF cytology is the gold standard for diagnosis, but poor sampling, inadequate sample volume (<10.5 mL), and inefficient handling may lead to false-negative results. Serial CSF sampling and collection of CSF at the site of symptoms (i.e., ventricular for cranial disease and lumbar for spinal disease) increase the diagnostic yield. CSF flow cytometry increases sensitivity to leptomeningeal spread of hematologic malignancies. Other CSF findings include elevated proteins and low glucose levels. Liquid biopsies utilizing assays that detect spinal fluid

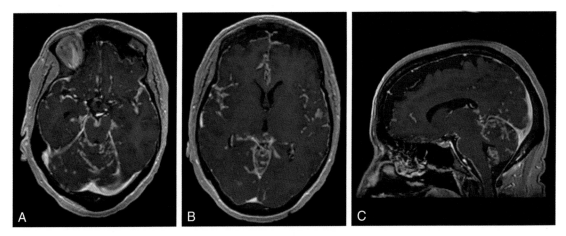

Fig. 8.2 A 61-year-old female with a history of adenoid cystic carcinoma of the nasal cavity, metastatic to the lungs and bone, presented with progressive generalized weakness, lightheadedness, gait unsteadiness, frequent falls, and nausea and vomiting. Brain MRI showed leptomeningeal enhancement along the cerebellar folia (A), cerebral sulci (B), and along the anterior and posterior surfaces of the brainstem and cervical spine (C). She was treated with whole-brain radiation (WBRT). Unfortunately, her central nervous system and systemic disease progressed shortly after completion of WBRT and she passed away.

circulating tumor cells or cell-free DNA are being developed for clinical use; some studies suggest that these technologies may be more sensitive than CSF cytology.

Oncological Management

The management of BM requires a multidisciplinary approach and depends on the patient's clinical and radiological status, and the type of the primary malignancy. Guidelines have been proposed by the Society for Neuro-Oncology (SNO), American Society of Clinical Oncology (ASCO), and American Society for Radiation Oncology (ASTRO). As most patients with BM have advanced systemic disease, the prognosis remains generally poor, with a median overall in the range of months in most patients. Diagnosis-specific graded prognostic assessment (DS-GPA) indices exist to help estimate survival in BM patients; they were developed by identifying major prognostic factors (performance status, age, presence of extracranial metastases), based on aggregated data of patients with BM across various tumor subtype cohorts. In general, management is aimed at palliation in patients with poor prognoses. More aggressive management is reserved for select patients with good prognoses (such as a young patient with excellent performance status and BM from hormone receptor/HER2-positive breast cancer with estimated median survival time of 25.3 months per GPA).

The role of surgery depends on the diagnostic need and extent of disease. Surgical resection may be necessary to establish a diagnosis in patients with no history of systemic malignancies or with multiple concurrent cancers. In patients with good functional status, controlled or absent systemic disease, and a single, surgically accessible brain metastasis, surgical resection may be indicated and associated with improved survival and lengthened functionally independent survival time. In those with multiple BM, surgical resection may be considered for the removal of a bulky, dominant lesion causing symptoms refractory to corticosteroids for palliation. In patients who develop hydrocephalus from diffuse LM, a ventriculoperitoneal shunt may be considered for CSF diversion. On the other hand, surgical resection can be deferred in patients with BM from radiosensitive tumors (i.e., small cell lung cancer, select germ cell tumors, hematological malignancies), or tumors with effective CNS-penetrant therapies, such as EGFR-mutant NSCLC and BRAF-mutant melanoma. Laser interstitial thermal therapy (LITT) is a less aggressive surgical approach, where tumor is ablated by laser-derived thermal energy emitted through a catheter. Although its established role is limited to radiation necrosis, it can be used to treat select recurrent BM.

Whole-brain radiotherapy (WBRT) is the historic standard for palliative radiotherapy in BM. It results in improvement in neurologic function, and decreased incidence of intracranial recurrence and neurologic death. However, WBRT is associated with increased neurotoxicity, particularly fatigue and neurocognitive dysfunction. Hippocampal avoidance WBRT (HA-WBRT) preserves the radiosensitive neural stem cells of the hippocampus and is associated with reduced decline in memory and improvement in quality of life compared to the standard WBRT in patients devoid of BM in close proximity to the hippocampi. The addition of memantine, an NMDA receptor antagonist, during the course of WBRT and up to 6 months afterward, has also led to prolonged time to cognitive decline.

The limitation of WBRT created an interest in studying treatment with more focused forms of radiotherapy, like stereotactic radiosurgery (SRS) or stereotactic radiotherapy (SRT), which consist of a single fraction of highly conformal, high-dose radiation (SRS), or multiple fractions of moderate doses of radiation (SRT). Multiple studies failed to identify a survival advantage to the combination of SRS and WBRT, or to WBRT, compared to SRS alone, despite improved local and distant brain recurrence rates. Thus, SRS alone is the preferred modality for patients with a limited number and small volume of BM, especially in older patients, and patients with progressive extracranial disease, as SRS is associated with less cognitive side effects and permits a more rapid transition to systemic therapies. Although SRS did not use to be an option in patients with more than 3 BM, more recent studies have shown comparable outcomes with SRS in patients up to 10 BM. WBRT is currently reserved for patients with numerous (>10) BM, or patients with diffuse symptomatic LM.

Historically, systemic therapies played little role in the direct treatment of BM, but rather for control of systemic disease. However, advances in immunotherapy and the development of targeted therapy agents that cross the blood-brain barrier have shifted this paradigm. In melanoma, the combination of the immune checkpoint inhibitors ipilimumab and nivolumab has been established as an efficient therapy of BM after significant CNS responses and clinical benefits and durable responses were observed in an open-label, phase 2 study. Results from the COMBI-MB trial of dabrafenib plus trametinib in $BRAF^{V600}$-mutant metastatic melanoma showed an intracranial response in up to 88% of patients. Although response occurred relatively quickly, there was limited benefit in progression-free survival.

Hence, this combination is used in symptomatic patients with $BRAF^{V600}$-mutant melanoma BM in need of a rapidly efficacious treatment. Other examples include EGFR inhibitors and ALK targeting agents in NSCLC. Osimertinib, a third-generation EGFR inhibitor has led to CNS response in up to 91% of patients with BM and LM from EGFR-mutant NSCLC, which translated into prolonged progression-free and overall survivals. Multiple agents targeting Her2, such as trastuzumab, and Her2 tyrosine kinase inhibitors, such as lapatinib, neratinib, and tucatinib, have been studied, alone or in combination with chemotherapy, in Her2-positive metastatic breast cancer, with CNS responses reaching 66% with some agents.

MENINGIOMAS

Meningiomas are the most common primary intracranial tumors in the United States, accounting for 39.7% of all primary CNS tumors according to 2015–19 data from the Central Brain Tumor Registry of the United States (CBTRUS). Around 35,000 new cases are diagnosed every year, and the estimated population prevalence is around 1 in every 100 adults aged 45 years or older. They are mostly benign, slow-growing neoplasms derived from the meningothelial cells of the arachnoid layer, although they can rarely occur within the ventricles or extracranial sites such as the lungs. Risk factors for their development include ionizing radiation and familial syndromes like neurofibromatosis type 2. The World Health Organization (WHO) classification scheme grades meningiomas as grade 1 to 3, based historically on mitotic rate and specific histological features. Grade 1 meningiomas, also called benign meningiomas, are the most common, accounting for 80% of all meningiomas, and carry a very favorable prognosis. On the other end of the spectrum, WHO grade 2 and 3 meningiomas are more aggressive and are associated with a 78% and 44% survival rate at 5 years, respectively. Specific molecular and genetic alterations have been recently identified to be associated with worse prognosis and higher risk of recurrence, even in low-grade meningiomas. Such alterations include CDKN2A/B loss, TERT promoter mutation, chromosome 1p loss, and loss of nuclear expression of H3K27me3. This has led to the inclusion of homozygous CDKN2A/B loss and TERT promoter mutation in allocating meningioma a grade 3, irrespective of the histological criteria of anaplasia.

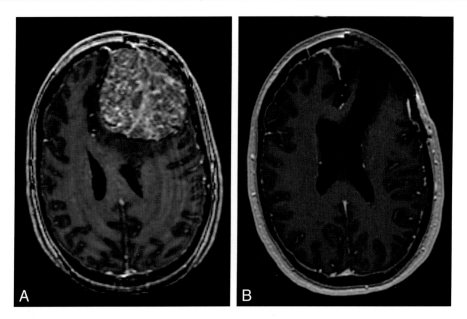

Fig. 8.3 A 24-year-old female, with no medical comorbidities, presented with progressive headaches awakening her from sleep, associated with recurrent nausea and vomiting, along with progressive loss of her vision. She was found to have a large extra-axial, dural-based, homogenously enhancing mass, in the left frontal lobe (A). She had a gross total resection of the mass, with pathology confirming anaplastic meningioma, WHO grade 3 (B). She was treated with adjuvant radiation.

Clinical Presentation and Diagnosis

Meningiomas may present with headaches, seizures, or focal neurological symptoms due to compression or invasion of adjacent structures. Oftentimes, they are incidentally found on neuroimaging. A radiographic diagnosis of meningioma can be suspected when there is evidence of a homogeneously enhancing, extra-axial, dural-based mass with a dural tail and CSF cleft (figure 8.3). Calcifications, hyperostosis, and overlying skull remodeling are often present. Peritumoral edema, heterogeneous enhancement, and intratumoral necrosis may suggest a higher-grade meningioma (i.e., WHO grade 2 or 3). The main differential diagnosis of dural-based lesions includes dural metastases, CNS lymphoma, hemangiopericytoma, sarcoidosis, or other inflammatory or infectious processes such as tuberculosis. In cases of diagnostic uncertainty or concern for high-grade features, biopsy or resection can establish the diagnosis.

New PET modalities have been developed to detect the expression of somatostatin receptor, which is expressed in 70% of meningiomas, using somatostatin analogs ^{68}Ga-DOTATATE and ^{90}Y-DOTATOC. These have not been implemented in the standard practice yet but can help distinguish tumor from healthy brain tissue and postoperative changes in challenging cases.

Oncological Management

Meningioma management depends on the presence of symptoms, the histologic grade of surgically resected meningiomas, and, for high-grade meningiomas, the extent of resection. Most incidental meningiomas can be safely managed with observation and serial brain MRIs until persistent radiologic or clinical progression, given their often slow or absent growth. In symptomatic patients, including those with tumor-associated headache, focal neurological deficits or seizures, or in patients with rapidly growing tumors, surgery is indicated for both therapeutic and diagnostic purposes. The extent of resection is an important prognostic factor, and is defined by the Simpson grade that ranges from complete resection of the enhancing mass, with dural and bone resection, to biopsy alone. SRS is an alternative to surgery for small tumors in elderly or critically ill patients.

Patients with grade 1 meningiomas can be observed, without adjuvant treatment, even if a gross total resection, defined by no residual enhancement on postoperative

MRI, has not been achieved. However, patients with grade 3 meningiomas, and those with partially resected grade 2 meningiomas require adjuvant radiotherapy, given the high risk of recurrence and high mortality rate.

Chemotherapy plays a limited role in the management of meningiomas, mostly as salvage therapy for refractory disease. Classical cytotoxic agents, including temozolomide, irinotecan, and hydroxyurea are not active. Recently identified promising agents include antiangiogenic compounds, such as bevacizumab and sunitinib, as vascular endothelial growth factor (VEGF) is often overexpressed in meningiomas. Somatostatin analogs and mTOR inhibitors have also been studied, given the strong and frequent expression of somatostatin receptors, and activation of the PI3K/AKT/mTOR pathway in meningiomas. However, all the listed agents have been evaluated in small patient cohorts, with varying outcomes, and are yet to be validated. Finally, pembrolizumab, an immune checkpoint inhibitor, has recently shown promising efficacy in recurrent high-grade meningiomas in a small phase 2 study, and various immune checkpoint inhibitors are currently explored in ongoing clinical trials.

GLIOMAS

Gliomas are the most common malignant tumors of the CNS and include astrocytomas, oligodendrogliomas, ependymomas, and a variety of rare histologies. Glioblastoma (GBM), a grade 4 glioma, is the most common and, unfortunately, the most aggressive subtype (Fig. 8.4). GBM makes up 14.2% of all primary CNS tumors and 50.1% of all malignant CNS tumors, with an age-adjusted incidence in the United States of 3.22 per 100,000 persons. The second most common gliomas are astrocytomas and oligodendrogliomas. While the classification and grade determination were mainly based on histology, the 2021 WHO classification of CNS tumors categorizes gliomas mainly on molecular basis. Astrocytomas and oligodendrogliomas are characterized by a mutation in the isocitrate dehydrogenase (IDH) gene, in contrast to GBM where IDH is wild type. The only recognized risk factor for the development of gliomas is prior ionizing radiation exposure to the head and neck area, while a history of atopic disorders (i.e., allergies, asthma, eczema, hay fever) can be a protective factor.

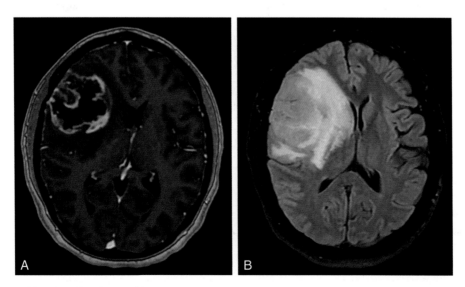

Fig. 8.4 A 55-year-old male, with history of hypertension, presented with 1 week of left facial droop, dysphagia, and dysarthria. He had a brain magnetic resonance imaging that showed a left frontal heterogeneously enhancing mass with central necrosis (A). The mass was surrounded by significant vasogenic edema, causing a mass effect on the adjacent brain parenchyma and left lateral ventricle (B). The mass was resected, and pathology was consistent with glioblastoma, O⁶-methylguanine-DNA methyltransferase promoter methylated. He was treated with radiation and concurrent temozolomide, followed by six cycles of adjuvant temozolomide, and is currently on observation.

Glioblastoma

Clinical Presentation and Diagnosis

As with BM and meningioma, GBM may present with headaches, seizures, or focal neurological symptoms. Due to the aggressive nature of the disease, symptoms may develop rapidly within the course of weeks. Brain MRI with and without contrast is the modality of choice for neuroimaging. The appearance can vary, but most often shows a supratentorial, heterogeneously enhancing mass with central necrosis and surrounding nonenhancing white matter signal that may be due to edema or infiltrating tumor (Fig. 8.4). Hemorrhage, cystic changes, and multicentric enhancement are frequently present.

Diagnosis requires pathological confirmation, in the form of a biopsy or surgical resection. A hypercellular tumor with severe atypia, necrosis, and microvascular proliferation are hallmarks for a grade 4 glioma. In the absence of grade 4 pathologic features in an IDH wild-type astrocytoma, such as necrosis and microvascular proliferation, effort should be made to identify the presence of EGFR amplification, and/or TERT promoter mutation, and/or gain of chromosome 7 combined with loss of chromosome 10, which establishes the diagnosis of GBM.

O^6-Methylguanine-DNA methyltransferase (MGMT) promoter methylation status is another important molecular marker in glioblastoma. The MGMT protein reverses alkylation of DNA, induced by alkylating chemotherapy agents, at guanine sites, and silencing of the MGMT promoter via DNA methylation results in its decreased expression. MGMT promoter methylation is reported in 30% to 40% of GBM and is associated with prolonged overall and progression-free survival, and better tumor response in patients treated with an alkylating agent.

Oncological Management

Management of GBM includes a combination of neurosurgery, radiotherapy, and chemotherapy. Referral to an experienced brain tumor neurosurgeon for maximum safe resection is imperative, as the extent of resection impacts survival. Gross total resection of the enhancing mass is associated with prolonged survival, and recent studies showed extended survival with a supramaximal resection including the enhancing mass and the surrounding nonenhancing disease. However, radical microsurgical resection is often limited by the invasive nature of the tumor and involvement of eloquent cortex. In the latter situation, a functional brain MRI can help optimize the surgical plan and achieve a maximal safe resection.

In 2005 Stupp et al. reported on the results of the European Organisation for Research and Treatment of Cancer (EORTC) and National Cancer Institute of Canada Clinical Trials Group (NCIC) trial and established the current standard of care for postoperative management of newly diagnosed glioblastoma. This consists of 6 weeks of focal irradiation (60 Gy divided into 2 Gy fractions per day, over the course of 6 weeks) with concurrent daily temozolomide, an alkylating agent, followed by six cycles of monthly adjuvant temozolomide. The regimen resulted in a median overall survival of 14.6 months, compared to 12.1 months for GBM patients treated with radiation alone. The 5-year analysis of the EORTC-NCIC trial confirmed that the greatest benefit of adding temozolomide was seen in those with MGMT promoter methylation. Although a prolonged (>6 cycles) treatment with adjuvant temozolomide has been suggested in patients with MGMT promoter methylated tumors, it has not been associated with improved progression-free or overall survival. No additional survival benefit has been reported with more frequent, daily dosing, of adjuvant temozolomide either. In select patients with MGMT promoter methylated GBM, the combination of temozolomide and lomustine, another alkylating agent, in the concurrent and adjuvant settings, was associated with improved overall survival compared to temozolomide alone in a randomized phase 3 trial. However, the sample size of patients was small in each treatment arm, and the effect was small in a univariate analysis.

Elderly patients usually have a worse prognosis and are less tolerant of radiation toxicity. A hypofractionated course of radiation (such as 34 Gy over 2 weeks, or 40 Gy over 3 weeks) can be considered and has shown to be noninferior to the standard 60 Gy radiation. Although no randomized study compares standard radiation plus temozolomide with hypofractionated radiation plus temozolomide, a phase 3, randomized study of patients 65 years and older with a newly diagnosed GBM and good performance status demonstrated increased survival with hypofractionated radiation plus temozolomide compared to hypofractionated radiation alone, especially in patients with MGMT promoter methylated tumors. For patients in whom combined chemoradiation may not be tolerated (due to comorbid conditions, poor functional status, patient preference, etc.), temozolomide monotherapy can be a reasonable treatment for those with MGMT promoter methylated tumors, whereas hypofractionated radiation therapy is a viable option for those with unmethylated tumors. This also applies to patients with immunosuppressive conditions.

Tumor treating fields (TTF) are also a standard-of-care option for glioblastoma. This modality consists of a portable device that provides low-intensity, intermediate-frequency, alternating electric field therapy, and disrupts mitoses selectively in dividing tumor cells. It is applied in the adjuvant setting, in addition to monthly temozolomide, and its daily application for more than 18 hours a day was associated with prolonged progression-free survival and overall survival compared to adjuvant temozolomide alone in a randomized clinical trial.

There is no standard of care for the treatment of recurrent glioblastoma. Options include neurosurgery for resectable recurrent disease, reirradiation (especially if the recurrence is distal from the original tumor), and/or systemic therapies such as temozolomide, lomustine, and bevacizumab. Bevacizumab is humanized VEGF antibody that is not associated with survival benefit but helps with improvement of peritumoral edema and control of related clinical symptoms. The combination of dabrafenib (BRAF inhibitor) and trametinib (MEK inhibitor) was associated with an overall response rate of 32% in patients with recurrent BRAF-mutant GBM in a phase 2, single-arm, study. Ongoing clinical trials are evaluating various targeted therapies, immunotherapies, newer chemotherapy agents, and other treatment modalities, and are encouraged by the NCCN guidelines.

Isocitrate Dehydrogenase–Mutant Gliomas

The IDH mutation was first incorporated in the classification of gliomas in the 2016 WHO classification of CNS tumors, and additional molecular alterations were identified to define the type and grade of IDH-mutant gliomas in the 2021 WHO classification of CNS tumors. The majority of IDH-mutant gliomas harbor a heterozygous point mutation in the IDH1 gene consisting of arginine-to-histidine substitution at codon 132 (R132H), although other point mutations in the IDH1 and IDH2 genes have also been reported. The presence of concomitant codeletion of the short arm of chromosome

1 and long arm of chromosome 19 (1p/19q codel), resulting from an unbalanced translocation between the two chromosomes, is required for the diagnosis of oligodendrogliomas, whereas astrocytomas lack the 1p/19q codeletion. Oligodendrogliomas are classified into WHO grade 2 and 3, the latter consisting of higher rates of cellular proliferation, vascular proliferation, and necrosis. Astrocytomas in adults can be of WHO grade 2, 3, or 4—a grade 3 tumor is histologically distinguished from grade 2 by increased cellular proliferation and pleomorphia, whereas a grade 4 tumor has the histological features of GBM. In addition, a homozygous deletion of CDKN2A/B gene automatically upgrades the tumor to an astrocytoma, IDH-mutant, WHO grade 4, as such deletion has been associated with significantly worse outcomes.

Besides prior exposure to ionizing radiation, risk factors for the development of IDH-mutant gliomas are poorly understood. IDH-mutant constitute about 4.4% among all CNS tumors, with an incidence rate of 0.25 per 100,000 for oligodendrogliomas, and 0.44 per 100,000 population for astrocytomas.

Clinical Presentation and Diagnosis

Most patients, particularly those with oligodendrogliomas, present with focal seizures, while about 30% of patients present with focal motor or sensory deficits. Given the slow-growing nature of these tumors, symptoms develop over the course of months before a diagnosis is established. On brain MRI, IDH-mutant gliomas appear as expansile, T2/fluid-attenuated inversion recovery (FLAIR) hyperintense lesions commonly located in the frontal lobes. Enhancement is rarely seen with grade 2 tumors, whereas grade 3 and 4 tumors can be partially enhancing. Cortical involvement and the presence of calcifications on susceptibility-weighted images (SWI) sequences are more characteristic of oligodendrogliomas. On the other hand, a T2/FLAIR mismatch sign, where a homogenous hyperintense signal on T2 sequence is countered with suppression of FLAIR signal in the lesion core compared to the rim, is highly specific for astrocytomas (Fig. 8.5).

Pathological confirmation, immunohistochemistry and other molecular testing are required for diagnosis. MGMT promoter methylation is present in about 85% of astrocytoma and 98% of oligodendrogliomas, but its clinical implications and associated response to alkylating agents have not been as clearly established as with GBM.

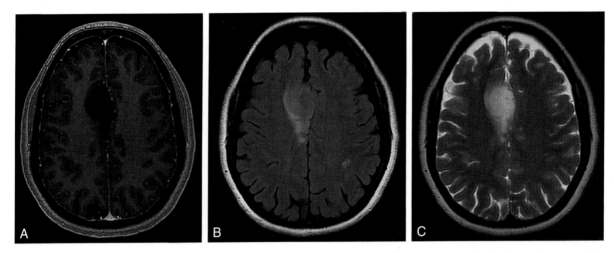

Fig. 8.5 A 53-year-old female, with no medical comorbidities, presented with an acute transient episode of numbness involving her left arm and leg. She had a brain MRI that showed an expansile, nonenhancing mass (A), with an apparent T2/fluid-attenuated inversion recovery mismatch (B and C). She had subtotal resection of the mass, and pathology was consistent with astrocytoma, IDH-mutant, WHO grade 3, without CDKN2A loss. She was treated with radiation followed by 12 cycles of adjuvant temozolomide. She is currently on observation.

Oncological Management

Surgical resection is recommended for diagnostic and therapeutic purposes. More extensive resection is associated with improved survival and improved seizure control. Gross total resection of the entire enhancing and nonenhancing disease is recommended if it can be performed safely, but recent data have suggested survival benefit for supramaximal resection (i.e., resection beyond the tumor margins). A follow-up brain MRI 1 to 2 months after the surgical resection allows for an accurate assessment of the extent of resection after resolution of the surgery-induced changes that might look similar to tumor on MRI.

Postoperative treatment varies by the tumor grade, extent of resection, age, and neurologic status of the patient. Young (<40 years old), asymptomatic patients, with a totally resected WHO grade 2 tumor, are considered low-risk patients and can be observed after surgery, without any further tumor-directed therapy. Otherwise, the remaining patients with WHO grade 2 tumors, and all patients with WHO grade 3 and 4 tumors should receive radiation and chemotherapy.

The treatment of WHO grade 2 gliomas is based on the NRG Oncology/RTOG 9802 study, where treatment with radiation followed by PCV chemotherapy regimen (procarbazine, lomustine, vincristine) was associated with improved survival compared to radiation alone.

The combination of radiation and PCV was also superior to radiation alone in WHO grade 3 tumors, regardless of the chronology of treatment (i.e., radiation followed by chemotherapy in EORTC 26951 study, or vice versa in RTOG 9402 study). In WHO grade 3 astrocytomas, radiation followed by adjuvant temozolomide was superior to radiation alone, and to radiation with concurrent temozolomide with or without adjuvant temozolomide in the CATNON study. Based on these data, the current recommended standard of care for high-risk WHO grade 2 tumors and for WHO grade 3 tumors consists of radiation followed by chemotherapy. The radiation dose is 45 to 54 Gy in WHO grade 2 tumors, and 59.4 to 60 Gy in WHO grade 3 tumors. Adjuvant chemotherapy options include six cycles of PCV or 12 cycles of temozolomide. No randomized trials have compared the two chemotherapy regimens, and the decision of using either regimen varies by institution, and is driven by the 1p/19q codeletion status for many, with PCV favored for IDH-mutant, 1p/19q-codeleted oligodendrogliomas, and temozolomide favored for IDH-mutant, 1p/19q noncodeleted astrocytomas, although temozolomide is a reasonable option for oligodendrogliomas as well. An ongoing CODEL study is evaluating differences in progression-free and overall survival between temozolomide and PCV following radiation in high-risk WHO grade 2 oligodendroglioma and WHO grade 3 oligodendrogliomas.

IDH inhibitors are newly developed agents that selectively inhibit IDH-mutant enzymes, and have been studied in treatment-naïve patients and patients with recurrent nonenhancing WHO grade 2 gliomas. Ivosidenib is an IDH1 inhibitor, approved for the treatment of subsets of acute myeloid leukemia and cholangiocarcinoma, and vorasidenib is a dual inhibitor of IDH1 and IDH2, designed for improved blood-brain barrier penetrance. Both have achieved antitumor activity in IDH-mutant gliomas, but vorasidenib had a better brain penetrance and achieved a more consistent inhibition of the mutant IDH enzyme. The efficacy of vorasidenib in increasing PFS and time-to-next-intervention was recently demonstrated in a phase 3, randomized, placebo-controlled, study in treatment-naïve patients with mainly nonenhancing, WHO grade 2, IDH-mutant gliomas, who had only received surgical resection as prior tumor-directed therapy. This positive study suggests a new treatment approach for newly diagnosed nonenhancing IDH-mutant gliomas, WHO grade 2.

Astrocytoma, IDH-mutant, WHO grade 4, is a new entity that was introduced in the 2021 WHO classification of CNS tumors. There are no available data that specifically address patients with such tumor. However, the current recommendation is extrapolated from GBM treatment, consisting of radiation with concurrent temozolomide followed by 6 cycles of adjuvant monthly temozolomide.

There is no standard of care treatment for progressive or recurrent IDH-mutant gliomas. As for GBM, options include neurosurgery, reirradiation, rechallenge with chemotherapy (temozolomide, lomustine, PCV), and/or bevacizumab. Novel perspectives, currently evaluated alone or in combination with chemotherapy or IDH inhibitors, include poly(ADP-ribose) polymerase inhibitors (PARPi), demethylating agents, IDH vaccine, and other immunotherapies.

MEDICAL COMPLICATIONS IN BRAIN TUMOR PATIENTS

The diagnosis of CNS tumors carries a high risk of medical and neurologic complications that develop as a direct effect from the tumor, or from its treatment (table 8.2). Management of these complications by primary care providers and internists can significantly improve the quality of life of life and potentially impact patients' survival.

Tumor-Related Epilepsy

Seizures affect up to 70% of patients with brain tumors and are the presenting symptom in up to 40%. The incidence is the lowest in CNS lymphoma and LM, and the highest in low-grade tumors, including IDH-mutant gliomas. This may be related to the more common cortical location and longer survival observed with IDH-mutant gliomas. IDH mutation also increases the production of 2-hydroxyglutarate, which structurally resembles glutamate, a potent excitatory neurotransmitter.

Despite the high risk of seizure development in patients with CNS tumors, there is no benefit from primary prophylaxis with antiseizure medications (ASM) in seizure-free patients, and the use of ASM should be limited to 1 to 2 weeks in the postoperative setting, as advised by a recent practice guideline update from the Society of Neuro-Oncology (SNO) and European Association of Neuro-Oncology (EANO).

There are no studies favoring specific ASM in brain tumor patients, and the choice of ASM should be individualized based on the type of seizures, medical comorbidities, toxicity profiles of the ASM, and concomitant therapies. Enzyme-inducing ASM should be avoided as they would interact with certain chemotherapy regimens. Levetiracetam is the most widely used ASM, due to its ease of use, limited to no interactions with other drugs, and its well-tolerated adverse event profile. Other nonenzyme-enhancing ASM options include lacosamide, lamotrigine, and valproate. Perampanel is a highly selective α-amino-3-hydroxy-5-methyl-4-isoxazolepropionic acid (AMPA) receptor antagonist, and might be theoretically effective in disrupting established glioma-neuron synapses in gliomas, leading to antitumor effect, in addition to seizure control; however, such benefit is yet to be validated.

Peritumoral Edema

Disruption of the blood-brain barrier is common with CNS tumors, causing extravasation of plasma fluids and proteins and subsequent vasogenic edema, increased intracranial pressure, and neurologic morbidity. Vasogenic edema is typically managed with corticosteroids. Dexamethasone is the preferred steroid given its potent glucocorticoid, antiinflammatory effect, lack of mineralocorticoid activity, and long half-life. It can be administered daily or twice daily, and the dose and duration of treatment should rely on the clinical symptoms rather than the radiographic extent of edema. An expert panel in 2019 from American Society of Clinical Oncology (ASCO) and

TABLE 8.2 **Workup and Management of Common Medical Complications in Brain Tumor Patients**

Complication	Clinical Presentation	Diagnosis	Management
Cerebral edema	Worsening of neurologic deficits arising from culprit brain mass Significant increases in cerebral edema can cause increased ICP and present as somnolence, confusion, headaches, nausea, vomiting, etc.	Clinical diagnosis Cerebral edema is visible on brain imaging (either head CT or brain MRI)	Corticosteroids (preferably dexamethasone) Treatment should be based on symptoms, not imaging
Endocrinopathies	Diabetes mellitus from high doses of steroids SIADH: encephalopathy, seizures, worsening focal neurologic symptoms Hypothalamus-hypophysis-adrenal axis deficits: in patients whose radiation field involves the hypothalamus and pituitary gland	High serum glucose levels Low serum sodium Standard laboratory testing for endocrinopathies based on symptoms, such as TSH, cortisol, testosterone, FSH, LH, and GH	Correction of hyperglycemia and hyponatremia Hormone replacement based on the endocrinopathy
Fatigue	Patient self-reported	Evaluation for treatable causes of fatigue, such as medications, depression, sleep disturbance, anemia, nutritional deficiencies, alcohol/substance abuse, and endocrinopathies	Limited data on beneficial interventions Reported benefit from exercise and corticosteroids Studies of psychostimulants (methylphenidate, modafinil, armodafinil) in brain tumor patients have failed to show significant benefit
Mood and other psychiatric disorders, including depression	Patient self-reported depression or reported by caregiver Psychosis, mania or irritability secondary to steroid use	Clinical diagnosis	Antidepressants or mood stabilizers (preferably ones that do not decrease the seizure threshold) Steroid wean

Neurocognitive Impairment	May be a presenting symptom or due to tumor growth. Can be seen after radiation, particularly after WBRT. Can also be seen in patients with long history of multiple chemotherapy regimens	Clinical diagnosis. Screening tests (MOCA, MMSE). Neuropsychological evaluation	Cognitive behavioral therapy, cognitive rehabilitation. Occupational and speech therapy. Modest benefit with donepezil. Prophylactic memantine for patients undergoing WBRT
Seizures	Depends on type of seizure (focal versus generalized) and location of the seizure nidus	Clinical diagnosis based on description of event. EEG is often not required	Antiepileptic drug (preferably nonenzyme-inducing agent)
Venous thromboembolism	DVT involving the leg typically presents with unilateral calf pain/tenderness and/or leg swelling. PE can present with shortness of breath, chest pain, and/or tachycardia	Venous ultrasonography. Chest CT angiogram with contrast	Management is guided by safety of anticoagulation. Anticoagulation is preferred treatment, but may be contraindicated in patients with active intracranial bleed or hemorrhagic brain tumors. DOAC and LMWH are safe and better than VKA

CT, Computed tomography; *DOAC*, direct oral anticoagulants; *DVT*, deep venous thrombosis *EEG*, electroencephalogram; *FSH*, follicle-stimulating hormone; *GH*, growth hormone; *LH*, luteinizing hormone; *LMWH*, low-molecular-weight heparin; *MMSE*, minimental status examination; *MOCA*, Montreal cognitive assessment; *MRI*, magnetic resonance imaging; *PE*, pulmonary embolism; *SIADH*, syndrome of inappropriate diuretic hormone; *TSH*, thyroid-stimulating hormone; *VKA*, vitamin K antagonists; *WBRT*, whole-brain radiation.

SNO recommended a starting dose of 4 to 8 mg for mild symptoms and 16 mg for moderate to severe symptoms. The main side effects of steroids include weight gain, irritability, insomnia, tremors, gastritis, and myopathy. Their prolonged use also increases the risk of osteoporosis and infections. Therefore the lowest clinically effective dose should be used, followed by a gradual taper, every 3 to 5 days over the course of 2 to 4 weeks, once clinical improvement is observed and maintained. In patients who need high doses of steroids for prolonged duration, or those who do not respond to steroids, alternative therapies like bevacizumab should be considered.

Infectious Complications

Treatment with radiation, chemotherapy, and steroids often leads to immunosuppression and increased risk of acquired infections. *Pneumocystis jirovecii* pneumonia (PJP) is a rare, but potentially fatal infection that may develop in lymphopenic patients in the setting of chemotherapy and prolonged steroid use. It can also be a complication in patients with GBM receiving radiation with concurrent temozolomide. Although PJP prophylaxis used to be recommended in patients during such treatment, recent emerging data did not find significant adjusted absolute reduction in PJP or survival benefit with prophylaxis in areas where PJP is rare like the US or Canada. However, PJP prophylaxis with trimethoprim-sulfamethoxazole is recommended in patients on steroid dose equivalent to dexamethasone 4 mg or greater for more than 4 weeks.

Immunosuppression also increases the risk of *Candida* infections, the most common manifestation of which is oropharyngeal candidiasis. Local treatment with nystatin, clotrimazole, or miconazole is recommended. Systemic antifungal agents are reserved for resistant or severe cases.

Venous Thromboembolism

Venous thromboembolism (VTE), including deep vein thrombosis and pulmonary embolism, is common in cancer, particularly with GBM, with an incidence of 20% to 30%, and is associated with a shorter survival. The risk is particularly increased in the postoperative period, and with age, body weight, tumor grade, and hemiparesis, as well as with larger residual tumor size. Vitamin K antagonists are not recommended due to their limited benefit in preventing recurrent VTE events, increased risk of intracranial bleed, and potential interactions with concomitant drugs. Treatment with low-molecular-weight heparin (LMWH) or direct oral anticoagulants (DOAC) is preferred. While concerns of increased risk of intracranial bleeding were initially raised with DOAC, recent data suggest very few intracranial hemorrhagic events, with a lower incidence to that of LMWH. Given the persistent risk of recurrent VTE, lifelong secondary thromboprophylaxis is needed. In patients with a recent or active intracranial or intratumoral hemorrhage, or other medical contraindications for pharmacological anticoagulation, inferior vena cava filters should be considered.

CONCLUSION

The prevalence of brain tumors and their complications is expected to rise with the diagnostic and therapeutic advances. Their management requires a multidisciplinary approach with the involvement of neurooncologists, medical oncologists, brain tumor surgeons, radiation oncologists, and vascular medicine specialists. Primary care providers and internists should be acquainted with their basic management, as they are at the forefront of diagnosis, care coordination, and management of complications.

"For the full bibliography list, please use the pincode on the inside front cover to access the electronic version of the text at ebooks.health.elsevier.com."

9

Infections of the Nervous System*

G. Kyle Harrold

INTRODUCTION

There are a seemingly insurmountable number of infections that can affect the nervous system. However, as in all areas of neurology, the principles of a neurologic history and exam are essential to diagnosis. Focusing on the localization of the syndrome and the patient's infectious risk factors (e.g., travel history, animal exposures, occupational exposures, immune status) narrows the differential diagnosis sufficiently to make infections of the nervous system approachable. This chapter highlights common infections of the nervous system, "do-not-miss" infections of the nervous system, and infections that are more prevalent in patients who are immunocompromised but is far from a comprehensive list of all possible nervous system infections.

CENTRAL NERVOUS SYSTEM

Meningitis

Meningitis refers to inflammation of either the pachymeninges (dura mater) or leptomeninges (pia mater and arachnoid) with infectious meningitis typically predominantly affecting the leptomeninges. Multiple types of organisms can cause meningitis and the spectrum of meningitis can range from a true neurologic emergency (bacterial meningitis) to a relatively mild presentation (some cases of viral meningitis).

*Based on Levin SN, Lyons JL. Infections of the nervous system. *Am J Med*. 2018;131(1):25–32. ISSN 0002-9343. https://doi.org/10.1016/j.amjmed.2017.08.020.

Bacterial Meningitis

The most feared type of meningitis, and perhaps most feared neurologic infection, is bacterial meningitis. Bacterial meningitis in the pre–antibiotic era had a mortality rate approaching 100%, but even in the modern era mortality from *Streptococcus pneumoniae* remains as high as 30%. Because mortality is so high, prompt recognition and initiation of treatment is vital. The classic triad of fever, neck stiffness, and altered mental status has been shown to be relatively insensitive, occurring in 41%–44% of patients, although having two of either fever, neck stiffness, altered mental status, or headache has been shown to have a sensitivity as high as 95%. Bacterial meningitis should be considered in any patient with at least two or more of those symptoms.

All patients suspected of having meningitis should have blood cultures drawn and undergo urgent lumbar puncture for CSF analysis to evaluate for meningitis and to attempt to isolate the causative organism. Lumbar puncture should only be delayed to obtain imaging (head CT without contrast) in the subset of patients at risk of herniation: those who are immunocompromised, have a history of mass lesion in the brain (e.g., tumor, stroke, focal infection), have new-onset seizures, have papilledema on examination, have an abnormal level of consciousness, or have a focal neurologic deficit. Opening pressure should be measured and CSF should be sent for cell count with differential, protein, glucose, gram stain, and culture at minimum. Multiplex PCR has also become increasingly available with high sensitivity and specificity for common organisms (including *Neisseria meningitides*, *S. pneumoniae*, *Haemophilus influenzae*) and the added benefit of rapid turnaround time. Cerebrospinal fluid values can be variable, but generally in bacterial meningitis the nucleated cell count is often >1000 cells/μL with a neutrophil predominance of ≥80%, protein is often elevated >200 mg/dL, and glucose is often decreased <40 mg/dL with a CSF to serum glucose ratio of ≤0.4.

Prompt initiation of treatment is crucial as soon as bacterial meningitis is suspected. Lumbar puncture should ideally be performed prior to antibiotic administration so as to not decrease the yield of the CSF culture, but antibiotics should not be delayed if lumbar puncture cannot be performed immediately. Empiric antibiotics should include a third-generation cephalosporin to cover for *Streptococcus* species, *N. meningitides*, and *H. influenzae*, the three most common causative organisms for community-acquired bacterial meningitis, as well as vancomycin to cover for cephalosporin-resistant *S. pneumoniae*. Ampicillin should be added to cover for *Listeria monocytogenes* in neonates, adults over age 50, and those who are otherwise immunocompromised. Antimicrobial therapy should be tailored based on Gram stain, culture, and/or PCR results.

In addition to antibiotics, patients suspected of having bacterial meningitis should be treated with dexamethasone *concurrently* with antibiotics based on data showing both a mortality benefit among patients with *S. pneumoniae* and a lower rate of hearing loss. Dexamethasone should only be continued if *S. pneumoniae* is found to be the causative organism, as dexamethasone was not found to be as beneficial in meningitis caused by other organisms. Dexamethasone should not be started *after* antibiotics have already been given, as this timing has been associated with worse outcomes.

Patients with bacterial meningitis are at risk for numerous complications and often require an ICU level of care with a multidisciplinary team including infectious disease, neurology, and neurosurgery. Neurologic complications to monitor for include increased intracranial pressure (from cerebral edema and/or hydrocephalus), seizure, ischemic stroke, venous sinus thrombosis, and subdural empyema. Patients who survive bacterial meningitis may be left with a spectrum of neurologic sequela including cognitive impairment, cranial neuropathies, hearing loss, and paresis.

In addition to meningitis, *Listeria* can additionally lead to a rhombencephalitis in 17% of cases, with progressive cranial nerve palsies, cerebellar signs, weakness, and decreased level of arousal. Development of abscess from *Listeria* is uncommon but does occur.

Viral Meningitis

Viruses are the most common cause of "aseptic" meningitis, which would be more accurately called nonbacterial meningitis. Viral meningitides tend to be much less severe than bacterial meningitis and are often self-limited. The typical presentation includes a combination of headache, neck stiffness, and/or photophobia.

All patients presenting with concern for viral meningitis should undergo lumbar puncture as there are no specific clinical features for viral meningitis, and it is prudent to rule out other causes, specifically bacterial meningitis. Typical CSF findings include moderate lymphocytic pleocytosis (in the range of 100–1000 cells/μL; may be neutrophilic early in the course), moderately elevated total protein (in the range of 100–1000 mg/dL), and normal or only mildly reduced glucose, although wide variations may be seen for each of these.

The most common causative viruses include enteroviruses, herpes simplex virus–2 (HSV-2), varicella zoster virus (VZV), and arboviruses. PCR testing for enteroviruses, HSV, and VZV are routinely available and should be performed. Multiplex PCR is also available but may be less sensitive and specific than the individual PCR tests so should be used cautiously. Primary infection with HIV can also present as a self-limited meningitis and can present before antibodies are present. Patients with risk factors for HIV infection should have HIV serum viral load tested.

Most causes of viral meningitis do not have specific treatments and self-resolve with supportive care. Patients with HSV or VZV meningitis should be treated with IV acyclovir, which can be transitioned to oral valacyclovir. There is stronger evidence to support treatment in immunocompromised patients, although the risk/benefit ratio is likely also favorable for immunocompetent patients. HSV-2 can cause a recurrent lymphocytic meningitis (Mollaret meningitis) characterized by repeated, self-limited attacks of meningitis. Suppressive valacyclovir is often used although one small randomized trial did not find a benefit and showed a higher risk of recurrence after stopping valacyclovir.

Fungal Meningitis

Yeast and fungi can cause a more indolent meningitis, typically presenting with days to weeks of meningismus and signs of intracranial pressure such as fever, headache, neck stiffness, photophobia, malaise, vomiting, and cranial nerve palsies. Cryptococcosis is the most common cause of fungal meningitis, although the endemic dimorphic fungi can also cause meningitis.

Cryptococcosis most commonly occurs in patients who are immunocompromised, with HIV/AIDS being the predominant risk factor, though patients without any known immunodeficiency can also develop cryptococcal meningitis. Typical CSF findings include lymphocytic pleocytosis, normal to elevated protein levels, low glucose, and elevated opening pressure, although the nucleated cell count and protein may be normal in patients with HIV. Culture is insensitive; diagnosis is typically made via testing the CSF for cryptococcal antigen. Treatment follows an induction, consolidation, maintenance paradigm (typically with amphotericin B and flucytosine followed by fluconazole) and should be done with infectious disease consultation. Patients are at high risk for elevated intracranial pressure and may require serial lumbar punctures or CSF diversion (e.g., ventriculoperitoneal shunt or lumbar drain).

Histoplasmosis, blastomycosis, and coccidiomycosis can each additionally present with meningitis within their respective geographic territories. These dimorphic fungi can additionally present with mass lesions and can cause a basilar meningitis and/or vasculitis leading to infarcts. Treatment typically involves at least 12 months of an antifungal agent.

Encephalitis

Encephalitis refers to inflammation of the brain parenchyma itself and is typically infectious or autoimmune in etiology. Infectious and autoimmune encephalitis can be very difficult to distinguish clinically. Fever, prominent findings on MRI, and/or marked CSF abnormalities may be a clue to an infectious rather than autoimmune etiology. Most infectious causes of encephalitis are viral, although in 60%–70% of viral encephalitides no virus is identified.

HSV Encephalitis

HSV is the most common cause of infectious encephalitis, accounting for 35%–55% of infections with an identified organism. Over 90% of HSV encephalitis (HSVE) results from HSV-1 with less than 10% from HSV-2, which is more associated with meningitis. HSVE is thought to result both from primary infection with

entry through the nose leading to infection of olfactory bulb neurons and retrograde spread to the mesial temporal lobes as well as from reactivation of latent virus in the trigeminal ganglia. HSVE typically presents with altered mental status, fever, headache, focal neurologic deficits, and/or seizures which develop over days. Focal neurologic deficits may include aphasia, apraxia, memory impairment, visual field impairment, cranial nerve deficits, hemiparesis, and/or ataxia.

Diagnosis of HSVE was historically made via brain biopsy, but in the current era is almost exclusively made by CSF PCR. All patients suspected of having HSVE should undergo lumbar puncture to evaluate for the HSV PCR, which is extremely sensitive and specific for HSVE. However, some experts have suggested that false negatives are more likely when the lumbar puncture is performed within 72 hours of symptom onset, in which case a repeat lumbar puncture should be performed. Additionally, the sensitivity of the HSV PCR decreases with time, to as low as 30% from 11 to 20 days after symptom onset and 19% from 21 to 40 days after symptom onset. CSF HSV antibodies are generally not useful and should not be sent in the acute setting. There are rare instances where they may be useful to make a delayed or retrospective diagnosis. General examination of the CSF typically shows a lymphocytic pleocytosis (which may be neutrophilic early in the course of the infection) of 10–500 cells/μL, red blood cells of 10–500 cells/μL, elevation in total protein that may be mild or in the 100s of mg/dL, and may show mild hypoglycorrhachia. MRI typically shows T2 and/or diffusion-weighted imaging (DWI) changes in the temporal lobes early in the course of the infection which may extend into other lobes of the brain (Fig. 9.1).

All patients suspected of having HSVE should be started on IV acyclovir as soon as the diagnosis is suspected. Delay in treatment initiation is the only modifiable risk factor shown to affect prognosis. There is no need to wait for lumbar puncture as starting acyclovir should not meaningfully affect the sensitivity of HSV PCR in the short term. Treatment is with IV acyclovir at a dose of 10 mg/kg (which may need to be adjusted for renal insufficiency) every 8 hours for 14–21 days. Even with treatment HSVE has a mortality rate between 6% and 15% and moderate to severe morbidity including cognitive deficits, aphasia, seizures, and/or weakness in 32–56%. Recently, it has become clear that as many as 27% of patients with HSVE will develop a secondary

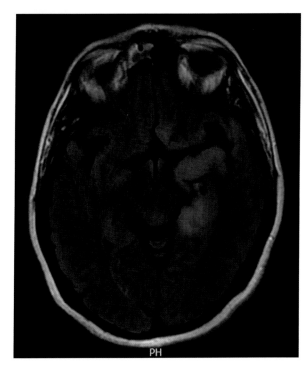

Fig. 9.1 Herpes simplex virus (HSV) encephalitis. Brain magnetic resonance imaging of a patient who presented with memory impairment, headaches, and fevers. Axial T2 fluid-attenuated inversion recovery imaging shows left hemispheric hyperintensity in the anterior and medial temporal lobe and mass effect approaching the midbrain. HSV DNA was detected in the cerebrospinal fluid by polymerase chain reaction. (From Levin SN, Lyons JL. Infections of the nervous system. *Am J Med.* 2018;131(1):25–32.)

autoimmune encephalitis, most commonly with positive NMDA receptor antibodies, within 2 months of their treatment for HSVE. These patients should be treated with immunotherapy as would any other patient with autoimmune encephalitis.

Arboviral Encephalitis

Arboviruses refer to viruses spread through the bite of an arthropod, typically a tick or mosquito. In the United States, the most common arboviral infection is West Nile Virus (WNV), which is transmitted via the bite of the *Culex* mosquito, with birds as the amplifying host. It has been reported in all 50 US states with almost 28,000 neuroinvasive cases reported through 2021. WNV leads to an asymptomatic infection in most people, a febrile illness in approximately 25%, and neuroinvasive disease

(encephalitis) in less than 1%. Among those who develop neuroinvasive disease, three syndromes are most common: meningitis, encephalitis, and acute flaccid paralysis, which can develop in isolation or in combination. Testing for WNV is via IgM in the serum and/or CSF. PCR-based testing has limited utility as the viremia generally clears early in the course of the infection. Among the almost 28,000 neuroinvasive cases reported through 2021, the mortality rate was 9%.

Powassan virus is an emerging tick-borne virus in the northern and northeastern US with cases also reported in Canada and Russia. Powassan is carried by the same tick, *Ixodes scapularis*, as Lyme disease but can be transmitted in as little as 15 minutes from time of tick attachment. In the United States, 189 neuroinvasive cases have been reported as of 2021 with a mortality rate of 13%. Powassan encephalitis can present with fever, encephalopathy, decreased level of arousal, seizures, and focal neurological deficits. Diagnosis is via IgM from the serum and/or CSF. Historically this has only been available in the United States through the CDC, but has recently become available through other clinical labs. PCR testing should be reserved for patients who would not be expected to mount an antibody response (e.g., those receiving anti-CD20 therapies like rituximab).

Other arboviral infections include Eastern Equine Encephalitis (EEE), which is rare (46 cases reported in the United States from 2012 to 2021), but has a mortality rate over 40%; La Crosse virus; and St. Louis encephalitis, although others also exist. Imaging in arboviral infections can be variable, although many patients will have symmetric deep T2-hyperintense lesions (i.e., T2 hyperintensity of the basal ganglia). No specific treatments beyond supportive care have been proven to be effective for any of the arboviral encephalitides.

Brain Abscesses

Infectious abscesses are typically bacterial, although other types of organisms, such as fungi and toxoplasma, can also form abscesses. Bacterial abscesses arise from contiguous sites of infection (i.e., otitis, mastoiditis, or sinusitis) in over 40% of cases, hematogenous spread of a distant infection in about 33% of cases, and are related to recent trauma or neurosurgery in 23% (14% and 9%, respectively). The most common organisms are *Streptococcus* (34%), *Staphylococcus* (18%), and enteric gram-negative rods (15%). Abscesses can cause variable neurologic deficits depending on their location in the brain and their size. Most patients (69%) have a headache, but only about half have fever or a focal neurologic deficit. Initial workup for an abscess is largely with urgent imaging, with contrast-enhanced MRI preferred over CT if available. Typical findings on MRI include peripheral enhancement and diffusion restriction. Lumbar puncture is typically not performed due to the theoretical risk of herniation (if there is a large mass lesion) and because CSF culture is insensitive. All patients with suspicion for brain abscess should have neurosurgical consultation as most patients should undergo neurosurgical aspiration or resection, although medical treatment alone can be considered for those with small abscess(es), who are clinically stable, and who have a known etiologic organism. Empiric treatment is generally with 4–8 weeks of a third-generation cephalosporin plus metronidazole with modifications based on risk factors (e.g., adding vancomycin if there are risk factors for methicillin-resistant *Staphylococcus aureus*). If clinically stable, empiric antibiotics can be delayed until after neurosurgical drainage to increase the yield of the culture, although many experts advise continuing anaerobic coverage regardless of the culture result as >30% of abscesses are polymicrobial. Although historically brain abscesses have had a mortality rate of 40%, modern series show this has declined to approximately 10%.

Neurocysticercosis

Cysticercosis is caused by the tapeworm *Taenia solium* and can lead to both neurocysticercosis and extraneural cysticercosis. Ingestion of undercooked pork leads to gastrointestinal tapeworm infection; ingestion of tapeworm eggs via the fecal-oral route is required for cysticercosis (although those with tapeworm infection are at risk for autoinoculation). The most important sequela of neurocysticercosis is epilepsy and neurocysticercosis is one of the leading causes of epilepsy globally. Although not endemic in the United States, it has been shown to be the cause of 2% of new-onset seizures. Neurocysticercosis can manifest in the brain parenchyma itself or can be intraventricular or subarachnoid and can be single or multiple. While parenchymal lesions are more associated with seizures, intraventricular lesions can lead to obstructive hydrocephalus and subarachnoid lesions can lead to communicating or obstructive hydrocephalus. Lesions progress through multiple stages, starting out as viable cysts,

then degenerating cysts, and finally as calcified lesions. Although they can present at any stage, most present during the degenerative stage. Diagnosis is largely based on a compatible clinical history and imaging, with visualization of a scolex within a cyst sufficient to make the diagnosis. Antibody, antigen, and PCR-based testing may also be useful, although antigen and PCR testing are not widely available. All patients with suspected or confirmed neurocysticercosis should undergo ophthalmologic exam for evaluation of ocular cysticercosis, which generally requires surgical removal. All patients should similarly be evaluated for evidence of hydrocephalus (obstructive or communicating), which may require neurosurgical intervention. Patients with viable or degenerating cysts may be candidates for treatment with antiparasitic therapy with albendazole or albendazole plus praziquantel depending on the burden of disease. All patients should receive corticosteroids *prior to*, concurrent with, and following antiparasitic therapy to decrease the risk of seizures.

Infectious Myelopathies

Infections of the spine are relatively infrequent but do occur. Infections can occur within the spinal cord itself or can be extramedullary, such as spinal epidural abscesses, and cause extrinsic compression of the spinal cord. A wide variety of infectious agents including viruses, bacteria, fungi, and parasites may cause spinal cord infection.

Among immunocompetent people, herpesviruses are the most common cause of viral myelitis with VZV and HSV being the most common. Both VZV and HSV can reactivate from the dorsal root ganglia and travel anterograde to cause rash or retrograde to, less commonly, cause myelitis. Both HSV and VZV myelitis can occur concurrently with typical HSV or VZV rashes (i.e., anogenital vesicular rash or dermatomal shingles rash, respectively) in which case the etiology of the myelitis can be presumed, but they can also occur without rash. HSV and VZV PCR may be useful but are more specific than sensitive. Both HSV and VZV myelitis should be treated with IV acyclovir. Other herpesviruses including CMV, EBV, and HHV-6 have also been associated with infectious myelopathy, typically in immunocompromised individuals. HIV infection is known to cause HIV-associated vacuolar myelopathy with the white matter of the dorsal columns and corticospinal tracts predominantly affected in a pattern similar to that seen in subacute combined degeneration from B12 deficiency.

Human T-cell lymphotropic virus type I (HTLV-I) is an important cause of infectious myelopathy worldwide, and particularly in specific populations within Central and South America, Africa, and Japan. It is transmitted vertically mother-to-child (likely predominantly through breastfeeding), via sexual contact, and via contaminated blood products. Although most people infected will remain asymptomatic, approximately 2%–4% develop HTLV-I-associated myelopathy (HAM; also known as tropical spastic paraparesis). HAM is characterized by slowly progressive hyperreflexia, spasticity, and weakness of the legs with resulting gait impairment. Patients often additionally describe urinary dysfunction, lower back pain, and sensory dysfunction. Progression is usually over years to decades. Imaging may be normal or may reveal cord atrophy without specific signal change in the cord. Diagnosis is made based on a compatible clinical syndrome and the presence of HTLV-I antibodies in the serum and CSF. HTLV-I proviral load in the CSF may be useful but is not clinically available. There are no proven disease-modifying therapies for HAM although there is preliminary evidence for mogamulizumab.

Syphilis, caused by *Treponema pallidum*, was historically a common cause of infectious myelopathy (tabes dorsalis), although this manifestation has become less common in the modern era. Tabes dorsalis, when it does occur, tends to occur in chronic, untreated infection and manifests with demyelination of the dorsal cord with resulting impaired proprioception and gait impairment. More common in the modern era, although still uncommon, is syphilitic meningomyelitis, manifesting as spastic weakness and generally responsive to treatment with penicillin. Early neurosyphilis can manifest as a meningitis, presenting with headache, neck stiffness, encephalopathy; ocular syphilis with uveitis, vitreitis, retinitis, and/or optic neuropathy; or otosyphilis. Patients with suspected early neurosyphilis should have lumbar puncture and if there is a CSF pleocytosis, elevated CSF total protein, or reactive CSF VDRL assay should generally be treated with IV penicillin.

Bacterial abscesses can occur in the spine and are most commonly located in the epidural space. Spinal epidural abscesses result from hematogenous spread of infection in approximately half of cases and from contiguous infection in approximately one-third of cases with

Staphylococcus aureus accounting for about two-thirds of cases. Epidural abscesses can cause both mechanical compression of the spine as well as ischemia via septic thrombophlebitis. Patients can present with pain, weakness, sensory changes, and bowel and/or bladder dysfunction. The triad of back pain, fever, and neurologic deficit may only be present in 13% of patients. MRI with contrast is the diagnostic modality of choice. CSF culture is insensitive and is generally only positive in patients with positive blood cultures, so CSF analysis is generally not recommended. All patients should have urgent neurosurgical consultation for consideration of surgical drainage which can be both diagnostic and therapeutic. Antibiotics should be tailored to the causative organism, if known. Empiric antibiotics should cover methicillin-resistant *S. aureus* and Gram-negative bacilli; usually vancomycin plus a third or fourth generation cephalosporin.

Infectious Causes of Stroke

The most important infectious cause of stroke is infective endocarditis (IE), where microorganisms, most commonly staphylococci or streptococci, form a vegetation on a cardiac valve. Pieces of this vegetation may embolize and occlude cerebral blood vessels, leading to ischemic strokes. Approximately 25% of patients with IE will have a clinically apparent stroke and a higher proportion have clinically asymptomatic strokes visible on imaging. The other major neurovascular complication of IE is mycotic aneurysm formation where the arteries themselves become infected and are high risk for hemorrhage. Both ischemic strokes from septic emboli and mycotic aneurysms carry a high risk of hemorrhage, so anticoagulation and antiplatelet therapy should generally be avoided in patients with either complication. A common clinical dilemma is when or if to offer cardiac surgery to a patient with neurovascular complications of IE due to the need for intraoperative anticoagulation. This decision is best made with multidisciplinary input from cardiac surgery, neurology, and infectious disease.

Any infection that causes a meningitis and, especially meningitis at the skull base (basilar meningitis), can also lead to ischemic strokes. This is particularly well described in bacterial and tuberculous meningitis. In tuberculous meningitis, antiplatelet therapy has been shown to reduce risk of ischemic stroke, although not mortality. VZV can also infect cerebral arteries and lead to ischemic strokes and/or hemorrhage, a syndrome termed VZV vasculopathy. VZV vasculopathy is often associated with a typical VZV rash, and especially with herpes zoster ophthalmicus, but there is no rash in almost 40% of cases. Diagnosis is generally via CSF PCR for VZV DNA or elevation of VZV IgG in the CSF (ideally with an increased CSF:serum IgG index). Patients should be treated with high-dose IV acyclovir and experts also recommend a short course of glucocorticoids to reduce inflammation although there is no trial data to support this recommendation.

Central Nervous System Tuberculosis

Although the incidence of tuberculosis (TB) in the United States has been decreasing, there are still almost 8000 new diagnoses annually, with almost 1700 of those presenting with extrapulmonary tuberculosis. Approximately 5% of those with extrapulmonary disease will have tuberculous meningitis, a severe neurologic infection resulting in death or permanent disability in about half of those affected. People living with HIV are at higher risk for tuberculous meningitis and for more severe disease. CNS TB most commonly presents as tuberculous meningitis which often starts subacutely with nonspecific symptoms such as fever, headache, nausea, and anorexia before progressing to focal neurologic symptoms such as cranial neuropathies, paresis, encephalopathy, and/or seizures. Imaging may show evidence of a skull base predominant meningitis (Fig. 9.2) and CSF analysis typically shows a lymphocytic pleocytosis with elevated protein and low glucose. CNS TB can also manifest with tuberculomas with or without meningitis. Tuberculomas can occur throughout the brain or spine and can be asymptomatic, cause neurologic deficits associated with their location, or cause seizures. Prompt recognition and initiation of treatment are important to minimize morbidity and mortality, but diagnostic evaluation of CNS TB is complex with multiple diagnostic tests with varying sensitivity and specificity available. Treatment of CNS is similarly complex with multiple complex considerations including choosing an adequate drug regimen and duration, ensuring adequate drug dosing, considering whether to add corticosteroids and at which dose/duration, and, in people living with HIV, when to start antiretroviral therapy. Additionally, patients with CNS TB are at risk for multiple complications including hydrocephalus, strokes, seizures, and paradoxical worsening. Because of the complexities of diagnosis and management of CNS TB, infectious disease and neurology consultation should be sought as soon as the diagnosis is being considered.

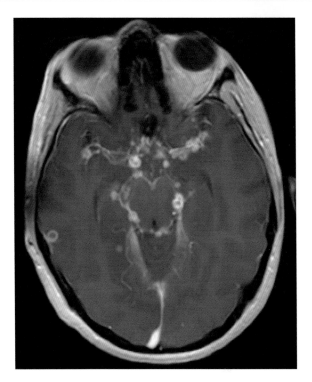

Fig. 9.2 Tuberculous meningitis. Brain magnetic resonance imaging of a patient who presented with nausea, vomiting, and progressive encephalopathy found to have CNS tuberculosis. Postcontrast T1-weighted MRI shows basilar leptomeningeal enhancement with multiple ring-enhancing lesions consistent with tuberculomas. With prolonged antituberculous treatment the patient had a good outcome. (From Levin SN, Lyons JL. Infections of the nervous system. *Am J Med.* 2018;131(1):25–32.)

PERIPHERAL NERVOUS SYSTEM

Radiculopathies
Lyme Radiculoneuritis

Although Lyme disease (caused by *Borrelia burgdorferi* most commonly in North America) is often considered in the differential of many neurological syndromes, the clinical spectrum of nervous system Lyme is likely much more constrained. In North America, the most common manifestations are lymphocytic meningitis and cranial neuropathies (most commonly facial neuropathy) followed by a painful radiculoneuritis (also known as Bannwarth syndrome), whereas in Europe (where *Borrelia garinii* and *Borrelia afzelii* predominate) painful radiculoneuritis is the most common manifestation followed by cranial neuropathies and lymphocytic meningitis. The lymphocytic meningitis, cranial neuropathies, and radiculoneuritis can occur in isolation or in any combination. Lyme radiculoneuritis typically starts with asymmetric radicular pain, which can be exquisite, and usually progresses to weakness and/or sensory loss of the affected nerve root(s). The joint guidelines from the Infectious Disease Society of America (IDSA), American Academy of Neurology (AAN), and American College of Rheumatology (ACR) recommend testing for Lyme only in the setting of meningitis, painful radiculoneuritis, mononeuropathy multiplex, or acute cranial neuropathies and recommend against routine Lyme testing in patients with typical amyotrophic lateral sclerosis (ALS), multiple sclerosis (MS), Parkinson disease, dementia/cognitive decline, new-onset seizures, or psychiatric disease and against routine testing in patients with nonspecific white matter lesions on brain MRI or in patients without epidemiologic risk factors for Lyme disease. Testing for nervous system Lyme disease should start with serum antibody testing. If CSF testing is performed, the test of choice is a CSF:serum antibody index. Lyme PCR should not be used due to its low sensitivity and specificity. If there is active nervous system Lyme, CSF analysis should show a lymphocytic pleocytosis and elevated protein; the absence of pleocytosis and protein elevation with a positive Lyme CSF:serum antibody index implies a previous, inactive nervous system infection. In North America, treatment is typically with 2–3 weeks of IV ceftriaxone, although in Europe there is more experience with oral doxycycline. A minority of patients develop posttreatment Lyme disease syndrome with persistent fatigue, cognitive difficulties, and musculoskeletal pain. Multiple clinical trials have evaluated the use of repeated antibiotic treatment for patients with posttreatment Lyme disease and have found no benefit but significant risk, so additional antibiotic therapy is not recommended in the absence of objective signs of persistent infection.

Herpes Zoster

VZV reactivation, also known as shingles or herpes zoster, occurs when latent virus in sensory ganglia reactivates and spreads down the sensory nerve causing dermatomal pain and rash. Herpes zoster can lead to necrosis of the sensory ganglia and nerve cells ultimately leading to sensory loss and neuropathic pain, in this setting referred to as postherpetic neuralgia. Herpes zoster is relatively common; approximately one-third of people in the United States are estimated to experience it during their lifetime, with age and immunocompromise being the major risk factors. Immunocompetent patients presenting with a painful dermatomal rash can generally be presumptively treated with oral antivirals (valacyclovir, famciclovir, or acyclovir) but immunocompromised patients should be considered for treatment with IV acyclovir due to higher risk of developing disseminated VZV. Those who develop postherpetic neuralgia should generally receive topical lidocaine and/or a gabapentinoid or tricyclic antidepressant as first-line treatment. Herpes zoster can reactive in the ophthalmic division of the trigeminal nerve leading to herpes zoster ophthalmicus (HZO), which can lead to multiple ophthalmologic complications including loss of vision. HZO should be treated with antiviral agents as shingles with consideration of using IV acyclovir if vision is threatened and should be comanaged with ophthalmology. Additional complicated presentations of VZV include acute retinal necrosis; herpes zoster oticus (Ramsay Hunt syndrome) with reactivation from the geniculate ganglion affecting the facial and vestibulocochlear nerves (cranial nerves VII and VIII) with resulting facial paralysis, ear pain, hearing loss, and vesicles in the auditory canal; meningitis; encephalitis; myelitis; and vasculopathy (as discussed earlier). These more complicated presentations of VZV reactivation should generally be treated with IV acyclovir.

Neuropathies

Infectious causes of peripheral neuropathy are less common but can occur. HIV infection is associated with a length-dependent distal symmetric polyneuropathy (HIV-DSPN) with a prevalence of almost 40% among people living with HIV. Some historically used antiretroviral treatments including zalcitabine, didanosine, and stavudine, are associated with a direct toxic neuropathy but these are not generally used in the modern era. The mechanism in the modern era is likely multifactorial with both direct and indirect viral effects. Hepatitis C virus is also associated with length-dependent sensory and sensorimotor polyneuropathy and less commonly with mononeuropathies and mononeuropathy multiplex. Hepatitis C virus is also associated with cryoglobulinemia which can lead to a medium or small vessel vasculitis which itself can cause a vasculitic neuropathy. Although uncommon in North America, leprosy, caused by *Mycobacterium leprae*, remains endemic in many countries within the tropics, especially India, Brazil, Indonesia, and Nigeria. Leprosy presents on a spectrum between tuberculoid leprosy characterized by few, well-demarcated, hypopigmented skin lesions with hypoesthesia and lepromatous leprosy with diffuse, less well-defined lesions, and skin thickening. Patients most commonly have mononeuropathy or multiple mononeuropathies although polyneuropathy has also been reported and there is often characteristic palpable nerve enlargement. Treatment is with prolonged multidrug therapy.

HIV NEUROLOGY

HIV Infection

HIV is associated with both primary and secondary neurologic sequela. HIV has been shown to invade the nervous system early in the acute infection; HIV RNA has been isolated from CSF as early as 8 days following exposure. Over half of patients evaluated with acute HIV have at least one neurologic finding on examination, most commonly cognitive deficits. About one-quarter of patients have symptoms suggestive of meningitis. These acute manifestations generally improve with antiretroviral therapy (ART). Patients with chronic uncontrolled HIV can develop a vacuolar myelopathy which appears similar to subacute combined degeneration associated with B12 deficiency. As above, a distal predominant sensory polyneuropathy (HIV-DSPN) is common in patients with HIV. Although historically neuropathy correlated with control of HIV, more modern series have not shown a correlation with viral load or low CD4 count. Perhaps surprisingly, multiple series have shown a correlation between neuropathy and higher CD4 counts, although ART has also been associated with symptomatic improvement. Apart from ART, treatment is largely symptomatic with neuropathic pain medications.

HIV-Associated Neurocognitive Disorder

HIV is associated with a spectrum of neurocognitive disorders including asymptomatic neurocognitive impairment (ANI), mild neurocognitive disorder (MND), and HIV-associated dementia (HAD), which are under the umbrella of HIV-associated neurocognitive disorders (HAND). Prior to the availability of ART, severe neurocognitive deficits (i.e., HAD) were relatively common among people with HIV, with an incidence of almost 6 per 100 person years; however, this decreased dramatically to 0.5 per 100 person years from 1994 to 2002 as ART became increasing effective and available. Although the incidence of HAD has decreased, HAND remains fairly common. Studies have reported variable prevalence in the modern era. One of the largest cross-sectional studies showed that 33% of people living with HIV had ANI, 12% had MND, and 2% had HAD with lowest ever CD4 nadir the strongest predictor of d eveloping HAND. Traditional cardiac and metabolic risk factors correlate with worse cognitive impairment so management of HAND should focus on ART as well as management of cardiac/metabolic risk factors.

Opportunistic Infections

When HIV is untreated (usually either prior to diagnosis or due to lack of adherence to antiretroviral therapy), people living with HIV are at risk for a variety of opportunistic infections depending on their CD4 count. People with other causes of immunosuppression such as hematologic malignancies, use of immunosuppressive mediations, or bone marrow transplant are at risk for similar infections.

Toxoplasmic Encephalitis

Among people with HIV and low CD4 counts, the most common central nervous system infection is toxoplasmic encephalitis, which typically occurs at CD4 counts under 100 cells/μL. Toxoplasmosis is spread through the fecal-oral route or via ingestion of undercooked meat and the seroprevalence varies widely from 11% in the United States to 80% in some areas of Europe, South America, and Africa. There is no specific clinical finding for toxoplasmic encephalitis with 55%, 52%, and 47% of patients having headache, encephalopathy, and fever, respectively. MRI typically shows ring-enhancing lesions with associated vasogenic edema which can occur throughout the brain but often have a predilection for the basal ganglia (Fig. 9.3). Diagnosis is challenging as there are no noninvasive diagnostic tests that are both sensitive and specific and definitive diagnosis requires brain biopsy. Commonly, the diagnosis of toxoplasmic encephalitis is presumptive and treatment is

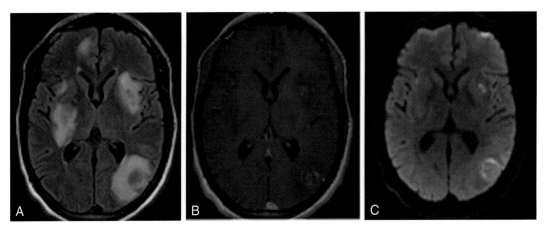

Fig. 9.3 Cerebral toxoplasmosis. Brain magnetic resonance imaging of a patient with uncontrolled HIV-1 infection who presented with seizures and altered mental status. Fluid-attenuated inversion recovery sequence (A), T1 postcontrast imaging (B), and diffusion-weighted imaging (C) reveal multiple heterogeneous, peripherally enhancing deep gray and juxtacortical lesions with areas of low diffusivity, surrounding vasogenic edema, and local mass effect. Toxoplasma immunoglobulin G from serum was positive, and the lesions improved with antitoxoplasmosis antimicrobials, confirming the diagnosis. (From Levin SN, Lyons JL. Infections of the nervous system. *Am J Med.* 2018;131(1):25–32.)

started empirically. If the patient clinically and radiologically responds to therapy then therapy is continued for the full course. If there is a lack of response then brain biopsy to evaluate for other diagnoses, specifically CNS lymphoma, is often considered. Treatment has historically been with pyrimethamine and sulfadiazine, but recently there has been increasing data to support and clinical experience with use of trimethoprim-sulfamethoxazole, which is generally less expensive and more available.

Progressive Multifocal Leukoencephalopathy

Progressive multifocal leukoencephalopathy (PML) is classically associated with HIV infection, typically with CD4 counts under 200 cells/µL but also occurs in the context of other causes of immunosuppression such as immunosuppressive therapies and hematologic malignancies. PML results from reactivation of the JC virus, which is present as a latent infection in up to 86% of adults. PML typically presents with progressive neurological deficits, which depend on the location of the lesions, and worsens over days to weeks. MRI shows single or multiple white matter T2 hyperintensities which typically demonstrate little to no mass effect or contrast enhancement but which may show a rim of diffusion restriction (Fig. 9.4). Diagnosis is typically made by positive JC virus PCR from the CSF, although the gold

standard for diagnosis is brain biopsy, which can be considered if a high index of suspicion remains despite negative CSF PCR. Treatment is focused on reversing the cause of immunosuppression; starting ART in people living with HIV or stopping immunosuppressive medications in people receiving them. There are no proven interventions specific for PML, although there has been emerging data and interest in the use of checkpoint inhibitors, interleukin-7, and virus-specific T-cell therapy.

COVID-19

Since the beginning of the COVID-19 pandemic, neurological symptoms were found to be common with COVID-19 infection with the most frequently reported including myalgias, headache, encephalopathy, and anosmia/dysgeusia. The pathogenesis of the neurological symptoms is thought to be multifactorial with contributions from ischemia/hypoxia, systemic inflammation, and microglial activation within the brain. Although low levels of viral RNA have been isolated from the brain, this has not been found to correlate with histopathological changes and may represent hematogenous contamination rather than direct viral infection of brain parenchyma. A UK biobank study found a reduction in gray matter thickness of the orbitofrontal cortex

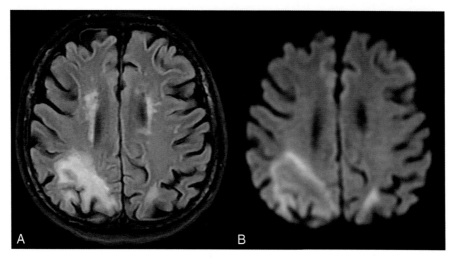

Fig. 9.4 Progressive multifocal leukoencephalopathy. Brain magnetic resonance imaging of a patient with progressive multifocal leukoencephalopathy who presented with weeks of progressive left-sided weakness. Fluid-attenuated inversion recovery sequence shows a large right and smaller left hyperintense white matter lesion (A) which both show a rim of diffusion restriction on diffusion-weighted imaging (B).

and parahippocampal gyrus among patients who had COVID-19, but similar findings have also been shown among patients with other causes of olfactory dysfunction suggesting that these changes may be related to anosmia from COVID-19 rather than a direct viral effect on the brain. Despite early media reports, the risk of ischemic stroke in patients with COVID-19 has been shown to be low, although concurrent COVID-19 and ischemic stroke have been associated with increased morbidity. Although Guillain-Barré syndrome has been reported in association with COVID-19, no causal link has been proven.

Persistent symptoms after infection with COVID-19, or postacute sequalae of SARS-CoV-2 infection (PASC), commonly referred to as long-COVID, is common with over half of patients having at least one persistent symptom 6 months after recovery from the acute infection. The most common neurological symptoms include brain fog, headache, paresthesias, altered taste and smell, and myalgias. Although some patients do improve over time, many patients continue to experience neurological symptoms and decreased quality of life over a year after their initial illness. Unfortunately there are as yet no proven biomarkers or targeted therapies for neurological PASC, although this remains an active area of research.

"For the full bibliography list, please use the pincode on the inside front cover to access the electronic version of the text at ebooks.health.elsevier.com."

10

Autoimmune Neurologic Disorders*

Giovanna S. Manzano and Daniel B. Rubin

INTRODUCTION

In recent years the field of neuroimmunology has grown as diagnostic assays for the detection of pathogenic autoantibodies have been developed and refined. Improved diagnostic assays have improved our understanding of the clinical and radiographic spectrum of some of these conditions. Yet, despite increased recognition, there remains a need for further biomarker development and standardization of management that could in turn support appropriate and timely initiation of treatment. The etiologic classifications of neuroimmunologic conditions are diverse: autoantibody mediated, paraneoplastic, inflammatory, para- or postinfectious, idiopathic, or iatrogenic (Table 10.1). An understanding of the pathophysiology of a given neuroimmunologic presentation can be helpful in determining the diagnosis, anticipating associated conditions, and determining appropriate treatment.

PATHOGENESIS

Autoantibody-Mediated Neuroimmunologic Disease

Autoantibody-mediated neuroimmunologic conditions are thought to reflect a maladaptive loss of self-tolerance. Such conditions include demyelinating central nervous system (CNS) disorders, such as myelin oligodendrocyte

glycoprotein antibody disease (MOGAD) and neuromyelitis optica spectrum disorder (NMOSD), autoimmune encephalitis and myasthenia gravis (MG), among others (see Table 10.1). Pathogenic autoantibodies may cause cellular dysfunction or injury through several different mechanisms, including receptor agonist or antagonist effect, antigen/receptor internalization, activation of the complement system, and antibody-dependent cell–mediated cytotoxicity. Broadly, pathogenic autoantibodies are classified as those that target surface antigens versus those that target intracellular antigens. Distinguishing the targeted antigen location helps to tailor treatment approach (e.g., anti-CD20 immunosuppressive therapies, such as rituximab, are more commonly used for autoantibody conditions targeting cell-surface antigens, whereas cytotoxic therapies, such as cyclophosphamide, are used to treat autoantibody conditions targeting intracellular antigens). It is recognized that the location of the targeted antigen type may correlate with prognosis. Receptor agonist and antagonist effect, including receptor internalization, are generally reversible. Thus neuroimmunologic conditions secondary to pathogenic cell-surface antigens may more favorably respond to treatment. Whereas, neuroimmunologic conditions mediated by pathogenic antigens that are intracellular, may cause damage that is less likely to be reversible. This is observed in practice when we examine the overall treatment responsivity of limbic encephalitis secondary to a cell-surface autoantibody to that of an intracellular autoantibody-mediated cerebellar degenerative syndrome.

It is important to note that not all detectable autoantibodies are pathologic. In some cases, detected autoantibodies may be a nonspecific marker of autoimmunity,

*Based on Rubin DB, Batra A, Vaitkevicius H, Vodopivec I. Autoimmune neurologic disorders. *Am J Med.* 2018;131(3):226–236. ISSN 0002-9343. https://doi.org/10.1016/j.amjmed.2017.10.033.

TABLE 10.1   Autoimmune Central Nervous System Diseases as Classified by Mechanism of Underlying Immune Dysfunction

Predominant Pathophysiology Disorders	T-Cell Mediated	Autoantibody Mediated	Granulomatous Disorders	Autoinflammatory Disorders	Iatrogenic
	Multiple sclerosis	SLE	Sarcoidosis	Behçet disease	Checkpoint inhibitors
	ADEM	Demyelinating disorders associated with anti-AQP4 (NMOSD) and anti-MOG antibodies	GCA	Monogenic periodic fever syndromes	CAR-T
	PACNS (PCNSV)	Miller Fisher syndrome (anti-GQ1b antibodies)	Granulomatosis with polyangiitis (Wegener granulomatosis)		
	Aβ-related angiitis	Bickerstaff encephalitis (anti-GQ1b antibodies)			
	Antibodies against intracellular antigens: ANNA-1 (Hu), ANNA-2 (Ri), ANNA-3, Ma1/Ma2, CV2/CRMP5, PCA1 (Yo), PCA-2, GFAP, amphiphysin, GAD65	Antibodies against cell-surface synaptic receptors and ion channels causing encephalitis (NMDA, AMPA, LGI1, CASPR2, GABA-A GABA-B, glycine receptor, mGluR1, mGluR5, DR2, DPPX), LEMS (VGCC), MG (AChR)			
	Sjögren syndrome				
	IgG4-RD				
	CLIPPERS				

Adapted from Rubin DB, Batra A, Vaitkevicius H, Vodopivec I. Autoimmune neurologic disorders. *Am J Med.* 2018;131(3):226–236; Zong S, Vinke AM, Du P, et al. Anti-GAD65 autoantibody levels measured by ELISA and alternative types of immunoassays in relation to neuropsychiatric diseases versus diabetes mellitus type 1. *Front Neurol.* 2023;14:111063. https://doi.org/10.3389/fneur.2023.111063. PMID: 3735746; PMCID: PMC10248002.ᵃ; Antoine JC, Absi L, Honnorat J, et al. Antiamphiphysin antibodies are associated with various paraneoplastic neurological syndromes and tumors. *Arch Neurol.* 1999;56(2):172–177. https://doi.org/10.1001/archneur.56.2.172; Dalmau J, Geis C, Graus F. Autoantibodies to synaptic receptors and neuronal cell surface proteins in autoimmune diseases of the central nervous system. *Physiol Rev.* 2017;97(2):839–887.

ᵃAutoantibodies to the intracellular synaptic antigen GAD65 may not be pathogenic.

Aβ, Amyloid-β; *AChR,* acetylcholine receptor; *ADEM,* acute disseminated encephalomyelitis; *AQP4,* aquaporin-4; *CAR-T,* chimeric antigen receptor T cell; *CLIPPERS,* chronic lymphocytic inflammation with pontine perivascular enhancement responsive to steroids; *GABA,* gamma-aminobutyric acid; *GCA,* giant cell arteritis; *IgG4-RD,* IgG4-related disease; *LEMS,* Lambert-Eaton myasthenic syndrome; *MG,* myasthenia gravis; *MOG,* myelin oligodendrocyte glycoprotein; *NMDA,* N-methyl-d-aspartate; *NMOSD,* neuromyelitis optica spectrum disorders; *PACNS,* primary angiitis of the central nervous system; *PCNSV,* primary central nervous system vasculitis; *SLE,* systemic lupus erythematosus; *VGCC,* voltage-gated calcium channel.

or a bystander autoantibody. Knowledge of the expected clinical syndrome and titer ranges of positivity that yield clinical significance are important to mind.

Paraneoplastic Autoantibody–Mediated Disease

As clinical awareness of various autoantibody-mediated neuroimmunologic syndromes evolves, we are better able to define the expected features of certain "classic syndromes" (Table 10.2). This improved recognition can help clinicians to then order appropriate diagnostic studies and ideally become more apt to initiate empiric treatment while still remaining in the investigative stage of assessment. Paraneoplastic neuroimmunologic conditions can occur in an individual with a known, preceding cancer diagnosis; however, it may also be that the development of a neuroimmunologic syndrome is what leads to the diagnosis of or precedes the development of an associated malignancy. Conditions such as autoimmune encephalitis, autoimmune cerebellar degenerative disease, and NMOSD are among neuroimmunologic conditions in which the etiologic driver is a present, prior, or a yet-to-be-detected malignancy. Similarly, the identification of a neuroimmunologic syndrome with a risk of associated malignancy should prompt cancer screening. As an example, a patient presently with a progressive cerebellar syndrome, found to test positive for anti–PCA1 (anti-Yo) autoantibodies, should then have a detailed evaluation for malignancy as ~90% of patients with anti–PCA1 cerebellar degeneration have an associated cancer. In such paraneoplastic conditions, the resultant immune dysregulation is believed to be triggered by the atypical expression of neuronal antigens by the associated malignancy leading to inappropriate

TABLE 10.2   Recognized Autoimmune Syndromes of the Central Nervous System

Classic Syndromes	Etiologies
Limbic encephalitis	Paraneoplastic or primary autoimmune (several autoantibodies), HSV, HHV6, syphilis
with faciobrachial dystonic seizures, hyponatremia	Anti-LGI1 antibodies
with abnormal behavior (psychiatric manifestations), movement disorder (dyskinesias), dysautonomia	Anti–NMDAR antibodies
Cerebellar ataxia (subacute cerebellar degeneration)	Paraneoplastic (anti-PCA1 [Yo]), autoimmune (mGluR1, GAD65), parainfectious and infectious (VZV, EBV, CJD), toxic/metabolic (ethanol, phenytoin, lithium, chemotherapy [cytarabine], vitamin E deficiency, gluten sensitivity), genetic (spinocerebellar ataxias)
Opsoclonus-myoclonus(-ataxia)	Anti–ANNA-2 (Ri), anti–ANNA-1 (Hu) antibodies, anti–GAD65 antibodies
Neuromyelitis optica	Anti-AQP4, anti-MOG disease
Cerebral cortical encephalitisMiller Fisher syndrome	Anti-MOG diseaseAnti-GQ1b antibodies
Stiff person syndrome	Anti–GAD65, antiamphiphysin, antiglycine receptor antibodies
Morvan syndrome (myokymia or neuromyotonia, dysautonomia, sleep disturbance, encephalopathy with visual hallucinations)	Anti-CASPR2 antibodies
Sensory ganglionopathy (neuronopathy)	Paraneoplastic (anti–ANNA-1 [Hu] antibodies), Sjögren syndrome, pyridoxine intoxication, platinum-based chemotherapy
Myasthenia gravis	Anti-AChR, anti-MuSK, anti-LRP4 antibodies
Lambert-Eaton myasthenic syndrome	Anti-VGCC antibodies

Adapted from Rubin DB, Batra A, Vaitkevicius H, Vodopivec I. Autoimmune neurologic disorders. *Am J Med.* 2018;131(3):226–236.
AChR, Acetylcholine receptor; *CJD,* Creutzfeldt-Jakob disease; *EBV,* Epstein-Barr virus; *HHV6,* human herpesvirus 6; *HSV,* herpes simplex virus; *MuSK,* muscle-specific kinase; *NMDAR, N*-methyl-D-aspartate receptor; *VGCC,* voltage-gated calcium channel; *VZV,* varicella zoster virus.

self-attack (e.g., limbic encephalitis caused by expression of the ANNA-1 [anti-Hu] antigen by small cell lung cancer).

Para- and Postinfectious Neuroimmunologic Conditions

In para- or post-infectious conditions, immune dysregulation is incited by an adaptive immune response to a foreign antigen that results in inappropriate targeting of similar appearing self-antigen. This is the proposed pathophysiologic mechanism of postinfectious Guillain-Barré Syndrome [GBS], classically following *Campylobacter jejuni* infection. Infectious processes may also heighten an inflammatory state leading to immune dysregulation as is thought to occur in para-infectious myopathies and postinfectious acute disseminated encephalomyelitis (ADEM). Infections may also play an inciting causative role in the development. of a subsequent, secondary neuroimmunologic disease as has been described for post–herpes simplex virus (HSV) *N*-methyl-D-aspartate receptor (NMDAR) limbic encephalitis. Clinical history and supportive evidence of CNS inflammation provide diagnostic support for these conditions. There may not be a present autoantibody, or other biomarker, to further diagnostic certainty of these para- or post-infectious entities.

Neuroinflammatory Conditions

Broadly, neuroinflammatory conditions are mediated by pro-inflammatory cytokines, no defined autoantibody is implicated. A prominent example of such a condition is neurosarcoidosis.. In neurosarcoidosis, TNF-alpha and other pro-inflammatory factors are thought to culminate in chronic inflammation and the pathologic formation of non-caseating granulomas. The clinical and radiographic manifestations of neurosarcoidosis are in turn quite variable given its heterogeneity as to where the disease may be present within the nervous system. A diagnostic search for neurosarcoidosis includes an evaluation of any systemic burden of disease, excluding alternative etiologies, and importantly evaluating for lymphadenopathy, which if biopsied may provide pathologic evidence of non-caseating granulomas, improving diagnostic certainty. The standard approach to treatment of neurosarcoidosis is administration of glucocorticosteroids. The exact dosing, duration, and when to escalate treatment and/or whether to start a steroid-sparing agent initially, are areas of active research.

Other prominent neuroinflammatory granulomatous diseases include those with underlying vasculitis, rheumatologic disease. Giant cell arteritis (GCA), also referred to as temporal arteritis, is among this group. Suspicion for GCA should be prompted by the development of a headache, vision change/loss, jaw claudication, with or without proximal joint pains in an individual older than 50 years of age, with elevated inflammatory markers (i.e., ESR, CRP). Glucocorticosteroids are again mainstay of treatment (see Table 10.1).

Lastly, autoinflammatory disorders, which are disorders of a dysregulated innate immune system, are within this category. These tend to be less common, but generally steroid responsive. Examples of such diagnoses include idiopathic hypertrophic pachymeningitis and chronic lymphocytic inflammation with pontine perivascular enhancement responsive to steroids (CLIPPERS). In some cases, steroid-sparing agents may be required for adequate treatment response. At, but often require steroid-sparing agents for disease control. At present, the management of these conditions is driven by retrospective series and anecdotal experience.

Iatrogenic Neuroimmunologic Complications and Neurotoxicities

Oncologic therapies and disease-modifying antirheumatic drugs (DMARDs) are iatrogenic exposures with risks of neuroimmunologic complications and toxicities. Chemotherapies may cause neurologic side effects such as peripheral neuropathy, headache, encephalopathy, seizures, and posterior reversible encephalopathy syndrome; direct toxicities, that is, leukoencephalopathies, are also possible from chemotherapy. Lastly, a risk of severe infection due to immunosuppression should be considered (e.g., progressive multifocal leukoencephalopathy (PML)). For these reasons, attention to and appropriate evaluation of new neurologic deficits/symptoms in patients receiving chemotherapies are pertinent.

Novel oncologic-directed immunotherapies, for example, immune checkpoint inhibitors (ICI) and genetically altered chimeric antigen receptor T cells (CAR-T cells), are among agents with potential to cause iatrogenic neurotoxicities. ICIs are a novel class of therapeutics designed to target the inhibitory pathways in the immune system that maintain self-tolerance and modulate the immune response. The checkpoint inhibitors ipilimumab (human antibody to CTLA-4) and pembrolizumab and nivolumab (PD-1 antagonists) all function to block pathways that normally suppress the activation and expansion of T cells, harnessing the host's native immune response against cancer. However, they have also unmasked a broad spectrum of immune-related neurologic adverse events (Table 10.3), the incidence of which may be as high as 1%. The array of potential peripheral and central neuroimmunologic complications from ICI exposure is vast. Expert consensus guidelines have been published to guide an understanding of diagnostic approach and severity grading of these neurotoxicities, referred to as immune-related adverse effects (iRAEs). Assessing the severity grading of a recognized iRAE guides management, as lesser grade iRAEs warrant watchful observation whereas higher grades iRAEs warrant treatment with corticosteroids and potentially second-line disease-directed therapies while withholding further ICI exposure as per the American Society of Clinical Oncology guidelines.

TABLE 10.3 Central Nervous System Disorders Associated With Immune-Mediated Treatments

Treatment Class	Medication	Clinical Syndrome
Anti–TNF-α	Adalimumab Etanercept Infliximab	Demyelinating disorders (CNS [including optic neuritis]PNS)
Anti–IL-6R	Tocilizumab	Demyelinating disorders, MS Cognitive Impairment with leukoencephalopathy
Anti–PD-1/L1	Nivolumab Pembrolizumab	Myasthenia gravis Encephalitis Demyelinating disorders PRES Stiff person syndrome
Anti–CTLA-4	Abatacept Belatacept Ipilimumab	Hypophysitis Ischemic stroke PRES Myasthenia gravis Guillain-Barré Syndrome

Adapted from Rubin DB, Batra A, Vaitkevicius H, Vodopivec I. Autoimmune neurologic disorders. *Am J Med.* 2018;131(3):226–236. *CNS*, Central nervous system; *MS*, multiple sclerosis; *PNS*, peripheral nervous system; *PRES*, posterior reversible leukoencephalopathy syndrome; *TNF*, tumor necrosis factor.

CAR-T cells are genetically modified T cells that have a fabricated antigen receptor from multiple sources engineered to a specific target cell antigen. A patient's own cells are isolated, genetically modified, cloned, and reinfused to redirect T-cell specificity to a specific tumor-associated antigen. Cytokine release syndrome (CRS) is a potential systemic side effect encountered with CAR-T-cell therapy, which results from T-cell activation, proliferation, and production of endogenous cytokines. Neurologic CRS manifestations may range from headache and confusion/delirium to seizures, cerebral edema, and coma. A standardized approach to assessment, as developed by the American Society for Transplantation and Cellular Therapy, guides appropriate triage and management of patients with immune effector cell-associated neurotoxicity syndrome (ICANS). Generally, prompt recognition and management of iatrogenic immunotherapy-related neurotoxicities, particularly iRAEs and ICANS, can lessen morbidity and mortality. However, despite improved recognition, we continue to lack reliable biomarkers to predict and prognostic toxicity risk and outcome. Thus a greater understanding of the pathogenesis of CNS-related adverse effects and how to evade development of these toxicities remains an active need.

DMARDs also carry risk of neuroimmunologic complications, such as the induction or exacerbation of demyelinating syndromes or the development of neurosarcoidosis-like presentations (see Table 10.3). Presently, expert consensus and anecdotal clinical experience guide current practice that emphasizes avoidance of the inciting agent and appropriate management based on the consequential phenotype developed.

EPIDEMIOLOGY

Age, race, or sex in which a neuroimmunologic condition may be more likely to occur is dependent upon the condition. Conditions that may be present in children include ADEM, Rasmussen encephalitis, MOG-AD, pediatric multiple sclerosis, particular autoimmune/paraneoplastic encephalitides such as anti–NMDAR encephalitis, and genetic conditions such as Aicardi-Goutières syndrome and hemophagocytic lymphohistiocytosis. In contrast, certain disorders, such as GCA and IgG4-related disease (IgG4-RD), occur almost exclusively in older populations. Some conditions, such as opsoclonus/myoclonus/ataxia, have both pediatric and adult forms. Similarly, MG has a bimodal age distribution of incidence, with peaks in age in late adolescence/early adulthood and in the elderly. Regarding associations with an individual's race, neurosarcoidosis is prevalent among individuals with African descent, whereas multiple sclerosis is more common in Caucasians. Autoimmunity, in general, is more prevalent in females than males; however, Behçet is the exception to this rule. Among neuroimmunologic conditions, NMOSD, multiple sclerosis, Susac, anti–NMDAR encephalitis, and GCA are female predominant. Whereas GBS, chronic inflammatory demyelinating polyneuropathy, ADEM, IgG4-RD, and MG in older patients are all slightly more common in males. No sex predilection exists in sarcoidosis or primary angiitis of the CNS.

EVALUATION

Patient History

Accurate and detailed assessment of a patient's presenting history is key for refining your differential diagnosis. Attention to the rate at which a condition occurred, and/or progressed is critical as this time course informs both the differential diagnosis and general approach to management. In general, demyelinating events tend to be either discrete occurrences (either monophasic or relapsing) or gradually progressive. Autoimmune encephalitides are commonly subacute in onset and progressive in the absence of appropriate treatment. Post- or parainfectious conditions tend to occur either concurrently or subacutely in the days to weeks following an infection. Iatrogenic neurotoxicities tend to develop subacutely, but acute toxicity is possible. Lastly, the great masquerader, neurosarcoidosis, may present acutely, subacutely, or gradually, with various stages severity at symptom onset.

In addition to attention to duration of onset and progression, identifying the clinical sympotomatology (i.e., how the condition is clinically and/or radiographically manifests), is the next step in localizing the pathology and categorizing its underlying etiology. Localization of neurologic signs and symptoms at the onset of an evaluation, with clinical course trajectory in mind, will help to inform which diagnostic studies are warranted. Lastly, demographic details and associated nonneurologic signs or symptoms will help to further refine the differential and management. It remains important to exclude potential mimickers, inclusive of toxic, metabolic, infectious, genetic, and iatrogenic etiologies, as well as to consider nonneuroimmunologic conditions when appropriate. There are several well-defined syndromes for which a thorough clinical history can lead to a plausible diagnosis (see Table 10.2); however, more frequently, clinical findings can be nonspecific and will require appropriate diagnostic studies for support.

Diagnostic Investigations

Serologic Tests

Similar to the need for a thorough yet focused history and physical examination, serum studies to exclude toxic, metabolic, and infectious causes are an essential component of the diagnostic approach to neuroimmunologic disease. Commonly, we consider excluding nutritional deficiencies, syphilis infection, toxins, among other studies, while also seeking to assess for any associated systemic conditions such as rheumatologic disease or malignancies (Table 10.4).

Imaging

The imaging modality and the area of the nervous system to image will be informed by clinical history and examination (Table 10.5). Most commonly, neuroimmunologic disease will require magnetic resonance imaging (MRI), at times with paired MR angiography when a vasculitis is among the differential. Non–contrast head computed tomography can be helpful in the acute setting to rule out mimickers; however, a follow-up MRI will be needed to better assess any white matter or gray matter abnormalities. It is important to note that for some subtypes of autoimmune encephalitis, many patients may present with a normal MRI. When the brain MRI is not informative but a neuroimmune process is suspected, a brain fluorodeoxyglucose-positron emission tomography (FDG-PET) should be considered for further evaluation. Some neuroimmunologic conditions may have characteristic features on FDG-PET brain imaging that may provide further diagnostic clues. For instance, isolated basal ganglia hypermetabolism is sensitive for the diagnosis of LGI1 autoimmune encephalitis. In addition to neuroimaging, it is at times equally important to obtain appropriate imaging to screen for associated systemic malignancies, particularly in cases of autoimmune encephalitis. Current practice for malignancy screening is to obtain computed tomography (CT) of the chest, abdomen, and pelvis, and either a testicular ultrasound for those of male sex or an ovarian

TABLE 10.4 Suggested Diagnostic Tests in Patients With Suspected Autoimmune Disorders of the Nervous System

Alternative Pathologies	Markers of Inflammation and/or Autoimmunity
CBC w/diff[a]	ESR[a]
Electrolytes, glucose[a]	CRP[a]
BUN/Cr[a]	ANA[a]
LFTs[a]	Anti-dsDNA[a]
Ammonia	ENA—anti-Ro/La[a]
Vitamin B12	ANCA[a]
Coagulation panel[a]	RHF, CCP
Thyroid function	Antiphospholipid antibodies
Cortisol	Myositis-specific antibodies
Toxicology screen[a]	Complement levels
Urinalysis and culture[a]	Cryoglobulins
Blood culture	IgG4 level
Serologies for syphilis	Anti-TPO and thyroglobulin antibodies
	ACE
SPEP with Immunofixation	HLA-B51
Serum flow cytometry	Anti-AQP4 and anti-MOG antibodies
	Autoimmune/paraneoplastic antibodies

Adapted from Rubin DB, Batra A, Vaitkevicius H, Vodopivec I. Autoimmune neurologic disorders. *Am J Med.* 2018;131(3):226–236. *ACE*, Angiotensin-converting enzyme; *ACPA*, anticitrullinated peptide antibodies; *ANA*, antinuclear antibody; *ANCA*, antineutrophil cytoplasmic antibody; *AQP4*, aquaporin-4; *BUN/Cr*, blood urea nitrogen/creatinine; *CBC*, complete blood count; *CRP*, C-reactive protein; *ENA*, extractable nuclear antigens; *ESR*, erythrocyte sedimentation rate; *LFTs*, liver function tests; *MOG*, myelin oligodendrocyte glycoprotein; *RF*, rheumatoid factor; *SPEP*, serum protein electrophoresis; *TPO*, thyroperoxidase.
[a]Denotes basic laboratory evaluations.

ultrasound of those of female sex. If there remains a high likelihood of an associated malignancy despite negative whole-body CT imaging and gonadal ultrasound, then a FDG-PET body scan recommended. Of note, outpatient colonoscopies and mammogram are additionally important as indicated. Expert consensus is to repeat malignancy screening for 2 to 5 years for conditions with potential risk of an associated malignancy.

Cerebrospinal Fluid Analysis

Cerebrospinal fluid (CSF) analysis is commonly indicated for further diagnostic investigation of neuroinflammatory, neuroinfectious, and neuro-oncologic conditions, as clinical history and radiographic tests can be similar. Recommended CSF studies include total cell count (in tubes 1 and 4), total protein, glucose, culture, IgG index and oligoclonal band testing (these require paired same-day serum samples), and appropriate autoantibody panels or infectious studies as warranted by the clinical context. Lastly, CSF flow cytometry and cytology are also recommended in many instances to exclude leptomeningeal malignant disease, as well as to better characterize a suspected neuroinflammatory process. As an example, flow cytometry in neurosarcoidosis may reveal a 5:1 ratio of CD4+ to CD8+ T cells in the CSF. Generally, CNS inflammation is supported by CSF demonstrating a pleocytosis, elevated protein, elevated IgG index, and/or CSF oligoclonal bands (Table 10.6); however, not all are required to be present for any given neuroimmunologic diagnosis.

Electroencephalography

Electroencephalography (EEG) is often informative when evaluating patients with altered mentation. Determination of new epileptic seizures and/or discharges in a patient with subacute neuropsychiatric decline without identifiable risk factors or prior history of seizures should raise suspicion for an autoimmune etiology among other possible differential diagnoses. Reassuringly, awareness of autoimmune encephalitis is improving such that previously signature late-stage EEG findings are less commonly seen (e.g., extreme delta brush on EEG in patients with NMDAR autoimmune encephalitis).

TREATMENT

Treatment Approach

Clinical suspicion for a neuroimmunologic process, particularly when supported by collected objective data, should prompt early and appropriate initiation of immunotherapy. The need for prompt immunosuppression and/or immunomodulation is justified by studies that detail poor outcomes secondary to treatment delay. As may be the case when testing requires send-out studies,

TABLE 10.5 Diagnostic Imaging Studies for Evaluation of Suspected Autoimmune Disorders of the Nervous System

Diagnostics	Finding	Potential Diagnosis
CT/CTA head	Vascular beading	Vasculitis
	Venous engorgement	AVM, fistula, VST
	Atrophy	Neurodegenerative process
CT chest, CT abdomen/pelvis	Mass	Malignancy
MRI brain	Mesiotemporal T2/FLAIR hyperintensities	Autoimmune/paraneoplastic limbic encephalitis, HSV, syphilis, HHV6
	White matter T2/FLAIR hyperintensities	MS, NMO, ADEM, neurosarcoidosis, Behçet disease, Sjögren syndrome, vasculitis, CAA-related inflammation, Susac syndrome, CADASIL, viral encephalitis, PML, neoplasms (gliomatosis cerebri, lymphomatosis cerebri, intravascular lymphoma), toxic exposures (methotrexate, cytarabine, toluene, heroin), leukodystrophies, mitochondrial disease
	Intra-axial rim enhancement	Metastases, abscess, glioma, infarction, contusion, demyelination, radiation necrosis
	Pachymeningeal enhancement	Syphilis, TB, fungal infection, neurosarcoidosis, IgG4-related disease, rheumatoid arthritis, idiopathic hypertrophic pachymeningitis
	Leptomeningeal enhancement	Intracranial hypotension, infectious meningitis, leptomeningeal carcinomatosis, neurosarcoidosis
	Nerve root enhancement	Guillain-Barré syndrome/CIDP, metastases, granulomatous disease, Lyme disease, CMV
MRI spectroscopy	Lactate peak	Metabolic abnormalities
Brain FDG-PET/CT	Medial temporal lobe *hypermetabolism* (patterns of cerebral glucose metabolism described in NMDAR and LGI1 encephalitis)	Limbic encephalitis
	Hypometabolic brain regions	Other forms of autoimmune encephalitis
Whole body FDG-PET/CT	Areas of FDG avidity	Malignancy, inflammation (e.g., sarcoidosis)
EEG	Extreme delta brush	NMDA encephalitis
	PSWC	CJD
	Periodic temporal discharges	HSV
	Diffuse slowing with triphasics	Metabolic encephalopathy

(continued)

TABLE 10.5 Diagnostic Imaging Studies for Evaluation of Suspected Autoimmune Disorders of the Nervous System—Cont'd

Diagnostics	Finding	Potential Diagnosis
Mammogram	Breast lesion (cancer)	Conditions associated with several antineuronal autoantibodies
Transvaginal US	Ovarian mass	Anti-NMDA encephalitis
Testicular US	Testicular mass (cancer)	Brain stem, limbic encephalitis, cerebellar degeneration
Dilated funduscopic examination and fluorescein angiography	Branch retinal artery occlusions with hyperfluorescence of the vessel wall	Susac syndrome
	Uveitis	Sarcoidosis, Behçet disease, other rheumatologic conditions
	Vitreous opacities, subretinal pigment epithelial infiltrates	Intraocular–central nervous system lymphoma
Temporal artery biopsy	Granulomatous inflammation	Giant cell arteritis
Labial salivary gland biopsy	Focal lymphocytic sialadenitis	Sjögren syndrome

Adapted from Rubin DB, Batra A, Vaitkevicius H, Vodopivec I. Autoimmune neurologic disorders. *Am J Med.* 2018;131(3):226–236.

ADEM, Acute disseminated encephalomyelitis; *AVM,* arteriovenous malformation; *CAA,* cerebral amyloid angiopathy; *CADASIL,* cerebral autosomal dominant arteriopathy with subcortical infarcts and leukoencephalopathy; *CIDP,* chronic inflammatory demyelinating polyneuropathy; *CJD,* Creutzfeldt-Jakob disease; *CMV,* cytomegalovirus; *CTA,* computed tomography angiography; *EEG,* electroencephalography; *FDG-PET/CT,* fluorine-18-fluorodeoxyglucose positron emission tomography/computed tomography; *FLAIR,* fluid-attenuated inversion recovery; *HHV6,* human herpesvirus 6; *HSV,* herpes simplex virus; *MRI,* magnetic resonance imaging; *MS,* multiple sclerosis; *NMDAR, N-*methyl-D-aspartate receptor; *NMO,* neuromyelitis optica; *PML,* progressive multifocal leukoencephalopathy; *PSWC,* periodic sharp wave complexes; *TB,* tuberculosis; *US,* ultrasound; *VST,* venous sinus thrombosis.

TABLE 10.6 Cerebrospinal Fluid (CSF) Studies Consistent With Central Nervous System (CNS) Inflammation

CSF Study	Result	Comments
Glucose	Normal	Hypoglycorrhachia (glucose <45 mg/dL) is more commonly seen in infectious and carcinomatous meningitis but can be observed in neurosarcoidosis, PACNS, and Neuro-Behçet disease.
Protein	Elevated	
WBCs	5–100	
IgG index	>0.66	Defined as: [CSF IgG ÷ CSF albumin] ÷ [serum IgG ÷ serum albumin]. Though the precise value considered positive is laboratory dependent and may vary, in general an IgG index >0.66 suggests the presence of CNS inflammation.
Oligoclonal bands	>2 (laboratory-dependent value)	The number of bands for positive result is defined by each laboratory; comparison with serum is mandatory. *Though classically associated with MS, CSF oligoclonal bands are a nonspecific finding of intrathecal immunoglobulin production unique to CSF and may be seen in a number of disorders.*
Autoimmune autoantibody panel	Positive	Detection of antineuronal autoantibodies strongly supports the diagnosis of autoimmune encephalitis. Albeit, seronegativity does not exclude the diagnosis.
New generation sequencing of microbial DNA	Negative	
Flow cytometry	Normal	This remains a field of ongoing investigations—potentially, characteristic cell type profiles may reflect particular neuroimmunologic diseases.
Cytology	Normal	
HSV1/HSV2 PCR	Negative	HSV PCR may be falsely negative in the first 24 hours of infection; repeat testing may be necessary.
VZV PCR and Ab	Negative	
IgH gene rearrangement	Absent	

Adapted from Rubin DB, Batra A, Vaitkevicius H, Vodopivec I. Autoimmune neurologic disorders. *Am J Med.* 2018;131(3):226–236.
Ab, Antibody; *HSV,* herpes simplex virus; *MS,* multiple sclerosis; *PACNS,* primary angiitis of the central nervous system; *PCR,* polymerase chain reaction; *VZV,* varicella zoster virus; *WBC,* white blood cell.

not all objective tests may result in a timely manner, and thus once sufficient clinical suspicion is present and benefits of empiric therapy outweigh potential risks, clinicians should administer treatment. Some treatments, such as B cell–depleting agents, plasma exchange, and/or intravenous immunoglobulin G (IVIg), may obscure serologic test results such that interpretation is questioned. Therefore it is important to send autoantibody tests that may be indicated as part of a patient's initial diagnostic workup prior to initiating these immunomodulating therapies. Storing extra specimens is often a useful approach.

In majority of neuroimmunologic conditions the mainstay of acute treatment includes glucocorticosteroids (e.g., intravenous methylprednisolone [IVMP] 1 g daily for 3–5 days followed by an oral steroid taper). Often, pairing with IVIg or therapeutic plasma exchange is appropriate, particularly in severe disease. In some cases, a corticosteroid trial may prove to be diagnostic, whereas, in others, a failure of steroid response does not always equate to misdiagnosis. It is therefore important to have an appropriate index of clinical suspicion before empiric treatment administration.

The duration of corticosteroids to follow acute high-dose steroids will vary by condition. For example, in multiple sclerosis, pulse dose IVMP is the mainstay of acute flare management, whereas, in MOGAD, a slightly prolonged steroid taper is suggested. In neurosarcoidosis an even slower prednisone taper is recommended. The choice of steroid-sparing agent is then dependent upon the diagnosed and/or suspected condition. Given iRAEs and immunosuppression, maintenance therapy should be initiated only in cases with a high index of clinical suspicion and a complete diagnostic workup has excluded alternative etiologies. Further details of maintenance regimens according to disease process are outside the scope of this chapter.

Lastly, it is important to note that in iatrogenic or paraneoplastic neuroimmunologic conditions, addressing the inciting cause is equally important as empiric immunotherapy. In iatrogenic causes such as ICI-induced neurotoxicity, removal of the offending agent, and, at times, avoidance of reexposure is necessary. In paraneoplastic cases, multidisciplinary collaboration is essential to treat the associated malignancy as well as to ensure appropriate modification to neurologic-directed treatment to provide adequate oncologic-directed therapy.

Treatment Risks and Safety Precautions

It is important to educate providers and patients alike regarding potential risks and required precautions that are necessary in the setting of immunotherapy. As with any new medication, the risk-to-benefit ratio should be adequately reviewed with the patient and/or the patient's surrogate decision-maker prior to administration. Obtaining informed consent is required for second-line immunotherapy agents.

Treatment with immunosuppressants may pose risks of infection, malignancy, and, in some cases, renal or hepatotoxicity. Pretreatment screening for prior indolent infections (e.g., tuberculosis, hepatitis C, hepatitis B) and an assessment of baseline blood counts and renal and liver function are standard. Additionally, pretreatment screening in patients with suspected or confirmed demyelinating disease requires testing for JC virus due to risk of PML. A complete list of suggested pretreatment screening tests is outlined in Table 10.7. If an indolent infection is discovered, referral to an infectious disease specialist should be considered to help address management and determine risk mitigation steps to permit safe administration of appropriate treatment.

TABLE 10.7   Suggested Pre-treatment Screening Studies and Baseline Evaluations Before Initiating Immunosuppressants

Infection Screens	Other Diagnostic Studies
Hepatitis B screening (HBsAg, anti-HBs, anti-HBc)*	CBC*
Hepatitis C screening (anti-HCV)*	BUN/Cr*
HIV antibodies,* PCR; T-cell CD4 count	LFTs*
TB testing (PPD/IGRA)*	hCG
JC virus antibody index	25-hydroxycholecalciferol (vitamin D) level
Strongyloides stercoralis, serology	Bone densitometry
Trypanosoma cruzi, serology	TPMT genotype
	CXR
	Ophthalmologic evaluation
	Immunoglobulin levels (IgM, IgG, IgA)

Adapted from Rubin DB, Batra A, Vaitkevicius H, Vodopivec I. Autoimmune neurologic disorders. *Am J Med*. 2018;131(3):226–236. *BUN/Cr*, Blood urea nitrogen/creatinine; *CBC*, complete blood count; *CXR*, chest x-ray; *HBc*, hepatitis B core; *HBsAg*, hepatitis B surface antigen; *hCG*, human chorionic gonadotropin; *HCV*, Hepatitis C virus; *HIV*, human immunodeficiency virus; *IGRA*, interferon-gamma release assay; *LFTs*, liver function tests; *PCR*, polymerase chain reaction; *PPD*, purified protein derivative; *TB*, tuberculosis; *TPMT*, thiopurine S-methyltransferase.
*Obtain in all patients.

Vaccination status should be assessed with immunization as warranted in accordance with established guidelines as detected by the Centers for Disease Control and Prevention. When able, timing of vaccinations should be planned to optimize potential vaccine response. This timing of vaccination may not always be feasible pending the acuity of a patient's presentation and need for treatment; however, there are instances when pretreatment vaccination is mandatory (e.g., meningococcal vaccination before complement inhibitors). Of note, overwhelming evidence supports that vaccines are not significant triggers of disease flares in patients with neuroimmunologic conditions. This has been recently relevant in the setting of the COVID-19 pandemic. Any question of the relation between a vaccination and subsequent neuroimmunologic disease should be reviewed with the appropriate specialist.

The impact on fertility is another potential consequence of immunosuppressants that requires a thorough discussion prior to administration. In cases when acute administration is not mandatory, every effort should be made to preserve fertility in patients when there is a plan to use a medication with high-impact risk on fertility (e.g., cyclophosphamide). Before and after initiation of maintenance immunotherapies, ongoing counseling regarding appropriate contraception remains necessary. Should a patient become pregnant while receiving an immunotherapy with teratogenicity or other fetal risk, then appropriate measures should be enacted to minimize potential harm to the developing fetus. There are some medications in which a nonchildbearing partner receiving immunotherapy can also confer risk to the fetus, as is the case for a male taking teriflunomide. Protocols are available for providers to enact in such instances. Similarly, should an individual receiving immunotherapy desire to become pregnant, a discussion regarding appropriate wash-out time should be reviewed. In some instances, the use of an immunosuppressant with less potential fetal risk is used as an interim approach during periods of planned conception.

CONCLUSION

Neuroimmunologic disorders continue to gain recognition, yet our understanding of their pathophysiology and best practices is continuously being investigated and revised. These conditions often have the potential for significant morbidity and, in some cases, mortality. Thus early recognition and prompt appropriate treatment are key. Education pertaining to clinical recognition, appropriate diagnostic investigations, and optimal management is essential to ensure providers are equipped to provide optimal care to this patient population, thereby portending a greater likelihood of favorable outcomes. In some conditions, halting of progression is the targeted outcome available given the current therapeutic landscape, whereas in others, reversibility of deficits is a reasonable goal. Research aimed at a better understanding of the pathophysiology and epidemiology of these diseases will help to expand our understanding to yield more effective management in the years ahead.

"For the full bibliography list, please use the pincode on the inside front cover to access the electronic version of the text at ebooks.health.elsevier.com."

11

Headache*

Paul B. Rizzoli, Melissa Darsey, Kathryn E. Hall, and William J. Mullally

INTRODUCTION

Headache is an almost universal human experience and is one of the most common complaints encountered in medicine and neurology. Ancient references to headache can be found in the Ebers papyrus (1200 BCE) and the discovery of trepination of 9000-year-old Neolithic skulls has provided evidence of the earliest headache treatment. Hippocrates described visual symptoms associated with a headache, and Aretaeus of Cappadocia crafted the earliest classification of headache in the second century AD. The evaluation of this condition may be straightforward or challenging, and, though often benign, headache may prove to be an ominous symptom. In this chapter we discuss the diagnosis and classification of headache disorders and principles of management, with a focus on migraine, tension-type headache, trigeminal autonomic cephalalgias, and various types of daily headache. The direct and indirect socioeconomic costs of headache to society are estimated at 14 billion dollars per year. All primary care providers will encounter the clinical problem of headache on a regular basis; early and accurate diagnosis and appropriate treatment will help to reduce pain and suffering and the economic burden.

EPIDEMIOLOGY

Almost everyone has experienced headache at one time or another. For migraine, the lifetime prevalence is about 30% of the population, with a female predominance. Depending on the methodology used, tension-type headache is even more common. At any one time, approximately 40% of the global population is experiencing tension-type headache, and for migraine the prevalence is about 10%. Migraine occurs most commonly between the ages of 25 and 55 years and is three times more common in females. Despite the fact that it causes significant disability, migraine remains underdiagnosed and undertreated.

Trigeminal autonomic cephalalgias are rare compared with migraine and tension-type headache. The most common trigeminal autonomic cephalalgia is cluster headache, with a population prevalence of 0.1% and a male-to-female ratio that has fallen over the years and is now thought to be about 2:1.

Chronic daily or near-daily headache, lasting for months to years, is widely reported in the literature but is not an official diagnosis in the most widely used classification system, the International Classification of Headache Disorders (ICHD). Chronic daily headaches of long duration include chronic migraine, chronic tension-type headache, hemicrania continua, and new daily persistent headache. Worldwide prevalence of chronic daily headache has been consistent at 3%–5%, most of which likely represents chronic migraine.

CLASSIFICATION

First published in 1988, the ICHD underwent its most recent revision in 2013. The classification, freely available online at https://www.ichd-3.org/, contains explicit criteria based on phenomenology for the diagnosis of many types of headache. By convention, headache

*Based on Rizzoli P, Mullally WJ. Headache. *Am J Med*. 2018;131(1):17–24, ISSN 0002-9343. https://doi.org/10.1016/j.amjmed.2017.09.005.

classification is based on the characteristics of the individual headache in the prior year, not the individual with the headache, though features specific to individuals may be used in helping to differentiate between two close diagnostic matches. The ICHD continues to evolve with an appendix system that allows for the introduction of proposed new headache types or new criteria for old headache types and for eventual removal of outmoded or unhelpful criteria.

PRIMARY VERSUS SECONDARY HEADACHE

The major division in the ICHD is between primary and secondary headache. A primary headache has no known underlying cause. The most common primary headaches include migraine, tension-type headache, and cluster headache.

Secondary headache is the result of another condition causing traction on or inflammation of pain-sensitive structures, resulting in headache. Headache due to psychiatric disease is also considered secondary. Headaches related to infection, vascular disease, and trauma are examples of more common secondary headaches. Studies have shown that only 2%–12% of patients with brain tumor will have headache as the sole presenting complaint. Most patients who present to their primary care provider for an evaluation have a primary headache disorder.

EVALUATION

Patient History and Evaluation

The first step in diagnosis is to obtain a detailed history of the patient's headache. This is of paramount importance in making the correct diagnosis. In fact, if diagnostic confusion remains, repeating the history intake is more important than any diagnostic study. Information gathered in the history is compared with the diagnostic criteria to create the best diagnostic match. The history records details about the headache, such as frequency, duration, character, severity, location, quality, and triggering, and aggravating and alleviating features. Age of onset is extremely important, and a family history of headache, often present in migraine, should be explored. Lifestyle features including diet, caffeine use, sleep habits, work, and personal stress are important to obtain.

Finally, details of any comorbid conditions, such as an associated sleep disorder, depression, anxiety, and an underlying medical disorder are also useful to record.

The examination in headache is based on the general neurologic examination. A funduscopic examination should be performed in every patient presenting for evaluation of headache. Additional features include examination of the superficial scalp vessels and neck vessels, dentition and bite, temporomandibular joints, and cervical and shoulder musculature. The ICHD classification considers pericranial muscle tenderness to be an important physical finding in the diagnosis of tension-type headache.

Diagnostic Evaluation

The diagnosis of migraine is based almost entirely on the history; there is no diagnostic test for migraine. Further, evidence suggests that, in the specific setting of a history suggesting migraine combined with a normal neurologic examination, imaging is overwhelmingly likely to be unremarkable. There remain, however, appropriate indications for imaging in the evaluation of headache. Imaging should be considered when various "red flags" are present that could indicate the presence of a serious underlying structural explanation for headache (Box 11.1). These red flags include indications, such as fever, night sweats, and weight loss, of an underlying systemic illness; focal neurologic signs or symptoms; sudden or thunderclap onset of headache; or headache onset over the age of 60. Notwithstanding, in practice, many patients, over the course of their years with headache, will end up undergoing imaging at least once, and most of these studies will be negative. On the one hand, negative imaging may be reassuring to the patient; on

---

BOX 11.1 Headache "Red Flags" That Could Indicate Need for Evaluation

- New headache in patients over the age of 60
- Abnormal neurologic examination, including papilledema and change in mental status
- New change in headache pattern or progressive headache
- New headache in the setting of HIV risk factors, cancer, or immunocompromised status
- Signs of a systemic illness (e.g., fever, stiff neck, rash)
- Triggered by cough, exertion, Valsalva maneuver
- Headache in pregnancy and/or postpartum period
- First or worst headache

the other hand, the cost for such imaging can reach one billion dollars per year.

Approach to Treatment

The approach to treatment of secondary headaches is focused on treatment of the suspected cause (e.g., treating the sinus infection). The treatment of some secondary headaches, such as posttraumatic headache, may default to the treatment of migraine because many posttraumatic headaches have the phenotype of migraine. The treatment of migraine and other primary headaches is not uniform but is proportioned to the severity of the symptoms and resulting disability. Mild and infrequent symptoms may be initially treated with lifestyle modification, stress management techniques, and over-the-counter abortive medications. Prescription medications may be added as warranted to help thwart disability and maintain function. A distinction is made between prescription abortive and preventive medication in the management of headaches. Abortive medications are prescribed to treat an individual attack, and preventative medications are used to reduce the frequency and severity of the individual attacks, with the goal of reducing disability.

PRIMARY HEADACHE

Migraine

Migraine is the third most prevalent disorder according to the 2010 Global Burden of Disease Survey and the seventh highest cause of disability worldwide. The main subtypes are migraine with and without aura (Box 11.2). An aura is a fully reversible set of nervous system symptoms, most often visual or sensory symptoms, that typically develops gradually, recedes, and is then followed by headache accompanied by nausea, vomiting, photophobia, and phonophobia. Less common symptoms of aura include speech/language symptoms, motor or brain stem symptoms, or retinal symptoms. If an aura contains multiple features, symptoms usually occur in succession of at least 5 or so minutes each, with a total symptom complex of 5–60 minutes. Thus visual symptoms, both positive, such as scintillations, and negative, such as scotomata, are typically noted at the outset, followed by development of sensory complaints, then a mixed dysarthric/aphasic language disorder, followed by gradual clearing. The headache usually begins within 60 minutes

---

> **BOX 11.2   International Classification of Headache Disorders, Third Edition (ICHD-3) Migraine Without Aura**
>
> A. At least five headache attacks fulfilling the criteria B–D
> B. Attacks last 4–72 hours
> C. With at least two of the following four characteristics:
>   1. unilateral location
>   2. pulsating quality
>   3. moderate or severe pain intensity
>   4. aggravation by or causing avoidance of routine physical activity
> D. At least one of the following during headache:
>   1. nausea and/or vomiting
>   2. photophobia and phonophobia
> E. Not better accounted for by another ICHD-3 diagnosis

---

after the resolution of the neurologic symptoms. Some patients will experience an aura, usually visual, without an accompanying headache, referred to as "typical aura without headache." Hemiplegic migraine is a rare subtype of migraine with aura that is characterized by unilateral weakness and may be familial or sporadic. Aura phenomena are likely linked to a characteristic spreading cortical depression, starting posteriorly and moving slowly across the brain surface, producing this orderly progression of neurologic symptoms.

The overall clinical picture of migraine may be divided into four phases: prodrome, aura, headache phase, and postdrome. The prodrome, which is present in up to 60% of patients, may precede development of the headache by hours to days and can consist of a multitude of symptoms, including depression, hyperactivity, cognitive changes, frequent urination, irritability, euphoria, neck stiffness and/or pain, and fatigue. Food cravings, such as for chocolate, may be present and result in these foods being blamed for triggering the attack when in fact the craving was simply part of the prodrome. A subset of patients will then experience an aura but not necessarily with each and every attack. The headache in migraine is typically, approximately 60%, described as unilateral and of moderate to severe intensity. Though an individual's headache attacks tend to be fairly stereotyped, many variations can be present. Finally, the headache may be followed by a postdrome, often referred to as a "headache hangover," characterized by impaired concentration and fatigue or feeling "washed out." Some patients alternatively report feeling refreshed and rejuvenated after an attack.

From a pathophysiologic standpoint, migraine is considered a genetically induced hypersensitivity of the brain to both internal and external homeostatic changes that can act as headache triggers. These triggers influence the trigeminovascular system, which contains both peripheral and central nervous system components. Stimulation of the trigeminovascular system results in release of neuropeptides and other substances that cause both local inflammation and distant amplification of neural circuitry in the brain stem, trigeminal nucleus caudalis, thalamus, and cortex, leading to central sensitization and symptom worsening along with reduced activity in central descending inhibitory systems and reduced ability to control or extinguish the headache attack.

Chronic migraine, defined as headache on more than 15 days per month for a period of more than 3 months, shows a persistent prevalence of approximately 3% of the population and forms up to 70%–80% of cases seen in a tertiary headache center. Implicit in the diagnosis is a process of transformation from a prior pattern of episodic migraine that can occur over months to years. Though the resulting headache pattern may lose many of its distinguishing features, typical migraine features on 8 days per month are required for the diagnosis (Box 11.3). Risk factors associated with transformation to chronic migraine include coexisting noncephalic sites of pain, mood and anxiety disorders, medication overuse, obesity, female sex, and lower educational status. It is, however, not possible to predict who will transform and whether aggressively treating a pattern of increasing-frequency migraine can reliably prevent transformation to chronic migraine.

Treatment Principles

Treatment of migraine has traditionally been divided between abortive management, designed to reduce or resolve an individual headache event, and preventive management, used to reduce the overall headache activity. Treatment early in the attack produces the best results. Features of the headache, including severity, speed of onset, and early associated nausea/vomiting, may influence the choice of agent. Efficacy is based on the treatment's ability to reduce symptoms and restore function.

Abortive medications include nonsteroidal antiinflammatory agents, combination analgesics, antiemetic medications, and corticosteroids. Opioid medications and butalbital compound are generally discouraged because of the risk of overuse and potential for rebound. More specific antimigraine agents include the selective 5-HT1B/D serotonin agonists, the triptans (Table 11.1), and ergotamine-containing preparations, such as intravenous/intranasal dihydroergotamine. Randomized controlled trials have revealed that standard dose

---

BOX 11.3 International Classification of Headache Disorders, Third Edition (ICHD-3) Chronic Migraine

A. Headache (tension-type-like and/or migraine-like) on 15 days per month for >3 months and fulfilling criteria B and C
B. Occurring in a patient who has had at least five attacks fulfilling criteria B–D for 1.1 migraine without aura and/or criteria B and C for 1.2 migraine with aura
C. On 8 days per month for >3 months, fulfilling any of the following:
  1. criteria C and D for 1.1 migraine without aura
  2. criteria B and C for 1.2 migraine with aura
  3. believed by the patient to be migraine at onset and relieved by a triptan or ergot derivative
D. Not better accounted for by another ICHD-3 diagnosis

TABLE 11.1 The Triptan Medications

Name (Brand)	Formulation	Half-life (h)
Sumatriptan (Imitrex)	PO (25, 50, 100 mg), SC (4, 6 mg),	
	Nasal spray/powder	2.5
Sumatriptan/ Naproxen sodium (Treximet)	PO (85/500 mg)	2/19
Rizatriptan (Maxalt)	PO and ODT (5, 10 mg)	2–3
Naratriptan (Amerge)	PO (2.5 mg)	5–8
Eletriptan (Relpax)[a]	PO (20, 40 mg)	4
Almotriptan (Axert)	PO (6.25, 12.5 mg)	3–4
Frovatriptan (Frova)	PO (2.5 mg)	26
Zolmitriptan (Zomig)	PO and ODT (2.5, 5 mg)	3

[a]Unlike others, metabolized by CYP3A4 system.

triptans provide freedom from pain at 2 hours in 18%–50% of patients and pain relief in 42%–76%. Combining the triptan with a nonsteroidal antiinflammatory drug enhances the effectiveness of the triptan.

Preventive medication is considered if the patient is suffering from headaches for more than 6 days, impaired for 4 days, or completely disabled for 3 days each month despite abortive treatment. In initiating preventive management, it is important to begin at a low dose, increase the dose slowly to help minimize adverse side effects, and continue for an adequate trial length of time, usually 3 months, so as not to miss a slowly developing therapeutic effect (Table 11.2). The management of chronic migraine can be challenging, and preventive agents used in combination may be of benefit. There are data to support the combination of topiramate and nortriptyline. Onabotulinumtoxin A administered every 3 months has demonstrated efficacy in reducing the number of headache days per month and is a US Food and Drug Administration–approved treatment.

Specific Treatments

Lasmiditan. Lasmiditan is a 5-HT1F receptor agonist that has been shown to block neurogenic inflammation and c-Fos expression in neural tissue but, unlike the triptans, without evidence of vasoconstriction in vascular tissue models in vitro. It has been FDA approved since 2019 for the acute treatment of migraine with or without aura at doses of 50, 100, and 200 mg. Lasmiditan works both centrally and peripherally on 5-HT1F receptors, and this likely explains central nervous system (CNS) adverse effects, including dizziness, fatigue, and somnolence. Based on these AEs, the FDA approval came with a warning against driving for 8 hours after each dose, the first time such a driving restriction has been included in an approval.

Calcitonin Gene–Related Peptide Antibodies. Extensive research has demonstrated that calcitonin gene–related peptide (CGRP) plays an important role in the development of migraine pain through the activation of the trigeminovascular system. Serum CGRP levels are elevated during migraine attacks, and intravenous administration of CGRP will trigger a migraine-like headache. CGRP antagonists are a class of drugs that work by blocking the activity of CGRP, thereby reducing the severity and frequency of migraines. CGRP monoclonal antibodies are administered via injection and are generally well tolerated with minimal side effects.

TABLE 11.2   Selected Traditional Oral Migraine Preventive Medications

Name	Daily Dose (mg)	Comments
Established Efficacy		
Candesartan	4–16	
Metoprolol	50–150	Question avoid in migraine with aura
Propranolol	80–240	Question avoid in migraine with aura
Topiramate	25–150	Avoid in pregnancy
Valproate sodium	250–1500	Avoid in pregnancy
Probably Effective		
Amitriptyline	10–100	Strong clinical impression of efficacy
Nortriptyline	10–100	
Atenolol	50–150	
Lisinopril	10–20	
Memantine	10–20	Generally well tolerated
Venlafaxine	37.5–150	Well tolerated and nonsedating
Others		
Cyproheptadine	2–8	Used in the pediatric population
Gabapentin	300–1800	Favorable AE profile
Verapamil	80–480	Migraine with prolonged aura, vestibular migraine

Based on AHS Consensus Statement 2021; Ailani J, Burch R, Robbins M. Matthew S. The American Headache Society consensus statement: update on integrating new migraine treatments into clinical practice. *Headache.* 2021.

There are two types of CGRP antagonists: monoclonal antibodies and small molecules. Monoclonal antibodies are large proteins that are administered via injection and work by binding to CGRP, preventing it from interacting with its receptors. Small molecules are orally active drugs that are able to penetrate the blood-brain barrier and directly inhibit the activity of CGRP receptors. The first CGRP antagonist to receive FDA approval for migraine prevention was erenumab, a monoclonal antibody that is administered via subcutaneous injection once per month, targets and blocks the CGRP receptor. Other CGRP monoclonal antibodies that have been approved for the prevention of migraine include fremanezumab, galcanezumab, and eptinezumab; they act by binding to the CGRP ligand. Small molecule CGRP antagonists that have been approved for the abortive treatment of migraine include ubrogepant and rimegepant, both of which are administered orally. Studies revealed pain freedom at 2 hours in approximately 20% of patients and pain relief in 61%. Zavegepant nasal spray for the acute treatment of migraine has been demonstrated to effect freedom from pain in about 23% of patients. Rimegepant taken every other day has also been approved for migraine prevention. Atogepant taken daily has proven to be extremely effective in reducing the frequency of migraine attacks. Clinical trials have shown that CGRP antagonists are effective at reducing the frequency and severity of migraine episodes and may have a lower risk of side effects compared to traditional migraine medications such as triptans. However, as with any medication, there may be potential risks and side effects associated with CGRP antagonists, and they may not be effective for all patients. The most common side effects are constipation and nausea (Table 11.3).

Neuromodulation Devices. A number of devices have come to market in recent years with FDA clearance for use in the acute and/or preventive treatment of migraine as well as other headache disorders. Before coming to market, devices like those discussed here must only receive clearance from the FDA as safe. This level of FDA approval is much less stringent than that for medication for which randomized controlled trials are required to demonstrate that the medication is both safe and effective. Because the FDA level of approval for devices emphasizes safety and is silent on whether the treatment is effective, insurance companies have traditionally declined coverage for devices under most circumstances. The advantages of devices, however, include that they are noninvasive, are associated with a low incidence of adverse effects, and may prove to be useful when standard treatment options are limited, such as in pregnancy, but data are lacking.

Cefaly, one of the earliest migraine treatment devices was FDA-cleared in March 2014. It is an external trigeminal nerve stimulator, specifically targeting the supraorbital branch of the trigeminal nerve. This device is placed between the eyebrows and attached to the skin by an electrode. The prevention mode is a 20-minute stimulation designed to be used daily, and the acute mode is a stronger 60-minute stimulation that is used when a migraine attack is starting or ongoing. Two small studies have shown efficacy in the abortive management of episodic migraine.

Single-pulse transcranial magnetic stimulation is another noninvasive migraine treatment modality. The device uses magnetic stimulation to interrupt pain transmission. It is currently not available but may return to market in the future.

TABLE 11.3 Currently approved CGRP monoclonal antibodies					
Drug Name	**Dosage (mg)**	**Route of Administration**	**Frequency**	**Half-life (days)**	**Differences**
Erenumab (Aimovig)	70 or 140	Subcutaneous injection	Monthly	28	The only CGRP monoclonal antibody that targets the CGRP receptor instead of the CGRP molecule itself
Fremanezumab (Ajovy)	225 or 675	Subcutaneous injection	Monthly or quarterly	32	Approved for both episodic and chronic migraines
Galcanezumab (Emgality)	120, 300	Subcutaneous injection	Monthly	27	Higher dose for cluster
Eptinezumab (Vyepti)	100, 300	Intravenous infusion	Every 3 months	27	The only CGRP monoclonal antibody approved for intravenous infusion. Onset of action 1–3 h

CGRP, Calcitonin gene–related peptide.

Gammacore, an externally applied vagal nerve stimulator device, has recently been cleared for use in the acute treatment of migraine. It had previously been used in the treatment of episodic cluster headache. Applied to the region of the sternocleidomastoid muscle, The device produces a sine wave shock or stimulus that stimulates the vagus nerve. Multiple "shocks" can be administered in succession for maximal benefit.

Remote electrical stimulation, via a device called Nerivio, has been studied for both acute treatment and preventive treatment of migraine. This device is placed on the patient's arm, and stimulation is provided for a period of 45 minutes. This technology utilizes a mechanism called conditioned pain modulation to ultimately inhibit pain sensation in the head.

One of the newer device options available now is a combined trigeminal and occipital nerve stimulator called Relivion. This device stimulates multiple nerve pathways for acute treatment of migraine effect.

While there are certainly advantages to devices for management of migraine, there are some disadvantages. One possibly prohibitive factor is cost. Some devices do require a monthly subscription, and often insurance does not cover these costs. The devices also may not offer sufficient ease of use; for example, a patient may not be able to use a device readily while at work in an office. Regardless, treatment of migraine with devices can be a valid option in a certain patient population and can be very effective at times.

Tension-Type Headache

Although typically not as severe as migraine, tension-type headache is far more common, with a lifetime prevalence in the general population of up to 80%. There is often a degree of associated disability, and this, combined with the high frequency, produces a significant socioeconomic impact. Tension-type headache is a dull, bilateral, mild-to-moderately intense pressure pain without striking associated features that may be categorized as infrequent, frequent, or chronic and is easily distinguished from migraine. Infrequent tension-type headache is thought to be the form of headache experienced by nearly everyone at one time or another and typically does not require medical management (Table 11.4).

Although there may be a genetic element in the development of tension-type headache, environmental factors likely play a larger role than they do in migraine.

Tenderness of pericranial muscles, coexisting mood disorders, and mechanical disorders of the spine and neck may be contributing factors.

Abortive and preventive medication management of tension-type headache may be considered, depending on the frequency and disability. Simple and compound over-the-counter analgesic agents with caffeine have shown efficacy. Preventive agents include tricyclic antidepressant medications and various muscle relaxants

Muscle relaxants are used largely based on anecdotal evidence. Selective serotonin reuptake inhibitors and selective norepinephrine reuptake inhibitors, advised in the past for this pattern of headache, have been shown to be ineffective. Monoamine oxidase inhibitor drugs have shown efficacy but are used infrequently, owing to potential side effects. Memantine, a glutamatergic N-methyl-D-aspartate receptor antagonist, has been studied in chronic tension-type headache and chronic migraine and may have some benefit. In patients with chronic daily headache having features of both tension-type headache and migraine, treatment may default to the preventive management of migraine, including, at times, the use of onabotulinumtoxin A.

Nonmedication management techniques, including physical therapy and other manual therapies, various local injections, counseling including cognitive behavior therapy, relaxation techniques, and biofeedback, may have limited benefit but have not been shown to be unequivocally effective in the treatment of headache. There is limited evidence of the benefit of acupuncture in the treatment of tension-type headache.

When tension-type headache is refractory, a blend of abortive and preventive pharmacologic management is used, along with nonpharmacologic modalities.

Trigeminal Autonomic Cephalalgias

Trigeminal autonomic cephalalgias are a group of headaches that are classified together as unilateral trigeminal distribution pain attacks, often associated with ipsilateral cranial autonomic features. These headaches lack the associated features that are seen in migraine and tension-type headache and are clinically distinct.

Cluster headache, often referred to as "suicide headache" because the intensity of the pain, occurs more commonly in men and is usually episodic, characterized by clusters of headaches over periods ranging from 2 weeks to 3 months. The pain is extremely severe, with one to eight episodes per day, often awakening the

TABLE 11.4 Trigeminal Autonomic Cephalalgia

TAC Type	Age of Onset (years)	Sex	Site of Pain	Typical Features	Frequency of Attacks	Duration of Attacks	Acute Treatment	Preventive Treatment
Cluster headache	20–40	M > F 4:1	Unilateral, often periorbital or temporal	Severe, excruciating pain; autonomic symptoms; restlessness	1–8 attacks/day	15–180 minutes	Oxygen inhalation, triptans, intranasal lidocaine	Verapamil, lithium, topiramate
Paroxysmal hemicrania	20–40	F > M 1:1 to 1.7:1	Unilateral, often periorbital or temporal	Severe, stabbing pain; autonomic symptoms	5–40 attacks/day	2–30 minutes	Indomethacin	Indomethacin
SUNA and SUNCT	40–70	F > M 1.14 –1.21:1	Unilateral, orbital or temporal	Very frequent, brief, excruciating pain; prominent autonomic symptoms	Multiple attacks/ day	6–600 seconds	Lamotrigine, topiramate, gabapentin	Lamotrigine, topiramate, gabapentin
Hemicrania Continua	Any age	F > M 2:1	Unilateral, continuous pain with exacerbations	Continuous moderate pain with superimposed severe exacerbations	Continuous	Continuous	Indomethacin; celecoxib	Indomethacin; celecoxib

SUNA, Short-lasting unilateral neuralgiform pain with autonomic symptoms; *SUNCT*, short-lasting unilateral neuralgiform headache attacks with conjunctival injection and tearing.

patient from sleep shortly after falling asleep. Features are stereotyped with attacks of severe unilateral orbital pain lasting 15 minutes to 3 hours, usually associated with ipsilateral autonomic symptoms (increased lacrimation, nasal congestion/discharge, partial Horner's syndrome) and producing a characteristic restlessness. Cluster episodes tend to recur annually at about the same time of year, though significant variation is reported. Approximately 20% of patients do not experience a remission of more than 3 months in a calendar year and suffer from chronic cluster headache.

Short-lasting unilateral neuralgiform headaches are rare, severe, side-locked, very brief sharp pains currently subcategorized as follows, depending on the pattern of associated autonomic features: either SUNCT with ipsilateral conjunctival injection and tearing or SUNA with those features or rhinorrhea and nasal congestion. Episodes last from 6 to 600 seconds and may occur multiple times during the day. Unlike the other TACs, which usually begin between the age of 28–34 years, the onset of SUNA is typically in the sixth decade.

Paroxysmal hemicrania is a rare severe headache disorder characterized by brief frequent side-locked orbitofrontal headache attacks with ipsilateral autonomic features. Attacks, usually with a duration of minutes, may appear on a background of chronic mild headache in up to one-third of patients. Both chronic and episodic paroxysmal hemicrania are described, and the chronic form is more common in females. Hemicrania continua is a persistent, lateralized, side-locked headache associated with ipsilateral autonomic features. Hemicrania continua and paroxysmal hemicrania share an often dramatic response to therapeutic doses of indomethacin and otherwise typically respond poorly to other treatments.

Other Primary Headaches

A number of primary headaches are categorized according to their relationship to specific triggers. They are considered to be primary when an underlying structural or inflammatory cause has been ruled out. Cough headache occurs more commonly in men and is precipitated by coughing, sneezing, laughing, bending, and straining. The pain is usually bilateral and short-lived and will generally respond to indomethacin. Headache associated with sexual activity occurs just before or at the time of orgasm. The headache has a male preponderance and usually lasts from minutes to a few hours but may persist for a longer period of time. Primary sexual headache often occurs in bouts followed by long periods of remission. Indomethacin is often effective as abortive treatment and may be taken prior to sexual activity. If episodes occur frequently, propranolol or another beta blocker can be used for prevention. Headache triggered by cold exposure, such as the commonly described ice cream headache, or by diving into cold water are referred to as cold stimulus headache. The pain will usually resolve within 30 minutes. Headache related to external cranial pressure or traction can be triggered by a tight headband or helmet or by placing the hair in a ponytail and will disappear within 1 hour after the stimulus is removed. Exercise headache may be precipitated by strenuous aerobic activity or weightlifting. The pain is often bilateral and throbbing in character but without typical migraine features. It is more likely to occur at high altitude and in warm weather. The headache is often comorbid with migraine, and each headache may last from 5 minutes to 48 hours. In older adults, cardiac cephalgia secondary to cardiac ischemia must be considered, and only approximately half of those cases have accompanying chest discomfort. For primary exercise headache, indomethacin and beta blockers have been reported to be effective. Hypnic headache occurs in adults over the age of 50 and is referred to as alarm clock headache. The pain typically awakens the patient from sleep between 2:00 and 4:00 a.m. on at least 10 days per month with each episode lasting from 15 minutes to 4 hours. There are no accompanying cranial autonomic symptoms or prominent migrainous features. Caffeine or indomethacin taken before sleep will often prevent the headache, and lithium may help refractory cases. Primary stabbing headache, previously referred to as the syndrome of "jabs and jolts" or icepick headache, is characterized by irregular stabbing pain lasting seconds into different parts of the head and ranging in frequency from occasional to multiple episodes per day. Indomethacin can be used when the episodes are occurring frequently. Nummular headache is characterized by pain that may be continuous or intermittent involving a small round or elliptical area on the scalp. The location is most often parietal, and there is typically accompanying alopecia and tenderness. Injection of a local anesthetic into the area is usually not effective, but there are reports of sustained relief with onabotulinum A injections. Gabapentin has been used with limited beneficial effects.

Thunderclap Headache

In 1986 Day and Raskin reported the case of a patient who over a period of 5 days suffered the sudden onset of three intense headaches that they described as thunderclap headaches. Evaluation revealed an internal carotid aneurysm, but there was no evidence of a subarachnoid hemorrhage (SAH). Cerebral angiogram showed diffuse vasospasm in the anterior and posterior circulation bilaterally.

A thunderclap headache is defined as a sudden, severe, explosive headache that reaches maximum intensity in less than 1 minute and lasts 5 minutes or longer. The location of pain may be occipital, frontal, or parietal, and while the character is "exploding" in half of the cases, it can also be stabbing, lancinating, pressure, or aching. Two-thirds of patients will experience nausea. A population-based study revealed an incidence of 43 per 100,000 persons per year. The lifetime prevalence in adults 55–94 years of age is 0.3%, and 30%–80% of thunderclap headaches are due to an underlying disorder.

Thunderclap headaches are classified as primary or secondary by the ICHD, third edition (ICHD-3), and primary thunderclap headache is filed in the Other Primary Headache Disorders category. When a patient presents with the sudden onset of an intense incapacitating headache, secondary thunderclap headache, symptomatic of underlying organic pathology, must always be the initial consideration, and immediate investigation is mandatory. The two most common causes are SAH followed by reversible cerebral vasoconstriction syndrome (RCVS). Other organic etiologies include intracerebral hemorrhage, cerebral venous thrombosis, arterial dissection, giant cell arteritis, third ventricle colloid cyst, sphenoid sinusitis, pheochromocytoma, acute angle closure glaucoma, pituitary apoplexy, CNS infection, ischemic stroke, and spontaneous intracranial hypotension. If organic pathology is not detected and the headache is not better accounted for by another ICHD-3 entity, then a diagnosis of primary thunderclap headache can be made. Thunderclap headaches that are precipitated by factors such as coughing, sexual activity, or physical exertion are classified as a primary headache secondary to the identified precipitating factor; true primary thunderclap headaches are rare.

Subarachnoid hemorrhage presents as a sudden isolated thunderclap headache, and 85% are the result of a ruptured aneurysm with a high mortality rate. Ten percent are perimesencephalic due to venous bleeding and have a generally benign prognosis. RCVS presents with recurrent thunderclap headaches over days to a few weeks and is the result of segmental narrowing of cerebral arteries. Exposure to vasoactive substances is often the trigger leading to dysfunctional regulation of vascular tone. Seizures, cerebral infarcts, and intracranial hemorrhage may occur, especially in younger patients, but RCVS has a benign self-limited course in 90% of patients with resolution of arterial vasoconstriction over 1–3 months.

The pathophysiology of secondary thunderclap headaches is specific to the underlying cause. The pathogenesis of primary thunderclap headache may be the result of hypersensitivity of the sympathetic nervous system. While vasoconstriction may contribute to the pain, it cannot be the only cause, as initial imaging in thunderclap headache with RCVS often reveals no evidence of vasospasm. In addition, persistent vasospasm noted on imaging may not be associated with a headache. Given the diverse etiologies of thunderclap headache, there are likely multiple factors contributing to the genesis of pain that have not yet been elucidated.

When a patient presents with a thunderclap headache, a detailed history and physical examination are required. A patient's report of the "worst headache of my life" may not actually indicate a thunderclap headache, as progression to maximum intensity within 1 minute and lasting for at least 5 minutes are required to make the diagnosis. The history must include potential precipitating activities, illicit drug use, medication (both prescription and herbal), and past medical history including headaches, hypertension, and hypercoagulable disorders. A postural headache may suggest spontaneous intracranial hypotension secondary to a cerebrospinal fluid (CSF) leak. A complaint of neck stiffness with the finding of nuchal rigidity on examination may indicate SAH. However, clinical evaluation alone is not sufficient to distinguish primary from secondary thunderclap headache. A noncontrast computed tomography (NCCT) scan of the head obtained within 6 hours of the onset of the headache has an almost 99% chance of detecting an SAH, a 98% chance at 12 hours, and a 93% chance at 24 hours. The ICHD-3 recommends a lumbar puncture if the CT scan is negative, but studies suggest that the chance of missing an SAH with a normal neurologic examination and a negative NCCT within 6 hours of the onset of the headache is extremely low. Beyond 6 hours an LP should always be performed.

A CT or magnetic resonance angiography of the head and neck should be obtained to rule out RCVS but may be normal in the first week. Patients who experience recurrent thunderclap headaches with normal vascular imaging initially should have repeat imaging performed at 3–4 weeks. When noninvasive imaging studies are not diagnostic and suspicion is high, conventional angiography can be considered and will reveal alternating segments of arterial constriction and dilatation referred to as a "string of beads." Vascular imaging will also detect cervical arterial dissection, and venous imaging with CT venogram or magnetic resonance venogram, cerebral venous thrombosis. Brain magnetic resonance imaging (MRI) will identify structural abnormalities such as hemorrhage or infarcts in patients who have focal neurologic symptoms or an abnormal examination. If a CSF leak is suggested by history, a gadolinium-enhanced study should be obtained to look for evidence of pachymeningeal enhancement.

Distinguishing RCVS from central nervous system vasculitis is essential and can be challenging. Thunderclap headache occurs in 94% of RCVS patients, will be recurrent in 87%, and 77% are provoked. CNS vasculitis rarely presents with a thunderclap headache. Neurologic signs and symptoms are more common in CNS vasculitis, and brain imaging studies are abnormal upon admission to the hospital, whereas initial imaging studies are abnormal in only 31% of RCVS cases. CSF analysis will reveal a pleocytosis in 90% of CNS vasculitis cases, but while the CSF is usually normal in RCVS, CSF leukocyte levels >10 may be detected, and a diagnosis of vasculitis cannot be made solely on the basis of CSF studies. High-resolution vessel wall MRI may detect arterial wall inflammation with contrast enhancement and narrowing, but contrast enhancement may also be seen in RCVS. Brain biopsy remains the gold standard for the diagnosis of CNS vasculitis but has inherent risks, and a false negative biopsy may occur as the result of segmental vessel wall inflammation.

Posterior reversible encephalopathy syndrome (PRES) appears to have significant overlap with RCVS, sharing clinical and imaging features. PRES is characterized by headaches, encephalopathy, seizures, and visual disturbances with evidence of vasogenic edema in the parieto-occipital regions best visualized by MRI. PRES can be precipitated by uncontrolled hypertension, preeclampsia, cytotoxic and immunosuppressive agents, and renal failure and may coexist with RCVS.

The treatment of thunderclap headache is dependent on the etiology. All vasoactive medications should be immediately discontinued. There is evidence to support the use of nimodipine, with or without vasospasm, for the headaches, and verapamil has also been used. Beta blockers and triptans should be avoided. Glucocorticoids should not be used, as they have been reported as an independent predictor of worse outcome. Persistent headache following thunderclap headache with RCVS may occur in up to 50% of patients and may also respond to the calcium channel blockers. While most patients completely recover, permanent neurologic deficits occur in up to 10%, and rarely death.

New Daily Persistent Headache

New daily persistent headache is an unusual and distinctive pattern of headache, first described in 1986, and is generally not well known outside of headache medicine. Though it is usually not particularly responsive to treatment, nonetheless it is important to recognize this pattern to advise patients correctly and avoid unnecessary testing. Once appreciated, the history is typically dramatic and pathognomonic: that of headache onset one day essentially out of the blue, becoming constant and unremitting. The headache may begin in the context of a viral infection and occurs more commonly in females. Patients can often recall the exact day that the headache began. Extensive evaluations in multiple patients have failed to disclose any clear cause, and the headache is currently classified as a primary headache disorder. Treatment protocols have been published, though the general experience is that the headache pattern is relatively refractory. Empiric treatment can be guided by the underlying phenotype.

SECONDARY HEADACHE

Numerous secondary headaches are cataloged by the ICHD. Categories include headache attributed to trauma, infection, vascular disease, or homeostatic disorders; toxic or withdrawal headaches; and headache due to nonvascular intracranial conditions. Inclusion in the list of secondary headaches is based solely on rigorous scientific literature support of the headache as having a secondary cause, and headaches are viewed as secondary if they begin or worsen in relation to the development of the pathologic condition and, further, if they clear or improve with amelioration of the condition.

Medication Overuse Headache

Medication overuse headache involves the tendency among some people to overuse abortive or analgesic medications in the management of migraine, leading ultimately not to the expected improvement but to the development of a more refractory headache pattern. With discontinuance and after a latency period, clinical improvement is described in approximately half of the patients. The mechanism is unclear, and the evidence for both the existence of and management of this often stigmatizing diagnosis is not rigorous. Therefore the value of sudden and complete removal of purportedly overused symptomatic medications is unclear and may produce unanticipated negative outcomes. An argument can be made that this diagnosis should viewed with more skepticism.

Postural Headache due to a Cerebrospinal Fluid Leak

A spontaneous CSF leak occurs when there is a rupture in the meninges, the protective layers surround the brain and spinal cord, leading to leakage of CSF. The CSF is a clear liquid that surrounds and protects the brain and spinal cord. Patients present with postural headaches that worsen when upright and improve when lying down. Other symptoms may include muffled hearing, pulsatile tinnitus, and rarely diplopia. The exact etiology is not always clear, but structural defects or anatomical variations in the skull base or spinal canal may make the meninges more susceptible to tearing. Certain connective tissue disorders, such Ehlers-Danlos syndrome and Marfan syndrome, can weaken the connective tissues that support the meninges, making them more susceptible to tearing or rupturing. Gadolinium-enhanced MRI typically shows enhancement of the pachymeninges, but in 20% of cases the MRI is normal, and then specialized imaging studies like computed tomography (CT) cisternography or myelography may be used to detect the site of the leak. Conservative management may include bed rest, hydration, and caffeine. If conservative management is not effective, then an epidural blood patch can be performed. Refractory cases may require surgical intervention.

Headache Associated With COVID-19

Approximately 50% of patients with a COVID-19 infection will present with headache. The headache occurs more commonly in younger patients and in those who have a history of migraine. The pain is typically constant, bilateral in location, and moderate to severe in intensity. The pain is usually pressure-like in character, and while it may be accompanied by nausea, photophobia, and phonophobia, the majority of patients do not experience migraine-like features, and the typical phenotype is that of a tension-type headache. The headache may persist beyond the acute phase, especially in patients who have a past history of headache, and new daily persistent headache has been described. Headache has also been reported in up to 30% of patients who have received a COVID-19 vaccine, mostly patients with a preexisting history of headache. Initial symptomatic treatment is with acetaminophen or nonsteroidal antiinflammatory medication.

CONCLUSION

Headache, a condition that has been described almost since the beginning of recorded history, is now an area of increasingly intense interest and focus. Fundamental improvements in our understanding of this common and, at times, debilitating condition are emerging. A flexible system of categorization of the various headaches allows for proper management in the present and sets the stage for advancement of future discoveries. A working knowledge of the presentation and management of the various headaches is important in many clinical settings, given how common and potentially debilitating these conditions can be.

"For the full bibliography list, please use the pincode on the inside front cover to access the electronic version of the text at ebooks.health.elsevier.com."

12

Facial Pain and Cranial Neuralgias

William J. Mullally, Paul B. Rizzoli, Melissa Darsey, and Kathryn E. Hall

INTRODUCTION

Facial pain, often referred to as orofacial pain, refers to any type of discomfort localized to the face, from the hairline to the lower mandibles, including the oral and nasal cavities. When all causes are considered, the prevalence has been estimated to be as high as 26% of the general population with 7% experiencing chronic pain. The differential diagnosis is extensive and includes structural pathology, both malignant and nonmalignant, inflammatory disorders, dental disease, infection, primary headache disorders, and neuropathic/neuralgic syndromes. Females are affected more frequently than males, and patients often are suffering from a concomitant chronic pain condition involving another area of the body. Underlying psychological disorders and a smoking history may be contributing factors. Because of the broad range of etiologic possibilities, the treatment of facial pain may fall into the purview of multiple disciplines including, dentistry, primary care, ophthalmology, otolaryngology, oncology, neurology, and neurosurgery. The International Classification of Headache Disorders, Third Edition (ICHD-3) focuses predominantly on the neurologic causes of facial pain, and while the International Classification of Orofacial Pain also addresses the dental disorders, neither classification includes the myriad of potential etiologic possibilities.

Paroxysmal painful disorders involving the face and head are referred to as the cranial neuralgias. The pain is usually unilateral, lancinating, and electric shock–like in character with each episode lasting a short period of time. While the cranial neuralgias are rare, a diagnosis must be made with alacrity, as the pain is disabling, often

the result of underlying compression or inflammation. It is important to distinguish neuralgic pain from neuropathic pain. With a neuropathy the pain is more often constant and burning in character, and there may be specific deficits in the distribution of the involved nerve. In addition to the persistent discomfort of neuropathic pain, there may be brief intermittent paroxysmal neuralgic discomfort. In evaluating a patient with neuralgic pain, it is important to determine whether the pain is idiopathic or the cause is structural, inflammatory, or infectious. In this chapter we will review facial pain and then the cranial neuralgias.

Disorders of Cranial Bone

While cranial bones are relatively insensate, blood vessels, muscles, skin, and the periosteum are highly pain sensitive. The typical pain is dull and aching in character and is always secondary to underlying pathology. The differential diagnosis may include multiple myeloma, Paget disease, fibrous dysplasia, metastatic disease, and scalp infection/osteomyelitis. Osteomas, consisting primarily of mature cancellous bone, are benign slow-growing tumors commonly affecting the craniofacial region. They may involve the skull, jaw, or sinuses and present with facial deformity and, at times, orofacial pain. Osteomas are usually solitary tumors, but multiple osteomas may develop in patients with Gardner syndrome, which is a type of autosomal dominant familial adenomatous polyposis. The diagnosis of cranial bone disorders requires palpation of the affected area and observing for tenderness, erythema, increased warmth, and evidence of a mass. Workup should include skull x-rays, computed tomography (CT) of the skull, and potentially a bone scan. Treatment is specific to the underlying cause. The pain of osteomas usually responds to aspirin or other nonsteroidal antiinflammatory medication. Indications for surgical treatment of osteomas include cosmetic disfigurement, progressive increase in volume, impingement on underlying structures, and limitation of function, which may occur with a tumor in the mandible.

Disorders of the Eye

Eye pain is a common cause of primary care and emergency room visits. When eye pain is accompanied by visual difficulty, the patient requires an emergent ophthalmology evaluation. Decreased visual acuity with accompanying eye pain occurs in acute angle closure glaucoma, scleritis, optic neuritis, orbital cellulitis, pituitary apoplexy, anterior uveitis, and keratitis.

Acute closed-angle glaucoma will cause retro-orbital and periorbital pain with severe central visual field defects accompanied by corneal clouding, fixed mydriasis, and conjunctival injection. Patients must receive immediate ophthalmologic treatment.

The sclera is the protective fibrous coating of the eye. The episclera is continuous with the cornea and covers the sclera. Scleritis causes severe boring eye pain that intensifies with movement of the eye and may precipitate a more generalized headache. The eye appears red with a bluish discoloration of the sclera, and vision is impaired. Episcleritis causes engorgement of superficial blood vessels but is not painful, and there is no accompanying visual loss or bluish discoloration. Scleritis is usually the result of an underlying rheumatologic disease, but infection must be ruled out. For noninfectious scleritis, initial treatment is with nonsteroidal antiinflammatory medication.

Optic neuritis causes orbital pain that increases with eye movement. Visual loss occurs over days, and on examination an afferent pupillary defect will be detected. Optic neuritis may be the result of multiple sclerosis or an underlying systemic inflammatory disorder. Patients should receive high-dose intravenous corticosteroids under the care of neurology and ophthalmology.

Pituitary apoplexy is a sudden infarction or hemorrhage of the pituitary gland within a pituitary adenoma and presents with the apoplectic onset of headache, eye pain, visual loss, and an oculomotor nerve deficit with ptosis, dilated pupil, and lateral eye deviation. Adrenal crisis occurs, and the patient requires immediate corticosteroid replacement. Patients with visual loss will require emergency neurosurgical intervention.

Orbital cellulitis presents with eye pain and swelling, diplopia with diminished eye movement, proptosis, visual loss, and ptosis. Associated paranasal sinusitis may be present, and treatment with intravenous antibiotics is indicated.

The uvea is the pigmented layer of the eye lying beneath the sclera comprising the iris, ciliary body, and choroid. Anterior uveitis, which is inflammation of the iris and ciliary body, presents with pain, photophobia, meiosis, and ciliary flush. This is often associated with underlying systemic inflammatory disorders such as sarcoidosis, rheumatoid arthritis, syphilis, reactive arthritis, or seronegative spondyloarthropathies. Treatment will depend on the cause. For noninfectious disorders, topical steroids and an immunosuppressant are indicated.

Infectious keratitis (inflammation of the cornea) due to herpes simplex virus, herpes zoster ophthalmicus, bacteria, or acanthamoeba causes eye pain, eye redness, photophobia, and visual loss due to corneal damage. Management by ophthalmology is indicated.

There are multiple disorders of the eye that cause pain without visual loss. The most common are corneal abrasions, hordeolum, and conjunctivitis. Dry eye syndrome may present with a burning discomfort.

Eye pain with ophthalmoplegia involving the oculomotor, abducens, and trochlear cranial nerves may occur as the result of an ischemic neuropathy usually due to diabetes mellitus, giant cell arteritis, or a systemic inflammatory disorder. The oculomotor nerve is most commonly involved, followed by the abducens nerve. The trochlear is rarely affected. The ophthalmoplegia lasts from weeks to months and then usually spontaneously resolves. Contrast-enhanced brain magnetic resonance imaging (MRI) and a magnetic resonance angiogram (MRA) should be performed, and the patient should also undergo testing to rule out giant cell arteritis.

Cavernous sinus thrombosis is a rare life-threatening disorder that presents with unilateral eye pain with proptosis, chemosis, and ophthalmoplegia. It may be the result of a facial infection, orbital cellulitis, sinusitis, pharyngitis, otitis media, surgery, or trauma. Fever will be present if there is an underlying infection. The oculomotor, abducens, and trochlear nerves and the first two divisions of the trigeminal nerve reside in the cavernous sinus, and involvement of several or all the cranial nerves located in the cavernous sinus may occur secondary to compression and inflammation. Contrast-enhanced brain MRI, MRA, and magnetic resonance venogram should be performed emergently. A lumbar puncture is required to exclude meningitis. Treatment is with parenteral antibiotics and anticoagulation.

Tolosa Hunt syndrome is a relatively benign idiopathic granulomatous inflammatory disorder of the cavernous sinus, superior orbital fissure, and occasionally the orbital apex. Symptoms include severe periorbital pain extending into the frontal and temporal regions. The pain increases with eye movement, and the oculomotor, abducens, and trochlear cranial nerves are involved, resulting in ophthalmoparesis and diplopia. Dramatic improvement usually occurs within 2–3 days after treatment with corticosteroids has begun. Untreated, symptoms will usually resolve within 8 weeks. Brain MRI with contrast and an MRA are indicated.

Trochlear headache presents with unilateral periorbital and frontal pain due to trochlear inflammation. The pain increases with eye movement and responds to nonsteroidal antiinflammatory drugs or a direct injection of a local anesthetic or steroid.

Heterophoria, heterotropia, and refractive errors may cause mild dull eye pain or frontal aching discomfort but not a severe headache.

Paroxysmal sharp stabbing pain into the eye lasting seconds is referred to as ophthalmodynia periodica and is an uncommon presentation of primary stabbing headache. While confined to the eye, the pain is not secondary to ocular pathology.

Rhinosinusitis

Although rhinosinusitis is often implicated as a cause of headaches, studies have shown that approximately 90% of patients who believe that they are suffering from "sinus" headaches fulfill the ICHD-3 criteria for migraine without aura. Chronic sinusitis persisting for more than 12 weeks rarely causes facial pain or headache. The location of pain is similar for both types of headaches, and migraine is often pressure-like in character and not uncommonly accompanied by nasal congestion and discharge. Both types of headaches can be precipitated by changes in barometric pressure, but whereas migraines last from hours to 1–2 days, a true sinus-related headache can persist for days to weeks. The pain from rhinosinusitis is secondary to inflammation of the sinus and nasal cavity, but pain is not the hallmark of the disorder, and only approximately one-third of patients experience facial pain or headache. Most infections are viral, and symptoms include nasal congestion,

postnasal drip, runny nose with discolored mucus, facial tenderness, and typical symptoms of an upper respiratory infection. With bacterial sinusitis, patients will be febrile and experience fatigue and pressure in the ears. Halitosis may be present. Sphenoid sinusitis is rare but more likely to cause a headache than infection in the other sinuses and is usually not accompanied by nasal congestion or discharge. The pain may be frontal, periorbital, temporal, or occipital in location. Thunderclap headache has been described with sphenoid sinusitis, and the pain may be accompanied by nausea and vomiting and photophobia. Complications include bacterial meningitis, subdural abscess, and cavernous sinus thrombosis.

Rhinosinusitis should be managed by ENT with antibiotics if a bacterial infection is suspected. A CT of the sinuses and a brain MRI may be required.

Dental Disease

Dental pathology, specifically caries and apical root infections, is the most common cause of lower orofacial pain. The character is usually constant and aching, but intermittent jabbing pain may occur. Diagnosis is facilitated by evidence of inflammation in the oral cavity and pain when palpating the affected tooth. Odontogenic pain is usually precipitated by intake of cold or hot liquids. Diseases of the oral mucosa may cause facial pain and disorders of the salivary glands due to sialolithiasis, sialadenitis, infection, Sjögren syndrome, or benign or cancerous tumors.

Burning Mouth Syndrome

Burning mouth syndrome (BMS) is a rare chronic disorder characterized by a burning sensation in the oral cavity without evidence of oral mucosal pathology. The tip of the tongue is usually involved, and there is often accompanying dysgeusia and a sense of dryness. It occurs more commonly in perimenopausal or postmenopausal females, and onset is spontaneous. With primary or idiopathic BMS a cause cannot be identified. Secondary BMS may be due to candidiasis, vitamin or nutritional deficiencies, diabetes mellitus, Sjögren syndrome, or psychosocial stressors. A small fiber neuropathy has been proposed as the potential etiology. If an underlying cause is not detected, then treatment may include topical lidocaine, capsaicin, alpha-lipoic acid, tricyclic antidepressant, gabapentin, pregabalin, venlafaxine, or duloxetine. Cognitive behavioral therapy may also be helpful.

Eagle Syndrome

Eagle syndrome, often referred to as stylohyoid syndrome, is a rare disorder that is the result of an elongated or disfigured styloid process. Neck movement can provoke orofacial and cervical pain by compressing adjacent structures, most commonly the glossopharyngeal nerve, but multiple cranial nerves can be stretched or compressed, accounting for the facial pain. The pain is usually unilateral, but bilateral discomfort may occur. It was initially described following tonsillectomy but usually there is no history of surgery. Impingement of the internal carotid artery will result in ipsilateral supraorbital pain and rarely transient neurologic symptoms. Surgical intervention may be indicated, but pain can often be managed with nonsteroidal antiinflammatory drugs, antidepressant medication, anticonvulsant medication, or transpharyngeal injections of a steroid and local anesthetic.

Gradenigo Syndrome

The classic triad of Gradenigo syndrome, also referred to as petrous apicitis, includes suppurative otitis media, abducens nerve palsy, and pain in the distribution of the trigeminal nerve. Patients present with retro-orbital and periorbital pain due to involvement of the trigeminal ganglion and diplopia due to a sixth nerve palsy. Ipsilateral peripheral facial weakness occurs if the seventh cranial nerve is affected, and rarely deficits of cranial nerves VIII, IX, and X are seen. Possible complications include meningitis and intracranial abscess. Both high-resolution temporal bone CT and brain MRI are required to evaluate the underlying pathology. Patients usually respond to high-dose antibiotic therapy, obviating the need for surgical intervention. In the postantibiotic era, the syndrome with the classic triad has become extremely rare.

Neck-Tongue Syndrome

Neck-tongue syndrome is characterized by episodes of severe sharp and stabbing pain lasting seconds to minutes in the neck extending into the occipital region. Unilateral auricular pain extending into the face may occur, and the discomfort is accompanied by numbness and dysesthesias of the ipsilateral tongue. Symptoms are precipitated by sudden rotation of the head and neck and typically occur in the pediatric and adolescent age group. The most likely cause is transient subluxation of the lateral atlantoaxial joint due to ligamentous laxity.

Cases have been observed to occur in families, suggesting a genetic predisposition. An MRI scan of the cervical spine and base of the brain should be performed. Most patients do not require treatment, but for persistent symptoms, cervical spine immobilization, spinal manipulation, and surgery to stabilize the spine have been used with reported success. Spinal manipulation is contraindicated if there is evidence of atlantoaxial instability, and there is the risk of vertebral artery dissection.

Carotid Artery Dissection

Carotid artery dissection is the result of a tear of the intimal layer of the carotid artery either occurring spontaneously or as the result of trauma. Blood flow to areas of the brain may be compromised, potentially resulting in an ischemic stroke, and dissection is the leading cause of stroke in younger patients. The tear results in an intramural hematoma causing stenosis of the vessel and thrombus formation. Traumatic dissections can occur as the result of a forcible whiplash injury, blunt trauma, or violent coughing or sneezing. Fibromuscular dysplasia, Marfan syndrome, and Ehlers-Danlos syndrome may increase the risk of spontaneous dissection, and it has been reported with Eagle syndrome due to direct contact on the carotid artery by the elongated styloid process. The presentation can be widely varied from a devastating stroke to simply a headache and facial pain on the side of the dissection. An ipsilateral Horner syndrome is often observed. CT angiogram or MRA of the neck including axial fat-suppressed T1-weighted images should be performed emergently if dissection is suspected. A head CT will detect a hemorrhage, but a brain MRI with diffusion-weighted images is required to determine whether there is evidence of an acute stroke. While the optimal treatment remains somewhat controversial, a direct oral anticoagulant for 3 months followed by 81 mg of aspirin daily for at least 3 additional months is the most pragmatic approach. Follow-up imaging of the vessels should be performed at 6 months. Endovascular carotid artery stenting has been performed on patients with symptoms of ischemic stroke and evidence of significant hypoperfusion on imaging, but controlled studies comparing it to the best medical therapy have not been performed.

Cervicogenic Headache

Headache and facial pain may occur as a result of disorders of the cervical spine. The pain is most commonly unilateral, nonthrobbing, and nonlancinating in character, beginning posteriorly then extending into the frontal region and face. Neck pain always accompanies the headache and may involve the shoulder and arm on the same side. Cervical range of motion is reduced, and provocative maneuvers will exacerbate the pain The pain affects males and females equally beginning in the fourth and fifth decades of life. While cervical structural disease, such as a herniated nucleus pulposus or degenerative disease, may be the cause, many patients have no detectable cervical spine pathology. In the elderly, cervical spondylosis is often the source of the pain. Physiotherapy is usually beneficial, and medication options include acetaminophen, nonsteroidal antiinflammatory medication, muscle relaxants, and tricyclic antidepressants. Acupuncture can be considered. If the pain does not respond to treatment, then MRI scans of the brain and cervical spine should be performed.

GIANT CELL ARTERITIS

Giant cell arteritis (GCA) is the most common systemic vasculitis in adults, and it occurs almost exclusively in patients over the age of 50, affecting females more than males. The granulomatous inflammation involves medium and large vessels, predominantly the temporal, ophthalmic, occipital, and vertebral arteries. The aorta and its proximal branches may also be involved and, rarely, intracranial vessels. Blood vessel inflammation can lead to stenosis, occlusion, or aneurysm formation. Headache is the presenting symptom in 80%–90% of patients, and the pain is usually unilateral, involving the temporal region with tenderness of the area, although any part of the head may be involved, and the pain may be bilateral. Other symptoms may include cramping pain in the jaw while chewing referred to as jaw claudication, malaise, fever, night sweats, and in 40%–60% of patients an accompanying rheumatologic condition, polymyalgia rheumatica, with pain and stiffness in proximal joints, typically the shoulders and hips. Patients who have a history of polymyalgia rheumatica alone have a 16%–21% chance of developing GCA especially if untreated. With GCA the sedimentation rate (ESR) and C-reactive protein (CRP) are usually significantly elevated, with CRP being the more sensitive test. However, 22.5% of patients who have GCA confirmed by temporal artery biopsy have a normal sedimentation, and 2%–14% of patients have a normal CRP. Four percent of patients with biopsy-confirmed GCA have both normal CRP and ESR. Blood work will often reveal anemia and thrombocytosis, and leukocytosis may also be present.

Doppler ultrasonography is a first-line diagnostic tool with a sensitivity of 69% and specificity of 82%, but techniques are constantly improving. The classic finding is the halo sign, which is a hyperechoic ring around the arterial lumen indicating thickening of the arterial wall due to inflammation. MRA is an alternative with a sensitivity of 73% and a specificity of 88%, and positron emission tomography has also been used with a sensitivity of 73%–92% and a specificity of 83%–85%. Temporal artery biopsy remains the gold standard for diagnosis with a specificity of 98% but a sensitivity of only 61% as the biopsy may miss skipped lesions in the artery. GCA is a medical emergency, as visual loss, stroke, and death may occur if treatment is delayed. Patients should be placed on prednisone 60 mg daily, and treatment should optimally be initiated prior to the biopsy to prevent visual loss due to ophthalmic artery occlusion. There is no advantage to using intravenous corticosteroids compared to high-dose oral corticosteroids. The IL-6 receptor alpha inhibitor tocilizumab is now used for maintenance of remission and reduction in the dose of glucocorticoids, but it is not effective in the acute phase, as it does not prevent optic neuropathy.

Raeder's Paratrigeminal Neuralgia

Raeder's paratrigeminal neuralgia is a unilateral deep, boring, nonpulsatile periorbital and retro-orbital pain accompanied by ptosis, meiosis, eyelid edema, and nasal congestion or rhinorrhea. Facial sweating is preserved. The syndrome is more common in males between the ages of 40 and 50 years, although onset has been reported in the second through eighth decades. The disorder may be idiopathic or secondary due to a parasellar mass, internal carotid artery aneurysm, head trauma, vasculitis, or sinusitis. Johan Raeder first described the syndrome in 1918, and it appears, based on our current knowledge of headache disorders, that the idiopathic form may actually be a trigeminal autonomic cephalgia, hemicrania continua, and not a distinct entity. Evaluation would include gadolinium-enhanced MRI of the brain and MRA. If the workup is negative, then a trial of treatment with indomethacin should be initiated beginning at 25 mg three times per day and increasing up to 225 mg/daily. Topiramate is also an option.

Temporomandibular disorder

Patients with temporomandibular disorder (TMD) present with unilateral facial pain that is usually dull or aching in character and accentuated by palpation or movement of the temporomandibular joint or muscles of mastication.

Intermittently, the patient may experience sharp stabbing pain in the temporomandibular region. Accompanying symptoms may include diminished excursion of the mandible on opening the jaw, deviation of the mandible suggesting subluxation and temporomandibular joint crepitations. Crepitations are significant only if there is accompanying pain, and restricted jaw movement is not required to make the diagnosis. The lower facial pain may extend into the temporal region, but the resultant headache does not have migraine-like features. TMD is more common in females, with a prevalence of 5%–15% in the general population and an incidence of 4% in adults. Risk factors for developing TMD include mood disorders, bruxism, migraine, tension-type headache, trauma, and other chronic pain conditions. Patients usually respond to a dental appliance and jaw exercises. Muscle relaxant medication such as orphenadrine or cyclobenzaprine or a tricyclic antidepressant medication, amitriptyline, or nortriptyline, may be beneficial. Surgical intervention should be considered as a last resort and only if MRI imaging of the temporomandibular joint is significantly abnormal. Botulinum toxin A injections into the masseter muscle may provide relief for up to 3–4 months.

Intracranial Lesions

Referred pain to the face may be the result of a mass lesion such as meningioma, schwannoma, neurofibroma, cholesteatoma, pituitary tumor, or nasopharyngeal cancer. The pain is caused by traction on or inflammation of meninges, cranial nerves, or blood vessels. The pain is most often dull, nonpulsatile, constant, and unremitting, aggravated by exertion and change in position, but intermittent neuralgic pain may occur. Headache and facial pain, however, are rarely the presenting symptom of tumor. Thalamic lesions such as stroke may cause unilateral burning facial pain accompanied by a dysesthetic sensation. Constant severe unilateral lower facial pain extending into the ear may be the presenting symptom of nonmetastatic lung cancer. If an underlying structural lesion is suspected, then an MRI of the brain with gadolinium should be performed. For unremitting lower facial pain without an obvious cause, a chest CT scan should be considered.

Primary Headache Disorders

The primary headache disorders are discussed in detail in another chapter, but clinicians must be mindful of the fact that the trigeminal autonomic cephalgias and migraine may present with middle and lower orofacial pain. It often takes years for a patient with cluster headache to be accurately diagnosed, and patients who report severe unilateral maxillary pain during an attack often undergo unnecessary dental procedures. Also due to the prominent autonomic symptoms, specifically nasal congestion and discharge, in association with the severe pain, many patients are subjected to sinus surgery. The interventions are not performed with any malice, as the treating clinicians are desperately trying to provide relief for their patients who are suffering from disabling head pain that is often referred to as the "suicide headache." Severe retro-orbital and periorbital pain occurs with cluster headache, paroxysmal hemicrania, and short-lasting unilateral neuralgiform headache (SUNA). Migraine headache may also be confined to the face on occasion, and "facial migraine" and "lower half headache" are well described in the literature but not listed as a distinct diagnostic entities in the ICHD-3 classification. With "facial migraine" the pain is confined to the lower face and accompanied by typical migrainous features, including nausea, photophobia, and phonophobia.

CRANIAL NEURALGIA

Trigeminal Neuralgia

In 1677, John Locke provided the first detailed description of trigeminal neuralgia, and a French physician, Nicholas Andre, in 1756 coined the term "tic douloureux," as the episodes of facial pain were associated with transient twitching of the facial muscles. The classification of trigeminal neuralgia has evolved over the years, and the most current criteria are listed in the ICHD-3 (Box 12.1). The classification includes subdivisions, and

---

BOX 12.1 Trigeminal Neuralgia Diagnostic Criteria in International Classification of Headache Disorders, Third Edition (ICHD-3)

Diagnostic criteria

Recurrent paroxysms of unilateral facial pain in the distribution(s) of one or more divisions of the trigeminal nerve, with no radiation beyond, and fulfilling criteria B and C

A. Pain has all of the following characteristics:
1. lasting from a fraction of a second to 2 minutes
2. severe intensity
3. electric shock–like, shooting, stabbing or sharp in quality
B. Precipitated by innocuous stimuli within the affected trigeminal distribution
C. Not better accounted for by another ICHD-3 diagnosis

a diagnosis of classical trigeminal neuralgia is made when there is evidence of neurovascular compression, usually by the superior cerebellar artery, on MRI/MRA sequences with nerve root atrophy or displacement. If the trigeminal neuralgia is due to compression from a mass or a demyelinating plaque, it is then referred to as secondary trigeminal neuralgia. If the etiology is unknown and imaging and electrophysiologic testing are normal, then the diagnosis is idiopathic trigeminal neuralgia. While most patients are pain free between the paroxysms of pain, some will experience continuous dull discomfort, which is officially referred to as trigeminal neuralgia with concomitant continuous pain. Figure 12.1 depicts the nerves of the face.

Trigeminal neuralgia is rare, with a lifetime prevalence of 0.3%. The disorder is slightly more common in females, and while most patients are over 50 years of age, patients with idiopathic or secondary trigeminal neuralgia may present at a younger age. Trigeminal neuralgia is sporadic, but up to 11% of patients have a family history. While cluster headache has been referred to as the "suicide headache" trigeminal neuralgia has been described as the "suicide disease" because of the excruciating pain. Episodes are paroxysmal, brief, lancinating and shock-like with repetitive attacks occurring over a period of usually less than 1 hour. The pain is almost always unilateral, more often right sided, and predominantly confined to the second and third divisions of the trigeminal nerve (Table 12.1). Bilateral trigeminal neuralgia should raise the possibility of a demyelinating lesion secondary to multiple sclerosis. Trigeminal neuralgia occurring in the distribution of the ophthalmic division of the trigeminal nerve occurs in fewer than 5% of affected patients and is often accompanied by mild autonomic symptoms, making the distinction between trigeminal neuralgia and short-lasting unilateral neuralgiform headache with cranial autonomic symptoms (SUNA) somewhat murky. Ninety-nine percent of patients with trigeminal neuralgia report triggers such as brushing teeth, chewing food, talking, shaving, applying makeup, touching the face, or exposure to a cold wind. After a series of severe paroxysmal attacks, patients often describe a refractory period during which the triggers no longer precipitate pain. It is interesting that SUNA patients also describe triggers but without a refractory period, and the age of onset is much later than with other trigeminal autonomic cephalgias. Patients with trigeminal neuralgia may experience random remissions from pain lasting from weeks to years.

The neurologic examination in classical and idiopathic trigeminal neuralgia is normal. With secondary trigeminal neuralgia, sensory loss in the distribution of the affected nerve will be present. The most common causes of secondary trigeminal neuralgia are multiple sclerosis and a cerebellar pontine angle tumor, and the onset of trigeminal neuralgia may precede the diagnosis of multiple sclerosis by years. Other secondary causes include epidermoid cyst, aneurysm, arteriovenous malformation, bony compression from an osteoma, and small infarcts in the brain stem. Diagnostic testing should include a gadolinium-enhanced brain MRI with thin cuts through the posterior fossa in combination with a time-of-flight MRA to look for vascular compression.

Regarding treatment, carbamazepine is the most effective medicine, bringing relief from the pain in approximately 80% of patients, but the beneficial effects tend to wane over time. Carbamazepine blocks sodium channels, stabilizing the membrane and reducing the hyperexcitability of the trigeminal nerve root and ganglion. The medicine has potential side effects, including drowsiness, dizziness, ataxia, bone marrow suppression, hepatotoxicity, and hyponatremia, and blood work should be performed prior to starting and then at regular intervals while the patient is on the medicine. Prior to beginning carbamazepine in Asian patients, genetic testing for the HLA B* 1502 allele should be performed due to the high risk of Stevens-Johnson syndrome, toxic epidermal necrolysis, and drug-induced hypersensitivity rash with eosinophilia and systemic symptoms. The initial dose should be 200 mg twice/day, and the dose can be gradually increased as tolerated and as necessary to 600 mg twice/day. A carbamazepine level will help to direct adjustment of the dose and avoid toxicity. Oxcarbazepine is also effective with the same mechanism of action as carbamazepine with dose range from 300 to 1800 mg/day in two divided doses. While oxcarbazepine is better tolerated than carbamazepine, there is a higher incidence of hyponatremia. Other medication options include gabapentin, pregabalin, lamotrigine, phenytoin, eslicarbazepine, topiramate, and baclofen. Onabotulinum toxin A injections have been used with reports of success. Patients presenting to the hospital emergency department with an acute exacerbation that is refractory to medication can be treated with intravenous fosphenytoin. Peripheral trigeminal nerve blocks of the affected trigeminal nerve branches using bupivacaine may provide temporary relief.

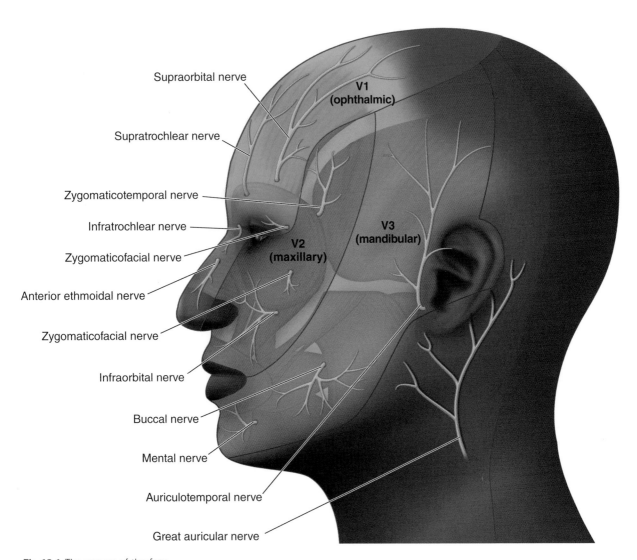

Fig 12.1 The nerves of the face.

TABLE 12.1	**Trigeminal Nerve Terminal Branches**	
Ophthalmic (V1)	Frontal	• Supratrochlear • Supraorbital

	Nasociliary	• Long ciliary
		• Infratrochlear
		• Posterior ethmoidal
		• Anterior ethmoidal
		  • External nasal
		• Sensory root of ciliary ganglion
		  • Ciliary ganglion

	Lacrimal	
Maxillary (V2)	In middle cranial fossa	• Middle meningeal

	In pterygopalatine fossa	• Zygomatic
		  • Zygomaticotemporal
		• Zygomaticofacial
		• Infraorbital
		  • Posterior superior alveolar
		  • Middle superior alveolar
		• Anterior superior alveolar

Mandibular (V3)	In middle cranial fossa	• Meningeal

	Anterior division	• To muscles of mastication
		  • Medial pterygoid/to tensor veli palatini
		  • Lateral pterygoid
		  • Masseteric
		  • Deep temporal
		• Buccal

	Posterior division	• Auriculotemporal
		  • Otic ganglion
		• Lingual
		  • Submandibular ganglion
		• Inferior alveolar
		• Mylohyoid
		  • Mental

A patient who has not responded to or not tolerated treatment with multiple medications would then be a candidate for invasive treatment. Stereotactic radiosurgery is performed by directing an external beam of radiation to part of the trigeminal nerve root. The response rate is 85% within 2 weeks to 2 months, and 33%–56% of patients are pain free at 4–5 years. Side effects occurring in 3% of patients include sensory loss and weakness of masticatory muscles; rarely, anesthesia dolorosa develops, which is a constant burning pain accompanied by numbness in the distribution of the damaged nerve. Percutaneous ablative procedures are also an option, including radiofrequency thermocoagulation, glycerol injection, or balloon compression targeting the trigeminal nerve branches or ganglion. Initial pain relief occurs in 90% of patients and is sustained in 53%–69% at 3 years. Twenty percent will experience side effects similar to those following stereotactic radiosurgery. Partial sensory rhizotomy with surgical section of the trigeminal sensory nerve root may provide sustained relief in 70%–80% of patients with side effects like those of the other ablative procedures. For classical trigeminal neuralgia, microvascular decompression is reported to have the greatest probability of pain relief with 68%–88% of patients pain free at 1–2 years postoperatively and 64% at 10 years. The procedure, which was pioneered by Peter Jannetta in the 1960s, requires a retromastoid craniotomy and then placement of synthetic material between the vessel and the nerve. Potential side effects at less than 2% include cerebrospinal fluid (CSF) leak, facial palsy, ipsilateral hearing loss, facial numbness, brain stem infarct, abducens or trochlear palsy, and death. Seventeen percent of patients suffer a transient aseptic meningitis.

Painful Trigeminal Neuropathy

Trigeminal neuropathy presents with numbness in the distribution of one or more branches of the trigeminal nerve and may be accompanied by constant burning pain with paresthesias and a dysesthetic sensation. Superimposed paroxysmal pain may occur intermittently, but the predominant discomfort is constant burning accompanied by allodynia and hyperesthesia. The etiology may be infectious, inflammatory, neoplastic, or posttraumatic following dental or facial surgery. Neuroablative procedures for trigeminal neuralgia may result in a painful trigeminal neuropathy.

A herpes zoster viral infection with a vesicular rash in the distribution of one or more branches of the trigeminal nerve will cause constant neuropathic pain; rarely, the infection occurs without the accompanying rash (zoster sine herpete). A diagnosis of postherpetic neuralgia is made if the pain persists for more than 3 months. When the rash and pain are in the distribution of the first division of the trigeminal nerve, the condition is referred to as herpes zoster ophthalmicus, which represents approximately 10% of all herpes zoster cases.

Isolated numbness and pain of the chin, referred to as mental nerve neuropathy or numb chin syndrome, often suggest an ominous diagnosis. In the absence of a precipitating cause, such as facial surgery or a dental procedure, patients will often be found to have an underlying malignancy, most commonly metastatic breast cancer.

Patients who present with a trigeminal neuropathy require an MRI of the brain with gadolinium. Additional testing will depend on the results. A herpes zoster infection should receive treatment with an antiviral agent (acyclovir, valacyclovir, or famciclovir) within 72 hours of the appearance of the rash. For symptomatic treatment of trigeminal neuropathic pain, a tricyclic antidepressant (amitriptyline or nortriptyline), gabapentin, pregabalin, or duloxetine, may be used. Onabotulinum toxin A may be an option, and topical lidocaine or capsaicin is sometimes effective.

Glossopharyngeal Neuralgia

Glossopharyngeal neuralgia (Box 12.2) causes pain very similar to that of trigeminal neuralgia, typically in the tonsillar region and back of the pharynx. The discomfort is unilateral and can extend into the ear and below the angle of the jaw. The paroxysmal electric shock–like attacks of pain last from seconds to 2 minutes and at times can occur in rapid sequence. The pain is typically provoked by swallowing, coughing, yawning, throat clearing, and speaking. Approximately 2% of patients suffer syncope in association with the pain due to a bradyarrhythmia secondary to vagal nerve involvement. The incidence is quite rare at 0.2–0.7/100,000, and it can occur in association with trigeminal neuralgia. The painful episodes occur in cycles lasting weeks to months and may increase in frequency and severity over time. Typically, glossopharyngeal neuralgia, like trigeminal neuralgia, is caused by neurovascular compression, most commonly

---

BOX 12.2 Glossopharyngeal Neuralgia Classification in International Classification of Headache Disorders, Third Edition (ICHD-3)

Description

A disorder characterized by unilateral brief stabbing pain, abrupt in onset and termination, in the distributions not only of the glossopharyngeal nerve but also of the auricular and pharyngeal branches of the vagus nerve. Pain is experienced in the ear, base of the tongue, tonsillar fossa, and/or beneath the angle of the jaw. It is commonly provoked by swallowing, talking, or coughing and may remit and relapse in the fashion of trigeminal neuralgia.

Diagnostic criteria

A. Recurring paroxysmal attacks of unilateral pain in the distribution of the glossopharyngeal nerve and fulfilling criterion B
B. Pain has all of the following characteristics:
   1. lasting from a few seconds to 2 minutes
   2. severe intensity
   3. electric shock–like, shooting, stabbing, or sharp in quality
   4. precipitated by swallowing, coughing, talking, or yawning
C. Not better accounted for by another ICHD-3 diagnosis

Note

Within the posterior part of the tongue, tonsillar fossa, pharynx or angle of the lower jaw and/or in the ear.

by the posterior inferior cerebellar artery but occasionally by the vertebral artery or anterior inferior cerebellar artery. Potential secondary causes include oropharyngeal, laryngeal, or skull-based tumor; parapharyngeal abscess; demyelinating lesion; carotid sheath trauma; or elongated Eagle syndrome. Evaluation includes contrast-enhanced MRI scans of the brain and anterior neck, and a time-of-flight MRA. Pharmacologic treatment is identical to that of trigeminal neuralgia. A topical anesthetic or a glossopharyngeal nerve block may provide temporary relief from the pain. Microvascular decompression or direct sectioning of the glossopharyngeal nerve can be considered for cases that are refractory to medical therapy.

Nervus Intermedius Neuralgia

Nervus intermedius neuralgia (Box 12.3), also referred to as geniculate neuralgia, is characterized by paroxysmal stabbing pain in one ear lasting from seconds to a few minutes. The pain can be precipitated by light touch or a cold wind against the posterior wall of the external auditory canal. Onset is in the sixth decade of life, and females are affected more often than males. The pain may be accompanied by increased salivation, tinnitus, rhinorrhea, hyperacusis, and a bitter taste.

Neuralgic pain may follow Ramsey Hunt syndrome, which is a herpes zoster viral infection causing a vesicular rash in the ear canal and ipsilateral facial paralysis. Zoster sine herpete has been reported in up to 30% of cases. If the pain persists for more than 3 months, it is referred to as postherpetic neuralgia of the nervus intermedius.

Continuous ear pain that may or not be accompanied by brief paroxysms and is a result of a disorder other than herpes zoster is referred to as painful nervus intermedius neuropathy.

An MRI of the brain with gadolinium should be performed to rule out a cerebellopontine angle tumor. Pharmacologic treatment of the neuralgic pain is identical to the treatment of trigeminal neuralgia. Microvascular decompression and nervus intermedius sectioning may be considered if the pain is refractory to medical therapy.

Superior Laryngeal Nerve Neuralgia

Superior laryngeal nerve neuralgia is a rare condition that usually begins in the sixth decade of life and is more common in males. It presents with severe unilateral paroxysmal pain in the anterior neck extending into the submandibular region and ear. Episodes are brief, lasting seconds to several minutes, but may occur up to

---

BOX 12.3 Nervus Intermedius Neuralgia Classification in International Classification of Headache Disorders, Third Edition (ICHD-3)

Previously used term
Geniculate neuralgia

Description
A rare disorder characterized by brief paroxysms of pain felt deeply in the auditory canal, sometimes radiating to the parieto-occipital region. In the vast majority of cases, vascular compression is found at operation, occasionally with a thickened arachnoid, but it may develop without apparent cause or as a complication of herpes zoster or, very rarely, multiple sclerosis or tumor. It is provoked by stimulation of a trigger area in the posterior wall of the auditory canal and/or periauricular region.

Diagnostic criteria
A. Paroxysmal attacks of unilateral pain in the distribution of nervus intermedius and fulfilling criterion B
B. Pain has all of the following characteristics:
   1. lasting from a few seconds to minutes
   2. severe in intensity
   3. shooting, stabbing or sharp in quality
   4. precipitated by stimulation of a trigger area in the posterior wall of the auditory canal and/or periauricular region
C. Not better accounted for by another ICHD-3 diagnosis

Notes
1. Pain is located in the auditory canal, the auricle, the region of the mastoid process, and occasionally the soft palate and may sometimes radiate to the temporal region or the angle of the mandible.
2. In view of the complex and overlapping innervation of the external ear, deriving from trigeminal (auriculotemporal), facial (nervus intermedius), glossopharyngeal, vagus, and second cranial nerves, attribution of neuralgias to a single nerve may not be easy in this body region when a specific neurovascular contact cannot be visualized.

10–30 times/day and are usually accompanied by an urge to swallow, which precipitates an exacerbation of the pain. Coughing, sneezing, yawning, blowing the nose, and head rotation may precipitate the pain. Patients are unable to speak during an episode. The superior laryngeal nerve is a branch of the vagus nerve and supplies sensory and motor innervation of the larynx and

the glottic reflex. Damage to the nerve may occur as a result of carotid endarterectomy or thyroidectomy. Tumor must be considered as a potential cause, and patients should be evaluated by otolaryngology. While the typical anticonvulsant medications that are used in the treatment of the neuralgic pain disorders may be of benefit, patients often respond to a 4% lidocaine spray or an injection of lidocaine and a steroid into the space between the thyroid cartilage and hyoid bone where the nerve traverses. Surgical superior laryngeal neurotomy is a consideration for refractory cases as a last resort.

Nasociliary Neuralgia

Nasociliary neuralgia is a rare syndrome characterized by paroxysmal stabbing pain along one side of the nose extending to the eye and frontal region and typically lasting from seconds to 1 hour. Episodes can occur two to three times per day. Patients may note hyperesthesia on the affected side of the nose, and the pain can be precipitated by touching the ipsilateral nostril. The pain may be accompanied by increased lacrimation and nasal congestion and/or discharge on the side of the pain. The nasociliary nerve is a branch of the ophthalmic nerve, and it divides into three branches, one of which is the anterior ethmoidal nerve, which in turn gives rise to the external nasal nerve. The neuralgic syndrome is usually the result of trauma to the external nasal nerve and has been reported following rhinoplasty. Idiopathic cases may also occur. Brain MRI and CT scan of the sinuses are usually negative. Lidocaine nasal spray may sometimes provide temporary relief, but most patients respond to nerve blockade with a local anesthetic. Medication options include a tricyclic antidepressant medication, gabapentin, pregabalin, or duloxetine.

Supraorbital and Supratrochlear Neuralgia

It is extremely difficult to differentiate supraorbital from supratrochlear neuralgia. Both the supraorbital and supratrochlear nerves, which are terminal branches of the frontal nerve, a branch of the ophthalmic nerve, provide sensory innervation to the skin of the upper eyelid and forehead with the supratrochlear nerve medial to the supraorbital nerve. Anatomic variations of both nerves are common. The pain is predominantly confined to the forehead above one eye and is usually constant with intermittent paroxysmal stabbing pain. The area is tender to palpation with slightly diminished sensation, and while the etiology is usually compression or trauma, there are rare cases of tumor as the underlying cause. A contrast-enhanced brain MRI scan or CT of the sinuses should be performed if there is clinical suspicion of an underlying structural abnormality. Patients usually respond to an anesthetic nerve blocks injected both medially and laterally to ensure coverage of both nerves. A lidocaine patch may be of some benefit, and patients can be treated with the typical medications that are used for neuralgic pain syndromes. Neurolysis, nerve stimulation, and decompressive surgery can be considered for refractory cases.

Infraorbital Nerve Neuralgia

While neuralgic pain in the distribution of the maxillary division of the trigeminal nerve is usually the result of trigeminal neuralgia or painful trigeminal neuropathy, there are rare instances in which direct facial trauma or tumor can damage a terminal branch of the maxillary nerve, the infraorbital nerve, resulting in a more peripheral neuralgic pain syndrome. Treatment options would include nerve block and the medications for neuralgic pain.

Auriculotemporal Neuralgia

Auriculotemporal neuralgia is characterized by moderate to severe unilateral pain involving the temporal and auricular regions. The pain occurs paroxysmally and is stabbing in character; approximately 50% of patients will have dull background discomfort. The area is often tender to palpation. The syndrome is rare and occurs most commonly in females in their early 50s. The auriculotemporal nerve is a terminal branch of the mandibular nerve that supplies sensory innervation of the auriculotemporal region and conveys parasympathetic nerve fibers to the parotid gland. Before a diagnosis of auriculotemporal neuralgia can be made, GCA must be ruled out, and a contrast-enhanced brain MRI should be performed to exclude the possibility of underlying structural disease. Patients may achieve complete relief with anesthetic blockade. Medication may also be beneficial, and options include gabapentin, pregabalin, duloxetine, or a tricyclic antidepressant.

Great Auricular Neuralgia

The greater auricular nerve provides sensory innervation to the preauricular region, mastoid, skin over the parotid gland, jaw angle, and posteroinferior pinna. The nerve arises from the anterior rami of spinal nerves C1 and C2, wraps around the sternocleidomastoid muscle, then divides into an anterior and a posterior branch. Damage to the nerve can occur due to surgical procedures or trauma precipitating recurrent neuralgic pain that is unilateral, paroxysmal, and stabbing in character. The pain can be provoked by neck rotation, palpation of the neck, neck positioning during sleep, and movement of the jaw. Great auricular neuralgia is rare, and anesthetic nerve blocks are usually effective in alleviating the pain.

Occipital Neuralgia

The greater occipital nerve emanates from the dorsal ramus of the C2 spinal nerve emerging at the base of the posterior skull, then ascending to the vertex of the head. The lesser occipital nerve arises from the C2 and C3 rami and innervates the lateral scalp to the top of the external ear. The third occipital nerve emanates from the C3 dorsal ramus and innervates the upper medial neck and lower occipital scalp (Fig. 12.2). The greater and lesser occipital nerves are purely sensory, but in addition to its sensory innervation the third occipital nerve provides motor innervation to the semispinalis capitis muscle. Occipital neuralgia (Box 12.4) is characterized by severe paroxysmal stabbing pain lasting seconds to minutes in the distribution of the greater, lesser, or third occipital nerves. Ninety percent of cases involve the greater occipital nerve, and the majority of the remaining 10% involve the lesser occipital nerve. The pain may extend over the ear to the temple and into the vertex of the head and frontal region. There is accompanying pain and tenderness at the base of the skull, and palpation precipitates a dysesthetic sensation. The pain is usually unilateral but may occur bilaterally. While it is not mentioned in the ICHD-3 criteria, many patients experience constant dull pain interictally. Temporary relief after the injection of a local anesthetic is required to make the official diagnosis. The etiology is usually nerve compression at one of several anatomic sites. Rare etiologic possibilities, such as Chiari malformation, upper cervical cord demyelination or cavernous malformation, and occipital nerve schwannomas, must be excluded, and patients should undergo brain and cervical spine MRI scans. Treatment should include anesthetic nerve blocks, intermittently combined with a corticosteroid,

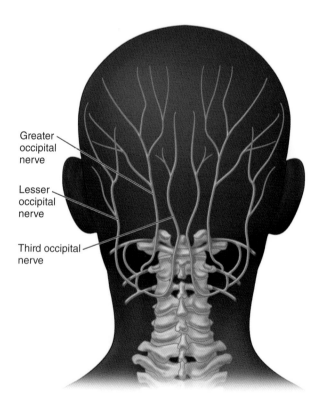

Greater occipital nerve

Lesser occipital nerve

Third occipital nerve

Fig 12.2 Occipital nerve.

BOX 12.4 Occipital Neuralgia Classification in International Classification of Headache Disorders, Third Edition

Description

Unilateral or bilateral paroxysmal, shooting or stabbing pain in the posterior part of the scalp, in the distribution(s) of the greater, lesser and/or third occipital nerves, sometimes accompanied by diminished sensation or dysesthesia in the affected area and commonly associated with tenderness over the involved nerve(s).

Diagnostic criteria

A. Unilateral or bilateral pain in the distribution(s) of the greater, lesser and/or third occipital nerves and fulfilling criteria B–D

B. Pain has at least two of the following three characteristics:
   1. recurring in paroxysmal attacks lasting from a few seconds to minutes
   2. severe in intensity
   3. shooting, stabbing, or sharp in quality

C. Pain is associated with both of the following:
   1. dysesthesia and/or allodynia apparent during innocuous stimulation of the scalp and/or hair
   2. either or both of the following:
      a. tenderness over the affected nerve branches
      b. trigger points at the emergence of the greater occipital nerve or in the distribution of C2

D. Pain is eased temporarily by local anesthetic block of the affected nerve(s).

incidence is low at 4.4 per 100,000 patient years with a lifetime prevalence of 0.03%. Most patients are female in their mid-40s. The pain is not typically accompanied by nausea, photophobia, or phonophobia or aggravated by exercise, and patients do not report accompanying autonomic or neurologic symptoms. The onset of pain often coincides with a minor dental, otolaryngologic, or surgical procedure and persists despite an uneventful full recovery. Coexisting depression and anxiety are common, and patients are often suffering from other chronic pain disorders. Persistent idiopathic facial pain is a diagnosis of exclusion, and patients require brain MRI and CT of the sinuses to look for evidence of a structural cause. Dental disease must be excluded, and laboratory testing must be done to rule out the possibility of an underlying inflammatory disorder. CT of the chest should be considered, as an occult lung cancer can on rare occasions present with facial pain. Treatment is quite difficult, as patients usually do not respond well to medication. Tricyclic antidepressant medication is the first-line treatment, followed by duloxetine or venlafaxine. If there is no response, then gabapentin or pregabalin should be used. Acupuncture and onabotulinum toxin A injections could then be considered. Patients should receive psychological support, and as with other chronic pain syndromes, cognitive behavioral therapy is beneficial in helping the patient deal with the constant discomfort and continue to function normally in daily life despite the ongoing pain.

Recurrent Painful Ophthalmoplegic Neuropathy

Recurrent painful ophthalmoplegic neuropathy (Fig. 12.3), formerly referred to as ophthalmoplegic migraine, is characterized by recurrent attacks of ophthalmoplegia in association with a headache ipsilateral to the side of the ocular cranial nerve paresis. The disorder is rare, with an incidence of 0.7/1,000,000 every year, and while it usually occurs in childhood, cases have been reported in adults. When a patient is old enough to describe the headache, it will often have typical migraine features with pressure to throbbing pain, nausea, and photophobia. The headache usually precedes the ophthalmoparesis by days to weeks, and the oculomotor nerve is most commonly involved. The abducens and rarely the trochlear nerve may be affected. Patients develop diplopia and, with oculomotor nerve involvement, ptosis and anisocoria with mydriasis on the affected side. There is usually full neurologic recovery within days, but after repeated attacks, some deficits

and medication. Patients often respond to gabapentin or pregabalin, and tricyclic antidepressants or duloxetine may also be effective. There are reports of patients responding to onabotulinum toxin A. Occipital nerve stimulation, radiofrequency neurolysis and decompressive surgery are reserved for refractory cases.

Persistent Idiopathic Facial Pain

Persistent idiopathic facial pain (Table 12.2), formerly referred to as atypical facial pain, is a chronic pain disorder in which patients experience dull, aching orofacial pain at least 2 hours daily for at least 3 months. Burning, throbbing, and stabbing discomfort are often described, and the pain ranges from mild to severe. There is often an observed disparity between a patient's calm emotional and physical state when they are reporting severe incapacitating pain. While the pain is predominantly unilateral initially, it may become bilateral over time. The

TABLE 12.2   Cranial Neuralgias

Name	Prevalence	Anatomy	Location	Characteristics	Triggers	Comments
TGN	0.03%–0.3% 0.1–0.2/1000	Usually in V2 or V3 divisions	Brief severe shooting pains in the midface or jaw region (V2 and V3)	Paroxysmal stabbing electric shock–like pain lasting seconds to 2 minutes occurring multiple times during the day	Triggers are present in 99% of patients. • Refractory periods present	Classical form is secondary to neurovascular compression usually at the root entry zone. Bilateral TGN can be seen in multiple sclerosis. If numbness is present with constant burning discomfort, then more likely trigeminal neuropathy than TGN
Nasociliary neuralgia-Charlin syndrome	Rare	Branch of the ophthalmic nerve (V1)	Pain in the eye, brow, and base of nose	Paroxysmal stabbing pain along one side of the nose for seconds to 1 hour, 2–3 times per day	Touching the lateral aspect of the ipsilateral nostril	May have associated autonomic symptoms
Supraorbital and supratrochlear neuralgia	Unknown but rare	Branch of the frontal nerve (V1)	Predominantly confined to the forehead above one eye and usually constant with intermittent paroxysmal stabbing pain	Dull pain with superimposed sharp or burning exacerbations		May be caused by trauma or compression
Infraorbital nerve neuralgia	Unknown but rare	Terminal branch of the maxillary nerve (V2)	Mid-maxillary region	Paroxysmal stabbing or constant pain		Usually related to direct facial trauma or other damage to a terminal branch of the maxillary nerve
Auriculotemporal neuralgia	Unknown but rare	Branch of V3	Ear, temple, and preauricular regions	Paroxysmal and stabbing, but 50% have a dull background pain		Can be difficult to distinguish from nervus intermedius, glossopharyngeal, vagus, and second CN neuralgias

	Prevalence	Nerve/Anatomy	Pain location	Pain character	Triggers	Notes
Glossopharyngeal neuralgia	Rare, 0.2%–1.3% of all neuralgias	Cranial Nerve (CN) IX	Ear, tonsillar fossa, base of the tongue, or beneath the angle of the jaw	Paroxysmal, brief, severe, stabbing pain involving remissions	Swallowing, coughing, talking, or yawning	Block available. Microvascular decompression for refractory pain
Nervus intermedius neuralgia	Rare	Branch of CN VII	Deep in the auditory canal	Paroxysmal, brief, severe, stabbing pain	Touching the ear or external auditory canal, air movement, cold temperature, jaw movement, noise	r/o Ramsay Hunt syndrome
Superior laryngeal nerve neuralgia	Rare	Branch of the vagus nerve	Unilateral, lancinating pain that radiates from the side of the thyroid cartilage to the angle of the jaw and sometimes to the ear		Swallowing and straining the voice	May be caused by surgery, tumor, infection, or trauma
Great auricular neuralgia	Rare	Great auricular nerve arises from the C2 and C3 nerve roots, innervates preauricular region and posterior jaw	Preauricular region Predominantly confined to the forehead above one eye and usually constant with intermittent paroxysmal stabbing pain	Neuralgiform dull pain with superimposed sharp or burning exacerbations	Head turning, neck touch, change of neck position during sleep, and jaw movement	May be idiopathic or the result of neck surgery, tumor, or prolonged compression
Greater occipital nerve	More common than the CN V neuralgias. One study puts prevalence at 1.2%.	From C2, travels through semispinalis and trapezius, supplying sensation to the posterior occipital region of the skull	Located in the unilateral or bilateral occipital region	Sharp, stabbing, electric or shock-like pain with a dull background pain	Tenderness over the nerve in the posterior occipital region and palpation may trigger a paroxysm of pain	Thought to result from chronic entrapment of the nerve by muscles of the neck and scalp
Lesser occipital nerve	As above	C2, C3	Pain in the posterior scalp, temporal region, periorbital and mandibular regions	Paroxysmal stabbing pain with associated constant dull aching, burning, or throbbing discomfort.	Suboccipital tenderness	Etiology similar to greater occipital neuralgia

TGN, Trigeminal neuralgia.

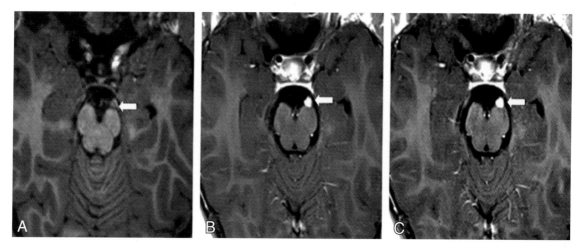

Fig 12.3 Recurrent painful ophthalmoplegic neuropathy. Images of axial precontrast and postcontrast T1-weighted images of the left third cranial nerve during an episode of recurrent painful ophthalmoplegic neuropathy (A, B). A recurrent episode 1 year later revealed similar findings (C). (From Sharifi A, Kayfan S, Clarke RL, Mehta A, Pfeifer CM. Recurrent painful ophthalmoplegic neuropathy: MRI findings in 2 patients. *Radiol Case Rep.* 2019;14:1039–1042.)

may persist. The etiology of the disorder is unknown, but on MRI imaging, focal thickening of the affected nerve and enhancement are often detected. Extensive laboratory testing to rule out a secondary cause and CSF analysis are normal. It has been proposed that the headache and ocular cranial nerve involvement are the result of a recurrent demyelinating inflammatory cranial neuropathy. Before arriving at the diagnosis, neoplasm, including schwannoma and head and neck cancer, lymphoma, aneurysm, infection, and neurosarcoidosis must be ruled out. While there are no randomized controlled trials addressing treatment, some patients improve with steroids, although the response is not dramatic. Beta-blockers, calcium channel blockers, topiramate, and tricyclic antidepressants were not effective in case reports, but patients using pregabalin reported symptomatic improvement.

Red Ear Syndrome

Red ear syndrome is a rare disorder that was first described by James Lance in 1994. Patients report intermittent attacks of burning of the external ear associated with erythema of the ear. Episodes are usually unilateral but may be bilateral in approximately one-third of cases. Symptoms last from seconds to several hours, and the pain can be precipitated by touching the ear, movement of the neck, exposure to hot or cold, hair brushing, chewing food, or exercise. The frequency varies from multiple episodes in a day to infrequent episodes that often occur in clusters. The median age of onset is 44 years with a slight female predominance. Red ear syndrome has been classified as being either primary or secondary. The primary form occurs in young patients, more commonly males, and is usually associated with migraine. The secondary form is more common in adult females, more likely to be provoked by triggers and is associated with upper cervical spine pathology or temporomandibular joint dysfunction. The pathophysiology of red ear syndrome is unknown, and there are peripheral and central theories. The peripheral theories suggest that the pain is the result of pathology in the upper cervical spine, specifically at C3, or in the temporomandibular joint. Central theories center on dysregulation of the trigeminal autonomic circuits. Red ear syndrome is often refractory to treatment, but some patients may respond to tricyclic antidepressants, propranolol, calcium channel blockers, gabapentin, or nonsteroidal antiinflammatory drugs. Anesthetic blockade of the great auricular nerve may be effective in some cases.

"For the full bibliography list, please use the pincode on the inside front cover to access the electronic version of the text at ebooks.health.elsevier.com."

13

A Review of Women's Neurology*

Mary Angela O'Neal

INTRODUCTION

The term "sex" refers to the different biological and physiologic characteristics of females, males, and intersex persons, such as chromosomes, hormones, and reproductive organs, whereas the term "gender" refers to characteristics that are socially or culturally constructed. Women's neurology uses a sex/gender lens to optimize clinical management, improving outcomes and minimizing complications of treatment. Women's neurology encompasses all neurologic diseases across a woman's lifespan with key sex/gender differences in reproductive planning, pregnancy, and menopause. This requires taking specific issues into account depending on where a woman is in her life cycle. These include reproductive concerns such as appropriate contraception and pregnancy planning, pregnancy and breastfeeding management, psychiatric issues, menopausal effects on the disorder, bone health, and healthy aging concerns. All of which require expertise in sex/gender-informed care.

EPILEPSY

Women's Issues in Epilepsy

Globally, 15 million females of reproductive potential are living with epilepsy with significant sex and gender influences that span their lifespan. A multitude of considerations result from the multidirectional interactions of exogenous and endogenous hormones, seizures, and

*Based on O'Neal MA. A review of women's neurology. *Am J Med*. 2018;131(7):735–744. ISSN 0002-9343. https://doi.org/10.1016/j.amjmed.2017.11.053.

antiseizure medications that together affect important aspects of a female's life, including menstruation, contraception, pregnancy, breastfeeding, and bone health. Practitioners must maintain knowledge of these specialized topics and provide regular counseling to optimize epilepsy care.

Catamenial Epilepsy

Seizure exacerbation during the menstrual cycle is common with catamenial epilepsy affecting one-third of women with epilepsy (WWE) of reproductive age, though a wide range of prevalence has been reported (10%–78%), reflecting early inconsistencies in its classification. Currently, catamenial epilepsy is defined as a doubling of seizures or seizures occurring almost exclusively during specific times of the menstrual cycle. This is attributed to the neuroactive properties of female sex steroids and their cyclical variation where estrogens mainly act as a proconvulsant, while progesterone and its metabolites have anticonvulsant properties. Three seizure patterns of catamenial epilepsy have been recognized, namely, perimenstrual (C1 pattern), periovulation (C2 pattern), and anovulatory cycles (C3 pattern), during which there is a heightened estrogen-to-progesterone ratio favoring a proconvulsant state (see Fig. 13.1 for catamenial patterns). In females with refractory seizures, catamenial epilepsy should be considered and investigated with a menstrual and seizure diary; if diagnosed, it has important management implications. Approaches include both hormonal and antiseizure medication (ASM) interventions and depend on pattern and patient preference. For instance, supplemental progesterone during the luteal phase in a C1 pattern, hormonal contraceptives for suppression of menstruation

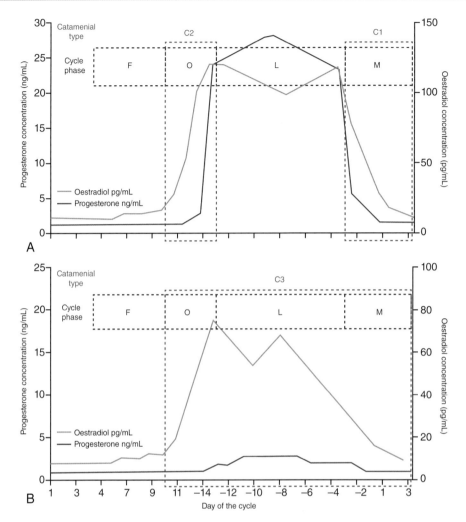

Fig. 13.1 Types of catamenial epilepsy. Day 1 is the first day of menstrual flow; day 14 is ovulation. (A) The C1 pattern represents perimenstrual seizure exacerbation, and the C2 pattern represents periovulatory seizure exacerbation. (B) The C3 pattern represents catamenial epilepsy in anovulatory cycles. *F,* Follicular phase; *L,* luteal phase; *M,* perimenstrual; *O,* periovulatory phase. (Reprinted with permission from Herzog AG, Klein P, Ransil BJ. Three patterns of catamenial epilepsy. *Epilepsia* 1997;38(10):1082–1088.)

to avoid cyclic variation, and increasing a background ASM dose or adding adjuncts such as clobazam or acetazolamide around the time of heightened risk are potential strategies.

Contraception

Contraceptive counseling should be offered to WWE of childbearing potential, as neurologists can positively influence the use of reliable contraceptive methods while incorporating patient preferences and maintaining epilepsy control. Interactions between various antiseizure medications and hormonal birth control can alter the efficacy of contraception and seizure stability. Specifically, hepatic enzyme-inducing medications through cytochrome P450 may induce metabolism of hormonal birth control, while estrogen induces glucuronidation, resulting in enhanced metabolism of lamotrigine and to a lesser degree valproate and oxcarbazepine (see Table 13.1 for ASM and contraception interactions). Copper and progestin intrauterine devices

TABLE 13.1   Interaction of Antiseizure Medications (ASMs) and Hormonal Contraceptives

Enzyme-Inducing ASMs	Enzyme-Inhibiting ASMs	ASMs With No Effect
Barbiturates	Valproate[a]	Brivaracetam
Carbamazepine	CBD	Clonazepam
Oxcarbazepine		Ethosuximide
Perampanel (>12 mg/d)		Lacosamide
Phenytoin		Levetiracetam
Clobazam		Gabapentin
Cenobamate		Tiagabine
Eslicarbazepine acetate		Vigabatrin
Felbamate		Zonisamide
Primidone		
Lamotrigine >300 mg/d[a]		
Rufinamide		
Topiramate >200 mg/d		

Data from Bui E. Women's issues in epilepsy. *Continuum* (Minneap Minn). 2022;28:399–427 and Reimers A, et al. Interactions between hormonal contraception and antiepileptic drugs: clinical and mechanistic considerations. *Seizure.* 2015;28:66–70.
Bold: strong enzyme inducers.
It is unknown whether pregabalin and stiripentol have an effect on hormonal contraceptives.
[a]Increased clearance with combined oral contraceptives.

(IUDs) have become the preferred recommended contraceptive method, as they are reliable and reversible and exert localized effects without systemic interactions or alterations of drug metabolism. In women who prefer an alternative method or in whom IUDs are contraindicated, other forms include the combined oral contraceptive pill, progestin-only formulations, and surgical nonhormonal measures such as vasectomy and tubal ligation. However, using these methods may have reduced efficacy or require dose adjustments due to increased clearance of either the contraceptive or antiseizure medication, depending on the combination.

Fertility

Fertility in WWE is challenging to study in isolation due to confounding psychosocial and biological causes. Biological reasons for infertility in WWE include central dysregulation of the hypothalamic-pituitary-ovarian axis, premature ovarian failure, and polycystic ovarian syndrome. Hepatic enzyme-inducing ASMs may contribute to menstrual dysfunction through increased metabolism of hormones, increased production of sex hormone binding globulin causing lower free bioactive hormones, and valproate (VPA) related effects of hyperandrogenism and weight gain. In WWE, polytherapy is consistently identified as a risk factor for infertility, while other factors have less reliably been reproduced, such as epilepsy severity, childhood-onset epilepsy, metabolic epilepsy, and lesional epilepsy (epilepsy characterized by a structural brain lesion as the underlying cause of recurrent seizures). Reassuringly, in the absence of preexisting risks of infertility, a recent study showed no difference in fertility rate or time to conception in WWE compared to controls, though avoidance of polytherapy and VPA may increase the chances of conceiving.

Assisted reproductive technology (ART) remains an option for WWE who are struggling with fertility and has similar reported efficacy as in the general population. However, associated risks from exogenous hormones that heighten the estrogen-to-progesterone ratio or interact with ASMs exist. The ART process may include administration of gonadotropins that stimulate ovaries, resulting in a large surge of estrogen, or involve direct administration of estrogen, both theoretically inducing a proconvulsant state. Current evidence for epilepsy management in this context is limited, but serum drug levels at baseline and during hormonal therapy, along with adjunctive pretreatment with clobazam, may be considered.

Preconception Care

In the United States, more than 50% of pregnancies in WWE are unplanned. This emphasizes the need for early reproductive counseling and family planning, as preparation can improve outcomes by mitigating the risk of seizure destabilization and teratogenicity. The best predictor of seizure control during pregnancy is indicated by baseline seizure frequency in the 9–12 months prior to conception and prepregnancy efforts should be aimed at optimizing stability. The risk of major congenital malformations (MCMs) with ASM exposure in pregnancy is two to five times higher than that in the general population; the risk is both drug and dose dependent, the highest risk being associated with polytherapy and high-dose VPA (≥1500 mg total daily dose). A transition to lamotrigine, levetiracetam, or oxcarbazepine should be

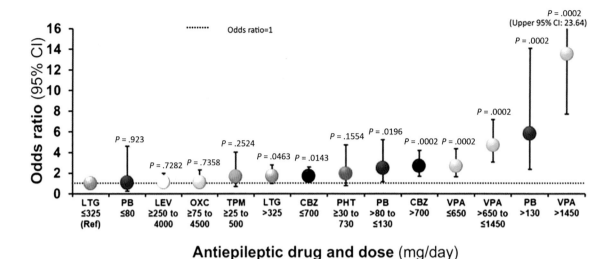

Fig. 13.2 Prevalence of major congenital malformations of antiseizure medication compared with lamotrigine ≤325 mg/d. *CBZ*, Carbamazepine; *CI*, confidence interval; *LEV*, levetiracetam; *LTG*, lamotrigine; *OXC*, oxcarbazepine; *PB*, phenobarbital; *PHT*, phenytoin; *Ref*, reference; *TPM*, topiramate; *VPA*, valproate. (From Tomson T, Battino D, Perucca E. Teratogenicity of antiepileptic drugs. *Curr Opin Neurol.* 2019;32(2):246–252.)

discussed, as these drugs have the lowest reported rates of teratogenicity observed across multiple international pregnancy registries (see Fig. 13.2 for the prevalence of MCMs with ASMs). Less is currently known about newer ASMs such as perampanel, eslicarbazepine, lacosamide, and brivaracetam. In addition to in utero exposure to VPA causing structural defects, VPA has been linked to impairment in cognitive and behavioral outcomes, also with a dose-dependent relationship. In considering a drug switch, shared decision must be employed to balance multiple factors, including patient preference, type of epilepsy, risk of seizure destabilization, and risks of teratogenicity and poor neurodevelopmental outcomes. A preconception drug serum level should be measured to establish a baseline for subsequent titrations as drug levels fall during pregnancy.

Periconceptional folic acid supplementation is recommended in all WWE of reproductive age to minimize risks of major congenital malformations, neural tube defects, and adverse neurodevelopmental outcomes. The optimal dosing has not been established, but folic acid typically is prescribed in the range of 1–4 mg daily at least 3 months prior to conception. A higher range of dosing may be considered for patients who are on VPA, carbamazepine, or polytherapy or who have a history of previous open neural tube defects. Recent evidence has demonstrated an association of high-dose folic acid and negative impacts including lower psychomotor scale scores and increased risk of cancer in children of mothers with epilepsy. Therefore, supratherapeutic dosing is not advised.

Pregnancy Care in Epilepsy

Pregnancy care for WWE involves balancing seizure control with in utero fetal drug exposure. Seizures in pregnancy have been associated with maternal injury and perinatal complications such as fetal hypoxia, preterm delivery, and low birth weight, while in utero ASM exposure has the potential for major congenital malformations, neural tube defects, and adverse neurodevelopmental outcomes. Therapeutic drug monitoring is an important tool that should be implemented if available to mitigate these risks with a baseline preconception level and then monthly monitoring following conception. Levels of all ASMs decrease due to physiologic changes in pregnancy, though the extent and timing are drug dependent. There is a prominent decline of levetiracetam and lamotrigine early in the first trimester, whereas clearance of oxcarbazepine and topiramate is greatest in the second trimester, and carbamazepine and lacosamide show minor changes (see Fig. 13.3 for ASM levels during pregnancy). As a general guideline,

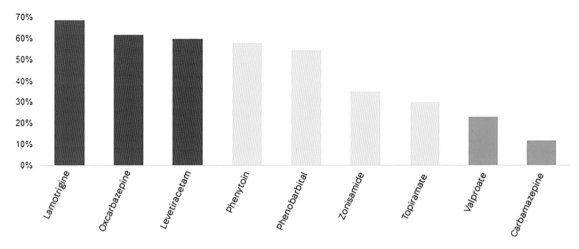

Fig. 13.3 Projected decrease of antiseizure medication concentrations during pregnancy if no dose changes are made. (Reprinted with permission from Li Y, Meador KJ. Epilepsy and Pregnancy. *Continuum (Minneap Minn)* 2022;28:34–54.)

if levels fall by >35% of preconception levels, women are at greater risk for breakthrough seizures, and a dose titration should be considered. If drug levels are not available, a dose increase of 30%–50% should be considered after the first trimester if it is a drug with a known pregnancy-associated decline, if the patient is on the lowest effective dose at the onset of pregnancy, or if the patient has a history of severe or breakthrough seizures. Reassuringly, the majority of pregnant WWE have a stable course that is attributable in part to carefully considered drug adjustments and monitoring.

Postpartum and Breastfeeding

WWE are particularly vulnerable to seizures in the postpartum period due to an increase in stress and sleep deprivation. Reported rates of hospital readmission and incidence of mental health comorbidities are also higher, emphasizing the importance of judicious follow-up for maternal health and well-being, including screening for postpartum depression. Anticipatory drug adjustments of ASMs changed in pregnancy are also required, as many ASM levels increase with return to prepregnancy physiology and metabolism.

Postpartum-specific epilepsy safety measures include ensuring maternal social supports, encouraging adequate periods of restful sleep (the National Sleep Foundation recommends at least 7 hours of sleep each night) with family helping with nocturnal feeds,

changing and feeding the infant near ground level, childproofing medications, using strollers rather than infant carriers, and avoiding cosleeping and bathing the infant alone.

Breastfeeding is safe and should be recommended to WWE, as it provides many benefits to infants and mothers. Transfer of antiseizure medications into breastmilk is an area that has been extensively studied with evidence showing minimal accumulation. In breastfed infants, serum drug concentrations for carbamazepine, oxcarbazepine, lamotrigine, levetiracetam, topiramate, valproic acid, and zonisamide remain low compared to maternal serum drug concentrations. If feasible, WWE should be reassured and encouraged to breastfeed without altering their antiseizure medication regimen.

Bone Health

Sex and gender disparities are prevalent in bone health, particularly in females over 50 years of age, who face higher rates of osteoporosis, risk of falls, and lifetime risk of fractures. Osteoporosis is four times more common in females, due to lower bone density and faster rate of bone loss, which can be exacerbated by postmenopausal estrogen decline. Risk of osteoporosis is further heightened by epilepsy and chronic exposure to ASMs, independent of drug mechanism of action; emerging evidence indicates that many ASMs accelerate osteoporosis onset, including those that induce cytochrome P450 as well as those that act via nonenzyme induction mechanisms. Therefore, WWE should be screened for vitamin D deficiency and bone loss and should be counseled on bone-protective measures such as weight-bearing exercises, avoidance of smoking and alcohol, and maintenance of a well-balanced and/or supplemented diet with adequate vitamin D and calcium. The current recommended intakes are 600 IU daily of vitamin D and 700–1300 mg daily of calcium, though WWE likely require higher doses, given the accelerated effects of epilepsy and chronic ASM use on osteoporosis incidence.

MENOPAUSE

Evidence on the effects of perimenopause (transitional phase leading to menopause) and menopause (cessation of menstruation for 12 consecutive months) in WWE is limited. Multidirectional interactions exist between changing endogenous hormone levels, exogenous hormonal replacement treatments, epilepsy, and ASMs, though to date no clear data have been established on ASMs in menopause. Females with catamenial epilepsy may experience seizure exacerbations during perimenopause as a result of greater hormonal fluctuations, followed by subsequent improvement with menopause. Additionally, WWE may transition to menopause at a younger age than the general population and with earlier onset with increased seizure burden. Menopausal WWE may desire symptomatic treatment, in which non–estrogen-based options are preferred (e.g., clonidine, selective reuptake inhibitors, serotonin-norepinephrine reuptake, vaginal lubricants). If hormonal replacement is used, a single estrogenic compound such as 17-beta-estradiol with natural progesterone is recommended, as according to current data, conjugated equine estrogens/medroxyprogesterone acetate has been associated with seizure exacerbation.

SLEEP

Sleep Disturbances in Women

Inherent sex differences of circadian rhythms between males and females have been reported, implicating a role of reproductive hormones in sleep physiology. This is further reflected in the higher prevalence of many sleep disorders in females, particularly during periods of hormonal change such as menstruation, pregnancy, or menopause.

Restless Leg Syndrome

Restless leg syndrome (RLS) is a sleep-related movement disorder that is frequently encountered in clinical practice and is twice as common in females. It is characterized by an uncomfortable urge and sensation to move the lower extremities that worsens at night when at rest. Studies of RLS pathophysiology have consistently identified central iron deficiency as a biological abnormality, which corresponds to symptom exacerbation during menses and pregnancy, when iron stores are reduced. It is also increased during menopause, during which estrogen and progesterone levels decline, though the role of sex steroids in RLS remains unclear. Pregnancy increases the risk of both debut and worsening of RLS with increasing prevalence in each trimester (8% in T1, 16% in T2, and 22% in T3), in part attributable to physiologic changes and blood volume expansion. Interestingly, higher parity is also associated with increasing risk of RLS later in life. Treatment in pregnancy should be aimed at replenishing iron stores and nonpharmacologic interventions (exercise, massage, avoidance of caffeine and stimulants, withdrawal of exacerbating drugs), but typically RLS resolves postpartum. According to the 2018 guidelines, if the ferritin level is <300 ng/mL and transferrin saturation is <45%, supplementation is recommended, though normal peripheral iron studies do not rule out central iron deficiency. Pharmacologic symptomatic strategies in nonpregnant females include $\alpha2\delta$ ligands (e.g., gabapentin or pregabalin) as first-line therapy, given that dopamine agonists may cause augmentation with long-term use.

Obstructive Sleep Apnea

Obstructive sleep apnea (OSA) is a sleep-related breathing disorder with repetitive airway closures, oxygen desaturation, and disrupted sleep. It is often overlooked in females, who more commonly report nonspecific symptoms of headache, depression, anxiety, fatigue, and insomnia in comparison to males, who characteristically present with snoring and apnea. The reported overall prevalence in females is 6%–19% (compared to 13%–33% in males) with a narrowing of the sex gap with advancing age, as evidenced by a significant increase in postmenopausal females. If undiagnosed, OSA can lead to negative outcomes, including worsening of cardiovascular, psychiatric, and neurologic disorders along with reduced quality of life. Specific risk factors in females include pregnancy, hyperandrogenism and polycystic ovarian syndrome, and menopause, with increased body mass index and hormonal alterations as contributors (see Fig. 13.4 for pregnancy-related physiologic changes that predispose females to OSA). Importantly, untreated OSA in pregnancy has been associated with poorer maternal-fetal outcomes. This emphasizes the importance of implementing screening tools and standardized evaluation of patients at risk with polysomnography or home sleep apnea testing. OSA is a treatable condition with a variety of interventions, though positive airway pressure therapy remains the gold standard if tolerated.

MIGRAINE

Definitions

Migraine without aura (MO) is defined by at least five episodes of unilateral throbbing headache with associated phonosensitivity and photosensitivity and nausea and/or vomiting of moderate to severe intensity lasting 4–72 hours that is not explained by another diagnosis. Migraine with aura (MA) requires at least two typical aura events usually visual, sensory, or language, lasting 15–60 minutes preceding the headache. The other criteria are the same as those of MO. Menstrual migraine (MM) is defined as migraine that occurs only in close relationship to the onset of menstruation, starting 2 days prior to 2 days after the first day of menses or withdrawal bleeding. Females with menstrually related migraine (MRM) have characteristics similar to those of females with MM, but migraines may occur at other times of their cycle as well.

Stroke Risk

Females who have MA have a small but real increased risk of stroke. Data have shown that the risk for stroke is 2.0–2.5 times greater in females with MA. This is not true for those with MO. The reasons for this increased risk are complex and may have to do with the pathophysiology of cortical-spreading depression, predilection for endothelial injury, migraineur's association with having patent foramen ovale, and genetic risks, as migraine is associated with neurologic disorders that

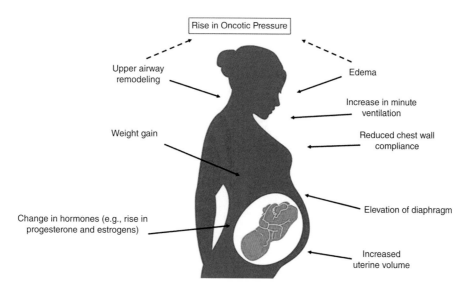

Fig. 13.4 Anatomic and physiologic changes during pregnancy that predispose females to sleep disturbances. During pregnancy, changes such as weight gain, increased uterine volume, and hormonal changes occur, which have been linked to the development of sleep disorders such as obstructive sleep apnea. (CC by 4.0) (From Martin H, Antony KM, Kumar S. Obstructive sleep apnea in pregnancy – development, impact and potential mechanisms. *J Women's Health Dev.* 2020;3(4):446–469.)

involve increased stroke risk (e.g., cerebral autosomal dominant arteriopathy with subcortical infarcts and leukoencephalopathy). These stroke risks increase with age and the presence of other traditional stroke factors such as hypertension and smoking.

Hormonal Contraceptives

Estrogen in combined hormonal contraceptives (CHC) confers an independent risk of stroke. For this reason, the American College of Obstetrics and Gynecology guidelines state that CHC should be avoided in females who have MA. This decision should be nuanced and individualized to determine the risks and benefits for a particular patient, including the indication and dose of CHC. For example, the need for CHC may be supported by a woman who has MA but no other traditional stroke risks and who needs estrogen for endometriosis.

MO is the more hormonally driven headache, so are those most likely to have either MM or MRM. In this subset of migraineurs, continuous CHC without placebo may be helpful to decrease the menstrual exacerbation of migraine and may be an excellent choice for females with MO who also want an oral contraceptive method. Other strategies include increasing the preventive medication dose premenstrually and mini-prophylaxis regimens (Box 13.1).

Pregnancy and Postpartum

Females who have MO, particularly those with a hormonal exacerbation, often have worsening in their migraine frequency during the first trimester. However, over 80% have a remission in their migraines by early in the second trimester. This time course is less predictable with females who have MA; where only 44% improve during pregnancy. Postpartum, there is often a migraine exacerbation due to changes in estrogen, sleep deprivation, and stress. Migraineurs have an increased risk for preeclampsia, and they should be counseled in this regard.

Females of reproductive age should be asked the key question "Are you planning pregnancy?" If they are, then a discussion about their migraine medication safety during pregnancy, the natural history of migraine during pregnancy, and postpartum and appropriate management of their headache disorder can ensue. During pregnancy, migraine management shifts to an increased use of nonmedical therapies (physical therapy, acupuncture, and stress management) and symptomatic medications (Table 13.2). This is due to both the expected improvement of migraines during pregnancy and the fact that most preventive medications carry some level of risk (Table 13.3).

Postpartum migraine management depends on the frequency and severity of headaches and whether or not the patient is breastfeeding.

BOX 13.1   Treatment of Menstrual Migraine

- Increase the dose of preventive medication premenstrually
- Use of either a nonsteroidal antiinflammatory medication or a long-acting triptan starting several days prior to the usual onset of the menstrual migraine and continuing through the at-risk period
- Hormonal strategies may include continuous combined hormonal contraception with suppression of menses

---

TABLE 13.2   Pregnancy and Breastfeeding Safety Data for Migraine Symptomatic Therapies

Generic Name	Level of Risk during Pregnancy	Breastfeeding, Hale Lactation Rating
Acetaminophen	Very safe	Compatible
Nonsteroidal antiinflammatory drugs	Very safe in the second trimester. Avoid in the third trimester.	Compatible
Metoclopramide	Very safe	Compatible
Prochlorperazine	Safe	Compatible
Dihydroergotamine	Avoid	Avoid
Magnesium IV	Safe when used for 1–2 days[a]	Compatible
Triptans	Safe	Compatible

[a]Cases of rickets have been reported when high-dose magnesium is used for more than this time period.

TABLE 13.3	Preventive Medications		
Drug Class	**Generic Name**	**Level of Risk in Pregnancy**	**Breastfeeding**
Beta-blockers	Atenolol	Avoid	Caution
	Propranolol	Probably safe (avoid at term)	Compatible
Antiepileptics	Gabapentin	Probably safe	Compatible
	Topiramate	Avoid	Caution
	Valproate	Never use	Avoid
Tricyclics	Amitriptylinc	Probably safe	Compatible
SNRIs	Duloxetine	Probably safe	Little data
	Venlafaxine	Probably safe	Little data, Caution
CGRP inhibitors	Ercnumab	No data	No data
	Fremane/umab		
	Galcanezumab		
Gepants	Rimegepanl	No data	No data
	Eptinezumab		
Vitamins	Magnesium	Safe	Compatible
	Coenzyme Q10		

CGRP, Calcitonin gene–related peptide; *SNRI*, serotonin and norepinephrine reuptake inhibitors.

Menopause

Females with hormonally exacerbated migraine may have an exacerbation during the menopausal transition. The approach to treatment is the same as that for any migraine patient. For females who have MA and need hormonal therapy for their vasomotor symptoms, estrogen therapy is deemed safe, especially the transdermal estrogen patch. This is because the amount of delivered estrogen is low, and for females younger than 60 years of age, the absolute risk of stroke from standard dose hormonal therapy is rare (two additional strokes per 10,000 person-years of use).

MULTIPLE SCLEROSIS

Definition and Prevalence

Multiple sclerosis (MS) is a demyelinating inflammatory autoimmune disease of the central nervous system that affects primarily the myelin sheath but also injuring the underlying axons. It is characterized by either relapses and remissions of neurologic deficits or a more progressive decline in neurologic function. In the United States, about 1 million people are affected by MS, with females affected three times more than males.

Contraception

Females with MS who do not want to become pregnant should be counseled on effective contraception. All contraceptive methods are available to these patients; therefore, the focus should be effective methods and ease of reversibility.

Prenatal Counseling

Prior to pregnancy there are multiple issues that should be discussed with females who are planning pregnancy. They should know that there is a small genetic risk such that if one partner has MS, the risk of an offspring developing MS is 2%–4%, and if both parents are affected, the risk is increased to around 20%. These females should be on both prenatal vitamins and vitamin D supplementation. (The recommended vitamin D3 dose is 4000 IU/day.) Females with MS need to understand that achieving disease stability prior to pregnancy is important, as those with stable disease are much more likely to have fewer relapses intrapartum as well as postpartum. Further, there needs to be a discussion about managing their disease-modifying therapy (DMT), as many patients require a washout (Box 13.2). In addition, there are specific concerns about discontinuation of natalizumab and fingolimod, as they carry a high risk of rebound of MS activity. Expert opinion now recommends continuing natalizumab treatment during pregnancy, timing administration in pregnancy to late first trimester to end around gestation week 32 with infusions every 6–8 weeks. Prepregnancy washout for natalizumab is not recommended.

BOX 13.2 Multiple Sclerosis Therapies: Washout Period/Label

- Interferons and glatiramer acetate
  - No washout
- Teriflunomide
  - 8 months or rapid elimination protocol
- Fingolimod
  - 2-month washout
- Dimethyl fumarate
  - No washout
- Alemtuzumab
  - 4-month washout
- Cladribine
  - 3-month washout
- Ocrelizumab
  - 6 months washout
- Natalizumab
  - 3 months washout

TABLE 13.4 Summary of the Pregnancy in Relapsing Multiple Sclerosis (MS) Trial

	MS RR	
	J Annual RR	P Value
Year before pregnancy	0.7	–
First trimester	0.5	0.03
Second trimester	0.6	0.17
Third trimester	0.2	<0.001
1–3 months postpartum	1.2	<0.001
4–6 months postpartum	0.9	0.17
7–9 months postpartum	0.9	0.15
10–12 months postpartum	0.6	0.59

RR, Relapse rate.

TABLE 13.5 Multiple Sclerosis Therapies

Treatment	Breastfeeding
Interferons	Compatible
Glatiramer acetate	Compatible
Fingolimod	Not compatible
Azathioprine	Not compatible
Methotrexate	Not compatible
Corticosteroids	Compatible
Teriflunomide	Not compatible
Dimethyl Fumarate	Not compatible
Natalizumab Rituximab	Yes, if needed. Caution: increased infant risks of infection, impaired vaccine response, and risk of disseminated disease from live vaccines

Pregnancy

Females with MS are not more likely to have pregnancy or labor complications. However, in a retrospective claims analysis in the United States, females with MS compared to those without MS were more likely to have infection, premature labor, cardiovascular disease, anemia/acquired coagulation disorders, neurologic complications, sexually transmitted diseases, acquired fetal damage, and congenital fetal malformations.

The pregnancy relapse in MS trial was the first prospective study of 254 women who were followed for up to 2 years after delivery. The trial showed that in the study cohort the annualized relapse rate (ARR) prepregnancy rate decreased in the third trimester. The relapse rate increased to 1.2 per year in the first 3 months postpartum, and in the year postpartum, the ARR did not significantly differ significantly from the prepregnancy rate (Table 13.4). Due to the increased incidence of postpartum relapses, a surveillance brain MRI in the first several months postpartum is recommended.

Breastfeeding

Exclusive breastfeeding has a protective effect, decreasing relapses in females with MS. Further breastfeeding confers significant benefits to both the mother and the child, so breastfeeding for females with MS should be encouraged. The decision about when to restart a DMT depends on the maternal risk for relapse and the safety of the particular DMT with breastfeeding (Table 13.5).

Menopause

Most studies show a transient worsening of disability associated with menopause, whereas a few have found that menopause has been associated with a possible worsening of MS disability.

There is an overlap of MS and menopausal symptoms, with exacerbations and pseudo-exacerbations triggered by hot flashes, and symptoms including increasing fatigue and cognitive disturbance may worsen in this setting. Hormone replacement therapy has shown inconsistent benefits.

SEX-SPECIFIC DIFFERENCES IN AUTOIMMUNE CENTRAL NERVOUS SYSTEM DISEASE

It has long been observed that the incidence and prevalence of autoimmune disorders in general are much higher in females than in males. Autoimmune disorders affecting the central nervous system are no exception, with females incurring the highest burden of autoimmune inflammatory CNS disease, MS, neuromyelitis optica spectrum of disorders (NMOSD), and autoimmune encephalitides. Fig. 13.5 shows the female-to-male ratio of patients affected by these disorders. Sex-specific considerations for the management of immunomodulatory and disease-modifying therapies during the reproductive years for MS were reviewed in the previous section. Here, we will discuss the sex-specific differences and considerations in the management of systemic lupus erythematosus and two paraneoplastic disorders: NMDA encephalitis and paraneoplastic cerebellar degeneration.

Systemic Lupus Erythematosus and Antiphospholipid Antibody Syndrome

Systemic lupus erythematosus (SLE) is an autoimmune disorder that can affect any organ system, with a wide spectrum of clinical presentations. It disproportionately affects females across all ages. Earlier data described the female-to-male ratio as 3:1 in the prepubertal stage, 8:1 in postmenopausal/older age group, and up to 15:1 in females of childbearing age. Constitutional symptoms such as fever, weight loss, and fatigue are features of the disease, occurring at various timepoints in the course of this chronic disorder. The involvement of the cardiovascular and central nervous systems can lead to life-threatening clinical presentations. Up to 50% of patients with SLE experience neurologic system involvement, and CNS involvement produces wide-ranging symptoms of neuropsychiatric disease (including cognitive and behavioral changes). Headache, seizures, and stroke syndromes are seen in the context of CNS inflammatory vasculitis in patients with SLE. A hypercoagulable state and increased risk of arterial and venous thrombosis are seen in SLE patients, especially those with antiphospholipid antibodies. (Antiphospholipid antibody syndrome, which is less common is discussed separately, in the following section.) This may increase the risk of thromboembolic events affecting all vascular beds (not just the brain) and significantly increases the risk of spontaneous miscarriages. The peripheral nervous system is also affected in SLE, but less commonly than the central nervous system, and various types of neuropathies (autonomic and sensorimotor mononeuropathies and polyneuropathies) affect SLE patients.

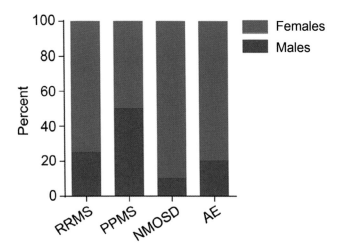

Fig. 13.5 Female/male ratio of multiple sclerosis (MS) subtypes, relapsing-remitting MS (RRMS) and primary progressive MS (PPMS), neuromyelitis optica spectrum disorder (NMOSD), and the most frequent neuronal antibody-mediated encephalitis subtype (anti-*N*-methyl-D-aspartate receptor encephalitis: age group 12–45 years). (Adapted from Gold SM, Willing A, Leypoldt F, Paul F, Friese MA. Sex differences in autoimmune disorders of the central nervous system. Semin Immunopathol. 2019;41(2):177–188.)

Preconception Counseling for Females With Systemic Lupus Erythematosus

Preconception counseling is of critical importance for female patients with SLE so that they understand whether pregnancy would incur an unacceptably high maternal or fetal risk. The main goals of the preconception visit are to review disease activity, perform a risk assessment, ideally adjust medications to where they are considered safe in pregnancy, and complete a workup for hypercoagulable disease. Patients with active renal disease (lupus nephritis) are advised to delay pregnancy until disease activity has been suppressed for 6 months to improve maternal outcomes. There are several published society guidelines to support pregnancy planning and management in women with SLE. Management of the CNS manifestations of SLE is with immunosuppressive and modulatory treatments, and both glucocorticoids and azathioprine are considered to have an acceptable risk profile during pregnancy. Hydroxychloroquine (HCQ), an antimalarial drug that is used in the management of patients with SLE, was recently shown in a large cohort study to be associated with a small risk of increasing the rate of various congenital malformations. Prior data showed no clear increase in birth defects, and the consensus remains that the benefits outweigh the risks for HCQ use during pregnancy in terms of reducing adverse pregnancy outcomes. This medication takes 3 months to become clinically effective, and it should be started well in advance of the planned pregnancy.

Pregnancy and Breastfeeding

Pregnancy is associated with an increased risk of relapse and flares in females with SLE. Previously described risk factors leading to an increased risk of relapse during pregnancy include active disease in the 6 months preceding pregnancy, any history of renal involvement, first pregnancy for the patient, and discontinuation of HCQ or other disease-modulating medications prior to pregnancy. Recently, a study found that preconception low levels of complement (C4) is an independent risk factor for disease relapse in pregnancy.

In addition to optimizing immunosuppressive medications and continuation of treatment with HCQ if prescribed, low-dose aspirin therapy is recommended for females with SLE at 12 weeks of GA for the duration of the pregnancy to minimize the risk of preeclampsia.

Specific considerations for patients with SLE who test positive for anti-ro and anti-la antibodies include establishing antenatal protocols for fetal cardiac monitoring, as the risk of heart block in neonatal lupus is the highest between 18 and 25 weeks of gestational age.

HCQ, aspirin, azathioprine, and glucocorticoids are safe to use during breastfeeding, and breastfeeding is encouraged in mothers with SLE. For detailed information regarding medication compatibility and safety with breastfeeding, the drugs and lactation database LactMed is a useful resource.

Antiphospholipid Antibody Syndrome

Antiphospholipid antibodies can be present in clinically asymptomatic individuals but are also implicated in the pathogenesis of primary antiphospholipid antibody syndrome (APLAS) or in secondary APLAS in association with other autoimmune disorders, most commonly SLE. APLAS is an autoimmune disorder that is defined by arterial and venous thrombotic events with or without pregnancy losses or morbidity with *persistent* detection of antiphospholipid antibodies. It occurs much more frequently in females than males with a ratio of 3.5:1. The antibodies that are most commonly associated with this increased thrombotic risk are lupus anticoagulant (LA), anti-beta-2-glycoprotein 1 antibodies (aβ2GP-1), and anticardiolipin antibodies (aCL). Stroke and transient ischemic attacks are the most common neurologic manifestations of APLAS, and these patients experience an increased risk of arterial and venous thrombosis. Interestingly, 50% of patients with Sneddon syndrome (rare thrombotic neurocutaneous vasculopathy defined by livedo reticularis and recurrent ischemic strokes) test positive for antiphospholipid antibodies. Management of APLAS in pregnancy with antithrombotic therapy is required. Whether antiplatelet therapy or anticoagulation is required depends on the patient's clinical history and pregnancy risk factors. It is recommended that pregnant patients with APLAS who have experienced any history of a thrombotic event receive antenatal therapeutic anticoagulation with low molecular weight heparin *and* antiplatelet therapy with low-dose aspirin to minimize risk of preeclampsia, followed by resumption of warfarin indefinitely in the postpartum period. For various clinical scenarios, this referenced guideline is a helpful resource.

OTHER AUTOIMMUNE AND PARANEOPLASTIC CENTRAL NERVOUS SYSTEM DISORDERS

Anti-NMDA Receptor Autoimmune Encephalitis

Anti-NMDA receptor encephalitis (AE) is an autoimmune inflammatory brain disorder characterized by the presence of antibodies against the NMDA (N-methyl-D-aspartate) receptor. It was first described in 2007 by Dalmau et al. It primarily affects females (up to 80% of patients reported in cohort studies in Western patient populations are female) and is considered to be the most common autoimmune encephalitis in female patients. It presents as a paraneoplastic disorder in up to half of patients, with the clinical CNS symptoms heralding the oncologic diagnosis in some cases. Ovarian teratoma is the most common neoplasm associated with this autoimmune encephalitis in females. Data on pregnancy in patients who are recovering from this disease or who present with anti-NMDAR AE for the first time during pregnancy are sparse. A case series and literature review that followed 11 patients (6 diagnosed during pregnancy and 5 who became pregnant during recovery) reported no maternal complications, but 6 of the babies were delivered prematurely. Maternal complications were seen in one-third of pregnancies reported in the literature review.

Paraneoplastic Cerebellar Degeneration

While it is considered a rare autoimmune disorder, paraneoplastic cerebellar degeneration (PCD) is one of the most common paraneoplastic disorders. In PCD, autoimmune antibodies attack the Purkinje cells in the cerebellum, producing an acute to subacute cerebellar dysfunction syndrome and subsequent neuronal degeneration. Anti-yo (PCA-1) antibodies that are associated with breast and gynecologic cancers were present in almost all patients in an earlier case series that characterized this disorder in a cohort of 55 female patients. The majority of these patients experienced a disabling neurologic syndrome that preceded the malignancy diagnosis. Other autoantibodies have been implicated in PCD, such as anti-hu, anti-tr, anti-ri, and anti-mGluR$_1$ antibodies. Management involves treating the oncologic cause and immunosuppressive therapy for the autoimmune neurologic disorder. The prognosis for these patients is poor, with the majority becoming significantly disabled. It has been noted that positivity for anti-yo antibody is associated with a more treatment-refractory course with a worse prognosis.

STROKE IN FEMALES

For males and females over 25 years of age, the global lifetime risk of stroke is 25%. Importantly, the incidence of stroke in the young (individuals < 55 years of age), and specifically young females, is on the rise in the United States and Europe. Existing data do not separate between sex and gender, and the observed sex-specific differences that are described in the literature for stroke patients likely include effects of both. It has been found that female stroke patients experience an increased rate of disability and mortality compared to their male counterparts. In addition to unique female-specific stroke risk factors, the degree to which various traditional cardiovascular risk factors influence stroke risk is different in females and males. Moreover, there are observed differences in the clinical presentation and management of stroke syndromes in females and in stroke outcomes. Here, we summarize sex-specific differences in stroke with special attention to stroke in pregnancy and the postpartum period and stroke risk with hormonal therapy.

Sex-Specific Differences in Modifiable Risk Factors for Ischemic and Hemorrhagic Stroke

It is important to recognize that there are key differences between sexes and in the well-known modifiable cardiovascular risk factors, namely, diabetes, obesity, hypertension, and atrial fibrillation. In females, a diagnosis of diabetes has a stronger association with the occurrence of stroke, especially Type I diabetes, with an increased risk of ischemic stroke developing at lower fasting blood glucose levels. A clinical diagnosis of obesity (body mass index > 30) and a higher waist-to-hip ratio has a stronger association with stroke risk in females than in males. Hypertension increases stroke risk in females at lower systolic blood pressures than males, has a stronger association with both ischemic and hemorrhagic stroke, and appears to develop at an earlier age in females than in males. The effect of hypertensive disorders of pregnancy and adverse pregnancy outcomes on developing chronic hypertension and increasing stroke risk is discussed in the next section. Female sex is a known risk factor for increased risk of recurrence of stroke events in the context of atrial fibrillation and is accounted for in the CHA_2DS_2-VASc score used clinically to aid decision-making regarding anticoagulation in secondary stroke prevention for patients with atrial fibrillation. Current data do not suggest a clear sex-specific difference in other modifiable stroke risk factors such as lipid profiles and level of physical activity.

Female-Specific Risk Factors for Stroke

Analogously to traditional cardiovascular risk factors, female-specific stroke risk factors can also be modifiable, such as exposure to estrogen-based hormonal therapy, parity (>5 pregnancies), and hypertensive disorders of pregnancy, or nonmodifiable, such as a shorter reproductive lifespan. A shorter reproductive lifespan is associated with an increased stroke risk. Both early (<11) menarche and late (>17) menarche double stroke risk, and early menopause is also associated with an increased stroke risk, with very early menopause (<40 years of age) considered to be an important stroke risk factor.

Exposure to hormonal therapy in the reproductive years has been associated with increased stroke risk, with the first meta-analysis of data to evaluate this association reporting an increased relative risk of stroke of 2.75 with oral contraceptive pill (OCP) use. More recent population data capturing time periods reflecting the use of combined OCPs with low-dose estrogen content reported a smaller increase in the risk of ischemic stroke than previously described, and no increased risk of stroke with the use of progestin-only contraceptive pills. It is of critical importance to account for other stroke risk factors, such as hypertension, smoking, and a diagnosis of migraine with aura, in estimating stroke risk in the context of OCP use. Smoking with OCP use increases the risk of stroke fivefold. Early data shows that migraine with or without aura and OCP use increases stroke risk by 5- to 17-fold with a much stronger association for migraine with aura and a higher frequency of aura conferring a higher risk of stroke.

Therefore, society guidelines recommend avoiding the use of combined OCPs in patients with migraine with aura if they are over the age of 35 or if they are younger than 35 and have a concurrent history of smoking. Initial clinical trials showed that hormone replacement therapy in menopause was associated with increased stroke risk. A recent population-based study also showed that the increased risk of stroke with hormonal replacement therapy use in menopause increases risk of all subtypes of stroke even after hormonal therapy discontinuation. However, further data are needed to address this question. Guidelines recommend the use of hormonal therapy for vasomotor symptom management in females younger than 60 years of age or within the 10-year time window from the start of menopause. The transdermal patch is considered to be low risk, as it contains a relatively small dose of estrogen.

Female-specific risk factors associated with pregnancy include assisted reproductive therapy (due to either multiple gestations or the use of ovarian stimulation, which increases the risk of thrombosis by 10%), cesarean section, metastatic choriocarcinoma, peripartum cardiomyopathy, and the hypertensive disorders of pregnancy.

In summary, the increased risk of stroke that is attributable to hormone therapy across the reproductive lifespan is a topic with multiple layers of complexity. Most large population registry analyses do not account for the dose or formulation of hormonal therapy, have limited information on medical comorbidities, and have other limitations beyond the scope of this chapter. Current clinical guidelines advise avoiding estrogen-based OCPs in females with migraine with aura and other stroke risk factors, such as smoking and hypertension, and to avoid estrogen replacement therapy in females over 60 years of age or beyond 10 years of menopause onset.

Ischemic Stroke in Females

Data show not only that females differ from males with regard to stroke risk factors, but also that there are observed sex-specific differences in ischemic stroke presentation, clinical management, and neurologic outcomes in the population typically affected by a higher ischemic stroke risk (patients over 55 years of age). Females present more frequently with nontraditional and nonfocal symptoms of arterial ischemic stroke, such as fatigue, headache, generalized weakness, altered mental status, and disorientation/confusion. Stroke mimics also tend to be more frequently observed in females, and these two clinical observations can lead to misdiagnosis and delays in acute neuroimaging and reperfusion therapy. In the US, female patients had longer delays to acute imaging, which affects candidacy for thrombolytic administration, and also had longer door-to-needle times. Stroke outcomes for females not only relate to premorbid functional baseline and rehabilitation efforts after the incident stroke, but also appear to be driven by key anatomic and spatial differences, as outlined in two recent studies, which showed that left hemispheric lesions in the thalamus, hippocampus, and occipital cortex conferred a more severe outcome in females than in males after adjusting for other variables such as age and premorbid functional baseline. There also appears to be an increased risk of poststroke depression in females after adjusting for all other confounding risk factors, as some recent data show.

In patients in their reproductive years, pregnancy poses a significant risk for both ischemic and hemorrhagic stroke. While pregnancy has been described as the ultimate physiologic stress test of the cardiovascular system, it is worth noting that stroke in pregnancy and childbirth is a leading cause of maternal disability and mortality. As with most cases of stroke in young patient populations, ischemic stroke etiology is not usually due to atherosclerotic disease or atrial fibrillation, but the most common etiologies are venous thromboembolism through a patent foramen ovale, preexisting cardiac disease, and hypercoagulable states. Studies have shown that ischemic stroke is most likely to be experienced in the peripartum and postpartum periods and may be the first presentation of a postpartum cardiomyopathy. Other ischemic stroke etiologies to be mindful of in pregnant females include spontaneous cervical artery dissection, which has a more than 5-fold increase in risk during pregnancy, and traumatic dissection in context of labor and delivery, in addition to intimate partner violence (pregnant and postpartum females are especially vulnerable to this). Acute neuroimaging such as a head computed tomography (CT) and head and neck CT angiography with the use of iodinated contrast should be performed in pregnant females with appropriate abdominal lead shielding to minimize fetal exposure to radiation. Gadolinium contrast is contraindicated in pregnancy and should not be used. With regard to acute reperfusion therapy in the context of ischemic stroke, thrombolytics such as alteplase and tenecteplase are not contraindicated in pregnancy and are large molecules that do not cross the placental barrier. A recent large retrospective analysis on national data in the United States concluded that mechanical clot retrieval in acute ischemic stroke can be safely performed in pregnant patients, and the American Heart Association/American Stroke Association's acute stroke management guidelines do not preclude pregnant patients from receiving acute reperfusion therapy.

Recent data suggest that adverse pregnancy outcomes (APOs) increase the risk of stroke in females and lower the median age of incident stroke. APOs are defined to include the hypertensive disorders of pregnancy (gestational hypertension, preeclampsia, and eclampsia), preterm delivery, small for gestational age infants, and placental abruption. It has recently been shown that the age for a first stroke was 58.3 years in females with no history of APOs, 54.8 years in women with a history of 1 APO, and as young as 51.6 years in patients with a history of two or more APOs. Clinical stroke risk factor assessments in females should include screening for a history of hypertensive disorders of pregnancy and adverse pregnancy outcomes, use of hormonal therapy, reproductive lifespan, parity, and other female-specific risk factors in addition to the standard practice of evaluating glycemic control, blood pressure control and lipid profiles.

Reversible Cerebral Vasoconstrictive Syndrome

Reversible cerebral vasoconstrictive syndromes (RCVS) refer to a group of disorders that clinically present with severe thunderclap headache and neuroimaging evidence of diffuse reversible foci of narrowing of the cerebral arteries. RCVS is 2–10 times more common in females than in males, and the $RCVS_2$ clinical scoring system that is used to aid in the diagnosis of RCVS incorporates female sex into its calculation. The pathophysiology underlying RCVS is not quite clear, and the "reversible" nature of this arterial narrowing does not always translate to reversible symptoms without neurologic sequalae in patients. Sustained arterial narrowing can lead to ischemic infarcts due to diminished perfusion. Intracerebral hemorrhage occurs in RCVS and is thought to be a reperfusion injury to the ischemic areas in the context of dynamic vasoconstriction and vasodilation, as is subarachnoid hemorrhage (SAH), which is presumed to be from the rupture of small arteries in the subarachnoid space. Importantly, RCVS is the most common cause of subarachnoid hemorrhage in pregnancy (compared to nonpregnant adults, in whom aneurysmal rupture underlies ~85% of SAH cases). Furthermore, the postpartum state accounts for one-fifth of all RCVS cases. Posterior reversible encephalopathy syndrome

(PRES) is another clinical syndrome that presents with severe headache and neuroimaging evidence of vasogenic edema of white matter classically involving the posterior parietal and occipital lobes. It may share a common pathophysiology with RCVS, and both disorders are more commonly observed during pregnancy complicated by preeclampsia.

Hemorrhagic Stroke in Females

Hemorrhagic stroke refers to intracerebral hemorrhage and subarachnoid hemorrhage. The most common causes of hemorrhagic stroke in patients over 55 years of age include hypertensive hemorrhages, rupture of vascular malformations, and cerebral amyloid angiopathy. Sex-specific differences in hemorrhagic stroke are less frequently studied and documented in the literature. Female patients in hemorrhagic stroke studies tend to be older with more severe stroke presentations, irrespective of the extent of the bleed, and sex does not appear to influence major outcomes such as death or major disability. However, with regard to vascular malformations, it has been observed that cerebral aneurysms are more common in females and twice as common in postmenopausal females. Female sex has been considered by some studies as an independent risk factor for aneurysm growth. Aneurysms are also more likely to rupture in female patients, even when correcting for other aneurysm-specific factors such as size and location.

Cerebral arteriovenous malformations (AVMs) clinically present with rupture in younger patient populations than cerebral aneurysms (between the second and fourth decades) and are observed in equal frequency between males and females. There are conflicting earlier data on whether the risk of cerebral AVM rupture increases with pregnancy and childbirth. In 2017 one study reporting on a North American cohort of females with cerebral AVMs found an annual hemorrhage rate of 1.3% in nonpregnant females versus 5.7% in pregnant females. A recent national audit of females with AVMs in the United States reported that pregnancy tripled the risk of AVM rupture compared to their nonpregnant counterparts.

It is also notable that while in the general adult population, hemorrhagic strokes account for a small proportion of all strokes (11%–13% are hemorrhagic, and the remainder are ischemic), 50% of strokes in pregnant females are hemorrhagic and 50% ischemic. This difference could be explained by the fact that strokes in pregnancy typically affect a younger patient population with fewer risk factors implicated in atherosclerotic ischemic stroke, in addition to the hypertensive disorders of pregnancy increasing the risk of hypertensive hemorrhages (as was noted above, RCVS and PRES can lead to intracerebral hemorrhage). Indeed, it has been noted that hemorrhages pertaining to vascular malformation rupture are observed more frequently during the pregnancy, whereas hypertensive hemorrhages are more common in the postpartum period.

Cerebral Venous Thrombosis

Females are three times more likely to suffer from cerebral venous sinus thrombosis (CVST) compared to males. This could be due to the increased presence of provoking factors in females such as acquired hypercoagulable states associated with hormonal therapy, pregnancy and peripartum, and autoimmune conditions such as APLAS. Pregnancy or postpartum in of itself should not be accepted as the sole underlying cause/trigger for CVST occurring during these periods and hematologic consultation and workup is indicated. The presentation of CVST can be quite insidious and subacute with a waxing and waning headache progressing over several weeks as the only clinical manifestation, so the index of suspicion for this diagnosis must be high. CVST can lead to cerebral edema secondary to venous congestion, ischemic stroke, and hemorrhagic infarction. Diagnostic neuroimaging should include vascular neuroimaging with contrast if no contraindications exist (head CT venogram or, ideally, brain MRI and MRV with T1 postcontrast sequences as this improves the sensitivity of the test). Treatment is typically with anticoagulation even in the presence of intracranial hemorrhage. Various considerations regarding management and choice of anticoagulant are beyond the scope of this chapter, however, note that anticoagulation is typically with heparin or low molecular weight heparin. Warfarin is used as a blood thinner in specific patient populations for longer-term anticoagulation (e.g., patients with disorders of acquired hypercoagulability such as antiphospholipid antibody syndrome); however, warfarin is contraindicated in pregnancy. Direct oral anticoagulants are also not safe to be used in pregnant females. It is advised that patients with a prior history of CVST around pregnancy or peripartum be treated with prophylactic low molecular weight heparin during future pregnancies up until 8–12 weeks postpartum. CVST in the context of "provoked" female-specific risk factors including hormonal therapy or pregnancy has been shown to be associated with better outcomes than CVST in males or older females presenting with CVST.

ALZHEIMER DISEASE

Alzheimer disease (AD) is the most common cause of dementia, affecting more than 6 million Americans, two-thirds of whom are female. Age is a known risk factor for development of AD, with the risk doubling for each decade after age 60. The Framingham study suggests that the difference in disease prevalence is due to a survivor bias, as males who survive beyond age 65 may have lower cardiovascular risk factors, which may explain the lower risk of dementia compared to females after the age of 80 years.

There are multiple potential biological mechanisms that may explain the sex difference in disease prevalence. These may include differences in genetic risk, hormonal effects, and psychiatric comorbidities as well as lifestyle/psychosocial factors affecting cognitive reserve.

Genetic Differences

The apolipoprotein E4 (APOE4) allele is the most potent genetic risk factor for late-onset sporadic AD. The APOE4 allele generates a dose-dependent risk of developing AD, where patients with the E4/E4 genotype have an increased risk of AD compared to the E4/E3 genotype. The apolipoprotein E (APOE) protein is widely distributed throughout the human body. In the brain, astrocytes primarily produce APOE. The APOE protein in AD plays an important role in amyloid-β protein transcription, production, aggregation, and clearance.

The risk associated with APOE4 is greater in females. Females who carry the APOE4 allele are more likely to develop mild cognitive impairment (MCI) than males. In addition, among patients with MCI, females with the APOE3/4 genotype are more likely to develop AD compared to males. In a meta-analysis of 27 studies with 58,000 participants, looking at patients with one copy of APOE4 allele, females were at increased risk to develop

AD at younger ages, 65–75 years. Further, female carriers had increased total tau in cerebrospinal fluid, a biomarker in AD indicative of neuronal injury volume. These data suggest that the APOE4 modulates the risk of AD in a sex-specific manner.

One study showed that there are sex-specific genetic covariances between resilience to developing AD and autoimmune traits such that the genetic predisposition toward resilience was associated with reduced genetic risk for autoimmune traits among females. This sex difference in the genetic architecture of cognitive resilience could be due to differences in hormones, sex chromosomes, or both.

Hormonal Effects

The Women's Health Initiative Memory study showed that postmenopausal females, ages 65–79, who had not had a hysterectomy, when treated with estrogen and progesterone compared to controls had a double risk of dementia. Subsequently, several studies have suggested that there may be a window during which hormonal therapy has a beneficial effect. This is in keeping with the findings that early menopause is associated with a higher risk of AD. This has also been corroborated in mice with AD, in which a reduction in circulating endogenous estrogen due to early menopause is associated with a proliferation of AD pathology. It is likely that these hormonal effects interact in complex ways with other AD risk factors.

CONCLUSIONS

This chapter has outlined some of the many factors to be considered in caring for female patients with neurologic disease. As we move toward more precision medicine, these sex-specific nuances are important to best care for our patients. In addition, sex differences in disease expression give important insights into disease pathophysiology and treatment in neurologic conditions.

"For the full bibliography list, please use the pincode on the inside front cover to access the electronic version of the text at ebooks.health.elsevier.com."

14

Parkinson disease and Parkinsonism*

Michael T. Hayes

Parkinson disease is a common neurologic disease. It is a progressive, degenerative disease manifested by motor and nonmotor symptoms. First described as a specific syndrome by James Parkinson in 1817 in "An Essay on the Shaking Palsy," the disease is estimated to affect 1 million people in the United States and 4 million people worldwide. The prevalence in industrialized countries is estimated to be 0.3%. It is rarely seen in patients under 40 years of age, but the incidence increases with age. It is estimated that perhaps 3% of the population over 80 years of age are affected. Multiple studies demonstrate that the onset of Parkinson disease occurs 2 years earlier, on average, in men than in women and that twice as many men as women will develop the disease. Epidemiologic studies have demonstrated few associations. Living in rural areas and exposure to pesticides (specifically paraquat) are risk factors. Smoking and coffee drinking appear to be protective.

CLINICAL PRESENTATION

Parkinson disease is manifested by motor and nonmotor symptoms. The classic findings of Parkinson disease are motor symptoms. These were described in a paper by Hoehn and Yahr in 1967 looking at 183 Parkinson patients. These symptoms include resting tremor, bradykinesia, postural instability, and rigidity. Parkinson disease frequently presents with tremor, usually unilateral. The tremor is typically seen in one extremity initially (sometimes involving only one finger or the thumb). The tremor is slower (4–6 Hz) than a classic essential tremor (8–10 Hz) and is most prominent when the limb is in a posture of repose (the term "resting tremor" is somewhat misleading, as complete relaxation frequently abolishes the tremor). The tremor is suppressed with movement. Less commonly, the head, jaw, and tongue may be involved. For some patients, the classic parkinsonian tremor is the only manifestation of the disease. This is referred to as tremor-predominant Parkinson disease. In our experience, these patients do eventually develop other symptoms of Parkinson disease, but after a period of time, sometimes a number of years.

Bradykinesia refers to slowing of movement and the simplification of complex motor tasks. Spontaneous movement is decreased. This is manifested in the "masked facies" (also known as hypomimia) of Parkinson disease. The blink rate decreases, and the eyes are more open, giving the appearance of staring. The facial muscles move less, so the face is less emotive. As the condition progresses, the mouth often stays slightly open. Speech becomes softer and monotone, with the words running together. Spontaneous swallowing is reduced, and the mechanics of swallowing are affected, resulting in sialorrhea. In Parkinson disease, sialorrhea is due not to increased saliva production but to an inability to efficiently handle saliva. Hand movements become more restricted. Finger tapping may have normal speed, but the amplitude of movement is decreased. Alternating movement becomes difficult, and there is frequent "freezing," that is, intermittent arrest of motor function. It becomes more difficult to do things such as stir with a spoon or brush one's teeth. Writing becomes cramped and small (micrographia). Eventually, the

*Based on Hayes MT. Parkinson's disease and parkinsonism. *Am J Med*. 2019;132(7):802–807. ISSN 0002-9343. https://doi.org/10.1016/j.amjmed.2019.03.001.

patient has difficulty rising from a chair. Changes in gait are noted, with a decrease in arm swing, usually asymmetrically. The length of the patient's stride diminishes, and arm swing may disappear altogether. The patient can no longer turn on a pivot but turns "en bloc," using multiple small steps to turn. Eventually, the patient may develop propulsion or retropulsion. The patient's trunk will "get ahead" of their feet, and they will need to take small running steps to regain their balance, which has been termed festination. As the disease progresses, this may result in the patient falling. Falling, however, generally occurs later in the disease. If a patient tends to fall early in the course of the disease, one should consider a diagnosis other than Parkinson disease.

Nonmotor symptoms of Parkinson disease have become better appreciated over time and can be as debilitating as the motor symptoms. Cognitive decline, depression, anxiety, dysautonomia, and sleep disturbances are all seen with Parkinson disease. Anosmia (loss of the sense of smell) occurs in as many as 90% of patients with Parkinson disease and may precede other symptoms by many years. Dysautonomia is present in virtually all Parkinson disease patients and includes constipation (also a very early symptom). Other gastrointestinal complaints include bloating, nausea, and abdominal discomfort. A study by Hardoff et al. showed slowed gastric emptying times, which were exacerbated by carbidopa levodopa. Orthostatic hypotension is a symptom that presents in some 50% of Parkinson patients; it results in increased debilitation and significantly affects the higher frequency of falling that is seen later in Parkinson disease. Urinary complaints, including increased frequency and urgency, are common. A study of early, untreated Parkinson patients showed abnormal urinary function in the storage phase of 84% of the patients studied. Depression and anxiety are comorbidities with Parkinson disease, present in approximately 35% of patients. Factors such as female sex, dependency, higher United Parkinson disease rating scale scores, and lower Mini Mental status scores may predispose patients to depression. Some data show different forms of depression related to sex. Women feel more melancholy, and men have more apathy and decreased libido. Anxiety occurs with depression or independently of depression. Apathy is seen with or without depression but is more common in patients with cognitive decline.

Dementia in Parkinson disease has a prevalence of 30%–40%. Cereda et al. looked at the onset of Parkinson disease and found that age, sex, and disease duration were independently associated with Parkinson disease, with higher rates of dementia found in men between 60 and 80 years of age. Hallucinations and paranoid ideation are also seen in Parkinson disease, generally in the setting of taking dopaminergic medications. When hallucinations and delusional thinking appear early or in the absence of medication, a diagnosis of Lewy body disease should be entertained.

DIAGNOSIS

A myriad of symptoms are associated with the diagnosis of Parkinson disease. However, many combinations of symptoms exist, and the absence of some symptoms does not necessarily exclude the diagnosis. Actually making the diagnosis, especially early in the disease, relies on the presence of certain cardinal symptoms. The diagnosis may be supported by the presence of certain symptoms or clinical criteria, while the presence of other specific clinical findings would argue against a diagnosis. Experience with the disease on the part of the clinician is helpful, and studies have suggested that experienced clinicians are more accurate in diagnosing Parkinson disease than occurs with the application of a set of diagnostic criteria.

The diagnosis is most strongly supported by the presence of the cardinal manifestations of Parkinson disease, including bradykinesia, rigidity (involuntary resistance to passive movements that are independent of velocity), and rest tremor. The symptoms are not necessarily unilateral but, in classic Parkinson disease, are clearly asymmetric. Not all the symptoms may be present, especially early on, in every patient with Parkinson disease, but the presence of all three clearly strengthens the case for the diagnosis.

The most powerful piece of evidence supporting the diagnosis of Parkinson disease is a clear-cut beneficial response to dopaminergic therapy. The response would be unequivocal with a very obvious improvement in symptoms or significant worsening of symptoms if the drug is withdrawn. If, by history, there is some doubt as to whether there is an improvement of symptoms, one can do an off/on evaluation. This is a test in which the patient comes in having not taken their medication at least for 12 hours. A clinical scale of motor function, most commonly the UPDRS III test, is administered. The patient is then administered their usual dose of dopaminergic medication (or perhaps a slightly higher dose), and a sufficient period of time is allowed for the medication to take effect. The UPDRS III test is then given again. For research purposes, a 30% improvement in score is considered a positive indication that the dopaminergic medication has an impact on the disease. An improvement that is at least close to that should be used as demonstration of clinical benefit in treating the individual patient. In fact, the absence of any significant effect of dopaminergic stimulation in a patient with at least moderate disease symptoms makes the diagnosis of Parkinson disease highly unlikely. However, unlike rigidity and bradykinesia, rest tremor is frequently not responsive to dopaminergic medication in any dose, so a lack of improvement and rest tremor with dopaminergic stimulation does not necessarily suggest that the condition is not Parkinson disease. Thus, for tremor-predominant Parkinson disease, the off/on test is less helpful.

Other clinical or historical features that support the diagnosis of Parkinson disease include the presence of a levodopa-induced dyskinesia, anosmia, and the presence of REM sleep disorder.

Some symptoms or clinical findings make the diagnosis of Parkinson disease less tenable. These may be symptoms that are occurring too early in the course of normal Parkinson disease, such as multiple falls or rapid progression of gait to the point of inability to walk within the first 5 years or severe dysphonia, dysarthria, or dysphagia early in the disease. Marked orthostatic hypotension or severe urinary incontinence early in the disease or the absence of any progression of motor symptoms for more than 5 years also make the diagnosis less likely. There are symptoms or signs that coexist with parkinsonian features that suggest a disease other than Parkinson disease. Cerebellar dysfunction, supranuclear gaze palsy, especially downgaze, progressive aphasia, cortical sensory loss, or limb apraxia all suggest a different diagnosis.

A Movement Disorders Society Task Force published a set of clinical diagnostic criteria for the diagnosis of Parkinson disease that takes into account all these factors.

While the diagnosis of Parkinson disease can be made on clinical grounds and in the majority of patients, some situations arise in which another form of testing can be helpful. A DaTscan or skin biopsy to evaluate for misfolded alpha-synuclein can be helpful in certain circumstances. The situations in which these tests might be helpful include patients with a prominent essential tremor and patients with significant tremor at rest and with action in whom a diagnosis of Parkinson disease versus essential tremor is unclear. Patients with early or very subtle symptoms, patients who show little improvement in their symptoms with dopaminergic stimulation, patients with less common parkinsonian symptoms such as "lower body" parkinsonism, and patients who develop parkinsonian symptoms in the setting of being on a potential dopamine-blocking drug all may be further assessed using these modalities.

DaTscan

The DaTscan is performed by intravenous injection of a radioligand, ioflupane, which binds to the presynaptic dopamine transporter protein. Single-photon emission computed tomography (SPECT) or positron emission tomography (PET) imaging of the radioligand is done, which images the activity in the caudate and putamen. The images can show lower striatal metabolism and binding potential in patients with parkinsonian disorders that are caused by a presynaptic lesion (decreased amounts of dopamine). In one study looking at patients with uncertain diagnoses, the DaTscan changed the pretest diagnoses of almost 40% of the patients and resulted in a change in medication therapy in 70%. To date, the DaTscan has not been used to differentiate Parkinson disease from progressive supranuclear palsy or multiple systems atrophy (which also have abnormal DaT scans), but advances in imaging may allow that in the future.

Alpha-synuclein Seed Amplification Assays

Seed amplification assays are a group of techniques that detect protein misfolding in proteinopathies. Some of these techniques are already accepted for demonstrating prions in the diagnosis of Creutzfeldt-Jakob disease. Similar protein amplification assays have been developed to detect misfolded alpha-synuclein in biopsy material. The assays have been performed on cerebrospinal fluid, skin biopsies, and olfactory mucosa. Because the test is sensitive to alpha-synucleinopathies, it can differentiate between Parkinson disease and Lewy body disease (alpha-synucleinopathies) and progressive supranuclear palsy (tauopathy) or between Lewy body disease and Alzheimer disease.

Because these studies detect a biomarker, they may be able to diagnose parkinsonian conditions prior to the patient developing clinical signs. This potential ability to diagnose these diseases earlier will be important in the development of potential future therapies affecting disease progression.

PATHOLOGY

The pathologic hallmark of Parkinson disease is depigmentation of the substantia nigra and locus coeruleus with neuronal loss in the pars compacta of the substantia nigra. Both apoptosis and autophagy are involved in the process. Neuronal loss is also seen in the basal nucleus of Meynert and the dorsal motor nucleus of the vagus nerve. In affected areas, Lewy bodies, which are eosinophilic cytoplasmic inclusion bodies containing alpha-synuclein, are noted. The primary cause of Parkinson disease remains unclear. How Lewy bodies are specifically related to the progression of the disease is not known. Current theories of how neuronal loss occurs in Parkinson disease include mitochondrial dysfunction, inflammation, abnormalities in protein handling, and oxidative stress (Figure 14.1).

PHARMACOLOGIC TREATMENT

The decision of when to treat a patient with Parkinson disease is made in collaboration with the patient. When symptoms affect the patient's quality of life (the ability to work or socialize), treatment is started. There is no compelling evidence that starting treatment early has any impact on the progression of the disease, and no

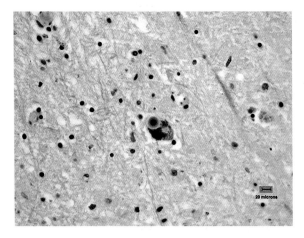

Fig 14.1 Lewy body. (Courtesy Dr. Mel Feany, Harvard Medical School.)

treatment confers neuroprotection. The decision to treat is based on the impact of symptoms.

Levodopa was the first effective medication for Parkinson disease and is still the most potent. Virtually all patients will use levodopa at some point during their disease. It is the immediate precursor to dopamine, which can cross the blood-brain barrier. It allows the depleted number of dopaminergic neurons to produce more dopamine and alleviate symptoms. It is usually paired with carbidopa, which blocks metabolism of levodopa in the periphery, increasing central nervous system bioavailability and lessening peripheral side effects, particularly nausea. Other side effects include hallucinations, delusions, somnolence, dystonia, and, prominently, dyskinesias. Dyskinesia (involuntary writhing movements) often limits the dose of carbidopa levodopa that can be used. Dyskinesias are estimated to occur in up to 40% of Parkinson disease patients within 4–6 years of starting carbidopa levodopa. For this reason, some practitioners will delay the use of carbidopa levodopa in favor of other agents (dopamine agonists), especially in younger patients. However, dopamine agonists are associated with a number of other unwanted side effects that will be described later in this chapter. Also, dopamine agonists are significantly less potent in ameliorating symptoms of Parkinson disease, and patients may sacrifice a better quality of life earlier in the disease in hope of putting off the onset of dyskinesias. Therefore, the decision of when to use carbidopa levodopa is made taking into account patient's age and symptom complex and, potentially, the effectiveness of other agents on their symptoms by medication trial. A number of controlled-release formulations of carbidopa levodopa using both short-acting and controlled-release carbidopa levodopa have been developed as well as a system of infusing carbidopa levodopa gel into the jejunum through a jejunal tube and a pump as a means of minimizing motor fluctuations and dyskinesias. The presence of motor fluctuations and dyskinesias are primary reasons why other medications or surgical interventions are considered.

Dopamine agonists (pramipexole, ropinirole, and rotigotine) stimulate dopaminergic receptors in the central nervous system, alleviating symptoms of Parkinson disease. While dopamine agonists improve symptoms, they are predictably less potent than levodopa. They are frequently used because they are less likely to cause dyskinesias, and they tend to have a longer half-life. The decreased risk of dyskinesias may be because they are less potent stimulators of the D2 receptors. The decreased specificity, in the way that they stimulate dopaminergic receptors, may be the cause of their increased risk of hallucinations, hypotension, somnolence (sometimes with sleep attacks), and leg edema and the risk of compulsive behaviors, such as compulsive sexual behavior, buying, or gambling. The risks of hypotension and hallucinations are higher in elderly patients, and it is prudent to try to use carbidopa/levodopa in the elderly, if possible, to avoid complications.

Catechol-O-methyl transferase inhibitors (entacapone) and monoamine oxidase aldehyde dehydrogenase B (MAO-B) inhibitors (rasagiline and selegiline) inhibit enzymes involved in the breakdown of levodopa and dopamine. They prolong the effect of carbidopa/levodopa. They may also increase the side effects of levodopa, specifically, hallucinations, dyskinesia, and nausea. In the case of the MAO-B inhibitors, there is a risk of interaction with multiple drugs, including antidepressants in terms of causing serotonin syndrome.

Anticholinergic medications (trihexyphenidyl and benztropine) are not effective in treating bradykinesia but may be effective in decreasing rigidity, dystonia, and tremor. In patients (generally younger ones) whose early disease manifestations are rigidity and tremor, these medications, even as the sole agent, may be effective. Side effects limit dosing and include dry mouth, dry eyes, urinary retention, memory issues, and hallucinations. These agents should be used with caution in the elderly.

Antipsychotics are sometimes necessary to treat the symptoms of hallucination and paranoid delusions that may occur in Parkinson patients. Traditional agents, such as haloperidol, increase parkinsonian symptoms. The best tolerated agents include quetiapine, clozapine, and pimavanserin. Depression is a frequent comorbid symptom in Parkinson disease. Treatment with tricyclic antidepressants, serotonin noradrenaline reuptake inhibitors, or serotonin reuptake inhibitors have all been used. Cognitive behavioral therapy has been reported to be helpful, but no large-scale trials have been done.

Table 14.1 lists commonly used medications for treatment of Parkinson disease.

FUNCTIONAL NEUROSURGICAL TREATMENT

Before the advent of medical therapy for Parkinson disease (primarily levodopa) in the early 1960s, some patients received lesions to the thalamus pioneered by Cooper and others. This therapy was used to suppress parkinsonian tremor. Through the 1960s and into the 1970s, surgical treatment of Parkinson disease was largely abandoned. Over time, the limitations of dopaminergic therapy became apparent. These included motor fluctuations, dyskinesias, and hallucinations. It was also found that a number of patients with significant parkinsonian tremor did not get any relief from dopaminergic medication. There was a resurgence of stereotactic ablative surgery to the thalamus and globus pallidus interna. Initially, with improved stereotactic technique, lesioning became a more widely used therapy. Initially, these lesions were made by using radiofrequency lesioning, which is similar to deep brain stimulation (DBS) insofar as it requires a stereotactic head frame and the introduction of an electrode intracranially. Patients are awake during this procedure so that clinical verification of the target can be done. While this technique is still used occasionally, it has been largely replaced by alternative techniques such as gamma knife, which uses a focused beam of ionizing radiation to create a lesion, or focused ultrasound, which uses intersecting beams of ultrasound to produce frictional energy to create a lesion. Neither of these techniques requires anesthesia or introduction of an intracranial electrode and is thus considered less invasive. Lesioning has the advantage of being a one-time procedure that does not require a sophisticated medical infrastructure to maintain it (as does DBS). It is also a cost-effective alternative, and for those reasons, it is utilized in less developed countries or may be appropriate for patients living in somewhat remote areas. Some patients may also choose one of the less invasive forms of lesioning because of concerns about surgical risks and anesthesia. Lesioning is currently used primarily for essential tremor but may be used for severe parkinsonian tremor. Pallidotomies (lesions in the globus pallidus interna) are occasionally done to treat dyskinesia as well as tremor.

DBS is the implantation of stimulating electrodes into certain deep nuclei of the brain. Each electrode has four contacts. This allows for shaping of the field in the vertical direction. The more modern contacts are also steerable, which allows shaping the field of stimulation in the horizontal direction. That, along with the ability to change the intensity, pulse width, and frequency of the stimulation allows significant freedom in the ability to control the shape and intensity of the stimulation field. Side effects

TABLE 14.1	Medications Commonly Used to Treat Parkinson Disease		
Medication	**Supplied**	**Dosage**	**Comment**
Dopaminergic Medication			
Carbidopa/levodopa	Multiple immediate-release and controlled-release formulations. Gel preparation for jejunal infusion	Start at 25/100 TID, titrating dose and dosing interval to symptomatic relief	Most potent medication but with short half-life. Dyskinesias more common
Pramipexole	Immediate and extended release formulations	Start at 0.125 mg TID, increasing weekly based on clinical response to total daily target dose of up to 1.5–4.5 mg	Less fluctuation of efficacy but less potent than carbidopa/levodopa. May develop compulsive behaviors. Fatigue and marked drowsiness are noted frequently
Ropinirole	Immediate and extended release formulations	Start 0.25 mg TID with gradual increases based on clinical response to daily total dose of up to 24 mg	
Rotigatine	Transdermal patch	2 mg patch daily, increase weekly based on clinical response, up to 8 mg/day	
COMT and MAO-B Inhibitors			
Entacapone	200 mg. Also supplied in combination drug with carbidopa/levodopa	Take with each dose of carbidopa/levodopa	COMT inhibitor
Rasagiline	0.5 mg, 1 mg	Take 0.5–1 mg daily	MAO-B inhibitor. Contraindicated with multiple drugs because of potential serotonin syndrome
Selegiline	1.25 mg, 5 mg	Take 5 mg daily, if tolerated increase to 5 mg BID	
Anticholinergics			
Benztropine	0.5, 1, and 2 mg	Starting with 0.5 mg BID, increase based on clinical response up to 2 mg TID	Use with caution in elderly patients. Dry mouth and urinary retention are side effects
Trihexyphenidyl	2 and 5 mg	Starting at 2 mg QD, increase based on clinical response up to 2 mg TID	
Treatment of Hallucinations and Delusions			
Quetiapine	25, 50, 100, 200, 300, and 400 mg	Start at 25 mg QHS and increase based on clinical response. Doses earlier in the day may be necessary	Rarely need to go above 400 mg/day total dose
Clozapine	25, 50, 100, and 200 mg	Start at 12.5 mg QD and increase based on clinical response up to 300–450 mg total daily dose	Close following of absolute neutrophil count is mandatory
Pimavanserin	10 and 34 mg	34 mg QD	
Amantadine	100 and 137 mg (long acting)	Start at 100 mg daily. 100 mg. BID is usual dose. Long-acting form is 137 mg daily	Used to treat dyskinesia and has mild dopaminergic effect by inhibiting reuptake of dopamine

COMT, Catechol-*O*-methyl transferase; *MAO-B*, monoamine oxidase aldehyde dehydrogenase B.

(diplopia, muscle tightness, paresthesias, speech difficulties) generally occur with stimulation in an unwanted area. DB has become a staple of treatment in patients with complications of medical treatment that include precipitous and unpredictable motor fluctuations and disabling dyskinesia or the presence of intractable tremor. The treatment effect looks similar to that of the ablative procedures, but exactly how the stimulation produces the effect is not known. DBS frequently allows a decrease in the dosage of medication, gives a smoother response throughout the day in terms of motor symptoms, and generally reduces dyskinetic movements. DBS does not affect the progression of cognitive decline or axial instability, which is to be expected, as dopaminergic medications also tend not to improve these symptoms.

Different surgical techniques may be used to implant the electrodes. The choice of technique is determined by the experience and training of the surgical team at the movement disorders program. In both cases. the target is defined by using a stereotactic ablative-based coordinates system or by direct visualization by imaging during the surgery. The majority of centers do the surgery with the patient awake with intraoperative physiologic mapping using microelectrode recording and macrostimulation to better define the appropriate target. Some centers do the procedure with the patient asleep using intraoperative MRI to confirm lead placement. This second type of procedure does not require physiologic mapping or intraoperative stimulation. The two types of surgery have shown similar clinical outcomes.

The ideal Parkinson disease candidate for DBS has tremor as a significant symptom, has difficulty with precipitous off symptoms, and has dyskinesias. They should otherwise be a good surgical candidate and not have any significant cognitive decline. At most movement disorder centers, a candidate is evaluated by a neurologist, neurosurgeon, neuropsychologist and, at some institutions, a psychiatrist. That group, after evaluating the patient, meets to discuss whether the patient is a good candidate, what the pros and cons are of each potential target for DBS, the type of procedure (awake or asleep or even if a lesioning procedure should be considered) to recommend and which device to use (there are currently three systems on the market). The recommendations are then presented to the patient who decides if they want to proceed. Once the procedure has been done there is about a 2- to 4-week wait (to allow postop swelling to resolve) and then programming starts. Because the deep brain stimulator treats the same symptoms as the Parkinson medications, medication changes need to be done in concert with programming to give optimal outcome. This is best done by practitioners experienced both in programming and medication management.

EXERCISE IN PARKINSON DISEASE

Neuroplasticity, the ability of the central nervous system to reorganize connections and functions in response to extrinsic and intrinsic stimuli, plays a significant role in the treatment of Parkinson disease as regards exercise therapy.

Exercise has been demonstrated to reduce the risk of developing Parkinson disease. The institution of an exercise regimen has been shown to extend that potential benefits through the life of the patient. Since then, multiple studies have been done to demonstrate the benefits of regular exercise on parkinsonian symptoms and pathophysiology. For instance, functional MRI studies have shown improved thalamocortical activity in patients involved in high-rate stationary bike exercise. Regular treadmill training has been shown to increase dopamine D2 receptor binding potentials, demonstrating a positive impact on neuroplasticity on dopamine pathways. Stationary cycling, specifically, as an aerobic exercise is safe (likely safer than a treadmill for patients with gait and balance issues) and has been shown to improve motor performance, cognition, and balance and to decrease depression. Resistance training has been shown to improve muscular strength, motor function, and endurance. Balance training of different types has shown to improve balance and gait function and been demonstrated to reduce the number of falls the patient suffers. Tai chi and yoga have been studied with Parkinson patients and have been shown to improve strength, flexibility, cognitive function, and psychological well-being.

Investigation into an "ideal" exercise regimen for Parkinson disease is ongoing, but institution of a regular exercise program early on in the disease improves function and quality of life and should likely include elements of resistance training, aerobic exercise like cycling, and exercise to improve flexibility.

Caregiver Burden

An area that is perhaps not given adequate consideration in the treatment of Parkinson diseases is the burden on the patient's caregivers. Informal caregivers, such as spouses and children, provide a significant amount of care to patients. This does affect the societal cost of Parkinson disease in terms of loss of work time, financial strain, and caregiver morbidity.

The presence of nonmotor symptoms, especially neuropsychiatric disturbances, contributes disproportionately to caregiver burden. Palliative care models are being developed to help with this, including supporting spiritual well-being (studies showed that the greatest social support outside of immediate family is that provided by spiritual and religious communities), a holistic look at patient and caregiver quality of life, and treatment of caregiver anxiety and depression. This is being done with an eye toward providing comprehensive patient care and caregiver psychological support.

DIFFERENTIAL DIAGNOSIS

Lewy Body Disease

Lewy body disease is akin to classic Parkinson disease, clinically and pathologically. Pathologically, in addition to Lewy bodies being found in the striatum, there is widespread involvement of Lewy bodies in cortical neurons, with a relative paucity of the neurofibrillary tangles and amyloid plaques associated with Alzheimer disease. The diagnosis is clinical and consists of the appearance of parkinsonian symptoms, dementia, and hallucinations and delusions, frequently fluctuating with periods of lucidity. If motor signs precede the onset of cognitive decline and hallucinations, patients are often diagnosed with Parkinson disease, but the cognitive symptoms generally follow the onset of motor symptoms fairly closely. In some patients, cognitive symptoms precede the motor symptoms. These patients may initially be diagnosed with Alzheimer disease. Patients with motor symptoms may initially respond to dopaminergic medication, although worsening hallucinations may be noted. Eventually, dementia and axial instability became the most limiting symptoms. As with Parkinson disease, rapid eye movement (REM) sleep disorder is common. Patients with Lewy body dementia are exquisitely sensitive to most neuroleptics, although quetiapine, pimavanserin, and clozapine may be tolerated.

Drug-Induced Parkinsonism

Parkinsonism as a side effect of certain medications is an underdiagnosed entity. It is due to postsynaptic blockade of dopamine receptors (especially D2 receptors). It occurs primarily with first-generation neuroleptics and many second-generation neuroleptics, and it may be seen with gastrointestinal prokinetics such as metoclopramide and domperidone. Although dopamine receptor blockade occurs within hours of taking the medication, the parkinsonian effect may not be seen for days to weeks. Half to three-quarters of these cases are evident within 1 month of starting the medication, and 90% of cases occur within 3 months. Symptoms include masked face, tremor, rigidity, and bradykinesia. Symptoms tend to be symmetric (unlike idiopathic Parkinson disease), but it may be difficult to differentiate between drug-induced parkinsonism and Parkinson disease. A dopamine transporter scan, while limited as a tool for diagnosing idiopathic Parkinson disease, as it is positive in other degenerative Parkinsonian disorders, may be useful in diagnosing drug-induced Parkinsonism, as it is normal in those cases. Treatment is reduction or discontinuation of the offending agents. Agents that are less likely to cause drug-induced parkinsonism (and are best tolerated in idiopathic Parkinson disease) include clozapine and quetiapine.

Progressive Supranuclear Palsy

Progressive supranuclear palsy, unlike the alpha synucleinopathy that is Parkinson disease, is a tauopathy. It may initially be diagnosed as Parkinson disease, as early symptoms include difficulty rising from a chair, tenuous gait, and changes in speech similar to those of Parkinson disease. With progression, it diverges clinically from Parkinson disease. Classically, the condition begins with progressive unsteadiness of gait and multiple falls. At some point, the patient develops difficulty with voluntary vertical eye movement. It is difficult to look down, and the patient has difficulty going downstairs. Later, there is difficulty with voluntary eye movements in all directions, with saccadic breakdown. In extreme cases, there are no voluntary eye movements, although if the patient fixates on an object and the head is slowly turned, full eye movement can be obtained. This demonstrates that the abnormalities of eye movements are indeed "supranuclear." Speech becomes soft and monotone and mildly dysarthric. The patient may develop axial dystonia, with the neck muscles becoming spastic. The patient may develop pseudobulbar affect. Dysphasia is sometimes seen. In our experience, there may be a transient response to carbidopa/levodopa, but overall, dopaminergic medications have no effect on symptoms. Anticholinergic medications may help with the dystonia, although botulinum toxin injections in focal dystonia are more effective. The patient may develop difficulty with decreased sleep, in particular decreased REM sleep. Dementia is less common in progressive supranuclear palsy. Treatment is supportive. The patient eventually becomes less mobile. A feeding tube is sometimes employed in patients with severe dysphagia.

The syndrome of pure akinesia with gait freezing has been demonstrated to be a variant of progressive supranuclear palsy. In this condition, patients develop a marked inability to initiate gait with their feet "frozen" to the floor. Other symptoms of progressive supranuclear palsy may not be present or may occur very late in the course.

Pathologically, there is atrophy of the dorsal midbrain, with neuronal loss and gliosis in the superior colliculus, subthalamic nucleus, red nucleus, periaqueductal gray, pallidum, dentate, and pretectal nuclei. Neurofibrillary degeneration and neurofibrillary tangles are noted, as is tau deposition.

Multiple System Atrophy

Multiple system atrophy (MSA) is a degenerative neurologic disease. As the name implies, multiple systems are affected. These include the extrapyramidal system, the cerebellum, and the autonomic nervous system. Subtypes of multiple system atrophy are determined clinically by their predominant symptoms. If extrapyramidal symptoms are more prominent, it is characterized as MSA-P (parkinsonian subtype). The parkinsonian symptoms are frequently preceded by urinary urgency, sexual dysfunction, orthostatic hypotension, and sometimes inspiratory stridor. REM sleep disorder is common. In the parkinsonian form, rigidity and akinesia are early symptoms, but the classic parkinsonian tremor is not seen. Orthostatic hypotension eventually becomes symptomatic in virtually all patients, and some cerebellar signs are generally noted. Dystonia is a prominent feature in a number of patients. Imaging will often show atrophy of the pons and cerebellum. Atrophy of the pontocerebellar fibers resulted in the "hot cross bun" sign seen on MRI, but this occurs so late in the disease that the diagnosis has been clinically obvious for some time.

Pathology shows proteinaceous oligodendroglial cytoplasmic inclusions containing misfolded alpha-synuclein. Along with these inclusions, olivopontocerebellar atrophy and striatonigral degeneration are prominent findings. There may also be involvement of the hypothalamus, dorsal nucleus of the vagus nerve, and noradrenergic and serotonergic brainstem nuclei.

Corticobasal Degeneration

Corticobasal degeneration is similar to Parkinson disease in that it has an asymmetric onset and asymmetric tremor and rigidity. It appears in middle to late life, as does Parkinson disease. With progression, the patient frequently develops apraxia of the affected limb, which is not typical of Parkinson disease. Myoclonus may be prominent in the affected limb. Dementia, sometimes profound, may develop. There is no response of the motor symptoms to dopaminergic drugs.

Gross pathology shows atrophy in the superior frontal gyrus, parasagittal gyri, and the superior parietal lobule. Unlike progressive supranuclear palsy, the brainstem is not obviously atrophic. The affected cortex shows astrocytic plaques containing tau proteins. Neuronal loss and gliosis are also seen in the globus pallidum, thalamus, and substantia nigra.

Normal Pressure Hydrocephalus

While the concept and management of normal pressure hydrocephalus continue to be a matter of some debate, it is in the differential diagnosis of patients with parkinsonian symptoms. Normal pressure hydrocephalus is a syndrome that manifests as some cognitive decline, urinary urgency progressing to incontinence, and gait difficulty and was first described in the 1960s. It is the abnormality of gait that most looks like Parkinson disease. Freezing on gait initiation is frequently seen, and the stride is short stepped with decreased arm swing. En bloc turning is also seen, as is also seen in Parkinson disease. Normal pressure hydrocephalus is, however, a symmetric disease. Tremor is not a part of the symptom complex. Tone is generally normal, and manual dexterity is unaffected. Rapid alternating movement is generally normal in the hands and feet. Imaging shows ventriculomegaly out of proportion to cortical atrophy. If the diagnosis is made, then treatment is generally placement of a programmable ventriculoperitoneal shunt.

"For the full bibliography list, please use the pincode on the inside front cover to access the electronic version of the text at ebooks.health.elsevier.com."

15

Dementia*

Anderson Chen, Kirk R. Daffner, and Seth A. Gale

INTRODUCTION

Dementia is any disorder in which decline from a previous level of cognition causes interference in a person's occupational, domestic, or social functioning. Generally, dementia should be considered to be an acquired syndrome, with multiple possible causes, rather than a specific disease. A syndrome is a pattern of symptoms and cognitive changes that are observed by others and/or experienced by the person, whereas the term "disease" refers to the pathophysiologic process and/or the neuropathology that underlies and gives rise to the syndrome. For example, a patient's experience and a family member's observation of a syndrome of slowly progressive decline in language over 2 years could be caused by various diseases, such as Alzheimer disease (AD), a slow-growing tumor in the brain's language cortex, or a frontotemporal dementia (FTD). In this way, it is useful to think of experiencing "dementia" as similar to experiencing chronic chest pain, in that they are both symptoms or syndromes that can have one or more underlying causes. This distinction may be most important to providers when they start to evaluate presenting dementia symptoms, as it is a reminder to keep one's differential diagnoses wide during the diagnostic process (Fig. 15.1).

Globally, there were at least 35 million older adults living with dementia in 2010 and more than 57 million in 2019. This number will continue to increase, with some global estimates predicting a dementia prevalence of more than 150 million individuals by 2050. Advancing age, genetic profile, and systemic vascular disease are major risk factors for developing dementia.

A traditional way to conceptualize the diseases that underlie dementia is to consider two broad categories: diseases that are neurodegenerative (which were classically considered irreversible) and those that are nonneurodegenerative (which, classically, were considered at least potentially reversible). This dichotomy is a helpful heuristic but is limited by oversimplicity. For example, patients with dementia can have multiple, concurrent, underlying diseases that can be neurodegenerative (e.g., dementia with Lewy bodies) and nonneurodegenerative (e.g., cerebrovascular disease, obstructive sleep apnea) which cumulatively account for the impairment in cognition and daily functioning. There are also diseases that can impair cognition without leading to a significant decline in individuals' daily functioning, either at diagnosis or subsequently. The terms "mild neurocognitive disorder" (from DSM-V) and "mild cognitive impairment" (MCI) are used variously to characterize these states.

Most dementia in older adults is caused by some degree of neurodegeneration. Some common degenerative diseases that cause dementia in older adults are AD, dementia with Lewy bodies, vascular dementia, frontotemporal lobar degeneration, and Parkinson's disease dementia.

Common causes of nonneurodegenerative MCI and dementia that can occur across the lifespan include vitamin deficiencies (e.g., B12, thiamine), hypothyroidism, normal pressure hydrocephalus, chronic alcohol abuse, chemotherapy-related cognitive dysfunction, infections

*Based on Gale SA, Acar D, Daffner KR. Dementia. *Am J Med*. 2018;131(10):1161–1169. ISSN 0002-9343. https://doi.org/10.1016/j.amjmed.2018.01.022.

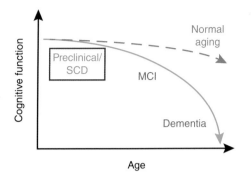

Fig. 15.1 Schema of dementia progression. *MCI,* Mild cognitive impairment; *SCD,* subjective cognitive decline.

(e.g., human immunodeficiency virus), intracranial masses (e.g., subdural hematomas, brain tumors), traumatic brain injury, and psychiatric illness (profound depression/anxiety).

Most frequently, patients or families will report initial symptoms of a dementia syndrome in primary care or family practice settings before having the opportunity to obtain specialized care. At these first touchpoints in the healthcare system, symptoms are sometimes presented to providers but then not further evaluated or ultimately diagnosed; these situations represent a missed opportunity for early interventions that can begin to improve patients' morbidity and other care outcomes. Estimates suggest that fewer than half of the expected patients with dementia are recognized in the primary care setting, and many who are identified do not receive diagnoses. The number of patients that are missed who have early changes of a dementia-causing disease rises substantially when you consider that these diseases may have years of a preclinical phase, during which some biological and pathophysiological changes occur in the brain that are not yet causing noticeable signs or symptoms.

Therefore it is important that primary care providers and other nonspecialists in cognitive disorders and dementia be familiar with the topics presented here. This is particularly true considering recent pharmacotherapeutic developments, particularly for cognitive impairment and dementia due to AD. Multiple steps within the healthcare system are often needed to determine the probable causes of dementia. Thus, if diagnoses of MCI or mild dementia are delayed well after symptom onset,

patients may receive proper care only after they have progressed to moderate stages of impairment, when treatments and care interventions are significantly less optimal.

For example, newer therapeutics such as lecanemab, a promising agent that was approved in 2023 by the US Food and Drug Administration to treat early AD, are likely to be effective only in milder stages of the disease. Failure to identify and diagnose dementia-causing diseases, especially at stages later than MCI, also leads to risks poorer patient understanding of the scope and expectations of treatment and higher rates of nonadherence to the schedule of any prescribed medications. Therefore, it is critical to consider screening guidelines to recognize symptoms, identify patients who are at risk, and provide early interventions, which will increasingly require tests for the biomarkers of AD and hopefully other diseases. Of note, the use of these newer AD therapeutics, which for now will likely be prescribed by neurology or psychiatry specialists, carries some risks of brain bleeds and edema, identified as amyloid-related imaging abnormalities (ARIA). Although these side effects are rarely consequential, additional studies are ongoing to help further characterize both risks and benefits, enabling more informed, personalized treatment discussions between providers and patients.

APPROACH TO EVALUATE FOR COGNITIVE IMPAIRMENT AND DEMENTIA

Screening Overview

There are currently no standardized guidelines on who needs to be screened for cognitive impairment and dementia. This contributes to the underdiagnosis and delayed diagnosis of dementia described previously. Notably, in the United States and around the world, delays in diagnosis are even more pronounced in certain subpopulations, with factors such as level of education, living alone, and being part of a minority racial or ethnic group likely playing a contributory role. Screening is also difficult because dementia has many different etiologies, so different risk factors that may prompt screening are more relevant for one or several causes of dementia but not all. Currently in clinical practice, screening for cognitive impairment and its sometimes associated psychiatric or motor symptoms often occurs later than is optimal and after the patient or family has raised subjective complaints and observations. Despite the current finding in the United States by the US Preventive Services Task Force that evidence is insufficient to assess the balance of benefits and harms of screening for cognitive impairment in all older adults, we advocate a shift to early identification of dementia risk factors and universal dementia screening in older adult populations.

Consideration of Dementia Risk Factors

While risk factors can be specific to the cause of the dementia, there are some risk factors to consider in primary care settings that are common to all diseases that cause dementia and can aid in decision-making about further evaluation. For simplicity, we will divide these risk factors into those that are nonmodifiable and modifiable and discuss accordingly.

Age is the most prominent nonmodifiable risk factor, as the incidence of dementia increases proportionally with age. For example, estimates from the past census in the United States suggest that among individuals with AD, the most common dementing illness, about 15% are between the ages of 65 and 74 years, almost 50% are between 75 and 85 years, and about 35% are 85 years or older. Differences in prevalence also occur along the lines of self-identified race and ethnicity. Many studies in the United States, for example, suggest that compared to their White counterparts, dementia prevalence is up to 1.5–2 times higher in Black and Hispanic individuals. This is supported by a summary of data reported annually by the Alzheimer's Association. The Association identifies two other nonmodifiable risk factors for dementia: low socioeconomic status and being a nonlocal language speaker. A family history of neurodegenerative dementia, especially of first-degree relatives, is another nonmodifiable risk factor and an appropriate consideration for screening and early provision of risk reduction recommendations.

Familial patterns of dementia are common, especially with AD, Parkinson disease, and FTD. Notably, there are currently minimal dementia "risk genes" available for testing in clinical settings in most countries, and genetic testing is not recommended for screening either by primary or specialist providers for most patients. In future years, recommendations for genetic testing may change when there is concern for AD, because carrying the apolipoprotein E-4 allele

(APOE-4) increases the risk of side effects with novel disease-modifying anti-amyloid antibody therapies, such as lecanemab. At the time of publication, however, there are no guidelines for referral for available genetic testing that consider the newly developed disease-modifying therapies for AD. In some selective families in which neurodegenerative disease has occurred in at least three individuals in two or more generations, with two of the individuals being first-degree relatives of the third generation (e.g., grandparent, parent, and child), it is reasonable to refer to a genetics program with counseling to consider testing.

Genetic testing results are increasingly available to individuals through direct-to-consumer testing; understandably, these have begun to affect care discussions in the clinic. Our experience is that test results showing a higher risk of AD, for example, motivates both patients and providers to develop treatment plans to increase patients' personalized, evidence-based brain health behaviors, which can mitigate important aspects of genetic risk over time.

There are 12 prominent modifiable risk factors to consider. These include five cardiovascular and cardiometabolic risk factors (hypertension, diabetes, obesity, physical inactivity, and smoking), three mental health risk factors (history of traumatic brain injury, depression, and alcohol use disorder), three social factors (social isolation, high air pollution, and low education), and hearing and vision impairment. As patients age, if cardiometabolic risk factors are not well controlled, the risk of vascular cognitive impairment, AD, and other neurodegenerative diseases increases significantly. In a prospective population cohort study with almost 230,000 patients, it was found that patients with controlled cardiometabolic risk factors over 9 years were less likely to develop dementia of any cause compared to their peers. In the same vein, it is critical to correct hearing and vision impairment to the extent possible in older individuals, especially those who are at higher risk of developing dementia. Modifiable dementia risk factors are essential clinical targets for interventions that should be discussed early and actively with patients and families.

Whether primary care providers or specialists identify nonmodifiable risk factors such as genetics or modifiable factors such as a sedentary lifestyle in older adults, it is essential that all providers adopt a proactive, prevention-oriented approach to dementia screening and risk reduction.

CLINICAL EVALUATION

Overview

The initial evaluation and diagnosis of possible cognitive impairment or dementia should include at least the following four elements: (1) a thorough clinical history, (2) a basic cognitive assessment and neurologic exam, (3) selective labs to screen for relevant metabolic/physiologic abnormalities (e.g., basic chemistries, thyroid panel, B12, Vitamin D), and (4) a structural brain scan, with MRI preferable to CT whenever possible. In certain patients, serologic studies such as antinuclear antibody, erythrocyte sedimentation rate, treponemal pallidum antibody or venereal disease research laboratory, HIV-ab, and heavy metal screen are warranted. Depending on the practice or workflow within different healthcare systems, these four elements may be carried out entirely within primary care or in collaboration between primary care and specialists when services are accessible.

Emphasis in the clinical interview should be placed on determining the pace of symptom onset (e.g., sudden/rapid or gradual) and symptom progression (e.g., decline over months or over years). For example, human prion diseases that cause dementia, such as Creutzfeldt-Jakob disease, typically have a rapid progression over weeks to months. Diseases such as AD and FTD, by contrast, usually progress gradually over years. In addition to asking about the nature of cognitive changes being experienced or observed (e.g., short-term memory changes, word-finding difficulty, calculating numbers), the clinical interview should include whether there have been changes in gait and balance, personality and emotional connection (e.g., changes in empathy, manners), autonomic symptoms (e.g., presyncope when standing, significant heart rate or blood pressure fluctuation), sleep behaviors (e.g., acting out dreams, vocalizations), visual or auditory misperceptions or hallucinations, and changes in smell and taste. See Table 15.1 for features of diseases that may involve dementia.

Cognitive Screening and Assessment

The Mini-Cog and Mini Mental Status Exam (MMSE) are two cognitive screening tools that are frequently used

TABLE 15.1	Signs and Features of Different Diseases				
	AD	**DLB**	**FTD**	**CJD**	**VCI**
Signs Affected					
Cognition	Always. Short-term memory usually first. Multiple cognitive domains often impacted.	Frequent. Most impact on visuospatial, attention. Memory deficits also seen in later stages.	Always. Language, speech, and executive function initially or as disease progresses.	Always. Rapid progression.	Always. Stepwise or slowly progressive decline. Attention, executive function.
Motor	Infrequent. Can be present in later stages.	Always. Present and early on. Tremors, masked facies, limb rigidity, shuffling gait.	Infrequent	Always. Myoclonus, extrapyramidal signs.	Frequent. Depends on area of damage to the brain.
Behavior and psychological	Sometimes. Delusions more common in later stages.	Frequent. Delusions in later stages.	Frequent. Loss of sympathy, empathy, and behavioral control.	Frequent. Mutism.	Frequent. Depends on area of damage to the brain.
Sleep	Sometimes. Can be present in later disease.	Frequent. Dream enactment and vocalizations.	Infrequent	Sometimes	Frequent. Depends on area of damage to the brain.

AD, Alzheimer disease; CJD, Creutzfeldt-Jakob disease; DLB, dementia with Lewy bodies; FTD, frontotemporal dementia; VCI, vascular cognitive impairment.

to assess older individuals at routine visits or when there is suspicion that a patient may have a cognitive disorder. The Mini-Cog is a three-step test that takes about 3 minutes to administer. The MMSE takes about 5 minutes. Some studies have supported comparable or improved sensitivity and sensitivity of the Mini-Cog compared to the MMSE in identifying MCI in community-dwelling older individuals.

A detailed mental status exam should assess multiple domains of mental function, including basic attention, memory, visuospatial abilities, executive function, and sociobehavioral aptitude. Although the 30-point MMSE can be used purely to determine whether further evaluation is warranted, it also remains a practical and helpful tool to provide enough information to help gauge the overall severity of cognitive impairment. Importantly, the MMSE is probably less informative in some populations, such as high-functioning and highly educated elders and those with low formal education. Other tests, such as the Montreal Cognitive Assessment (MoCA), offer a broader assessment of cognitive domains than the MMSE, providing more details that can sometimes help with differential diagnosis of the dementia-causing disease. Some evidence points to the MoCA as also being more sensitive than the MMSE for the early detection of cognitive impairment caused by a neurodegenerative disease. Importantly, tests such as the MoCA and MMSE are helpful in contributing to a diagnosis of dementia but are not sufficient to diagnose or exclude a dementia syndrome; results must be considered along with the other elements of evaluation, including clinical history of cognitive or daily functioning changes and imaging. Further cognitive testing, including neuropsychological evaluation, may be helpful in cases in which screening tests or clinical impression are equivocal.

In the United States, some patients are screened for cognitive concerns during their Medicare Annual Wellness Visit (AWV), which is focused on preventive care in older adults. During an AWV, any cognitive screening tool can be used by the primary provider. Current guidelines suggest the use of either the Mini-Cog, the General Practitioner assessment of Cognition (GPCOG), or the Memory Impairment Screen (MIS). Our experience in the United States is that there is currently limited knowledge and practice experience with the MIS and GPCOG.

Considering that there is also currently limited evidence to recommend any type of cognitive screen during an AWV, we suggest different screening strategies for primary care providers depending on practice setting. If the provider is in a resource-rich practice setting with timely access to knowledgeable specialists who can continue with dementia evaluations and management, a Mini-Cog should be sufficient as a screen to determine the need for a repeat screen or referral to a specialist. Other commonly used screening tests that also capture the person's status of daily functioning include the Eight-Item Informant Interview to Differentiate Aging and Dementia and the Blessed Dementia Rating Scale. Both are also brief scales that can be completed by family members and sometimes patients to help identity those who need more attention or evaluation. If the provider is in a more resource-limited practice setting, we recommend using the MoCA or MMSE to fulfill multiple functions, including as an initial screen, as an assessment to aid with diagnosis, as way to track disease progression over time, and potentially to gauge patient responses to care interventions. Providers should be mindful that the Mini-Cog may have a specificity of only approximately 73%; therefore, patients who screen negative on the Mini-Cog should continue to be evaluated at least on an annual basis.

Most aspects of evaluation that were mentioned here can be conducted both in person and through virtual visits. Some older adults seem to prefer virtual care; individuals who are frail and have multiple illnesses may find it difficult and perhaps traumatic to have to present for in-person care. Care partners and family members sometimes prefer virtual care, which we find is frequently the case for patients with moderate to severe dementia. Therefore developing the ability to gather as much clinical information in a virtual format will prove to be helpful, such as being able to perform a telephone- or video-based MoCA.

Neuroimaging

If a patient is screened positive from the Mini-Cog and has a clinical history of concern for, or observations of, cognitive changes over 6 months or more, the patient may benefit from neuroimaging. Having additional risk factors for dementia may also contribute to a decision about neuroimaging. Where possible, a brain MRI is preferable to a CT scan. Brain MRIs must be interpreted in the context of an abnormal cognitive screen and a history of cognitive changes or decline. That is, cognitively normal older adults without early dementia can also have brain lesions detected on MRI or volume loss (atrophy). It is common but not necessary for patients with early AD to have MRI patterns of generalized cortical atrophy (atrophy in most regions), with some predominance of atrophy in the medial temporal lobe, surrounding and including the hippocampi. There is not a consistent MRI finding to aid with diagnosis of Parkinson Disease dementia. For FTD, there is often prominent atrophy in the frontal and temporal regions on MRI, with dominance in the right hemisphere for behavioral variant of FTD (bvFTD) and the left hemisphere for the Primary Progressive Aphasia variant of FTD. MRIs with focal tissue loss in a region that reflects a prior stroke or that has significant white matter changes are common in vascular dementia.

It is clinically challenging to differentiate cognitive changes associated with normal, healthy aging from changes due to early neurodegenerative disease. The continuum from normal cognitive aging to dementia is detailed in Table 15.2. Differentiating normal aging from subjective cognitive decline (SCD), MCI, and major neurocognitive disorder or dementia relies on both detailed history taking and performance on objective clinical tests such as a MoCA. It is important to understand that, according to the DSM5, MCI is synonymous with *mild neurocognitive disorder*, and major neurocognitive disorder is synonymous with dementia. Regarding cognition, understanding the basics of major cognitive domains, which include attention, executive function, social cognition, learning and memory, language, and visuospatial function, is also useful for both history taking and interpreting the results of cognitive testing. For example, if clinicians identify specific examples of changes in cognition in one or more of these domains or in daily functioning for a single patient, they can reason in a measured way about whether and how much that patient has declined.

Understanding patients' motor function, which can include balance, muscle tone, strength, and abnormal movements (e.g., tremor, twitching, and myoclonus), can augment one's clinical reasoning when coupled with clinical history and the identification of a patient's cognitive deficits.

DEMENTIA CLASSIFICATION CONTINUUM

The mildest form of cognitive concern is SCD. In this state, patients notice cognitive changes, but their objective cognitive scores, such as those on the MoCA, are within normal limits, and their functioning in daily activities remains entirely independent. When even subtle cognitive deficits are detected objectively on testing but the patient remains independent in all activities, the condition is labeled mild cognitive impairment. In MCI, a MoCA score is frequently between 18 and 26 out of 30. Once cognitive decline begins to affect activities of daily living (ADLs), whether instrumental ADLs (IADLs), such as managing finances or medications or preparing meals, or basic ADLs, such as using the bathroom, maintaining personal hygiene, or eating, the patient is considered to have a major neurocognitive disorder or dementia; MoCA scores typically are less than 18. Table 15.3 provides a summary of how to conceptualize these different clinical presentations and lists of activities that are included in IADLs and basic ADLs.

Within the syndrome of dementia (major neurocognitive disorder), one helpful model for staging severity is the tripartite classification of mild, moderate, and severe. In this model, the staging is based on clinical information

TABLE 15.2   Characteristics of Subjective Cognitive Disorder (SCD), Mild Cognitive Impairment (MCI), and Dementia

	SCD	MCI	Major Neurocognitive Disorder (Dementia)
Subjective Complaints	Present	Often present	Often Present
MoCA	Normal (above 26)	18–26	Frequently below 18
Instrumental activities of daily living	Independent	Independent	Dependent
Activities of daily living	Independent	Independent	Dependent

MoCA, Montreal Cognitive Assessment.

TABLE 15.3   Specific Activities Associated With Instrumental Activities of Daily Living (IADL) and Basic Activities of Daily Living (ADL)

IADL	ADL
Ability to use the phone	Bathing
Shopping	Showering
Food preparation	Dressing
Housekeeping	Walking
Laundry	Using the toilet
Independent transportation	Eating
Ability to take medications	Getting in and out of bed
Ability to handle finances	Getting in and out of chair

rather than any cognitive testing or laboratory or imaging markers. A patient with mild dementia typically has lost independence in one or more IADLs but is independent in basic ADLs. With moderate dementia, patients are dependent on others for all IADLs and dependent for some basic ADLs. With severe dementia, patients are fully dependent on others for ADLs.

While it is not possible to predict the timeline of any one patient's progression through these stages, the model can be helpful for caregivers to understand more about what changes they may look out for. Since a majority of longitudinal care for dementia in the United States and globally is provided by primary providers and there are not enough subspecialty dementia experts (e.g., neurologists, geriatric psychiatrists, geriatricians) to provide initial or ongoing care, it is important for primary providers to be comfortable with the basics of classifying dementia severity and to be familiar with available and appropriate recommendations for the major stages. Of course, if specialists are available for either an initial consultation or longitudinal care, a referral to examine all evidence for the neurologic disorder and to help elucidate the cause, is sensible when these conditions of SCD, MCI, or dementia are identified.

EVALUATION OF COGNITIVE COMPLAINTS: CLINICAL PEARLS

A noteworthy clinical pearl is that many older adults have impairment in some aspect of their motor function, hearing, or vision acuity. These can sometimes be mistaken as clear evidence of a cognitive or neurologic disorder, or they can be the dominant cause of a cognitive complaint or errors on testing. For example, older patients may have the ability to perform normally on cognitive testing and in everyday life but score below normal on the MMSE due to hearing impairment. These common changes with aging are especially confounding to providers who do not know the patient well. Of course, the physical limitations of visual or hearing deficits are themselves independent risk factors for the development of dementia and should be addressed. Generally, providers should be attuned to potentially false positive cognitive screens or misdiagnosis of a cognitive disorder in these circumstances. As was mentioned earlier, the MoCA does have versions that are validated for individuals with significant hearing or visual impairment, which can be utilized.

It is often difficult to decide whether to evaluate cognitive complaints in the older population beyond obtaining a clinical history and administering a brief cognitive screen. From the perspective of a primary provider for the initial presentation of cognitive concerns, if a patient or the patient's care partner(s) endorse new psychiatric symptoms associated with the cognitive concerns, frequent unexplained falls, or drastic changes in weight, we do recommend further evaluation or referral to a specialist, as each has a strong correlation to many dementia-causing diseases.

Some common cognitive concerns include forgetting names, having trouble keeping track of daily events, taking longer than before to complete mentally complex tasks, experiencing word-finding difficulty, having trouble with mental calculations, and being unable to recall recent salient events. More concerning complaints include frequently getting lost or uncharacteristically misplacing household items, especially when attempts to organize have fallen short. Sometimes a false belief (i.e., a delusion), such as a belief that someone has entered the house and stolen an item that is now missing or a belief that a family member who has died is still alive, can be the initial presentation of early dementia, though it is more commonly seen in later stages. In contrast, apathy and disengagement are commonly seen in early mild dementia.

Wandering behaviors, which may manifest as regularly returning from a routine walk or drive later than usual, can lead to patients getting lost, and this should be considered an issue to be addressed urgently. Actions may include escalation of care to an inpatient hospital admission if there are clear, immediate safety concerns. Wandering and other unsafe behaviors are mostly observed in later stages of dementia but can sometimes occur in early stages. Psychiatric symptoms can range from development of depressive or anxious symptoms to becoming more irritable or even agitated.

NEURODEGENERATIVE DEMENTIAS

Alzheimer Disease

AD is the most common neurodegenerative cause of dementia in middle-aged and older individuals. Dementia due to AD has a global prevalence of 5%–6% of all individuals age 65 and above and up to 30% in those over age 85. About 5% of all Alzheimer dementia occurs before age 65, which is conventionally termed "early-onset." The disease typically begins with slowly progressive memory decline, although behavioral, visuospatial, or language symptoms can dominate early in less common variants, which are most often observed in early-onset cases (under 65 years old). The mean survival after symptom onset in AD tends to be 10–12 years.

Current models of AD include a preclinical stage, in which the first changes of AD biology may occur up to 20 years or more before onset of symptoms. The pathophysiologic process is characterized by the gradual accumulation of beta-amyloid-rich neuritic plaques and a buildup of tau protein into so-called neurofibrillary tangles throughout the brain. Beta-amyloid protein is dominant in the hardened, neuritic plaques and also exists in toxic, soluble forms that are found in the brain. These two findings define AD pathologically (see Fig. 15.2). Notably, based on autopsy studies of AD patients, it is very common to find other pathologies cooccurring with AD, including cerebrovascular disease and Lewy body disease, even if patients do not exhibit symptoms that clearly reflect those brain changes.

Early on in symptoms, patients may have subtle, everyday forgetfulness or occasionally repeat stories; they can also exhibit irritability, apathy, or low mood. (See the later discussion about mild behavioral impairment.) Patients or family members often first notice cognitive symptoms before any decline in daily functioning, which defines a stage described as MCI. (See the earlier section on evaluation and diagnosis for discussion about the MCI/dementia continuum.) As the

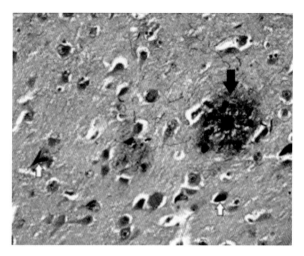

Fig. 15.2 The defining histopathology of Alzheimer disease in the hippocampus (Bielschowsky silver stain). Shown is a neuritic plaque (*black arrow*) rich with beta-amyloid protein and neurofibrillary tangles (*white arrows*), which contain tau-protein aggregates. (Courtesy Gad A. Marshall. MD, Brigham and Women's Hospital, Boston, MA.)

disease advances, brain MRI can show medial temporal lobe atrophy, involving the hippocampi, surrounding structures and diminished brain tissue in other regions (see Fig. 15.3). A fluorodeoxyglucose positron emission tomography (FDG-PET) scan classically shows bilateral temporoparietal hypometabolism, reflecting dysfunction of synapses and neural networks in these regions.

As disease-modifying medications to treat AD emerge in clinical care beginning in 2023, patients are increasingly being tested for biological markers (biomarkers) to identify the underlying amyloid and tau pathologies. This testing is currently carried out mostly by neurology or psychiatry specialists, but the practice may generalize to primary care settings over time. In the last decade, biomarkers have helped to catalyze a shift in the conception of AD from a clinical-pathologic condition, in which diagnoses are confirmed only after death, to a clinical-biological condition, in which diagnoses by biomarkers are confirmed during life. In the coming years, this shift toward a biologically centered understanding and treatment of AD will continue, with relevant impacts on patients, care partners, providers, insurance carriers, and healthcare systems alike.

Currently, Alzheimer biomarkers both help to confirm a diagnosis that is made clinically (i.e., one based on symptoms, cognitive testing, and sometimes MRI

Magnetic Resonance Imaging (MRI)

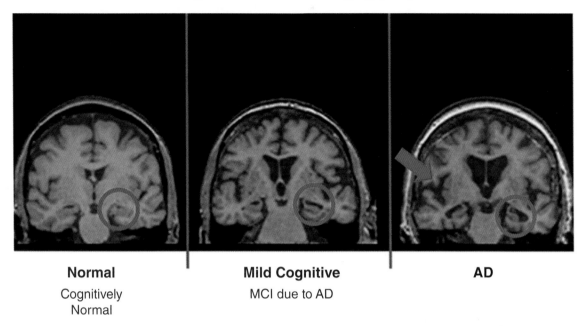

Normal
Cognitively
Normal

Mild Cognitive
MCI due to AD

AD

Fig. 15.3 Detecting changes in brain structure by MRI in Alzheimer disease (AD) over time. The red circles show the medial temporal lobe (hippocampi and surrounding structures) in three patients of comparable age: one cognitively normal, one with mild cognitive impairment (MCI) due to AD (mild atrophy), and one with AD dementia (moderate atrophy) (left to right; T2 fluid-attenuated inversion recovery coronal sequences). The red arrow shows additional cortical atrophy in the inferior frontal lobe in the patient with AD dementia.

scans) and ensure that patients' brains have the relevant targets for novel, disease-modifying medications. Cerebrospinal fluid tests are a commonly used Alzheimer biomarker and may be abnormal even early in the preclinical phase, when levels of the 42-residue long beta-amyloid protein (Aβ42) begin to decrease and levels of phosphorylated tau protein increase. PET scans that reveal amyloid plaque deposition (amyloid PET) and tau protein aggregates (tau PET) are biomarkers with emerging use in clinical care but have been limited by their financial cost. The earliest detection of AD may be by blood-based markers (BBMs) of tau and amyloid. At the time of publication, the evidence for clinical utility of BBMs to diagnose and track AD is still emerging and they are rarely used in clinical care. Expert opinion currently discourages the use of BBMs in a nonspecialist setting. Thus, apart from blood tests, AD is best detected by amyloid/tau PET, CSF-based biomarkers, or a combination of MRI and FDG-PET, both early on and through all stages of the disease (see Fig. 15.4).

Recent clinical and translational research has focused on early detection and therapeutic targeting of the underlying pathology. At the time of this chapter's writing, two medications that remove amyloid protein from the brain and that seem to slow the rate of decline of cognition and daily functioning in patients with MCI and mild dementia due to AD show promise. To be specific, one (lecanemab) has received full FDA approval, and another (donanemab) is likely to be reviewed relatively soon. These and other medications will likely soon be prescribed by specialists in clinical AD care throughout the United States and globally. If patients are thought to have probable MCI or mild dementia due to AD by their clinical evaluation, that is sufficient reason to refer to a specialist so that they may be considered for these medications.

Older medications, including cholinesterase inhibitors (i.e., donepezil, rivastigmine, galantamine) and an NDMA-receptor antagonist (memantine), which have been used globally for over 20 years, are still prescribed

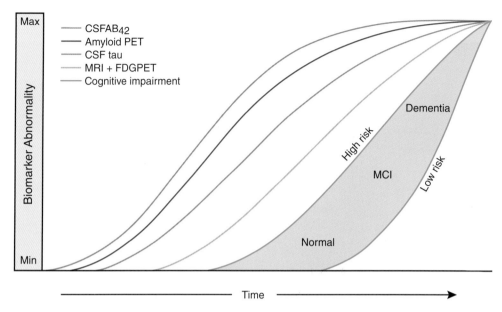

Fig. 15.4 Revised dynamic biomarkers of the Alzheimer disease pathologic cascade model-20212. (Reprinted with permission from Elsevier., Jack CR Jr, Knopman DS, Jagust WJ, Petersen RC, Weiner MW, et al. Tracking pathophysiological processes in Alzheimer's disease: an updated hypothetical model of dynamic biomarkers. *Lancet Neurol.* 2013 Feb;12(2):207–16. doi: 10.1016/S1474-4422(12)70291-0. PMID: 23332364; PMCID: PMC3622225.)

for patients at all stages of AD. Although these medications do not alter patients' inevitable decline in cognition or daily abilities, they may improve cognitive and behavioral symptoms for periods of 6 months to several years. There are also medications available for symptomatic treatment of depression, anxiety and other neuropsychiatric symptoms associated with AD, which are discussed later in the chapter. Substantial evidence suggests that regular aerobic exercise, adherence to a Mediterranean-style diet, and participation in socially and cognitively stimulating activities can decrease one's risk of AD and affect the rate of progression along the disease continuum.

Frontotemporal Dementias

The frontotemporal dementias are a group of neurodegenerative diseases linked by the selective degeneration of the frontal and temporal lobes. FTDs are relentless, devastating diseases in which the dominant symptoms usually include changes in some or all of social behavior, speech, language, and motor function. Overall, FTDs are much rarer than AD. Although the age range for FTDs can be anywhere from the second to the tenth decades of life, it is a relatively common cause of early-onset dementia (symptoms prior to age 65). In fact, the FTDs are the second most common disease causing early-onset

dementia after AD, accounting for close to 20% of all cases. In older age, FTDs are the third most common type of neurodegenerative disease, behind AD and dementia with Lewy bodies (an alpha-synucleinopathy).

The exact prevalence of FTDs is an ongoing subject of research but is likely between 1 and 17 patients per 100,000 overall, decreasing to 1–4 per 100,000 in patients over the age of 70. FTDs are most commonly diagnosed in middle age (age in the 50s), with ~13% of cases occurring before age 50.

The FTDs are dementia syndromes that most commonly arise from a group of underlying pathologies, unified by the term "frontotemporal lobar degeneration" (FTLD). FTLD includes at least three distinct pathologic subtypes: transactive responsive DNA-binding (TDP-43), tau protein, and fused-in-sarcoma. As discussed in this chapter's introduction, different syndromes (or clusters of symptoms) can arise from the same underlying pathology or pathologic subtype. The symptoms and signs that patients demonstrate largely depend on which brain regions are most affected. Knowing the pathology subtype may be more relevant when we have reliable biological markers to identify FTD or treatments that modify FTLD pathology, which are active goals of research.

The most common FTD syndromes that arise from underlying FTLD include the behavioral variant of FTD;

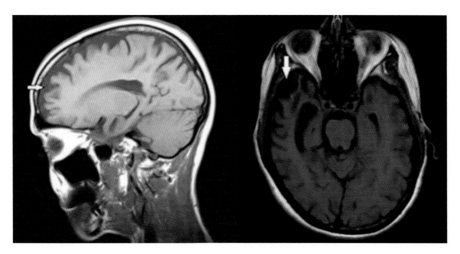

Fig. 15.5 Frontotemporal lobar degeneration. Left: Brain magnetic resonance image of a 58-year-old female with 1.5 years of personality change, loss of social graces, and behavioral disinhibition. Note the global atrophy, with frontal lobe predominance (*white arrow*), characteristic of behavioral variant frontotemporal dementia. (Courtesy: Seth Gale, MD). Right: Evidence of focal anterior temporal lobe atrophy (*downward white arrow*), characteristic of a subtype of primary progressive aphasia caused by frontotemporal lobar degeneration. (From Gale SA, Acar D, Daffner KR. Dementia. *Am J Med*. 2018;131(10):1161–1169.)

language variants, which include nonfluent agrammatic and semantic variant primary progressive aphasia; corticobasal syndrome; and progressive supranuclear palsy syndrome. Less commonly, patients show signs and symptoms of one of these syndromes and amyotrophic lateral sclerosis together, which constitutes an FTD/amyotrophic lateral sclerosis spectrum syndrome.

Behavioral variant FTD is characterized by early personality changes (i.e., decline in social comportment and empathy), disinhibited and/or compulsive behaviors, and executive dysfunction (i.e., mental inflexibility). Patients with primary progressive aphasia initially develop speech and language problems, which could be gross articulatory speech errors, impairments in syntax, the loss of word meaning, or word-finding difficulties or pauses in conversation. This can present with impairments in speech output and syntax (nonfluent, agrammatic variant) or in understanding the meaning of words (semantic variant). MRIs can show focal frontal or temporal lobe atrophy in these conditions (see Fig. 15.5). In corticobasal syndrome, which usually arises from either FTLD or AD, the initial symptoms frequently include asymmetric parkinsonism (e.g., limb rigidity, slowed movements); limb apraxia; executive dysfunction; behavioral changes; and, in subsequent years, aphasia, "alien limb" phenomenon, frequent falls, and impairments in gait. Progressive supranuclear palsy syndrome is usually characterized by axial rigidity, postural instability with

early falls, and vertical gaze palsy, with subsequent progressive motor and cognitive decline. Some subtypes of progressive supranuclear palsy can also have prominent cerebellar ataxia and apraxia of speech. Importantly, while we name these syndromes based on symptoms to fit a classification scheme, it is common for patients to exhibit a mixture of symptoms seen across the different syndromes, especially as the FTD progresses. For example, patients who have the core symptoms of behavioral variant FTD sometimes have or develop a progressive language difficulty (aphasia) as well.

Unfortunately, current medical treatment for FTDs remains supportive, as there are no interventions that modify the course of the disease. Medications such as antidepressants and antipsychotics can be used to relieve neuropsychiatric symptoms and dopamine-modulating therapy for motor symptoms; response to dopaminergic medications is usually poor.

Several neurodegenerative diseases are characterized by the pathologic accumulation of aggregates of a protein called alpha-synuclein in neurons and other nervous system cells. These diseases include dementia with Lewy bodies, Parkinson disease, and multiple system atrophy.

Dementia with Lewy bodies is probably the second most common degenerative dementia after AD. It mostly affects patients in their 60s to 80s, with a prevalence among older adults that is estimated to be 0.1%–2% and an incidence of 0.1%. Its core clinical features include fluctuating cognition with pronounced variations in attention and alertness, recurrent well-formed visual hallucinations, dream enactment behaviors during rapid eye movement (REM) sleep (known as REM sleep behavior disorder, or RBD), and one or more features of parkinsonism (slowing of limb movements, tremor at rest tremor, or limb rigidity). It is very common for RBD, which can include body movements, emotional expressions, or audible verbalization of dream content, to be the initial symptoms of dementia with Lewy bodies. RBD can occur 15 or more years before other symptoms. Primary providers should be attuned to older individuals' and their care partners' reports of new sleep behaviors and then continue vigilance in screening for changes in gait, variations in alertness and attention and involuntary movements to help with early identification of the disease. Patients with dementia with Lewy bodies, like those with AD, may be first identified and then often cared for longitudinally in primary care, which makes education about its evaluation and management critical to meeting the needs of this growing disease population. Medications such as melatonin for sleep behaviors and cholinesterase inhibitors (e.g., rivastigmine, donepezil) for cognition and fluctuation of arousal can have moderate symptomatic benefit in dementia with Lewy bodies.

The motor, cognitive, and sleep symptoms of dementia with Lewy bodies can also be features of Parkinson disease and the dementia associated with Parkinson disease, called Parkinson disease dementia. Conventionally, the term "Parkinson disease dementia" is used to describe dementia that develops in the setting of well-established Parkinson disease and occurs at least 1 year, but typically 5 or more years, after the onset of parkinsonism.

Multiple system atrophy is a less common alpha-synucleinopathy that manifests with any combination of parkinsonism, signs of cerebellar dysfunction (vertigo, gait ataxia, and a quivering voice), pyramidal signs (increased tendon reflexes, spasticity or weakness of the limbs), and dysautonomia (significant orthostatic hypotension, sexual dysfunction, and heat/cold intolerance). Severe forward neck flexion (antecollis) and hand or foot dystonia are common. More than half of patients with multiple system atrophy develop nonmotor symptoms, including inspiratory stridor, dysautonomia,

and RBD, months or years prior to motor symptoms. Dysautonomia is also common with dementia with Lewy bodies and Parkinson disease. Although cognitive difficulties may be minimal or negligible in multiple system atrophy, at least some impairment is present in up to half of patients. Deficits are predominantly in executive functioning, and less commonly involve memory, apraxia, and spatial difficulties.

Parkinsonism, which includes symptoms of slowed limb movements (bradykinesia), rigidity or stiffness in the limbs, tremor, and unstable posture or gait changes, is common among many dementia syndromes. Therefore any additional symptoms and clinical history along with the parkinsonism that are characteristic of a certain disease are key to determining a diagnosis. Parkinsonism as a syndrome either is driven by a primary neurodegenerative disease, as is seen in the alpha-synucleinopathies and the FTDs, or arises "secondary" to other brain injuries, as in stroke, small-vessel cerebrovascular disease, or repeated concussion or traumatic brain injury (as in chronic traumatic encephalopathy) (Table 15.4). For example, the clinical syndrome of chronic traumatic encephalopathy usually begins years after repetitive concussions or subconcussive injuries from sports or war combat, is progressive for more than 2 years, and may include parkinsonism, cognitive decline, behavioral changes with aggression and suicidality, and emotional dysregulation.

Limbic-Predominant Age-Related TDP-43 Encephalopathy

Limbic-predominant age-related TDP-43 encephalopathy (LATE) is a disease that is most associated with individuals past 80 years of age and is characterized by a progressive amnesia that eventually affects other cognitive domains, such as executive function and language. The brain changes that underlie this dementia-causing disease are called LATE-neuropathologic change (or LATE-NC). Providers should be mindful that older adults with predominantly memory loss may have LATE, given its prevalence of up to 20% in individuals above age 80. It is also common for LATE-NC to develop with AD as well, as a mixed underlying disease pathology. Notably, it is normal for older individuals with some cognitive impairment, especially beyond 80 years of age, to develop multiple brain pathologies; therefore the cooccurrence of LATE, AD, cerebrovascular disease, and dementia with Lewy bodies is quite high.

TABLE 15.4 A Summary of Common Clinical Symptoms, Pathology, Imaging, and Clinical Pearls

Disease	Clinical Symptoms	Pathology/Imaging	Clinical Pearls
Primary Neurodegenerative			
Dementia with Lewy bodies	Cognitive fluctuations, visual hallucinations, symmetric parkinsonism	Deposition of Lewy bodies (alpha-synuclein deposits) throughout the cortex subcortex. PET/SPECT may show hypometabolism in the temporoparietal/visual cortex.	Cognitive improvement with cholinesterase inhibitors. Increased sensitivity to atypical neuroleptics, with markedly increased parkinsonism.
Parkinson disease	Asymmetric rest tremor, rapid eye movement sleep behavior disorder, limb rigidity, shuffling gait, later-onset dementia	Dopaminergic neuron loss in substantia nigra (midbrain), Lewy bodies (alpha-synuclein deposits). MRI can have overall mild atrophy.	Cognitive deficits can improve with levodopa. DBS improves motor symptoms, variable impact on cognition.
Progressive supranuclear palsy syndrome, frontotemporal lobar degeneration	Multiple early falls, axial rigidity, eye movement abnormalities, dysarthria, dementia	Tau protein inclusions in brainstem, cortex. MRI often with midbrain atrophy.	Differentiate from Parkinson disease by early gait difficulties, erect posture, eye movements.
Corticobasal basal syndrome, frontotemporal lobar degeneration	Progressive, asymmetric rigidity and apraxia, limb dystonia, myoclonus, alien limb phenomenon, mild cognitive impairment	Tau protein inclusions in neuropil threads and astrocytic plaques in cortex, basal ganglia, brainstem (called corticobasal degeneration). MRI can have asymmetric, cortical atrophy in parietal lobe.	Has both cortical (apraxia, alien limb) and extrapyramidal (rigidity, dystonia) signs.
Secondary Parkinsonism			
Chronic traumatic encephalopathy	Early decreased attention, depression/mood swings, irritability; later incoordination, tremor, pyramidal and extrapyramidal signs	Superficial cortical layers with neurofibrillary (tau) tangles. MRI can show diffuse axonal injury, diffuse atrophy, petechial hemorrhages.	Follows repeated traumatic brain injury from boxing, contact sports, blast injuries. Early intervention for mood disorder, cognitive rehab. Vascular parkinsonism.
Vascular parkinsonism	Often has leg > arm rigidity; may have emotional incontinence (pseudobulbar palsy), pyramidal signs (hyperreflexia)	MRI with large strategic or multiple small lacunar infarcts in basal ganglia/circuits.	Risk increases with chronic hypertension, hypoxic-ischemic brain injury.

DBS, Deep-brain stimulation; *MRI*, magnetic resonance imaging; *PET/SPECT*, positron emission tomography/single photon emission computed tomography.
Adapted from Gale SA, Acar D, Daffner KR. Dementia. *Am J Med.* 2018;131(10):1161–1169.

The clinical symptoms of LATE can mimic those of AD, even while LATE-NC itself does not include AD-related amyloid and is isolated to limbic structures that affect mostly memory function. Brain MRI often has predominant atrophy of the medial temporal lobes, which includes the hippocampi, and can be similar to that in AD. The pathology of LATE demonstrates the presence of TDP-43 proteinopathy in limbic structures, sclerosis of the hippocampus (as suggested in the "limbic-predominant" disease label), and global brain atrophy.

It remains to be seen whether older patients with mixed pathologies that include LATE will benefit from novel, Alzheimer-specific disease-modifying medications. There are currently no treatments for LATE, and there are no specific reliable biomarkers for LATE to identify its presence, whether alone or among other brain pathologies.

NONNEURODEGENERATIVE COGNITIVE IMPAIRMENT/DEMENTIAS

Nutritional

Dementia can arise when patients develop a deficiency or derangement of vitamin levels or nutrients. Nutritional deficiencies due to malnourishment, such as severe thiamine (vitamin B1) deficiency, can cause an acute disease called Wernicke encephalopathy in its earliest phases and Korsakoff syndrome if it converts to a chronic memory disorder. This disease is seen most often in chronic alcoholics and those with poor nutritional intake. Wernicke encephalopathy usually presents abruptly as neurons that are deficient in thiamine undergo necrosis. Classically, the triad of symptoms include gait ataxia, delirium, and ophthalmoplegia, but fewer than 20% of patients present with all three signs. Korsakoff syndrome may become apparent weeks later when the disorientation and delirium of Wernicke encephalopathy subsides and one can detect severe anterograde amnesia and less prominent retrograde amnesia. The treatment for Wernicke encephalopathy is intravenous thiamine, which must be administered before glucose, as glycolysis itself consumes B1.

Apart from thiamine deficiency, there are other deficiencies that cause neurologic problems. Vitamin B12 deficiency is frequently linked to worse cognitive performance in older adults, and there is an association between low B12 levels and the risk of MCI. There is epidemiologic evidence that even relative vitamin D deficiency is associated with a higher incidence of all dementia syndromes. Other nutritional deficiencies that can rarely lead to cognitive impairment and dementia include niacin deficiency (pellagra) and folic acid deficiency, which can arise from malabsorption caused by certain medications, including trimethoprim, methotrexate, primidone, and chronic phenytoin.

Toxic

Any medication taken in excess or in combination with certain other medications can cause cognitive deficits; this occurs by either direct or indirect neurotoxic effects. Medications with strong anticholinergic properties, such as some tricyclic antidepressants, cyclobenzaprine, and oxybutynin, are particularly implicated. Exposure to toxic chemicals (e.g., organophosphate pesticides), air pollutants, and heavy metals can all cause dementia syndromes that often are nonprogressive but may also increase the risk of developing neurodegenerative dementia in the future. Lead, mercury, arsenic, and manganese poisoning have all been implicated in dementia syndromes. For patients with any disorder along the spectrum from subjective cognitive decline to dementia, it is good practice to review medications to minimize those that have anticholinergic properties; the anticholinergic drug scale is one helpful tool to use in primary care to enable more informed risk/benefit decisions about these medications with older patients.

Metabolic

Hypothyroidism can contribute to or be the primary cause of cognitive impairment or, rarely, dementia. Symptoms of hypothyroidism can include apathy, memory and attention problems, and depression. Severe hyperthyroidism or autoimmune thyroiditis can present with psychosis, psychomotor slowing, and lethargy. Given how common thyroid abnormalities are, it makes sense in primary care to screen for thyroid abnormalities with a basic thyroid panel and to be aggressive about treatment or referral when needed, especially for patients with or at high risk for cognitive disorders. Metabolic disorders such as chronic uremia, hepatic disease of various etiologies, parathyroid disorders, chronic hemodialysis (so-called dialysis dementia), and hypercortisolism/Cushing syndrome can all cause varying degrees of cognitive deficits. In addition, chronic respiratory insufficiency, congestive heart failure, exposure to chemotherapies such as certain immune-checkpoint inhibitors and CAR T cells, severe obstructive sleep apnea, cancer or paraneoplastic disease, and hematologic conditions, such as sickle cell anemia, can all lead to disabling cognitive impairment.

VASCULAR COGNITIVE IMPAIRMENT AND DEMENTIA

Cerebrovascular disease of differing etiologies is a common cause of cognitive impairment. These different vascular causes can be subsumed under the broad label of vascular cognitive impairment (VCI). Analogous to the conversion of MCI to mild dementia when patients experience difficulties in daily functioning, VCI can worsen and lead to vascular dementia.

Etiologies are myriad and include clinically evident stroke or multiple strokes, small-vessel ischemic disease (historically known as Binswanger disease), rare hereditary diseases such ascerebral autosomal dominant arteriopathy with subcortical infarcts (CADASIL), and cerebral amyloid angiopath. VCI probably accounts for between 15% and 35% of all dementia, making it likely the second most common disease causing dementia behind AD. If we consider all mixed-type dementias, in which vascular cognitive impairment cooccurs with AD, dementia with Lewy bodies, or other diseases, the prevalence of VCI is substantially higher. Systemic vascular risk factors, such as hypertension, diabetes, smoking, and hypercholesterolemia, are also major risk factors for VCI. Coronary artery disease, atrial fibrillation, and myocardial infarction are also independent risk factors for developing VCI.

One major etiology is poststroke (or multiinfarct) VCI. Cognitive deficits may start abruptly after the stroke or appear more subacutely, and the decline can sometimes plateau after weeks or months. Poststroke VCI is a strong risk factor for eventual vascular dementia. If patients have recurrent strokes that either cause symptoms or are covert ("silent"), their cognitive impairment will often worsen, a consequence of accumulated brain injury. Sensorimotor signs, such as subtle to overt weakness on one side of the body or a limb, facial asymmetry, or a visual field deficit, can be accompanying clues in poststroke causes of VCI.

In small-vessel ischemic disease, a common cause of VCI, the small arterioles in the deep white matter

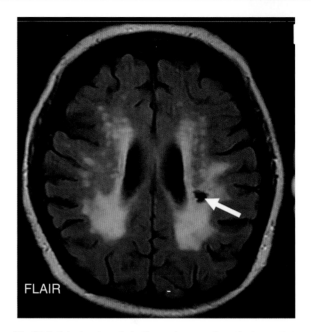

Fig.15.6 Arteriosclerosis in the cortex: small cortical penetrating arteriole occlusion, which is a contributor of cerebrovascular disease.

occlude over many years, demonstrated by large areas of hyperintense (white-appearing) lesions on MRI (see Fig. 15.6). In patients with small-vessel ischemic disease, it is common for symptoms to manifest gradually or subtly over time without overt neurologic events. Symptoms of small-vessel ischemic disease can include slowed speed of processing thoughts, dysarthria or subtle speech changes, memory and complex attention difficulties, and sometimes psychomotor slowing or apathy. Severe small-vessel ischemic disease can lead to urinary incontinence, lower extremity–predominant parkinsonism, and significant functional decline.

Cerebral amyloid angiopathy (CAA) is a condition that describes the pathologic accumulation of amyloid protein in cerebral vessels, which can cause microbleeds and larger hemorrhages. This diagnosis is often made by MRI and sometimes after a cerebral bleed causes focal neurologic signs or symptoms. From neuropathologic results, the prevalence of CAA seems to be up to 50% in patients with AD while closer to 20% in general older adults without identified cognitive impairment, even if some do have early underlying neurodegenerative disease. With CAA, patients can often have recurrent, transient ischemic attack–like symptoms, sometimes called transient focal neurologic episodes, including weakness, numbness, or paresthesia, often experienced as moving through contiguous body regions. Cognitive impairment in CAA is directly correlated with the number and location of bleeds; patients with more than one microbleed have up to a 70% risk of developing vascular dementia in 5 years or less. The coincidence of CAA and AD is frequent, with autopsy studies showing moderate to frequent neuritic plaques (AD) in most patients with cerebral amyloid angiopathy.

The key to treatment when any degree of VCI is identified, whether by evident symptoms and/or on a brain MRI, is vigilance in minimizing systemic vascular disease that can worsen impairment by causing further cerebrovascular injury. This translates to aggressive management of hyperlipidemia, hypertension, and diabetes. VCI can be treated with neuropharmaceuticals as well, including acetylcholinesterase inhibitors (e.g., donepezil, galantamine).

DISCUSSION: MIXED DEMENTIA AND COGNITIVE BURDENS

Despite much advancement in clinicopathologic correlation, it remains difficult in most dementia evaluations to account for all underlying causes of the dementia. That is, most dementia syndromes are complex and arise from a mixture of pathologies, whose effects are likely additive to the neurocognitive decline.

For example, it is common for an older dementia patient who exhibits only the slowly, progressive memory decline of AD, with no overt signs or symptoms of vascular dementia or dementia with Lewy bodies, to ultimately show some pathologic burden of all three diseases on autopsy. Furthermore, dementia patients of all ages and all causes are vulnerable to further cognitive decline when afflicted with any condition that is known to worsen cognitive function. These include sleep disorders such as obstructive sleep apnea, medications with cognitive side effects, concussions, and depression. For all these reasons, it is paramount to aggressively treat all known and even suspected underlying contributions to a cognitive disorder, including all medical-psychiatric conditions described here, and to be vigilant about promoting good brain health behaviors.

NEUROPSYCHIATRIC SYMPTOMS OF COGNITIVE IMPAIRMENT/DEMENTIA AND MILD BEHAVIORAL IMPAIRMENT

It is not unusual for mood or behavior changes to be the initial symptoms, or prodrome, of a dementia-causing disease. Diseases such as AD or VCI can present with one or more of these neuropsychiatric symptoms (NPS) and only over time cause the more overt, recognizable symptoms of cognitive impairment, motor, or gait changes. It is important for providers to be aware of the possibility that NPS can be early symptoms of dementia, even while it challenging to differentiate these from primary psychiatric disorders in the older population.

Mild behavioral impairment (MBI) is a diagnosis that captures this prodrome of NPS, which has also been labeled the behavioral and psychological symptoms of dementia (BPSD). MBI requires that behavioral or mood symptoms are new and are present for more than 6 months before cognitive symptoms. Behavioral symptoms that predate or occur along with cognitive symptoms can include neurovegetative symptoms (e.g., apathy, low mood), affective symptoms (e.g., anxiety, irritability), and disinhibition. Over time, a patient with MBI who is diagnosed with dementia would then be considered to have NPS or BPSD.

NPS by definition refers to noncognitive symptoms related to patients with dementia. It is frequently thought of as a more inclusive term than BPSD, as it encompasses clinical states before the development of dementia. NPS also entails the reality that underlying disease pathology may directly cause noncognitive symptoms. In the literature, behavioral and psychological symptoms of dementia (BPSD) have referred more specifically to symptoms of agitation—including aggression, screaming, and acting out—in any patient with a dementia diagnosis. One should note that while the terms BPSD and NPS are used interchangeably, BPSD is used mostly in Europe and NPS in the US. The classifications and definitions of these terms will likely continue to evolve. Our purpose is to highlight symptoms in dementia patients that are likely to prompt providers for further intervention. Here, we will use BPSD as a convention, as it more commonly captures symptoms of agitation, aggression, and irritability.

Dementia affects 1.6% of the US population, and as the nation ages, this is expected to double to 3.3% by 2060. Most patients with a dementia diagnosis will develop BPSD symptoms. BPSD development and exacerbation are frequently salient contributors to the escalation and cost of care. It is important to be able to discern BPSD early in the disease course, as early intervention can reduce caregiver burnout and reduce further decline in cognition and functioning. Common BPSD symptoms include aggression, agitation, psychosis, apathy, and mood symptoms. If these symptoms occur in the context of a patient with a dementia diagnosis and all medical causes have been ruled out, a diagnosis of BPSD or NPS is appropriate. BPSD progression is nonlinear and fluctuates from mild to severe symptoms even if overall an individual's clinical state worsens over time. As was discussed previously, the overall construct of MBI is premised on the reality that neuropsychiatric symptoms of a dementia syndrome, including depression, anxiety, apathy, and social withdrawal, can occur at least 6 months and up to 2 years or more before cognitive impairment, at which point it will be considered BPSD. Thus, if a patient has new-onset neuropsychiatric symptoms and does not have demonstrated cognitive impairment or a dementia diagnosis, it is prudent for providers to be more vigilant with cognitive screens to help facilitate early dementia syndrome identification and interventions. Once the diagnosis of dementia has been made in patients with MBI, up to 75% or more will exhibit agitative symptoms within 10 months.

Management of BPSD/NPS

Nonpharmacologic BPSD treatment should always be considered as part of first-line treatment and should be continued to be trialed and refined in treatment planning. Psychotherapy modalities such as cognitive behavioral therapy, supportive therapy, mindfulness, and psychodynamic therapy have all been shown to be helpful for affective symptoms such as depression and anxiety, though the content and modality will need to be tailored to the patients' current cognitive abilities. The DICE (describe, investigate, create, and evaluate) method is another useful clinical approach to help patients, care partners, and providers tackle BPSD symptoms in a systematic way. One should also be mindful that untreated affective symptoms can worsen clinical presentations of BPSD.

In considering pharmacologic BPSD treatment, it is important to note that two medications have been approved by the FDA in the United States for specific diseases. Brexpiprazole is an atypical antipsychotic

approved in May 2023 for the treatment of agitation associated with Alzheimer disease dementia. Pimavanserin, a serotonin-based antipsychotic, was approved in 2016 for the treatment of hallucinations and delusions associated with Parkinson disease psychosis. These indications for these medications have not been approved on other continents to date.

One framework to decide when to prescribe a medication for BPSD is to determine if the symptoms are "emergent, urgent, or, nonurgent. Emergent BPSD signifies that the patient is at immediate risk of harm to self and others. Urgent means that the patient's symptoms will escalate soon without intervention, but providers have a few days to implement a change. Nonemergent BPSD signifies that the provider has weeks to months, but the patient is suffering. There are many different medications that can be used. In emergent settings, the patient may be too agitated for oral medications, and sometimes intramuscular (IM) options may be appropriate in these circumstances, including IM olanzapine, haloperidol, and benzodiazepines. In urgent situations, medications to consider in order of our preference include aripiprazole, risperidone, and prazosin; ECT can also be considered urgently. In a nonemergent situation, some frequently used medications include escitalopram and sertraline. We refer readers to another of our publications for more detail on the clinical nuances and scenarios of when it is best to use these medications.

As important as knowing which medications to choose, one should know which to avoid in the treatment of BSPD in particular clinical situations. Other than in an emergent setting, there is no convincing evidence for the use of benzodiazepines. There is also no convincing evidence for valproic acid or for quetiapine broadly for BPSD across dementia-causing diseases, despite their common use. Quetiapine and clozapine have demonstrated modest benefits for neuropsychiatric symptoms and hallucinations in the alpha-synucleinopathies. Importantly, other atypical antipsychotic medications aside from pimavanserin should be avoided in the alpha-synucleinopathies, as they can worsen motor symptoms and increase the risk of neuroleptic malignant syndrome. Broadly, for all dementia-causing disease in older adults, olanzapine should be avoided where possible because of its anticholinergic and metabolic side effects.

Cognitive enhancers should also be considered for BPSD treatment. These medications are not likely to ameliorate current BPSD symptoms significantly, but they can delay the onset of new BPSD symptoms. Generally, they should not be discontinued unless there is convincing evidence that their use is leading to BPSD exacerbation or intolerable side effects.

CONCLUSION

Cognitive impairment and dementia continue to be major contributors to the global burden of disease. In this brief review, we provided an overview of epidemiology, classification, screening, and evaluation of these disorders with a focus on primary care settings. We then highlighted selected syndromes among dozens that arise from dementia-causing diseases. Dementia is a chronic condition that requires longitudinal care, ongoing counseling, and psychosocial support for patients and families by dedicated medical providers, social workers, and many others. Efforts to preserve daily functioning abilities and quality of life should be the driving aim of dementia management across the lifespan. The medical world is about to embark on an exciting new era of disease-modifying therapies for AD, and it is hoped that novel treatments for other diseases will follow. In this era, clinicians in primary care are positioned better than ever before to diagnose, understand, and manage a range of neurologic and neuropsychiatric symptoms of dementia, which can both improve the quality of life for current patients and their care partners and reduce dementia risk for all older adults.

"For the full bibliography list, please use the pincode on the inside front cover to access the electronic version of the text at ebooks.health.elsevier.com."

16

Introduction to Neuropsychological Assessment and Intervention

Ananya Ruth Samuel, Gretchen Reynolds, Kim C. Willment, and Seth A. Gale

INTRODUCTION TO NEUROPSYCHOLOGY

What is Neuropsychology?

Neuropsychology lies at the intersection of the fields of neurology, psychology, and psychiatry. Placed under the umbrella of clinical psychology, this discipline focuses on understanding brain-behavior correlates through performance-based measures used to assess cognitive functioning. The neuropsychological evaluation plays an essential role in diagnosis and treatment planning through a biopsychosocial framework. Neuropsychology as a field that emerged in the early 19th century to study focal brain lesions and their impact on day-to-day functioning. With the advent of neuroimaging, neuropsychology continues to aid in connecting structural findings to cognitive functioning, assisting with differential diagnosis, prognosis, and risk predictions, and treatment planning has become more of a focus.

Training in Neuropsychology

Clinical neuropsychologists are licensed clinicians with a doctoral degree (Ph.D./Psy.D.) in clinical psychology, and additional postdoctoral training in clinical neuropsychology. Neuropsychologists receive training in functional neuroanatomy, neurobiology, psychometrics, statistics, psychopharmacology, neurologic illness/injury, therapeutic interventions, and clinical psychology. After completion of their doctoral degree and postdoctoral fellowship, neuropsychologists can opt to pursue board certification through governing boards in their region or country, such as the American Board of Professional Psychology in the United States. This certification consists of credential review, written and oral examinations, and submission of practice samples for review. Although board certification is not required for a clinician to practice neuropsychology, it is recommended by the American Academy of Clinical Neuropsychology in the United States and other professional psychology boards to promote standardized quality of training and delivery of services.

Neuropsychological Assessment and Intervention

Historically, neuropsychology has focused on the assessment of brain-behavior relationships and the diagnosis of neurologic disorders. Neuropsychological assessments are standardized measures of cognitive functioning that identify and characterize the severity of deficits while also serving to track changes over time. Scores from the assessments provide an estimate of the person's cognitive functioning relative to a normative group with a similar demographic background, often based on age, education, sex, and occasionally also ethnic or racial identity, although more work is needed to expand and update available normative data to best serve increasingly diverse patient populations. Additionally, neuropsychological assessments inform treatment planning, as the neuropsychologist provides specific recommendations to optimize cognition and daily functioning. Furthermore, neuropsychologists provide patients with personalized and targeted suggestions for interventions and rehabilitative services that are informed by assessment findings.

In this chapter, we explore several topics relevant to neuropsychology, including an introduction to cognitive domains assessed through a neuropsychological evaluation; a brief overview of cognitive screening tools, standard assessment procedures, and referral questions; and a discussion of evidence-based neuropsychological interventions.

NEUROPSYCHOLOGICAL ASSESSMENT

Cognition: Neuroanatomy and Cognitive Domains

Cognition has been described as a multifaceted process of acquiring, perceiving, and processing information. Until the late 19th century, cognition was conceived of as a single construct called "intelligence." Over time and through rich observations and empirical study, cognition has come to be understood as a complex collection of mental processes with intricate nuances that separate how the mind perceives, calculates, decides, and functions. In our modern understanding, cognition is divided into various domains, including language (both receptive [input/acquisition of information, comprehension] and expressive functions [oral and written output]), memory and learning (encoding, storage, and retrieval), attention/executive function (e.g., problem-solving, organization, decision-making), visuospatial abilities, and social cognition. These processes work both narrowly and interdependently to provide a basis for human cognition and behavior. Cognition can also be measured and understood based on the type of stimulus that initiates a mental process, which can be divided into verbal (speech- and/or linguistic-mediated) and nonverbal functions (visually mediated). Neuropsychological assessment aims to characterize performance across these various cognitive domains and map patterns of strengths and weaknesses onto brain-behavior relations. Following is an overview of the five major cognitive domains that are often assessed in a neuropsychological evaluation along with the brain regions and networks associated with each of these domains (Box 16.1 and Fig. 16.1).

BOX 16.1   Functions of the Cerebral Cortex

Frontal Lobe
Voluntary movement and motor control
Attention and working memory
Executive functions (e.g., planning/organization, decision-making, problem-solving, cognitive flexibility)
Expressive language/speech production (left)
Memory encoding and retrieval
Motivation
Personality

Temporal Lobe
Memory (all stages)
Auditory processing
Receptive language/language comprehension (left)
Affective prosody (right)
Emotional regulation

Parietal Lobe
Tactile sensation
Visual-spatial attention and perception (right)
Mental rotation and visual construction
Reading (left)
Calculation (left)

Occipital Lobe
Visual processing

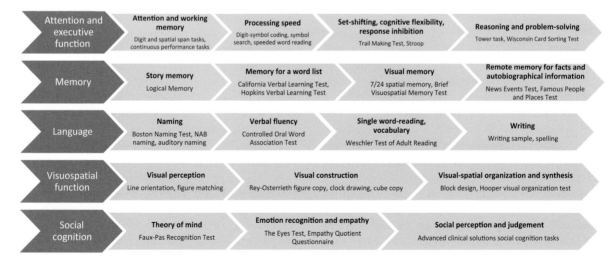

Fig. 16.1 Cognitive domains and examples of commonly used neuropsychological measures.

Attention and Executive Functioning

Attention is the foundation for most cognitive functions, including memory, processing speed, and executive function. Attention is a complex function that includes a variety of processes that support one's ability to focus on specific aspects of information to the exclusion of other information and distractors. The brain areas that are primarily associated with attention include the frontal and parietal lobes, specifically the dorsolateral prefrontal cortex, the posterior parietal cortex along the intraparietal sulcus, and other associated subcortical regions that connect with each other and with cortical regions. The literature on cognition and behavior has divided attention broadly into four hierarchical components: selective attention, sustained attention, divided attention, and alternating attention/cognitive flexibility. Given its complexity, attention is measured by various tests that are specific to this domain (e.g., digit and spatial span tasks, continuous performance tasks) as well as by interpretation of one's responses and types of errors on many tests across the neuropsychological assessment that can be affected by difficulty in regulating one's attention.

Executive functioning is a product of higher level attentional processes that support more complex cognitive tasks, including but not limited to working memory, problem-solving, planning, organization, inhibition, and self-monitoring/regulation. The brain regions that are associated with these functions primarily include the frontal lobe and its interconnected subcortical structures, including the prefrontal cortex, basal ganglia, and thalamus. Deficits in executive functions have significant implications for daily functioning and can affect both cognitive functioning and social/interpersonal functioning. For example, executive function deficits can manifest as reduced self-control and emotional dysregulation, which lead to emotional lability, irritability, or impulsivity.

Memory

Neuropsychological evaluations assess three major processes involved in memory, which are primarily mediated by frontal and temporal lobe structures, including the hippocampus and entorhinal cortex. The three stages of memory include encoding (ability to learn new information), retention/consolidation (ability to hold or store this information over time), and retrieval (ability to freely recall the learned information after a delay). Neuropsychological tests are designed to characterize memory at each of these levels to assist in differential diagnosis; these tests often include assessment of both verbal and nonverbal memory. Evidence of poor retention/consolidation often implicates dysfunction of medial temporal lobe structures and is commonly seen in early Alzheimer disease. By contrast, memory deficits primarily at the levels of encoding and retrieval with intact storage (retention/consolidation) may indicate more disruption in the frontal lobe and its connections that are more involved in attention/executive function. Broadly, encoding and retrieval deficits are nonspecific and can be seen various conditions, including vascular dementia or frontotemporal dementia, and in many other medical and neuropsychiatric conditions, including mood disorders, traumatic brain injury (TBI), and Parkinson's disease.

Language

Assessment of the patient's language functioning begins during the clinical interview, in which the clinician is attentive to any receptive or expressive language difficulties. If there is concern about a possible language disorder due to errors in naming objects, substitution of unintended words in a conversation, word-finding pauses, articulation difficulty, and/or difficulty comprehending language, a more systematic approach is taken to assess specific areas of impairment during a formal evaluation. The brain regions that are associated with language reception and production include the left hemisphere-dominant perisylvian (the region around the sylvian fissure) language network, which consists of parts of the frontal, temporal, and parietal lobes, including the inferior frontal gyrus, premotor cortex, and upper temporal lobe. Nonverbal aspects of language, such as facial expression, posture, and use of objects, are often mediated by the right hemisphere of the brain. Many aspects of both expressive and receptive language are assessed during neuropsychological evaluation, including but not limited to reading, writing, verbal comprehension, naming, repetition, and verbal fluency.

Visual-Spatial Functioning

Visual-spatial functioning encompasses one's ability to locate an object while processing the distance, depth, and direction of the object in relation to self or other objects and the ability to represent and mentally manipulate objects. Most spatial cognitive functions are associated with the posterior part of the parietal lobe as well as occipital lobe, with the ability to coordinate fine motor movements with visual abilities (visual construction) also associated with the frontoparietal networks. Assessment of visual-spatial functioning in neuropsychological evaluation includes characterization of visual construction as well as the ability to understand and process essential inputs to the visual system (visual perception) along with more complex functions like spatial orientation, mental rotation, and visual-motor integration.

Social Cognition

Although not routinely assessed in depth on formal testing, social cognition is an important aspect of one's health and overall functioning. Deficits in this domain are important in predicting and analyzing the ability to form and maintain interpersonal relationships. The brain areas that are involved in social cognitive functioning include the medial and anterior parts of the prefrontal cortex, the junction of the temporal and parietal lobes (temporoparietal junction), the fusiform gyrus, the posterior cingulate cortex, and the amygdala. Assessment of social cognitive functioning includes evaluation of theory of mind, social judgment, recognition of affect and empathy, and interpersonal behavior.

FROM THE PRIMARY CARE PROVIDER TO THE NEUROPSYCHOLOGIST: A STEPPED MODEL OF CARE

Referrals

Determining the appropriate referrals for a neuropsychological evaluation is particularly important, given the limited number of providers and the cost of services. The appropriateness of referrals tends to be optimized when referrals are triaged through specialists, such as neurologists or psychiatrists, although educating nonspecialists about how neuropsychological evaluations may be beneficial and for which patients will improve the judicious use of this often limited service. When possible, primary care providers (PCPs), including internists and family practitioners, are encouraged to make referrals as soon as they identify cognitive impairment in a patient. However, it is vital to strike a balance between early detection of and intervention for cognitive impairment and making the most efficient use of neuropsychology's specialized skills and often limited personnel

resources. Patients or family members might first notice changes from an individual's baseline in cognitive, emotional, and/or social and interpersonal functioning. Some common markers of potential cognitive decline include short-term memory problems (e.g., repeating oneself in conversation, difficulty recalling recent events), executive dysfunction and confusion (e.g., difficulty with planning, organization, problem-solving; frequently misplacing items; trouble following directions), word-finding difficulties, navigational challenges (e.g., getting lost in familiar places), personality changes (e.g., increased irritability, disinhibition, or apathy), and decreased ability to carry out daily activities, such as driving, managing finances, organizing one's medications and appointments, and self-care.

Currently, neuropsychology as a field is shifting toward a stepped model of care approach. Within this framework, PCPs and other providers can consult with a neuropsychologist as a Step 0. At this level, the provider is recommended to first administer a brief cognitive screener if any of the changes in cognition or daily functioning mentioned previously are noticed and then proceed to consult with a neuropsychologist if the results from the cognitive screen are concerning enough to warrant additional workup. In the United States, the Annual Medicare Wellness Guidelines suggests the use of cognitive screeners such as the Memory Impairment Screen (MIS), Mini-Cog, or the General Practitioner Assessment of Cognition (GPCog) to screen for cognitive concerns.

Other commonly used screeners include the Mini-Mental State Examination (MMSE); the Montreal Cognitive Assessment (MoCA), which is available in 36 languages; the Rapid Cognitive Screen; the Neurobehavioral Cognitive Status Examination; and CNS Vital Signs. These screeners are brief and do not provide the depth and breadth of information that are required to come to a diagnostic conclusion. However, tools such as the MoCA and MMSE can be used as a first step to identify cognitive impairment, assist in determining the need for further evaluation and testing, and support tracking of cognition over time. Both the MMSE and MoCA broadly assess the cognitive domains that are evaluated in a full neuropsychological evaluation, such as attention/orientation, memory, language, and aspects of visual-spatial ability. However, the MoCA is more sensitive for detection of executive dysfunction. A cutoff of 26 and 29 (out of 30) are commonly used to detect mild cognitive impairment (MCI) on the MoCA and MMSE, respectively. Furthermore, if the patient's activities of daily living are affected along with a score of <24 on the MMSE or <26 on MoCA, a diagnosis of a dementia syndrome should be considered, regardless of the underlying cause and etiology. Notably, MoCA and MMSE can also be used by nonspecialist providers to characterize deficits at specific stages of memory function, such as encoding and storage, which is useful in starting to differentiate some common conditions. Both tests have a memory component in which a list of three to five words is presented orally and asked to be recalled several minutes later. Inability to recall these words immediately after they are presented may suggest difficulty with encoding, which often affects subsequent retrieval after a delay. Both encoding and retrieval are attentionally mediated memory processes, and deficits at these levels are not necessarily indicative of a "true" memory storage problem, as is often seen in Alzheimer disease, for example. To tease apart memory encoding/retrieval deficits from storage loss, it is helpful to provide cues for any words that the patient is unable to freely recall at the delay. The MoCA includes suggested cues for both category and multiple choice, while the MMSE does not, in which case the examiner may consider providing cues to help with qualitative interpretation of results, even though the score will not change. If the patient is unable to retrieve or recognize the words they encoded even after suggested cues, this might be more suggestive of a "true" deficit in memory retention or storage as often observed in Alzheimer disease.

If concerns arise about the possibility of cognitive impairment based on patient and/or family report, clinician concern, and/or abnormal score on a cognitive screener, the next level of care may include Step 1, which entails brief neuropsychological evaluation (60–90 minutes long) or Step 2, which is a comprehensive neuropsychological evaluation (typically 90–180+ minutes long) at the discretion of the neuropsychologist. During this step of the stepped care model, the neuropsychologist collects and reviews prior medical data, including the PCP's cognitive screener scores and observations and the reason for referral, to build a tailored neuropsychological battery of tests to effectively characterize the patient's current cognitive functioning. On the day of the evaluation, the neuropsychologist typically conducts an initial interview with the patient and family (~45–60 minutes) before proceeding with ~1–3+ hours

of cognitive testing (Step 1 or Step 2). These components are often completed on the same day with breaks as needed, or they may be split across two sessions.

The most common referral questions for neuropsychologists include characterizing cognitive strengths and weaknesses, assisting with diagnostic clarification and treatment planning, establishing a baseline of cognitive function, and monitoring cognition over time. Specific patterns of strengths and weaknesses establish a kind of cognitive profile for a given patient, and stereotypical patterns and profiles can be associated with specific clinical syndromes and disorders. For this reason, it is crucial that the referring provider communicates the specific reason and circumstances for referral. A clear and specific reason for referral enhances the utility of neuropsychological evaluation, as the neuropsychologist is then able to provide the personalized and targeted recommendations that are most beneficial for the patient and the referring provider. Another important consideration is the patient's level of impairment and ability to tolerate neuropsychological evaluation. For example, comprehensive neuropsychological evaluation may not be clinically indicated for patients with very low scores on cognitive screeners and evidence of severe, global impairment due to floor effects (i.e., lower limits on what deficits testing is reliable in identifying); such testing may be of limited diagnostic utility in this population. Rather, these patients may be best served by tracking cognition via regular screening in ongoing follow-up with their providers.

Factors Affecting Test Performance

At Step 0, when the cognitive screeners indicate a possibility of cognitive impairment, it is important for the provider to consider confounding and/or modifiable factors that might affect the patient's test performance. If any of these factors seem likely to interfere significantly with the patient's ability to participate in a neuropsychological evaluation, it is recommended that they be resolved prior to Step 1.

Sleep

There is strong evidence for an association between sleep and cognitive function in adults, with poor sleep causing functional difficulties, especially in older adults. Apart from the long-term effects of sleep on cognition, there are also short-term effects that might affect the patient's performance on neuropsychological tests. Poor sleep quality and quantity in the prior day and week can have an adverse effect on cognitive functioning with a negative impact on attention, processing speed, and executive function. Sleep disorders such as untreated obstructive sleep apnea are also associated with cognitive impairment, primarily affecting attention, executive function, and aspects of memory, which may improve with regular treatment, including sustained compliance with CPAP over several months. Therefore, PCPs are recommended to address any significant sleep-related problems, such as marked insomnia or sleep apnea, prior to referring the patient for a neuropsychological evaluation whenever possible. In addition, addressing sleep problems might resolve or mitigate the patient's cognitive complaints, minimizing the need for a neuropsychological evaluation.

Mood

Mood and anxiety disorders can negatively affect attention/executive function, memory encoding and retrieval, and processing speed. Furthermore, these conditions can have downstream effects on motivation to engage in testing, which would affect the neuropsychologist's ability to characterize cognitive functioning accurately and comprehensively. Therefore, assessment of affective symptoms is regularly included as part of a neuropsychological evaluation via clinical interview and self-report questionnaires (e.g., the Beck Anxiety and Depression Inventories, PHQ-9, GAD-7). However, in situations in which the patient is experiencing severe depression, anxiety, or active psychosis, neuropsychological testing might not be advised until a decrease in symptom severity is noted. More immediate measures to target and stabilize affective symptoms would be recommended in such a situation.

Polypharmacy

Polypharmacy is common among medically complex patients and older adults, and the impact of polypharmacy on cognition can be significant, depending on the dosages and interactions between medications and comorbid conditions. Some known effects of polypharmacy on cognition include memory problems, attention difficulties, and slowed processing speed. Benzodiazepines and medications with high anticholinergic burden are known to have cognitive side effects, and a higher anticholinergic burden has been identified as a risk factor for MCI in older adults. If there is concern

for cognitive impairment in a patient treated with these or other medications with cognitive side effects, it is recommended that the provider reevaluate and simplify the medication regimen if possible and observe for any resolution or reduction of cognitive complaints prior to referring for neuropsychological evaluation. As a practical consideration, most insurances carriers in the United States do not cover neuropsychological services when known medication side effects or other common abnormalities in laboratory testing can explain better than a brain disease what may be contributing to or causing the cognitive changes.

Current Substance Use

Neuropsychology plays an important role in characterizing cognitive symptoms that may occur in the context of substance use disorders. However, because of the impact of substances on cognition, it is recommended that these patients achieve at least 6 weeks of abstinence prior to undergoing neuropsychological evaluation. More generally, patients are encouraged to abstain from taking any cognition-altering substances for at least 2 days prior to the neuropsychological evaluation to allow for the most accurate results. If sudden abstinence might pose a threat to the patient's overall health and functioning, providers may work with the patient to make sure abstinence can be safely achieved before proceeding with the evaluation.

Medical Necessity

In addition to insurance carriers in the United States not covering the cost of neuropsychological services when a patient has active psychosis, has specific lab abnormalities, or is taking medications that have clear cognitive side effects, neuropsychological evaluations must be determined to be medically necessary. Therefore referrals for academic performance-related testing and/or evaluation of certain neurodevelopmental disorders are often not covered unless there are medical comorbidities or atypical aspects of the condition that meet a standard of medical necessity. For example, it has been determined that neuropsychological evaluation is not required to diagnose autism spectrum disorder (ASD) or attention-deficit/hyperactivity disorder (ADHD) and therefore is deemed not medically necessary by insurance carriers. Of note, given the steady increase in the prevalence and/or increase in symptoms of these neurodevelopmental disorders in the past few years, during and following the COVID-19 pandemic, it is increasingly important that individuals with ASD and/or ADHD be diagnosed in a timely manner and supported with tailored interventions. To start the diagnostic process for these conditions, a detailed developmental history, including collateral information from family members or others where possible, and use of standardized questionnaires and observation tools may be conducted by a psychiatrist or psychologist. If diagnosis remains unclear after an initial psychiatric or psychological evaluation, particularly for patients with medical and psychiatric comorbidities or lack of response to treatment, neuropsychological evaluation can play an important role in clarifying differential diagnosis and informing treatment and support services for the individual and their families.

Performance Validity and Symptom Validity

Before interpreting the test results or sometimes before proceeding with a comprehensive neuropsychological evaluation, neuropsychologists must first determine the validity of the data that were collected through assessing patient effort and engagement via behavioral observations and objective measures of performance and symptom validity. As part of a standard neuropsychological evaluation, tests known as performance validity tests (PVTs) and symptom validity tests (SVTs) are included in the test battery. PVTs measure the validity of actual task performance; SVTs measure the accuracy of symptomatic complaints on self-report measures. There are stand-alone PVTs and SVTs that can be administered along with other tests in the neuropsychological battery as well as embedded measures of performance validity that are collected as part of tests measuring other cognitive processes such as memory and attention. If there is concern about variable or low engagement and effort during testing, neuropsychologists try to understand the reasons a person might not be performing at their optimal level and address these before proceeding to further testing or perhaps elect to defer evaluation to a later date. Additionally, there are situations in which a person may feign or malinger during testing for reasons that may be known or unknown to providers. In such cases, PVTs and SVTs are utilized to detect the likelihood of low effort, feigning, and/or malingering. These may be crucial when patients are seeking an evaluation for claims of disability due to cognitive impairment and/or for other forensic or legal reasons, given higher rates of malingering in these cases than in others.

Normative Data and Cultural/Linguistic Considerations

Normative data in neuropsychology refers to a collection of test scores from a representative sample that establishes a baseline distribution for performance on a measure. This data serve as reference points to compare a particular patient's performance to that of a relevant comparison group. Normative data is the basis for objective measurement and enables an accurate comparison of any one patient's cognitive functioning in reference to healthy controls or to patients with similar conditions. Normative data can be presented in various forms, such as percentile ranks, z-scores, T-scores, standard scores, or scaled scores (Fig. 16.2).

Given the use of normative comparisons in neuropsychology, there are some limitations to the interpretation of test scores for certain groups of individuals. The majority of the commonly used neuropsychological tests in the United States were constructed and normed with monolingual, US-educated, English-speaking individuals, thereby limiting their reliability and validity for individuals with divergent backgrounds, given the wide range of cultural and linguistic factors that can affect test performance. These factors include an individual's primary language, bilingualism or multilingualism, quality and level of education, level of acculturation, socioeconomic status, communication style, and familiarity with test materials. Due to the increasing sociocultural diversity within the United States and other parts of the world, a growing number of neuropsychologists specialize in working with populations characterized by specific factors that are not aligned with those for whom traditional, normative tests were constructed. There is a dire need for expansion of such neuropsychological expertise and services as well as more comprehensive training in cross-cultural neuropsychology for all clinicians. Ideally, patients will complete testing in their first or primary language, which may require the services of an interpreter. It is very helpful for providers who refer for neuropsychological evaluation to note the patient's first or primary language in the referral to ensure that interpreter services, if available, can be requested in advance. When possible, neuropsychologists work closely with medical interpreters, even while cross-cultural assessment continues to develop within the field with a need for more collaborative and focused effort in this area. Given the importance of the language in which tests are administered, some standardized tests are now

Standard Scores

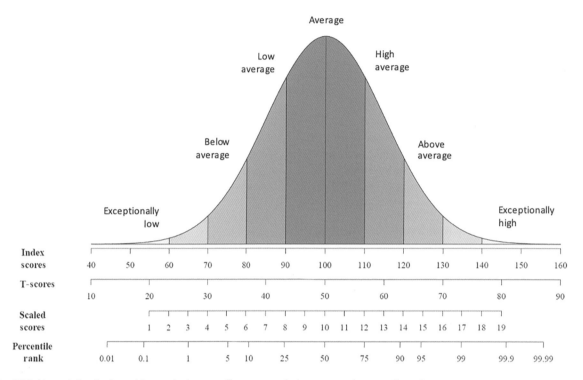

Fig. 16.2 Normal distribution with standard scores, T-scores, scaled scores, and percentile ranks.

available in many languages that can often be tailored to a patient's preferred language. Other test measures are thought to be more universal and less culturally biased toward one dominant culture, although there remains a critical need for further development of tests and normative data for use with diverse populations. Limitations in use of some normative data in working with socially, culturally, and linguistically diverse populations also highlight the value of baseline neuropsychological testing, especially when a patient is at high risk for a decline. Baseline testing allows for comparison of an individual's performances over time, with the individual's own data providing more reliable and valid reference points for evaluating for decline.

NEUROPSYCHOLOGICAL REPORTS

Upon completion of a neuropsychological assessment, the neuropsychologist analyzes and evaluates the collected data. This includes scoring all the administered tests, comparing the patient's scores to selected normative data, and then conceptualizing the overall cognitive profile in the context of the patient's developmental, medical, and psychiatric history based on information gathered during the clinical interview and chart review. The neuropsychologist then writes a comprehensive report that takes into account all biopsychosocial factors and usually describes or summarizes test results, diagnostic impressions including discussion of potential etiologies and contributing factors, and often personalized recommendations for treatment and care for the patient and family.

Interpreting Scores and Report Summaries

In the test results and summary sections of the report, the neuropsychologist might add a table with test scores or briefly discuss the scores in a narrative format. The table typically includes raw scores as well as demographically adjusted normative scores and standardized descriptive labels such as "exceptionally high," "above average," and "below average." These labels themselves do not indicate impairment, as the neuropsychologist interprets these results within the patient's specific biopsychosocial context and estimated baseline abilities to characterize impairment. It is also important to note that while most test scores fall on a normal distribution curve, some tests, such as the commonly used Boston Naming Test, have a skewed distribution that cannot be interpreted on a normal curve. With these factors in mind, the summary and/or impressions section of the neuropsychological report should synthesize the overall interpretation of test results within the specific clinical context. The referring provider is encouraged to reach out to the neuropsychologist at any time to clarify or discuss any component of the evaluation or to follow up with regard to diagnosis and treatment planning. The last section of a neuropsychological report often contains tailored recommendations for the patient, family, and treatment team, including suggestions for any further workup or evaluation based on assessment findings, designed to optimize the patient's daily cognition and functioning, as described in detail in the next section.

NEUROPSYCHOLOGICAL INTERVENTION

Feedback Sessions

Upon completion of the neuropsychological evaluation, the first step of intervention often consists of patient follow-up with the neuropsychologist to review test results and recommendations. These feedback sessions are typically conducted by the neuropsychologist in person or increasingly via telehealth with the patient as well as any family members or relevant care partners. In certain specialty clinics, such as a center dedicated to memory disorders or cognitive and behavioral neurology, the patient may elect to follow up directly with the referring neurologist to discuss neuropsychological test results and recommendations in the context of their ongoing clinical follow-up. If connection to such a clinic does not exist, it is the responsibility of the neuropsychologist to follow up with patients directly to discuss results and recommendations from the evaluation. There is also emerging evidence of the value of embedding neuropsychological services, including both assessment and intervention, into primary care and geriatric medicine clinics to optimize clinical care and access.

In addition to discussing diagnostic impressions, feedback sessions largely focus on providing support for the patient and family and reviewing personalized recommendations, which often include a combination of compensatory strategies to optimize daily cognition; psychoeducation, which may touch upon brain-behavior relationships; healthy lifestyle behaviors; and psychological treatment approaches (e.g., cognitive-behavioral and/or mindfulness strategies) as well as suggestions for other relevant workup or follow-up with other providers (e.g., sleep study, neurologic or psychiatric follow-up) and any suggested plan for repeat neuropsychological evaluation. Provision of written communication aids during feedback may support retention of information for patients and families. Moreover, emerging research suggests that neuropsychological feedback sessions are associated with enhanced patient satisfaction, understanding of one's condition, and improved coping, self-efficacy, mood, and quality of life.

Neuropsychological Rehabilitation

Beyond postevaluation feedback sessions, neuropsychologists are well suited to offer rehabilitation for patients in both individual and group settings. These clinical services can support the teaching and development of cognitive, mindfulness-based, and lifestyle strategies and can enhance self-efficacy and emotional well-being. They are often combined with elements of cognitive-behavioral therapy in a holistic treatment approach to optimize daily cognition and functioning. Cognitive rehabilitation strategies are often categorized as restorative (designed to improve the cognitive ability itself) or compensatory (designed to optimize function by using workaround strategies), with newer treatments increasingly incorporating metacognitive strategies as well. Rehabilitation is often conducted by neuropsychologists, clinical psychologists, and/or speech/language pathologists where available. In the following sections, we will offer a broad overview of neuropsychological rehabilitation, with a focus on cognitive training and mindfulness approaches as well as general recommendations and evidence basis for multidomain and lifestyle interventions.

Cognitive Training

Healthy older adults. Among healthy older adults, multicomponent cognitive training interventions have generally been shown to improve targeted cognitive abilities (e.g., near transfer) to a greater extent than untrained abilities (e.g., far transfer). Although different from traditional cognitive training delivered via paper-and-pencil methods, computerized cognitive training among older adults may also provide benefits to aspects of cognition, including working memory, executive function, and processing speed. Regarding mechanisms, there is some evidence that cognitive training among older adults may enhance global and regional cerebral blood flow and connectivity within the default mode and central executive brain networks and increase functional connectivity between the hippocampi and frontal and temporal regions, promoting memory function.

Mild cognitive impairment. Among older adults with MCI, cognitive training interventions are feasible; have yielded small to moderate effects on global cognition, executive function, and memory; and may promote neuroplasticity. However, it is unclear whether these improvements transfer to cognition and functioning in daily life, are maintained at long-term follow-up, or alter the disease course in MCI. Also of note, while there is some evidence basis for facilitator-mediated cognitive training in the treatment of MCI, there is scientific consensus that there is currently insufficient evidence that commercially available online "brain-training" programs prevent the onset of cognitive impairment or slow decline in MCI. That said, the application of digital cognitive training programs is an area of increasing research and clinical interest, particularly since the expansion of telehealth services during the COVID-19 pandemic.

In looking at specific interventions in MCI, cognitive training approaches with focus on episodic memory strategies and mnemonic training as well as computerized memory–attention training, have shown promise in improving memory. In addition to memory training, speed-of-processing training may improve processing speed, attention, and working memory among older adults with amnestic MCI, which may support driving abilities and lower dementia risk. Relatedly, emerging research has suggested the potential of "gamified" cognitive training, which has improved episodic memory and motivation among adults with amnestic MCI. Moreover, multidomain and multicomponent cognitive training, including lifestyle changes, may yield modest cognitive benefits in MCI. Recent reviews have emphasized the need for studies with larger samples, adequate control groups, and long-term follow-up.

Beyond potential improvements in cognition, there is preliminary evidence that cognitive training may also improve depression, anxiety, and possibly quality of life among adults with MCI, though most studies have been small and otherwise limited with some mixed effects. One important limitation is the fact that many studies have included participants with minimal anxiety and depression at baseline. This remains an essential area for future research, particularly considering that potential improvements in mood following cognitive interventions could be conceptualized as evidence of far transfer if mood symptoms are not explicitly targeted as part of the training.

Other neurologic/neuropsychiatric conditions. In addition to MCI, cognitive training interventions have shown promise for a variety of neurologic and neuropsychiatric populations, including TBI, stroke, cancer, multiple sclerosis (MS), Parkinson's disease, and substance use, among others. First, the Cognitive Rehabilitation Task Force (CRTF), a special interest group effort by the American Congress of Rehabilitation Medicine based in the United States, has highlighted emerging evidence for the clinical use of cognitive rehabilitation to target cognitive and socioemotional deficits after TBI or stroke, with a particular focus on comprehensive holistic rehabilitation. This treatment combines cognitive training with strategies to promote self-awareness and improve interpersonal and emotional functioning and is delivered individually and in group format. More specifically, among adults with history of TBI and stroke, the CRTF has recommended use of direct attention training as well as metacognitive training to target attention deficits and promote the transfer of skills to daily life, with an additional recommendation for use of clinician-directed, multimodal computerized training to improve attention, memory, and executive function. Indeed, cognitive rehabilitation may improve aspects of attention and subjective memory immediately posttreatment in stroke patients, for example, but there is a need for additional research to determine whether these benefits translate to daily life or persist over time.

Regarding other medical and neurologic populations, cognitive training has yielded benefits in verbal memory and processing speed among adults with cancer-related cognitive impairments. Likewise, cognitive rehabilitation may improve working memory, verbal memory, and executive function immediately after treatment, with smaller potential benefits in mood, among nondemented patients with Parkinson's disease; additional studies are needed to determine the generalizability of these findings to daily life. In MS, strategy-oriented cognitive rehabilitation has not been shown to enhance objective cognitive measures but does seem to improve self-perceived cognition. In at least one study, this improvement persisted at a 9-month follow-up, highlighting the potential of cognitive rehabilitation to support self-efficacy. There is also preliminary evidence that memory rehabilitation strategies (e.g., associative verbal learning with supported elaborative processing, extra processing and retrieval time, explicit support to make associations) may benefit individuals with alcohol-related cognitive impairment, though more rigorous research is needed.

As one specific example of a cognitive rehabilitation program, Goal Management Training (GMT) is a standardized protocol that targets executive function and has yielded small to moderate benefits on various cognitive abilities, including executive function, working memory, long-term memory, daily functioning, and mental health. In studies of GMT, objective cognitive gains are largely maintained at follow-up, typically at least 6 months posttreatment, among a variety of neurologic populations, including individuals with acquired brain injury, as well as those with substance use disorders, MS, spina bifida, cerebrovascular disease, and ADHD and healthy, cognitively normal older adults.

In summary, cognitive rehabilitation, delivered individually or in group format, has the potential to benefit for individuals with cognitive symptoms in aspects of cognition, mood, and quality of life, including healthy older adults, adults with MCI, and various neurologic and neuropsychiatric populations, including those with history of TBI, stroke, MS, Parkinson's disease, substance use disorders, and cancer-related cognitive impairment, though there is a need for further research to elucidate generalizability and longevity of effects. Even so, cognitive rehabilitation warrants consideration as part of tailored treatment planning for adults with cognitive concerns and may be offered by speech/language pathologists and/or clinical neuropsychologists in hospital-based settings or private practice.

Mindfulness-Based Interventions

Mindfulness is broadly defined as present-focused, nonjudgmental awareness, which may cultivate emotion regulation and enhance psychological health via improved attentional awareness and control, reduced rumination, and increased tolerance of affective distress. Mindfulness-based practices may also build cognitive reserve, which is the developed abilities of the brain, acquired through such activities as education and occupation, lifelong learning, and engagement in leisure activities, that allow individuals to better cope with cumulating brain pathology and optimize daily functioning. Studies also suggest that mindfulness can promote structural and functional changes in brain regions that are implicated in attentional and emotional regulation, though additional research is needed.

Mindfulness interventions have yielded positive effects on mood, quality of life, and cognition among adults, with mixed preliminary findings among older adults. Moreover, mindfulness-based interventions have been shown to be feasible and acceptable to middle-aged and older adults (~ages 45–85 years) with subjective cognitive decline and MCI, with mixed effects on global cognition in MCI in exploratory studies. Mindfulness-based interventions have also shown potential benefits for specific cognitive abilities in MCI, including improved reaction time, attentional control, and verbal memory, though with some variability across studies.

Mindfulness-based interventions may positively affect the disease course in MCI through various direct and indirect mechanisms, including potential direct impacts on brain structure and function, inflammatory processes, and gene expression, and indirectly through effects on stress and mood. The potential impact of mindfulness on improving the connectivity between brain regions in defined networks is of particular interest, given evidence that reduced activity in some networks, namely, in the default mode network in MCI and early Alzheimer disease, has been linked to disease progression. Among adults with MCI, emerging research suggests that mindfulness-based interventions may enhance functional connectivity within default mode network regions (posterior cingulate cortex, bilateral medial prefrontal cortex, left hippocampus), improve brain network efficiency (in the insula, right cingulate gyrus, and left superior temporal gyrus), and potentially reduce hippocampal atrophy, which is a commonly used marker of disease progression in Alzheimer disease.

Beyond potential cognitive benefits, there is preliminary evidence that mindfulness-based interventions may also improve mood, coping skills, and quality of life in MCI, perhaps by promoting acceptance of aging and cognitive changes and cultivating a stance of nonjudgment and curious observation of present experiences and thoughts. That said, more research is needed to better understand mechanisms of change and to clarify whether observed effects are specific to mindfulness rather than to psychoeducation, for example, which is an often-used control group.

In addition to MCI, mindfulness-based interventions have shown promise in improving aspects of cognition, mood/anxiety, and quality of life in several neurologic and psychiatric populations, including individuals with Parkinson's disease, MS, depression, anxiety, and cancer-related cognitive impairment. From a cognition standpoint, mindfulness- and acceptance-based interventions have yielded moderate to large effects on attention and memory at immediate posttreatment in MS, though more rigorous studies are needed to replicate findings and determine the longevity of effects. Preliminary studies have shown similar findings for individuals with Parkinson's disease, with the potential of mindfulness to improve aspects of attention and executive function, particularly among those with higher compliance to prescribed home practice. Likewise, mindfulness-based strategies and psychoeducation have been found to improve attention and executive function, respectively, among adults with cancer-related cognitive impairments. Mindfulness-based interventions may also enhance aspects of executive function, namely, cognitive flexibility, among individuals with generalized anxiety disorder and depression.

In sum, preliminary research suggests that mindfulness-based interventions over weeks to months may improve specific cognitive abilities, including aspects of attention, executive function, and memory, and enhance emotional functioning and quality of life for adults, older adults, and adults with various neurologic and psychiatric conditions. Additional studies with larger samples, adequate control groups, and long-term follow-up are needed. From a neuropsychological perspective, mindfulness-based strategies offer a low-risk intervention strategy with the potential to enhance emotional and cognitive well-being as individuals learn skills to manage stress and hone attentional abilities, with implications for improving daily cognition and quality of life and enhancing enjoyment of daily activities. Practically, mindfulness-based strategies may be incorporated as part of individual psychotherapy, be delivered via group therapy, and/or be self-paced through a variety of available books and online materials, the latter approach likely being best suited to motivated and higher functioning individuals and/or those with a supportive care partner or team at home.

Multidomain and Lifestyle Interventions

In addition to suggestions for cognitive training and/or mindfulness interventions, neuropsychological recommendations frequently highlight the importance of healthy lifestyle behaviors for adults of all ages, particularly for those with history of vascular risk factors and/or who are otherwise at risk for dementia. During feedback sessions, neuropsychologists often provide psychoeducation about the importance of healthy lifestyle behaviors to optimize cognition and brain health and may incorporate motivational interviewing strategies to enhance the adoption and maintenance of these behaviors within the context of brain health.

The importance of engaging in healthy lifestyle behaviors and managing vascular risk factors is most often discussed in the context of dementia prevention. A recent study reported that approximately 40% of dementia cases in the United States were associated with 12 modifiable risk factors, particularly among Black and Hispanic individuals (low education, hearing loss, TBI, excessive alcohol use, smoking, depression, social isolation, diabetes, air pollution, hypertension, obesity, and physical inactivity, with the strongest impact from the latter three). Considering this and the lack of strong evidence to date that pharmacological therapies for MCI are significantly effective or will alone be sufficient for care, there is increasing interest in preventive, nonpharmacologic interventions. These include lifestyle modifications, such as exercise, diet, cognitive and social engagement, and aggressive and early control of cardiovascular risk factors such as hypertension. For example, a large population-based case-control study found that moderate exercise in midlife or late life was associated with a reduced risk of MCI. Moreover, physical exercise has yielded positive effects on cognition among individuals with MCI, though there is a need for additional large, well-controlled trials to determine the specific qualities of effective exercise, including type, dose, and intensity.

Besides exercise, there is emerging interest in the impact of diet on cognition, with preliminary evidence showing that the MIND diet, which focuses on intake of green leafy (and other) vegetables, berries, whole grains, olive oil, nuts, beans, poultry, and fish, may enhance cognition and reduce the risk of cognitive decline and dementia in older adults, possibly by decreasing oxidative stress and inflammation. Notably, results of studies implementing the MIND diet for prevention of cognitive decline in older adults have been mixed, and more research is warranted. Additionally, recommendations to increase social, cognitive, and community and cultural engagement are relevant, as these factors may also reduce dementia risk.

To date, there have been a few randomized controlled trials that have employed multiple "brain-healthy" behaviors in cognitively normal older adults and/or those who are at risk for dementia, with varying success. In one large study, a 2-year multidomain intervention (prescribed diet, exercise regimen, cognitive training, and vascular risk monitoring) improved or maintained cognition among older adults who were at risk for dementia (ages 60–77 years) relative to a control group who received general health advice. In that study, the FINGER study, treatment effects were also observed in BMI, diet, and physical activity. That said, in a different 3-year trial of older adults, a multidomain intervention (physical activity, cognitive training, nutritional advice) or omega-3 supplementation, either alone or in combination, had no effects on cognition relative to placebo, highlighting the importance of continued research in this area.

SUMMARY AND FUTURE DIRECTIONS

Neuropsychology as a field has evolved to encompass a wide range of assessment and intervention approaches to support patients and families in optimizing cognitive and emotional health while continuing to assist in differential diagnosis, treatment planning, and close tracking of cognition over time. Moving forward, there is a need to expand available normative data to support increasingly diverse patient populations and a need to continue to update assessment tools for measuring cognition. The COVID-19 pandemic highlighted the value and feasibility of tele-neuropsychology, which will likely continue to be a valuable option for some patients and allows for flexible, hybrid approaches to evaluation (e.g., completion of initial interview and some testing virtually with completion of additional in-office testing on a separate day if clinically indicated). Unfortunately, availability of neuropsychological services is often limited and therefore involves long wait times. This has highlighted the need for a stepped model of care to triage the patients who will most benefit from neuropsychological assessment. Monitoring of cognition can start in the PCP or nonspecialist office with regular questioning of patients and care partners on any observed changes in daily cognitive or behavioral functioning. Whenever possible, nonspecialist providers can also incorporate cognitive screeners as a valuable first step when there is concern about possible cognitive decline, either reported by the patient or family or observed by the physician. Any available datapoints from cognitive screeners allow for broad tracking of cognition over time while also helping to inform the neuropsychological battery for patients who are referred for more comprehensive evaluation. Relatedly, many clinics are incorporating integrated clinic models, with close collaboration and consultation between neuropsychologists and other treatment providers to streamline the initial diagnostic workup and optimize patient care. As part of a clinical workup, neuropsychological evaluation can assist with differential diagnosis and facilitate early detection of neurologic and neuropsychiatric diseases, which is of critical importance to allow for preventive treatment approaches and connection to supportive resources. This is becoming increasingly important with the advent of potential disease-modifying treatments for early Alzheimer disease, for example.

Regarding neuropsychological interventions, cognitive training and mindfulness-based interventions warrant inclusion as treatment approaches for adults, older adults, and adults with various neurologic and neuropsychiatric conditions with the potential to benefit aspects of cognition, mood, and quality of life. Emerging research in MCI suggests that cognitive training may benefit global cognition, memory, working memory, and executive function, while mindfulness may enhance aspects of attention, psychomotor function, and possibly memory. Similarly, cognitive training and mindfulness interventions have shown preliminary promise in enhancing cognition (i.e., aspects of attention, memory, and executive function) and mood among individuals with history of TBI, stroke, Parkinson's disease, MS, depression, or anxiety and those with cancer-related cognitive impairment, among others. These treatments are generally considered feasible and low-risk; however, there remains a need to clarify whether the improvements transfer to daily life, are maintained over time, or significantly affect the disease course. Both mindfulness and cognitive training interventions may reduce stress and promote structural and functional changes in brain regions associated with cognitive control, attention and emotional regulation, and memory, though the underlying mechanisms are not yet well understood. Beyond cognitive training and mindfulness, multidomain lifestyle interventions have shown preliminary promise in reducing cognitive decline among older adults who are at risk for dementia.

Looking ahead, there remains a need for high-quality research to elucidate the effects of cognitive training, mindfulness, and lifestyle interventions on cognition and mood in healthy, neurologic, and psychiatric populations. Questions remain regarding optimal treatment duration and frequency, longevity of effects, impact on disease trajectory, and underlying mechanisms. It will also be important to determine whether current outcome measures best capture the impact of these interventions or need to be expanded. Clinically, patients with subjective or mild cognitive symptoms (due to various etiologies) may be especially well suited to engage in mindfulness or cognitive interventions, perhaps in addition to lifestyle modifications and/or pharmacologic strategies. Indeed, emerging research has highlighted the value of multidomain interventions (e.g., combinations of cognitive stimulation/training and mindfulness, neurofeedback, exercise and diet modifications, music therapy), which may improve cognition and increase gray matter volume and cerebral blood flow in adults with MCI, for example.

It has also been suggested that future research consider modifications of conventional mindfulness-based approaches to tailor treatment for older adults and neurologic populations, such as conducting mindfulness-based interventions with patients and supportive partners and/or combining elements of mindfulness with aging-related education. In addition, other mind-body interventions, such as yoga, tai chi, qigong, biofeedback, meditation, music-guided imagery, and dance, are feasible in adults with cognitive complaints, having the potential to benefit aspects of cognition (e.g., attention, executive function, verbal memory), mood, and possibly underlying physiology (e.g., levels of insulin-like growth factor–1).

Moving forward, there will likely be continued emphasis on holistic neuropsychological rehabilitation, including incorporation of emotion regulation strategies and cognitive-behavioral therapy into cognitive rehabilitation programs. Already, there is evidence that combined approaches may yield benefits on mood and quality of life among individuals with acquired brain injury, while CBT as well as cognitive rehabilitation and training may improve subjective cognition among adults with cancer-related cognitive symptoms. Another emerging area of work is the potential of virtual reality rehabilitation programs, which have shown some initial benefit on cognition among adults with TBI as well as MCI.

There remain important challenges of (1) how to translate and scale research findings into optimal treatment delivery systems in clinic- and community-based settings and (2) how to foster motivation for adoption and maintenance of cognitive rehabilitation strategies, mindfulness practices, and healthy lifestyle behaviors in daily life among individuals who are not involved in research. One such approach may be to frame these interventions in the context of brain health and cognitive and emotional well-being and draw on principles from motivational interviewing to support person-centered, values-based change, ideally with the support of a clinical psychologist or neuropsychologist, at least initially, to foster goal setting and treatment engagement.

Taken together, neuropsychological interventions, including cognitive training, mindfulness-based approaches, and lifestyle and combined or multidomain interventions, represent promising, low-risk treatment strategies that have the potential to improve cognition and mood, reduce stress, and enhance brain structure and function for a variety of healthy, at-risk, neurologic, and psychiatric populations. Future research, including the study of combined treatment approaches and the use of longitudinal designs, may clarify effects and underlying mechanisms, including the potential impact of these treatments on disease trajectories, to further inform and tailor clinical recommendations for neuropsychological intervention.

"For the full bibliography list, please use the pincode on the inside front cover to access the electronic version of the text at ebooks.health.elsevier.com."

17

Spinal Cord Disorders: Myelopathy*

Shamik Bhattacharyya and Sultana Jahan

INTRODUCTION

Myelopathy is a clinical syndrome caused by spinal cord dysfunction. Practitioners across different specialties from emergency medicine to trauma surgery, to neurology, to internal medicine encounter patients with myelopathy. Despite being anatomically small, the spinal cord can be pathologically affected by many disease etiologies, which often leads to uncertainty about the appropriate steps for diagnosis, investigation, and treatment. In this chapter, the clinical syndrome of myelopathy and then the specific causes of spinal cord disease will be reviewed.

ANATOMICAL STRUCTURE

Anatomically, the spinal cord starts at the cranio-cervical traction and descends to about the L1 level. The spinal cord is surrounded by the bony vertebral column and descends through the vertebral canal. Motor nerve roots exit the spinal cord ventrally, while sensory nerve roots enter the spinal cord in the dorsal or posterior aspect (Fig. 17.1). The motor and sensory nerve roots combine at the level of the intervertebral foramina to exit as spinal nerves. In the spinal cord, gray matter (containing neuronal cell bodies) is located centrally. Ascending and descending white matter tracts surround the central gray matter.

While many tracts exist in the spinal cord (Fig. 17.2), for the practicing clinician, three of these white matter

*Based on Bhattacharyya S. Spinal cord disorders: myelopathy. *Am J Med*. 2018;131(11):1293–1297. ISSN 0002-9343. https://doi.org/10.1016/j.amjmed.2018.03.009.

projections are especially significant for localization of injury.

- Lateral corticospinal tract: In the spinal cord the corticospinal tract is located laterally and provides mostly *ipsilateral* control of motor neurons.
- Posterior or dorsal columns: These white matter tracts are located dorsally in the spinal cord and mediate *ipsilateral* perception of vibration and joint position sense.
- Spinothalamic tracts: These tracts are located anterolaterally and conduct *contralateral* perception of pain and temperature.

Note that, for the sensory tracts, the distinction between the different types of sensation and their pathways is not exclusive. Touch sensation, for example, is conducted through both dorsal columns and spinothalamic tracts. The spinal cord is especially important for control of autonomic functions such as bladder or bowel sphincter control. These essential tracts are located centrally. The upper cervical spinal cord is also critical for controlling respiratory function (through innervation of the diaphragm by the phrenic nerves).

The vascular supply of the spinal cord differs between the anterior and posterior aspects. The anterior two-thirds of the spinal cord, including the corticospinal tracts and the spinothalamic tracts, are supplied by the anterior spinal artery. Posteriorly, there are paired posterior spinal arteries that supply the posterior columns. The spinal arteries form an anastomotic network that is reinforced through radiculomedullary arteries (segmental arteries that enter through the spinal intervertebral foramen and end in the spinal cord). One of the largest feeder arteries for the anterior spinal artery is the Artery of Adamkiewicz. Venous drainage of the spinal cord is

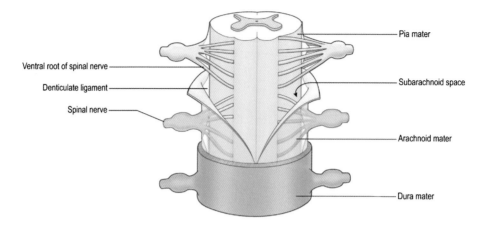

Figure 17.1 The spinal cord is covered by meningeal layers. Motor nerve roots exit the spinal cord ventrally, while sensory nerve roots enter the spinal cord dorsally (back of the projected image). (From *Neuroanatomy: An Illustrated Colour Text*, Sixth Edition.)

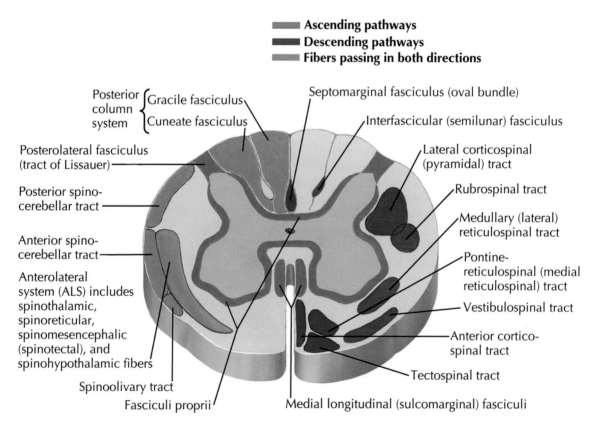

Figure 17.2 Axial cross section of the spinal cord showing ascending and descending white matter tracts. (From *Netter Collection of Medical Illustrations: Nervous System, Part II – Spinal Cord and Peripheral Motor and Sensory Systems.*)

through both segmental radicular veins and through longitudinal channels.

CLINICAL SYNDROME

Myelopathy is a clinical diagnosis, and ascertaining consistent symptoms and signs are key to the diagnosis. Common symptoms of spinal cord dysfunction are bilateral weakness in the arms or legs, gait disorder especially described as stiff and slow, numbness with paresthesia, urinary urgency or hesitancy, and bowel sphincter dysfunction. These symptoms are, however, not specific for spinal cord dysfunction and, hence, can be missed. For example, weakness in the legs can also potentially be caused by a brain lesion or from compression of lumbosacral nerve roots. There are some symptoms that are more indicative of spinal cord dysfunction. Many patients with spinal cord disease experience a band of tightness across the trunk that is often described as a plastic wrap or a squeezing sensation. This sense is typically circumferential across the trunk. The authors have met many patients who were brought to the emergency room with a concern about cardiac ischemia because of the tightness across the chest from a thoracic cord lesion.

Neurological examination provides more specificity to the diagnosis of myelopathy. Injury to the corticospinal tracts causes the upper motor neuron syndrome of weakness, spasticity, and increased deep tendon stretch reflexes. In acute spinal cord injury, there is usually flaccid paralysis that gradually converts over the space of days to weeks to spastic weakness. Neurological examination generally discloses sensory loss to different sensory modalities when the spinothalamic and dorsal columns are affected. There are patterns to the neurological examination that are especially suggestive of spinal cord dysfunction:

- *Lhermitte sign*: With the patient in a sitting position, the examiner flexes the neck forward to elicit electric sensation down the spine or into the arms. When flexing the neck forward, simultaneously flexing the hips can improve the sensitivity of the technique (Fig. 17.3).
- *Sensory level*: Sensation to pinprick, light touch, or temperature is best assessed at specific dermatome levels (Fig. 17.4). A sensory level is defined as the most caudal level at which both pinprick and light touch are preserved. The sensory level can be different on either side of the body. For example, sensory level on the right side can be at the T10 level (at the level of navel) while being T4 level on the left (at the level of the nipple line). Anatomically, the spinal cord lesion *does not* have to be at the same location as the clinical sensory level. In the prior example of T10 sensory level on the right and T4 sensory level on the left, the causative spinal cord lesion can potentially be in the cervical spinal cord. The sensory level indicates that the spinal cord lesion could be present at that level or at a level above.
- *Hemicord syndrome (Brown Sequard syndrome)*: This syndrome is caused by a lesion affecting one-half of the spinal cord. Because of the anatomy of the spinal cord, lesion of one-half of it causes ipsilateral weakness and loss of sensation to vibration/joint position *and* contralateral loss of sensation to

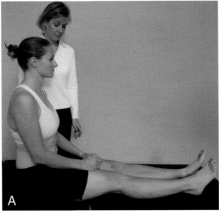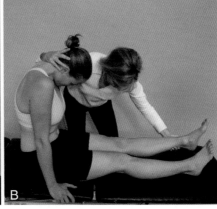

Figure 17.3 The Lhermitte sign is elicited by having the patient sitting (A) and then flexing the neck forward (B). Flexing the hip shown in B can further improve sensitivity of the sign. (From *Orthopedic Physical Assessment*, Chapter 3, 164–242.e6.)

Distribution of sensory dermatomes

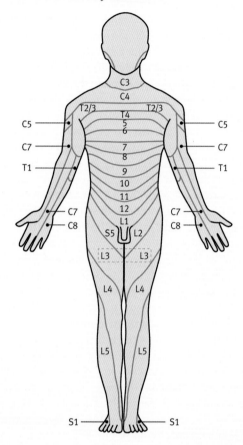

Figure 17.4 Dermatomes on the anterior surface of the body. Note that after C4 dermatome, the rest of the cervical dermatomes are represented in the arms. (From Lee J, Thumbikat P. Pathophysiology, presentation and management of spinal cord injury. *Surgery*. 2015;33(6):238–247.)

pinprick/temperature. To give a specific example, a thoracic cord lesion on the right would be expected to cause weakness in the right leg and loss of temperature/sharp sensation in the left leg. This dissociated and crossed pattern is highly suggestive of a spinal cord disorder. While not specific, laterally placed lesions causing the hemicord syndrome are often found in multiple sclerosis relapses.

- *Central cord syndrome*: The syndrome consists of bilateral weakness in arms greater than weakness in legs, bladder and bowel dysfunction, and variable sensory loss. Typically, central cord syndrome is associated with spinal cord trauma usually superimposed on preexisting spinal spondylotic disease.

IMAGING

After clinical diagnosis of myelopathy, the next steps focus on finding the cause. Generally, patients with myelopathy require spinal imaging. The preferred modality is magnetic resonance imaging (MRI), which can image the spinal cord, nerves, and surrounding soft tissue structures. MRI can show acutely threatening compressive lesions that need urgent intervention. In addition, the pattern of spinal cord lesion abnormality can sometimes suggest a cause. The ability to find lesions in the spinal cord on MRI is dependent on the resolution of the MRI. Hence, while full spine MRI can show all the spinal segments, the images are of lower resolution and miss small lesions. Imagining the spinal segment where the likelihood is highest of a lesion is generally preferred. For structural screening MRI, gadolinium intravenous contrast is not needed. When there is suspicion of inflammatory or neoplastic cause, intravenous gadolinium contrast can improve sensitivity and specificity.

In special circumstances, patients may need other imaging techniques. X-ray and computed tomography (CT) imaging show implanted metallic hardware better than MRI. Metallic hardware results in distortion of images in MRI. CT myelography is a procedure in which a CT scan is obtained after intrathecal injection of radiopaque contrast. Myelogram is useful for sensitive characterization of the subarachnoid space such as when there is suspicion of cerebrospinal fluid leak or to better characterize the relationship between spinal nerves and prior implanted hardware. X-ray of the cervical and lumbar spine can also be obtained in different postures such as with the neck or lower back flexed and extended. Dynamic views of the spine are obtained when patients complain of symptoms only in a specific posture and often show dynamic spinal alignment instability missed on static views (such as subluxation of a vertebral body on neck flexion).

SPECIFIC CAUSES OF MYELOPATHY

Finding a cause of myelopathy requires integrating clinical symptoms and signs, laboratories, and imaging—a process that can feel difficult especially to nonneurologists. An effective way to approach the differential diagnosis of myelopathy is to categorize by time course of symptom evolution from onset to nadir: hyperacute (less than 6 hours), acute (6–48 hours), subacute (over 2 days to 3 weeks), and chronic (longer than 3 weeks). In the following sections, some of the more common causes of myelopathy based on time of onset rather than a full exhaustive list of all possibilities will be briefly discussed.

Hyperacute Causes of Myelopathy

For rapid onset of myelopathy over the space of minutes to a few hours, the highest suspicions are for spinal cord trauma and spinal cord vascular injury. Trauma is typically elicited by history. However, in some instances, the history is unclear or unavailable. This is especially true for multifocal trauma, such as in car accidents, in which patients may not recollect the full extent of injury and multiple concurrent evaluations are typically ongoing. Patients who have had loss of consciousness such as from syncope or seizures also may be unable to tell if they have had spinal injury. Hence, every patient with suspected trauma should be screened neurologically. When spinal cord injury is suspected, the patient should urgently be placed in a hard cervical spine collar until further evaluation by imaging. Missing this simple but critical step can result in progressive cervical spinal cord injury. In patients with preexisting cervical spondylotic changes, relatively moderate accidents such as tripping down the stairs and falling may lead to traumatic spinal cord injury.

When there is no history of trauma, hyperacute evolution of spinal cord injury over minutes to hours is associated with vascular injury. More frequently, vascular injury to the spinal cord is from ischemic stroke. Unlike in the brain in which ischemic strokes are associated with embolism, spinal cord ischemic strokes typically occur from local vasculopathy such as from manipulation of a radicular artery during aortic surgery or occlusion of a radiculo-medullary artery from spinal degenerative disease. Spontaneous spinal cord infarcts can occur in older and younger individuals often with minor preceding risk factors such as heavy lifting or working in the yard. On clinical examination, when the anterior spinal artery is affected, patients have relatively preserved vibratory sense with impaired strength and pinprick sensation (anterior cord syndrome). This clinical pattern in the context of a hyperacute time evolution

strongly suggests spinal cord ischemic stroke. MRI of the spinal cord can show minimal abnormalities initially that then evolve. Cerebrospinal fluid testing typically is noninflammatory. Less frequently, spinal cord vascular injury occurs from hemorrhage usually associated with underlying vascular malformations such as cavernous malformations.

Acute and Subacute Causes of Myelopathy

Myelopathy with acute and subacute time courses is often from inflammatory or toxic causes. For example, transverse myelitis typically presents with an acute or subacute time course. Inflammatory myelopathy is a broad category, and some of the more common causes are discussed in the following:

- Multiple sclerosis is the most common primary autoimmune neurological disorder in the United States. This is a disease that typically causes relapsing and remitting clinical attacks from inflammatory demyelinating lesions in different locations in the brain and spinal cord. Most patients with multiple sclerosis have spinal cord lesions, and many patients with an eventual diagnosis of multiple sclerosis first present with myelitis. Hence, in any patient with myelitis (Fig. 17.5), multiple sclerosis is typically investigated for by obtaining a brain MRI, which can show asymptomatic demyelinating lesions, and cerebrospinal fluid testing, which can show presence of oligoclonal bands indicative of chronic inflammation. Lesions in the spinal cord associated with multiple sclerosis relapses tend to be small and eccentric in location.
- These observations about typical clinical relapses apply to younger patients with inflammatory attacks in the initial years of their disease course. Older adults diagnosed with multiple sclerosis often complain of slow progressive myelopathy such as a gait disorder with bladder dysfunction. Further MRI imaging discloses multiple demyelinating lesions likely present for years and subsequently causing progressive multiple sclerosis. These alternate presentations are both within the clinical spectrum of multiple sclerosis.
- Neuromyelitis optica (NMO): This is an example of antibody-mediated fulminant myelitis. Patients typically present with severe disability from longitudinal spinal cord lesions. NMO is also associated with severe optic neuritis. Antibodies to the water channel Aquaporin-4 are found in about 80% of

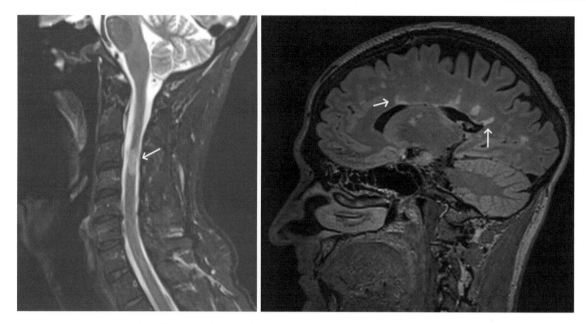

Figure 17.5 Sagittal T2-weighted image (*left*) shows cervical cord hyperintense lesion at C3–C4 level (*arrow*) in a patient with myelitis. Brain magnetic resonance imaging (*right*) shows multiple demyelinating lesions (*arrows*) that were clinically asymptomatic but indicative of diagnosis of multiple sclerosis. (*Original unpublished image.*)

patients with NMO, which can also be comorbid with other autoimmune disorders such as systemic lupus erythematosus or Sjögren syndrome. The diagnosis of NMO is important to distinguish because of multiple newly approved immunomodulatory medications specific to seropositive NMO that are effective in preventing relapses and accrual of disability.

- Transverse myelitis: The term "transverse myelitis" indicates any form of inflammatory myelitis when a more specific cause, such as multiple sclerosis or NMO, is not known. With time and increase in knowledge of specific diseases causing myelitis, transverse myelitis has become a diagnosis of exclusion when no other cause is found after a comprehensive evaluation. The term "transverse" is misleading as well, and patients may have partial myelitis without affecting all the ascending and descending tracts of the spinal cord and yet be called "transverse myelitis." Nonetheless, a significant population of patients with myelitis will have no other potential causes found. Some common antecedent events in patients with transverse myelitis include infections such as

upper respiratory infections or vaccinations. In many cases, what triggers transverse myelitis is unclear, and patients are followed longitudinally for evidence of other chronic, relapsing diseases.

- Infectious myelitis: Infections may injure the spinal cord directly (infectious myelitis) or trigger autoimmune response that causes spinal cord inflammation (postinfectious myelitis). In individual cases of myelitis accompanying infection the disease mechanism can be unclear, though the type of myelitis and accompanying symptoms provide clues. Enteroviruses (D68 and D71), West Nile virus, and flaviviruses are associated with the clinical syndrome of acute flaccid myelitis (flaccid weakness with decreased reflexes). Lyme disease–associated myelitis typically also has accompanying radiculitis (sudden sharp shooting pain in a spinal nerve distribution) or meningitis. Varicella zoster virus myelitis usually follows a clinical episode of shingles marked by radiculitis and dermatomal rash. Bacterial spinal cord abscess is rare but can occur in otherwise immunocompetent individuals and progress rapidly over hours to days.

Chronic Causes of Myelopathy

In contrast to myelopathy that is hyperacute or subacute, more slowly progressive myelopathy has a large heterogenous group of causes. These disease processes include structural changes, metabolic dysfunction, neoplasms, or genetic etiologies. Some of the more common causes are outlined below:

- Cervical spondylotic myelopathy: This is the most common cause of nontraumatic spinal cord injury in the United States. Cervical spondylosis typically occurs from a combination of factors including disc desiccation, disc protrusion, ligamentous laxity, calcification, and joint hypertrophy. These changes result in narrowing of the vertebral canal and radiographic finding of cervical spinal stenosis. An important clinical observation is that many patients with MRI findings of moderate or even severe cervical spinal stenosis are clinically asymptomatic and remain asymptomatic for years. In patients who eventually become symptomatic, they typically complain of numbness/tingling in the hands with decreased dexterity, stiffness of gait, and imbalance. Bladder and bowel sphincter dysfunction are unusual in the early stages of the disease. The lower extremity symptoms are from spinal cord dysfunction, while the hand symptoms are from a combination of myelopathy and cervical radiculopathy. These symptoms in an older adult are often overlooked and can be missed for years. Axial neck pain in cervical spondylotic disease is generally from musculoskeletal causes, and severity of neck pain is not predictive of the presence or absence of myelopathy from spinal cord compression.

- Neurological examination typically shows findings of myelopathy, such as spasticity and increased reflexes in the legs, along with mixed findings of radiculopathy and myelopathy in the arms. If left undiagnosed, cervical spondylotic myelopathy can potentially progress to severe weakness and inability to walk. Hence, in most adults with a new diagnosis of chronic myelopathy, cervical spinal imaging is often the first step (Fig. 17.6). Spondylotic changes in the thoracic spine can occur but are much less frequent compared to the cervical spine.

- Vitamin B12 deficiency: Vitamin B12 is an essential cofactor for multiple enzymatic processes. Deficiency occurs from restrictive diets or from decreased

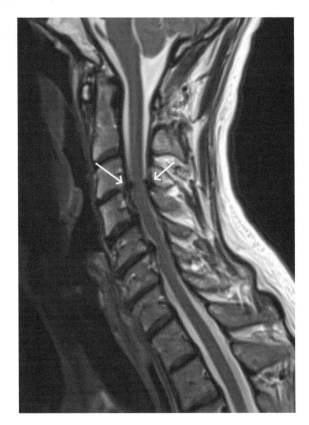

Figure 17.6 Sagittal T2-weighted image showing severe cervical spinal stenosis at C3–C4 level (indicated by *arrows*) in a patient with slow progressive gait disorder. (*Original unpublished image.*)

absorption such as in pernicious anemia (autoimmune gastritis affecting the parietal cells in the stomach) or following gastrointestinal surgery. Vitamin B12 deficiency is associated with the clinical syndrome of subacute combined degeneration. Generally, patients complain initially of paresthesia progressing to sensory ataxia. Clinical examination generally shows spasticity and increased reflexes. Significant weakness is uncommon as is bladder or bowel dysfunction. Diagnosis is made by laboratory testing of blood vitamin B12 level with a value below 200 pg/mL abnormal. Patients may clinically be symptomatic even with low normal levels between 200 and 300 pg/mL. In such patients, serum methylmalonic acid and homocysteine levels are tested. Elevated levels of both these metabolites are indicative of potential vitamin B12 deficiency. In addition to myelopathy, patients also have macrocytic anemia (which can be mild) and cognitive slowing. All three clinical features—myelopathy, anemia, and cognitive slowing—do not have to be present to the same degree in each patient. There is considerable clinical variation.

- Radiation-induced myelopathy: The spinal cord can become injured when exposed to significant degrees of ionizing radiation for treatment of cancer. The risk of spinal cord injury increases with increasing doses of radiation, especially in older protocols used to treat diseases like Hodgkin lymphoma. More recent oncologic radiation protocols strive to minimize exposure of the spinal cord to radiation. Unlike the brain, acute radiation to the spinal cord does not typically cause significant symptoms aside from Lhermitte sign. Over time spanning months to years following radiation, patients can experience slow progressive myelopathy in the radiation field (delayed radiation myelopathy). The diagnosis is primarily made clinically. MRI of the spinal cord may initially be normal or show changes from evolving injury. Similarly, cerebrospinal fluid does not have specific findings to suggest the diagnosis.

- Hereditary spastic paraplegia: This is a large group of genetic disorders marked by slow progressive myelopathy from a genetic source. There are over 70 genes implicated in genetic myelopathies, and inheritance pattern ranges from autosomal dominant to autosomal recessive to X-linked. Patients typically present with slow progressive gait spasticity worsening over years as the primary clinical feature with variable degrees of sensory loss, weakness, and bladder/bowel dysfunction. The age of onset can vary from infancy to late adulthood. Genetic testing panels exist, but many patients are clinically diagnosed with genetic myelopathy without a causative genetic mutation identified on screening panels. Some patients with hereditary spastic paraplegia additionally also have cognitive dysfunction, peripheral neuropathy, optic neuropathy, hearing loss, and other symptoms.

CONCLUSION

Myelopathy is a clinical condition caused by impaired function of the spinal cord. Initial priority should be to rule out traumatic causes or acutely compressive lesions. Myelopathy can be further subdivided based on the acuity of the symptom evolution, and this framework can lead to an appropriate differential diagnosis. In most instances, neuroimaging typically with MRI and possibly cerebrospinal fluid examination, will be necessary to determine the precise cause.

"For the full bibliography list, please use the pincode on the inside front cover to access the electronic version of the text at ebooks. health.elsevier.com."

18

Myopathy*

Orly Moshe-Lilie and Mohammad Kian Salajegheh

INTRODUCTION

Myopathies are a heterogeneous collection of disorders characterized by the abnormal structure or function of skeletal muscle. Such disorders are frequently encountered in primary care practices; however, recognizing and diagnosing these conditions can be challenging. In this review, we will discuss the symptoms and common patterns of weakness that should raise suspicion for an underlying muscle disease in adults and review common red flags that should prompt clinicians to consider referral to a neuromuscular specialist. We also introduce the basic elements of a head-to-toe approach to the neuromuscular examination, discuss differential diagnosis for these conditions, offer a diagnostic framework for early detection and workup, and review treatment plans for myopathies.

PATIENT PRESENTATION

As with most neurologic disorders, the key to diagnosing a myopathy begins with taking a careful and thorough history. Patients often report negative symptoms, such as fatigue, weakness, and loss of muscle bulk, or may endorse positive symptoms, such as muscle pain (myalgia), stiffness, cramps, contractures, or even muscle enlargement (pseudohypertrophy), which can be seen in dystrophinopathies and some limb-girdle muscular dystrophies (LGMD). An important point to remember

is that some of these symptoms are nonspecific and may reflect nonmyopathic conditions, including other neuromuscular disorders (e.g., motor neuron disease and neuromuscular junction disorders); cardiopulmonary, rheumatologic, and orthopedic disorders; medication or toxin effects; deconditioning; and even depression. In contrast, discrete patterns of muscle weakness or atrophy, myotonia or paramyotonia, and recurrent myoglobinuria may be highly suggestive of a form of myopathy. It is worth noting that some nonneuromuscular conditions involving the cardiovascular system (cardiac arrhythmia, early placement of a pacemaker or implantable cardioverter-defibrillator, congestive heart failure), respiratory system (dyspnea on exertion or orthopnea), skin (rash over the face or joints), or eyes (early cataracts or ptosis, without an identifiable cause should trigger suspicion for possible myopathic disorder. Moreover, recognition of classical skin manifestations in dermatomyositis (DM) that may precede muscle weakness can be useful clues in early detection and treatment of this inflammatory myopathy. These include a heliotrope rash (purplish discoloration of the eyelids and associated periorbital edema), Gottron's papules (violaceous lichenoid scaly rash over the extensor surfaces of the hands, fingers, and elbows), "V-sign" or "shawl sign" (describing a macular erythematous rash over the face, neck, anterior chest, or upper back), and "mechanic's hands" (thickened cracked skin over the dorsal and volar aspects of the hands). Dysmorphic features and early cognitive impairment, alongside myopathy, should raise concern for an underlying congenital or other hereditary myopathy such as myotonic dystrophy.

The evaluation of a patient with suspected myopathy should include a discussion of the onset and duration

*Based on Domingo-Horne RM, Salajegheh MK. An approach to myopathy for the primary care clinician. *Am J Med*. 2018; 131(3):237–243. ISSN 0002-9343. https://doi.org/10.1016/j.amjmed.2017.10.016.

of symptoms and the progression over time, including developmental milestones and early childhood history. Certain congenital, metabolic, and mitochondrial myopathies may present at birth or in early childhood, primarily with issues such as failure to thrive, delayed motor milestones, cognitive issues, seizure, ophthalmologic disorders, and contractures. A family history of similar symptoms or confirmed diagnosis of muscle disease and the pattern of inheritance are also key for diagnosing inherited myopathies and focusing on the differential diagnosis, targeted genetic testing, and proper family counseling. Autosomal dominant myopathies include myotonic dystrophy type 1 and 2, LGMD type 1 (or D), facioscapulohumeral muscular dystrophy (FSHD), and oculopharyngeal muscular dystrophy (OPMD). Autosomal recessive myopathies include LGMD type 2 (or R) and metabolic myopathies. X-linked pattern of inheritance would prompt consideration for dystrophinopathies (Duchenne muscular dystrophy and Becker muscular dystrophy) as well as Emery-Dreifuss muscular dystrophy. Maternal (non-Mendelian) inheritance pattern would point to mitochondrial myopathies. Some hereditary myopathies may not present until adolescence or adulthood, and it should be noted that the absence of a positive family history does not exclude the diagnosis of a genetic disorder. Inflammatory myopathies, such as polymyositis and DM, and toxic myopathies may occur at any age, whereas sporadic inclusion body myositis (sIBM) often presents in late adulthood.

A discussion regarding the tempo of symptom, onset or worsening in relationship to other illnesses, potential provoking or exacerbating factors, and initiation or regimen modification of medications may also provide diagnostic clues in evaluating patients with presumed muscle disease. For example, periodic attacks of weakness following a carbohydrate-rich meal may be suggestive of hypokalemic periodic paralysis. Weakness following intense activity or with fasting may raise the possibility of a metabolic myopathy, and onset of weakness after the initiation of a lipid-lowering agent points to the possibility of toxic myopathy from the agent or, rarely, an immune-mediated necrotizing myopathy. It is important to note that the presence of neuropathy should not dissuade clinicians from the diagnosis of myopathy. A patient may have an underlying polyneuropathy (e.g., from diabetes), or the causative factor for myopathy could also lead to neuropathy. Refer to the subsection discussing statins and other toxic myopathies

for common drug-induced presentations. Acquired conditions (vasculitis and amyloidosis) or even inherited conditions (myofibrillar myopathies) may also be included here.

COMMON PATTERNS OF WEAKNESS

It is critical for clinicians to determine the pattern and distribution of deficits in patients who complain of muscle weakness. Ten basic patterns of muscle weakness have been described by Barohn and colleagues and have been taught to countless medical trainees and practicing physicians. Despite broad advancements in specialized testing over the years, the ability of the clinician to recognize and categorize patients by these basic patterns of weakness can greatly improve diagnostic accuracy with more-targeted, ancillary testing.

Fixed weakness of the proximal (limb-girdle) musculature is the most common, and therefore least specific, pattern of weakness in patients with underlying myopathies. Patients with limb-girdle weakness of the upper extremities may describe difficulties in raising their arms up to lift objects overhead, whereas those with proximal weakness of the lower limbs may describe difficulty rising from a chair without pushing off with their arms. The majority of acquired myopathies present with this basic pattern of proximal weakness, whereas hereditary myopathies are a heterogeneous group of disorders with a broader spectrum of clinical presentation of weakness, including predominantly proximal weakness, distal weakness, or both, and even asymmetric weakness (Fig. 18.1).

Distal-predominant weakness can occur in various early- or late-onset distal myopathies, with either anterior or posterior distal leg compartment pattern of weakness. These include anterior tibialis weakness, leading to a dropped foot of later onset as in Udd and Welander distal myopathies, or earlier onset in Nonaka distal myopathy. Gastrocnemius muscle weakness can be present in disorders of early to mid-adulthood such as Miyoshi myopathy, which typically begins with weakness and atrophy of one or both calves, as well as in some anoctaminopathy-5 (ANO-5) related muscle disease. Myotonic dystrophy type 1 and myofibrillar myopathy with cardiomyopathy also present with distal predominance. While in these conditions, the distal predominant weakness may raise the possibility of, or be mistaken for, polyneuropathy, the absence of distal sensory loss is against the latter diagnosis.

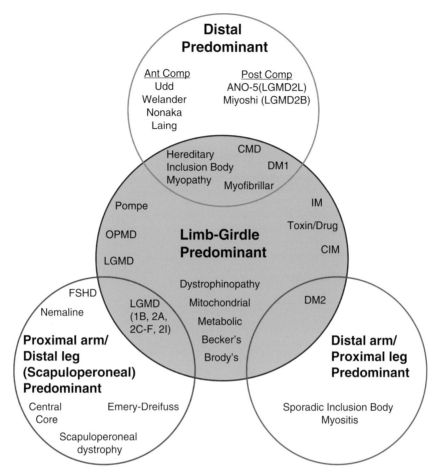

Fig. 18.1 Common patterns of weakness. *ANO-5*, Anoctaminopathy-5; *CIM*, Critical illness myopathy; *CMD*, Congenital muscu-lardystrophy; *DM*, Myotonic dystrophy; *FSHD*, Facioscapulohumeral muscular dystrophy; *IM*, inflammatory myopathies; *LGMD*, limb-girdle muscular dystrophies; *OPMD*, oculopharyngeal muscular dystrophy.

A scapuloperoneal distribution affecting the proximal arms and distal legs may be appreciated in patients with FSHD, scapuloperoneal dystrophy, Emery-Dreyfuss, late-onset acid maltase deficiency (Pompe), and nemaline and other hereditary myopathies and may be associated with additional scapular winging and an asymmetric pattern of limb weakness and atrophy.

The pattern of distal arm and proximal leg weakness is not a common presentation for myopathies but is pathognomonic for sIBM, particularly when asymmetric, and predominantly involving wrist and deep finger flexors and knee extensors while somewhat sparing hip flexors and arm abductors.

Other associated clinical patterns are summarized in Table 18.1. Patients with weakness of the cranial-innervated musculature may present with ptosis, ophthalmoplegia, facial weakness, dysarthria, and dysphagia. Certain combinations of these features should raise concern for the possibility of an underlying myopathy, such as a mitochondrial disorder, congenital myopathies, myotonic dystrophy, or OPMD. Besides myopathy, other neuromuscular conditions need to be considered in patients with these features. These include neuromuscular junction (NMJ) disorders such as myasthenia gravis, in particular if the weakness is fatiguable (worsens and improves with activity

TABLE 18.1   Associated Clinical Patterns

Bulbar	Facial	Neek Extensor (Head Drop)	Cardiac	Respiratory	Stiffness/Inability to relax
Pompe	Ptosis	INEM	LGMD	CMD	Myotonia (improved with exercise)
LGMD	Nemaline	Nemaline (SLONM)	Nemaline	Muscular dystrophy	K-sensitive myotonia
Emery-Dreifuss	CMD (central core)	Inflammatory	Myotonic dystrophy	Myotonic dystrophy	HyperPP
Myotonic dystrophy	Myofibrillar	Hyperparathyroidism	Dystrophinopathy	Metabolic	Myotonic congenita
OPMD	Myotonic dystrophy	Myotonic dystrophy	Emery Dreifuss	Inflammatory	Paramyotonia (worsened by exericse)
Mitochondrial	Ptosis with ophthalmoparesis	Metabolic	Metabolic		Paramyotonia congenita
IBM	Mitochondrial	FSHD	Mitochondrial		Brody disease
Inflammatory	OPMD		Anderse-Tawil		With fixes weakness
	CMD (centronuclear, multicore)		Inflammatory		Myotonic dystrophy
	Without ptosis				Myotonic congenita
	FSHD				

Hereditary Myopathies.
Acquired Myopathies.

CMD, Congenital muscular dystrophy; FSHD, facioscapulohumeral muscular dystrophy; HyperPP, hyperkalemic periodic paralysis; IBM, inclusion body myosis; INEM, isolated neck extensor weakness; LGMD, limb girdle muscular dystrophy; OPMD, oculopharyngeal muscular dystrophy; Pompe, acid maltase deficiency; SLONM, sporadic late-onset nemaline myopathy.

and use, respectively), motor neuron disease (MND) such as amyotrophic lateral sclerosis, in particular if progressive, with asymmetric limb weakness and atrophy alongside upper motor neuron signs (spasticity, increased deep tendon reflexes, exaggerated jaw jerk or positive Babinski sign).

Neck extensor weakness can be due to isolated neck extensor myopathy or may be seen with some acquired myopathies, such as inflammatory myopathies (rare cases of DM, polymyositis, and sIBM), sporadic late-onset nemaline myopathy, hyperparathyroidism, and amyloidosis as well as some hereditary disorders such as FSHD, myotonic dystrophy, and metabolic myopathies (such as primary carnitine deficiency).

Patients who experience muscle stiffness and trouble with muscle relaxation following contraction

(myotonia) or exposure to cold temperature may have a hereditary myopathy affecting muscle ion channels including muscle channelopathies (e.g., myotonia congenita and paramyotonia congenita) or myotonic dystrophy. Episodic weakness, in particular following triggers such as carbohydrate-rich or potassium-rich meals or rest after prolonged exercise, may also be suggestive of muscle channelopathies (e.g., hypokalemic or hyperkalemic periodic paralysis and paramyotonia congenita). Weakness during exercise (exercise intolerance) may be seen with certain metabolic myopathies or mitochondrial disorders, in particular if accompanied by muscle pain or myoglobinuria. In the absence of the latter, particularly with fatiguable weakness of ocular and bulbar muscles, one should consider NMJ disorders in the differential diagnosis.

Readers are encouraged to refer to the listed references, as an exhaustive discussion of muscle disorders is beyond the scope of this review.

RED FLAGS

Early recognition of certain worrisome features should prompt physicians to initiate rapid workup and treatment, as well as consideration for referral to a neuromuscular specialist. Rapid progression of muscle weakness, in particular in the presence of dyspnea and dysphagia, should be considered a neuromuscular emergency and should trigger referral to the emergency department. Determining the etiology of this presentation requires a detailed neuromuscular evaluation as well as targeted diagnostic testing. The possibilities to consider include NMJ disorders (e.g., myasthenic crisis), MND (usually from neurotrophic viruses such as enteroviruses or West Nile virus), Guillain–Barré syndrome and its variants, or acute myopathies (including inflammatory, toxic, and some inherited forms). These conditions may be potentially life-threatening if left unrecognized or when therapy escalation is delayed. The majority of these acute myopathies present with a limb–girdle pattern (symmetric, proximal more than distal weakness), without sensory changes or ophthalmoplegia, allowing for their differentiation from the other listed conditions.

Rapid development of dyspnea should raise concern for early respiratory muscle involvement, interstitial lung disease (ILD), or cardiomyopathy, seen in certain forms of autoimmune and inflammatory myopathies such as antimelanoma differentiation-associated gene 5 (MDA-5) DM, overlap syndromes such as antisynthetase syndrome (with anti-JO-1, PL7, or PL12 antibodies) and necrotizing myopathies (as with antisignal recognition particle antibody). Pronounced skin involvement with milder involvement of skeletal muscles prompts consideration for TIF1-γ subtype of DM. Some of these conditions, in particular with rapid and unintentional weight loss, may be part of a paraneoplastic syndrome and should prompt exploration for underlying malignancy. Another worrisome feature would be the presence of early signs of dysphagia that could accompany some of the listed conditions, presenting with difficulty swallowing pills, coughing when drinking fluids, cutting solid foods into smaller pieces, or the need for prolonged chewing. This should prompt immediate diagnostic evaluation of swallow function and dietary modification to prevent aspiration.

Changes in urine color and generalized myalgia or muscle swelling should raise concerns for rhabdomyolysis and necessitate prompt evaluation of serum electrolytes (for hyperkalemia) and serum muscle enzyme levels (e.g., creatine kinase, CK), with the need for prompt correction of the serum electrolyte imbalance or aggressive hydration to protect the kidneys (usually for CK 10,000 U/L), respectively.

A HEAD-TO-TOE APPROACH

Clinicians often develop their own methods for examination over time, and there is no "right way" to conduct a neurologic assessment, provided that the key components are included in an efficient, focused manner that maximizes diagnostic yield and minimizes patient discomfort. In our practice, we tend to take a head-to-toe approach to strength testing, evaluating for patterns of weakness that may help to narrow down a differential diagnosis of disease or exonerate a primary muscle disorder as a cause for symptoms (Table 18.2). Muscle power can be tested manually or by observation of functional ability in patients who are unable to cooperate with formal examination or in those who demonstrate intermittent voluntary activation on strength testing. It is important for the clinician to grade the strength of cranial-innervated, proximal, and distal limb musculature in a systematic manner so that future intra- and interrater comparative assessments can be considered reliable.

LABORATORY TESTING

The CK level is the most useful initial laboratory study in the evaluation of the patient with suspected myopathy. CK activity is elevated in approximately 70% of patients with DM and in the majority of cases with antisynthetase-associated myositis and immune-mediated necrotizing myositis. Based on diagnostic criteria, it should always be elevated in cases of polymyositis. Notably, CK levels may vary depending on the myositis type, patient demographics, stage of disease, and other systemic conditions, and levels do not always correlate with the severity of clinical weakness.

It is important to recognize that CK may be normal in patients with myopathy (as in those with very

TABLE 18.2 Head-to-Toe Approach to Testing	
Body Segment	**Assessment**
Cranial-innervated musculature	Listen for speech quality and tone/dysarthria Identify ptosis Test eyelid closure strength/ability to bury lashes Inspect eye movements/ophthalmoplegia Test mouth closure/ability to smile/puff out cheeks Ask the patient to whistle/drink from a straw Inspect lateral tongue movements against resistance Test palatal elevation Ask the patient to cough Inspect for facial/tongue fasciculations Inspect for muscle atrophy
Cervical-innervated musculature	Test neck flexion/extension Shoulder abduction/external lateral rotation Look for scapular winging Test arm, wrist, and finger flexion/extension Test finger abduction/adduction Evaluate grip strength and inspect for grip myotonia Inspect use of accessory respiratory muscles Inspection for presence of upper limb fasciculations Inspection for muscle atrophy
Thoracic-innervated musculature	Look for scoliosis or lordosis Ask the patient to sit upright Inspect use of accessory respiratory muscles Inspect for presence of truncal fasciculations Inspect for muscle atrophy
Lumbar-innervated musculature	Ask the patient to stand from a low seat without arms Look for Gower sign Ask the patient to climb 1–2 steps Test hip flexion/extension, abduction/adduction Test knee flexion/extension Test ankle dorsi/plantarflexion, inversion/eversion Inspect gait and ability to walk on toes and heels Inspect for presence of lower limb fasciculations Inspect for muscle atrophy/(pseudo)hypertrophy

slowly progressive conditions such as sIBM, patients with profound muscle atrophy, or those who are on corticosteroid therapy). CK may be elevated in some patients without myopathy (e.g., after heavy physical exertion or in some endocrinopathies such as hypothyroidism). Certain ethnic and demographic groups are also prone to CK levels at the upper end or in excess of normal laboratory ranges without myopathy, including African Americans and military recruits. Laboratory values should therefore be interpreted on an individual basis and correlated clinically. In general, patients with nonspecific symptoms, a normal neurologic examination and needle electromyogram (EMG), and normal to mildly elevated CK levels (up to three times normal) are less likely to have an underlying myopathy. CK isoenzymes testing can be considered to differentiate between muscle and liver pathology, in particular if there is concern for the latter.

It may be beneficial to check aldolase levels in a patient with suspected myopathy but normal CK. In approximately 10% of cases with a predominantly perimysial muscle pathology, such as DM, antisynthetase

TABLE 18.3 Antibodies Found in Myositis

Myositis-Specific Antibodies	Common Presentation
JO-1	DM/PM, ASyS (ILD, polyarthritis, Raynaud's, mechanic's hands)
PL-7, PL-12	DM/PM/CADM, ASyS, or ILD predominant
EJ	DM/PM, ASyS
OJ	DM/PM, ASyS, or ILD predominant
KS	DM/PM, ILD
Mi-2	DM, prominent muscle involvement, nailfold lesions, common in Hispanics
TIF-1γ (anti-p155)	DM/JDM/CADM, prominent skin involvement, cancer associated
MJ (p-140)/NXP-2	DM/JDM/CADM, calcinosis, prominent skin involvement, intestinal vasculopathy
MDA5/CADM-140	DM/CADM, severe ILD, cardiopulmonary syndrome, mucocutaneous ulcerations
SAE	DM, ILD (in Asia)
A-5	DM, dysphagia
SRP	PM, necrotizing myopathy
HMG-CoA reductase	PM, necrotizing myopathy
Myositis-Associated Antibodies	**Common Presentation**
PM-Scl	PM/DM-overlap syndrome
KU	PM/DM-overlap syndrome
RNP	PM/DM-overlap syndrome
Other	**Common Presentation**
Ro52	PM/DM
Ro60	PM/DM
Su/Ago2	PM/DM

ASyS, Antisynthetase syndrome; *CADM*, clinically amyopathic dermatomyositis; *DM*, dermatomyositis; *ILD*, interstitial lung disease; *JDM*, juvenile dermatomyositis; *PM*, polymyositis.
Anti–small ubiquitin–like modifier activating enzyme (A-5); EJ glycyl tRNA synthetase (EJ); 3-hydroxy-3-methylglutaryl coenzyme A (HMG-CoA); Jo-1 histidyl tRNA synthetase (JO-1); KS asparaginyl tRNA synthetase (KS); MJ/NXP-2 nuclear matrix protein 2 (NXP-2); melanoma differentiation-associated gene 5 (MDA5); OJ isoleucyl tRNA synthetase (OJ); PL-7 threonyl tRNA synthetase (PL-7); PL-12 alanyl tRNA synthetase (PL-12); signal recognition particle (SRP); TIF1γ transcription intermediary factor (TIF1γ).

syndrome, and mixed connective tissue disease, aldolase elevation may be seen despite normal CK levels. It is worth remembering that, among its three isoenzymes, while aldolase A is predominantly present in muscles, aldolase B and C are present in other tissues, including liver and brain. Elevated aspartate aminotransferase and alanine aminotransferase levels may also be seen in the context of muscle disease; however, they are not specific markers, and in particular, if accompanied by an elevated gamma glutamic transferase, the source is liver rather than muscle. A less helpful enzyme is lactate dehydrogenase, which, while elevated in the presence of dermatomyositis and other muscle disease, could also be seen in the context of damage to other tissue, requiring testing for its various isoenzymes to determine the source.

Myositis-specific autoantibodies (MSAs), which are defined as autoantibodies that are found exclusively in patients with autoimmune myopathies, have gained more importance over the years for the diagnosis of various forms of myositis (Table 18.3). Some MSAs are associated with a unique clinical phenotype, and in some cases, their presence alongside the expected phenotype may negate the need for a muscle biopsy for diagnosis. Myositis-associated autoantibodies may also be found in DM, polymyositis (PM), and/or overlap syndromes (Table 18.3); however, they are not specific for myositis or these specific disorders. Their presence is suggestive of muscle involvement in the setting of systemic lupus erythematous, scleroderma/systemic sclerosis, Sjögren syndrome, and other systemic autoimmune rheumatic diseases.

Additional laboratory studies that could be considered in the evaluation of patients with myopathy to identify underlying conditions leading to weakness or myopathy include serum electrolytes, thyroid function tests, inflammatory markers (ESR and CRP), rheumatologic markers (ANA, RF, CCP, SSA/SSB), HIV testing, parathyroid hormone test, and urinalysis.

When suspicion for a metabolic or mitochondrial myopathy exists and other than genetic testing and/or muscle biopsy biohistochemical studies discussed below, one could consider testing for resting serum lactate and pyruvate levels and calculated lactate-pyruvate ratio, serum and/or urine amino acids levels, carnitine profile and acyl-carnitine levels, fibroblast growth factor 21 (FGF-21), or growth differentiation factor 15 (GDF-15), depending on clinical suspicion for the type of metabolic myopathy. The forearm nonischemic exercise stress test could also be helpful in the diagnosis of some forms of glycogen storage disease, in which one would see elevation of serum ammonia levels, post exercise, without an accompanying rise in serum lactate levels.

A SPECIAL WORD ON STATINS AND OTHER TOXIC MYOPATHIES

Certain medications are known to cause CK elevations and lead to the development of iatrogenic toxic myopathies. Perhaps most recognized among these myotoxic medications are the HMG-CoA reductase inhibitors (statins) and other lipid-lowering agents. The development of a toxic myopathy in the setting of statin use has been well described in the literature and may include the development of myalgias, CK elevations, muscle weakness, and even rhabdomyolysis (which can, in rare instances, be fatal). Generally, these symptoms are relatively mild and will reverse with discontinuation of the offending agent. In patients without rhabdomyolysis and after the symptoms of myopathy have resolved, a rechallenge with a less myotoxic statin can be successful. A small subgroup of patients exposed to statins, however, may go on to develop anti–HMG-CoA receptor (HMGCR) immune-mediated necrotizing myopathy (IMNM), requiring immunomodulatory or immunosuppressive therapy. While rare, this condition must be considered and more fully evaluated (by muscle biopsy or antibody testing) when a patient's CK elevation and/or muscle weakness does not improve (or even worsens) after discontinuation of the statin. It should be noted that not all patients with anti-HMGCR IMNM have prior exposure to statin drugs, and while these patients are generally younger, their overall clinical presentation is similar to the classic phenotype. While also rare, it would be important to exclude an underlying malignancy in older patients with anti-HMGCR IMNM, irrespective of their exposure to statins, by obtaining a CT scan of the chest, abdomen, and pelvis and other age-appropriate cancer screening.

Certain drugs may cause a toxic myopathy along with neuropathy, leading to "neuromyopathy," such as amphiphilic drugs (chloroquine, hydroxychloroquine, and amiodarone) and antimicrotubular drugs (colchicine and vincristine), presenting with muscle weakness and concomitant sensorimotor neuropathy, or retroviral agents (zidovudine and others), leading to development of painful sensory neuropathy in additional to proximal muscle weakness. Common presentations of toxic myopathies associated with certain medications are summarized in Table 18.4. Alcohol could lead to chronic polyneuropathy with extended use as well as myopathy from its chronic effects or even acutely following binge drinking.

GENETIC TESTING

Genetic testing is key for the definitive diagnosis of hereditary myopathies. Historically, the most cost-effective way to order these tests has been the combined use of clinical and electrodiagnostic features as well as muscle biopsy findings to determine the gene(s) to be targeted for testing. With the advent of next-generation sequencing becoming more affordable and available, a greater number of genes can be tested concurrently within panels. The downside to this has been the increased chance of identifying variants of uncertain significance (VUS), which may pose a challenge in determining their pathogenicity and relationship to the patient's presentation and using it for reaching a definitive diagnosis. Referral to a neuromuscular specialist may help to avoid sending unnecessary tests and help in determining the clinic significance of these VUSs.

ELECTRODIAGNOSTIC TESTING

An EMG should be considered in all patients with suspected myopathy. Nerve conduction studies are typically normal in cases of myopathy; however, they are useful in

TABLE 18.4	Toxic Myopathies
Common Presentation	Drugs
Necrotizing myopathy	Statins, other cholesterol-lowering Cyclosporine Propofol Labetalol Alcohol
Inflammatory myopathy	Immune checkpoint inhibitors Tyrosine kinase inhibitors (Imatinib) Phenytoin Interferon alpha Tumor necrosis factor inhibitors Cimetidine Hydroxyurea D-Penicillamine
Amphiphilic myopathy	Amiodarone Chloroquine, hydroxychloroquine
Necrotizing myopathy	Colchicine Vincristine
Mitochondrial myopathy	Zidovudine, other antiretrovirals
Hypokalemic myopathy	Omeprazole Diuretics Laxative Toluene Alcohol abuse Corticosteroids
Critical illness myopathy	Nondepolarizing neuromuscular depolarizing agents Corticosteroids

that they can exclude a coexisting or mimicking neuromuscular condition, such as a neuropathy, a motor neuron disease, or a disorder of neuromuscular junction transmission. Findings on needle electromyogram examination include the presence of increased spontaneous activity as evident by fibrillation potentials and positive sharp waves, suggestive of muscle membrane irritability that can be seen with active inflammatory or toxic myopathies and some hereditary myopathies. Low-amplitude, short-duration, polyphasic motor unit action potentials with early recruitment, called myopathic units, are suggestive of myopathies. Needle EMG testing may also demonstrate myotonic discharges, which would be supportive of the clinical diagnosis of a myotonic disorder. In the absence of the latter, one

should remember that these discharges may be seen with other neuromuscular conditions and with use of certain medications. Needle EMG can also be used to determine which muscles are best suited for biopsy, if indicated, in particular in the absence of objective findings of muscle weakness on exam. Motor neuron disease, which in certain cases can mimic myopathy, can also be tested for and excluded by a needle electrode examination. It should be noted that a normal EMG does not exclude the presence of myopathy, as the study may be normal in certain patients.

MUSCLE BIOPSY

Muscle biopsy has been thought of as the cornerstone for diagnosing myopathies. Other than in cases where the etiology is clear from the initial evaluation (presence of a myotoxic agent or hyperthyroidism), hereditary with genetic confirmation, or inflammatory myopathies with a positive MSA correlating with the phenotype, a muscle biopsy may be necessary. In addition to determining the presence of an inflammatory myopathy, it may, in some cases, demonstrate features helpful in the diagnosis of specific hereditary forms, in particular when genetic testing has reported a variant of unknown significance, or the genotype and phenotype do not clearly match. Examples of stains and histochemical studies routinely performed include, but not limited to, hematoxylin and eosin stains that form the basis of analysis; modified Gomori trichome stain that best shows ragged red fibers in mitochondrial diseases or some inclusions; nicotinamide adenine dinucleotide dehydrogenase stain, to differentiate oxidative and nonoxidative fibers and helpful in showing myofibrillar architecture and target fibers; cytochrome c oxidase and succinate dehydrogenase stains, which distinguish positive-staining (brown) fibers, with normal mitochondrial activity, from the abnormally negative-staining (blue) fibers without mitochondrial activity; and periodic acid–Schiff stains, which are useful in the diagnosis of glycogen storage disease. Spectrophotometric enzyme assays can also be useful in investigating for mitochondrial myopathies, looking for reduced activities of individual respiratory chain complexes. Neuromuscular specialists can assist in guiding surgeons and neuropathologists prior to biopsy, in regard to both the most appropriate sites for biopsy and any special preparations, stains, or techniques that may be needed for a specific histologic diagnosis.

MUSCLE IMAGING

Imaging of skeletal muscles can be helpful in identifying patterns of involvement, optimal muscle to biopsy, signs of muscle edema or fatty infiltration and muscle atrophy. These are best appreciated by ordering T1-weighted images as well as fat-suppressed T2-weighted or short-tau inversion–recovery (STIR) images. These findings, however, are not specific for an underlying cause and can be seen with both acquired and inherited myopathies. It should also be noted that the presence of muscle edema may be seen with muscle injury or an active neurogenic process and is not necessarily indicative of an inflammatory myopathy.

BASIC PRINCIPLES OF TREATMENT

In general, supportive therapy is key in the management of most hereditary and acquired myopathies. This includes appropriate referrals to occupational and physical therapy for exercise and rehabilitation, mobility aids, and adaptive equipment; prosthetics for appropriate orthotic devices); dietetics/nutritional experts for dietary support to help with weight gains or losses, or dietary modifications for some metabolic myopathies; speech and swallow therapy, otolaryngologists, and/or gastroenterologists in cases of dysphagia; orthopedic spine surgeons (in severe cases of kyphoscoliosis or lumbar hyperlordosis, ankle and foot deformities, tendinopathies, and scapular winging; endocrinologists, cardiologists, pulmonologists, rheumatologists, and respiratory therapists based on the presence of, or suspicion for, endocrines issues (e.g., in myotonic dystrophy), heart failure or arrhythmias, dyspnea and diaphragmatic weakness, interstitial lung disease, or connective tissue disorders. Providers should also consider referring their patients to a sleep specialist for evaluation for sleep-related breathing disorders such as obstructive sleep apnea, seen in many myopathy patients, and REM sleep disorders associated with some hereditary myopathies, including dystrophinopathies, myotonic muscular dystrophies, FSHD, spinal muscular atrophy, and metabolic and mitochondrial myopathies.

In general, if considering an exercise program after diagnosing a patient with a specific type of myopathy, a provider should first identify whether there is cardiac and/or pulmonary involvement and obtain specialist consultation and clearance prior to exercise initiation if needed. Recommendations should first be for no more than a low-intensity program, following a baseline strength evaluation, with periodic follow-up examinations for surveillance monitoring. Low levels of aerobic exercises have demonstrated significant improvements in maximal oxygen uptake, isometric force, and functional scores in inflammatory myositis patients as well as FSHD, LGMD, Becker muscular dystrophy, and myotonic dystrophy. There is insufficient evidence to determine the effects of short- or long-term high-intensity aerobic exercise in these populations, and in theory, high-intensity aerobic exercise may increase the risk of muscular damage. Resistive exercises, designed to build muscles and improve strength through repetitive contractions against a resistive force (utilizing resistive bands, dumbbells, etc.), have been shown to be well tolerated and to improve peak torque in patients with chronic myositis other than sIBM (for which the results were mixed). Physical therapists often encourage aquatic therapy for patients with myopathy, as water buoyancy may assist with exercise mobility; however, further investigation is needed, and safety may be a concern in patients with notable weakness. Recommendations for passive stretching and/or positioning (utilizing splinting) by providers and physical therapies should be made on an individual basis in cases involving soft-tissue contractures, as there is no firm evidence that doing so would improve range of motion or preserve function in all cases.

Currently, there are no effective cures or disease-modifying treatments for most hereditary myopathies in adults. One exception is an enzyme replacement therapy with alglucosidase alfa, first approved by the FDA in 2006 for infantile-onset Pompe disease (also known as acid-maltase deficiency, GSD II). In 2010, the FDA approved a similar alglucosidase alfa therapy for late-onset Pompe patients, after the Late Onset Treatment Study, a randomized double-blind, placebo-controlled trial, demonstrated improvements in the 6-minute walk tests and percent predicted forced vital capacity in the treatment group. For other metabolic disorders, dietary modifications and/or oral supplementations are generally utilized, such as high-protein diet or oral galactose for some patients with impaired carbohydrate metabolism; carbohydrate-rich diet and replacement of long-chain fatty acids by medium-chain fatty acids for patients with impaired lipid/fat metabolism; NS coenzyme-Q 10, carnitine, and other supplements in some mitochondrial disorders, with partial positive effective.

Some patients with Duchenne muscular dystrophy who have a certain genetic mutation may be candidates for exon-skipping therapies aiming to slow the progression of or stabilize the disease. Exciting strategies are underway aiming to treat the disease, such as gene repair or replacement or therapies aiming to restore the production of a different but functional version of dystrophin.

For most inflammatory and autoimmune myopathies, immunosuppressive or immunomodulatory therapy remains the treatment of choice. First-line therapies that are used for inflammatory myopathies include oral prednisone alone or in combination with second-line immunosuppressive drugs such as methotrexate or azathioprine if weakness does not resolve or if it worsens upon attempts at steroid taper. Intravenous immunoglobulin has been approved by the FDA as first-line agent in DM and appears to be an effective agent in statin-induced IMNM. It is also a well-accepted second-line agent for most other disorders, alongside mycophenolate mofetil, cyclosporine, and tacrolimus (in particular in cases of ILD). Rituximab and cyclophosphamide are considered third-line agents in most refractory cases and/or in those with ILD. Methotrexate should be avoided if ILD is suspected, as it may cause pulmonary toxicity leading to pulmonary fibrosis and worsening of the lung involvement. Autoimmune necrotizing myopathies, however, may be resistant to single-agent immunosuppression therapy, requiring chronic immunosuppression with multiple agents.

Currently, there are no proven treatments to delay or stop progression of weakness in sIBM, an acquired disorder that inevitably leads to significant disability. However, there are ongoing investigative efforts to develop some form of treatment for sIBM. A 2-year extended clinical trial for patients with sIBM demonstrated safety and well-tolerability of long-term treatment with bimagrumab (a human monoclonal antibody developed to treat pathologic muscle loss and weakness); however, it failed to meet its primary endpoint, as patients did not demonstrate meaningful functional benefit. A study published by Greenberg and colleagues demonstrated the presence and persistence of highly differentiated muscle-infiltrating cytotoxic T cells in patients with inclusion body myositis (IBM). The authors highlighted the potential limitations of previous treatment strategies that have shown limited efficacy, such as those involving broad, nonselective lymphocyte depletion, and pointed to the potential value of targeting the highly differentiated cytotoxic T-cell population as a potential favorable approach to treatment of IBM in the future.

In cases of toxic myopathies, removing the offending agent usually leads to clinical improvement, and patients may require only supportive therapy until they recover unless the patient has gone on to develop a statin-induced IMNM with treatment outlined previously.

CONCLUSIONS

Patients who present with myopathies are encountered frequently in primary care practices. Although myopathic disorders may be diagnostically challenging, it is important for the general medical practitioner to have a high level of suspicion for an underlying disorder of muscle, to recognize common patterns of weakness, generate a basic differential diagnosis, initiate an appropriate workup, and recognize when to refer patients for specialized testing and neuromuscular evaluation. It is also very important to take notice of red flags and to plan emergent assessment and therapy when they are encountered.

"For the full bibliography list, please use the pincode on the inside front cover to access the electronic version of the text at ebooks.health.elsevier.com."

19

Approach to the Diagnosis and Management of Peripheral Neuropathy*

Christopher T. Doughty and Reza Sadjadi

INTRODUCTION

Peripheral neuropathy is among the most common neurologic problems encountered by primary care clinicians, as it affects up to 8% of adults over the age of 55. Despite its frequency, however, peripheral neuropathy can be challenging to recognize and evaluate because of its many diverse forms and presentations. Distal symmetric polyneuropathy (DSP) is the most common form and is often encountered in the primary care setting as the most common systemic complication of diabetes mellitus.

The clinical presentation of neuropathy can include weakness, sensory abnormalities, and autonomic dysfunction. Accordingly, the primary care clinician must be comfortable using the neurologic examination—including assessment of motor function, multiple sensory modalities, and the deep tendon reflexes—to recognize and characterize neuropathy. Although the causes of peripheral neuropathy are numerous and diverse, careful review of the medical and family history coupled with limited, select laboratory testing can often efficiently lead to an etiologic diagnosis.

One-quarter to one-half of patients will remain idiopathic even after thorough workup, and at least one-fifth of patients will carry two or more risk factors. Therefore sound clinical reasoning is required in deciding how far to direct a workup in newly diagnosed

patients. Moreover, the recommended testing can vary dramatically for other phenotypes of neuropathy (e.g., mononeuropathy multiplex). It is essential that one's clinical approach to evaluating a patient with suspected neuropathy can identify these divergent patterns. In this chapter, we focus largely on the presentation and evaluation of DSP, but we also offer suggestions for recognizing and evaluating other presentations.

Disease-modifying therapies for neuropathy are limited at present. Most patients still benefit from counseling on lifestyle changes that can help them to avoid foot injuries and ulcerations and prevent falls. Many patients also require symptomatic treatment for neuropathic pain, including such options as gabapentinoids, tricyclic antidepressants, serotonin-norepinephrine reuptake inhibitors, and sodium-channel blocking anticonvulsants.

CLINICAL PRESENTATION

Peripheral nerves consist of sensory, motor, and autonomic fibers. There are accordingly numerous complaints that can prompt the clinician to consider neuropathy (Table 19.1). Patients usually present with sensory signs or symptoms before motor or autonomic symptoms prevail. Sensory nerve fibers can be broadly divided into large-diameter fibers that mediate vibratory sensation and proprioception and small-diameter fibers that mediate pain and temperature sensation. Symptoms of neuropathy will vary based on the relative involvement of large fibers and small fibers; most, but not all, neuropathies affect both fiber types, often resulting in both negative (i.e., loss of sensation) and positive symptoms (e.g., pain, tingling). Neuropathic pain occurs in one-third of patients with peripheral neuropathy. Positive sensory

*Based on Doughty CT, Seyedsadjadi R. Approach to peripheral neuropathy for the primary care clinician. *Am J Med*. 2018;131(9):1010–1016. ISSN 0002-9343. https://doi.org/10.1016/j.amjmed.2017.12.042.

TABLE 19.1	Symptoms and Signs of Neuropathy	
	Symptoms	**Signs on Examination**
Motor	WeaknessCramps	Weakness Atrophy Fasciculations Areflexia
Large fiber sensory	Numbness Imbalance, falls Ataxia Paresthesias	Loss of vibratory sensation and/or proprioception Pseudoathetosis Sensory ataxia Areflexia
Small fiber sensory	Numbness Pain	Loss of pain and/ or temperature sensation
Autonomic	Postural dizziness Dry mouth, dry eyes, dry skin Early satiety Coldness or flushing Impotence Bladder dysfunction	Orthostatic hypotension Skin changes Loss of hair Hyperemia or cold, pale feet

symptoms include paresthesias—described as tingling, pins and needles, or feeling as if a limb is "asleep"—and dysesthesia—described as stabbing, bee stinging, burning, or sharp shooting sensations. Some patients will describe hyperesthesia, an accentuated sensation of tactile stimulation, or allodynia, the perception of normally nonpainful stimuli as painful. Patients with allodynia may describe intolerance to bedsheets overlying their feet or pain brought on by the breeze from a window fan. Patients with neuropathic pain often report that the pain is worst at night when they are trying to fall asleep. By contrast, pain on the soles of the feet that is worst with the first steps out of bed in the morning should prompt consideration of plantar fasciitis, an important entity in the differential diagnosis of painful neuropathy.

While patients do not often complain about negative sensory symptoms, it is important to recognize imbalance due to sensory loss and evaluate fall risk. On average, an increase in falls can be detected in patients with peripheral neuropathy 3 years before diagnosis. Patients usually cannot differentiate between motor and sensory symptoms

when they describe gait dysfunction. It is not uncommon for patients to describe weakness when, in fact, a loss of proprioception is the primary deficit responsible.

Autonomic symptoms are often underrecognized but are common and can have a great impact on quality of life. The most common autonomic symptoms include manifestations of sweating and vasomotor dysfunction, such as coldness, burning, or flushing in the feet. Dry mouth, dry eyes, and dry skin are also common. Orthostatic intolerance, gastroparesis, constipation, diarrhea, neurogenic bladder, and sexual dysfunction can all occur and can be associated with disability and reduced quality of life. However, these are all potential targets for symptom management. Patients do not often intuitively connect these symptoms with their neuropathy, so asking about and identifying these symptoms proactively is critical. This will provide an opportunity to intervene and improve patients' quality of life.

Rarely, autonomic symptoms may be the most prominent or only symptoms indicating neuropathy (Table 19.2). This narrows the differential diagnosis of the underlying cause somewhat. Autonomic neuropathy is particularly common in patients with polyneuropathy associated with diabetes and can occur independently from sensorimotor neuropathy. Patients may occasionally present with pure parasympathetic failure, leading to vagal denervation of the heart with a resultant rise in resting heart rate and loss of heart rate variability or even exercise intolerance. Autonomic dysfunction in diabetic patients has been consistently associated with an increased risk of mortality; patients are at risk for arrhythmia, left ventricular dysfunction, and silent myocardial infarction.

In taking a history from a patient, delineating the pace of progression is critical. When symptoms of neuropathy develop acutely, over days to a few weeks, the differential diagnosis is narrowed significantly (Table 19.2). Hyperacute onset of symptoms (e.g., sudden wrist drop) in the absence of compression or trauma raises concern for a vasculitic process and merits urgent evaluation. Conversely, patients may not recognize long-standing symptoms or signs as being related to their presenting complaint. Asking about childhood clumsiness or poor athleticism, high arches, or ill-fitting shoes may reveal unrecognized signs of a chronic and perhaps hereditary neuropathy.

Cervical myelopathy and lumbosacral radiculopathy/lumbar spinal stenosis are two important considerations in the differential diagnosis of patients presenting with numbness, weakness, and/or gait dysfunction. The presence of neck pain, low back pain, radiating limb pain, and/or significant bowel or bladder dysfunction should prompt consideration of these alternatives, as these would be atypical of distal symmetric polyneuropathy.

EXAMINING PATIENTS WITH SUSPECTED NEUROPATHY

Characterizing the Distribution of the Neuropathy

The examination of patients with symptoms that are concerning for peripheral neuropathy should focus on defining the anatomic distribution of findings and the extent of motor signs, sensory impairment, and absence of reflexes. The differential diagnosis for the causative process will vary based on these classifications. In a length-dependent process such as DSP, there is diffuse involvement of multiple nerves with symptoms and signs affecting the most distal segments first. This leads to the so-called stocking/glove distribution of findings. Symptoms or signs in the legs usually reach the knees or just above before symptoms or signs occur in the fingers. A non–length-dependent pattern and/or asymmetry may indicate a secondary process for which the differential diagnosis is different and the required workup changes.

Other common patterns include mononeuropathy, such as median neuropathy at the wrist (i.e., carpal tunnel syndrome), and radiculopathy, which is commonly caused by degenerative disease in the cervical or lumbosacral spine. Signs and symptoms will be restricted to the distribution of a single nerve, myotome, or dermatome in such cases.

The presence of multiple concurrent mononeuropathies—termed mononeuropathy multiplex—may suggest a vasculitic etiology (Table 19.2). This can be seen in diabetes or systemic vasculitis, but sometimes patients develop peripheral nervous system vasculitis in isolation or before systemic involvement is evident. Other nonvasculitic acquired conditions (e.g., amyloidosis) or inherited conditions (e.g., hereditary neuropathy with liability to pressure palsies) can cause mononeuropathy multiplex, but due to the relatively rapid and progressive course and potentially irreversible neurologic disability, it is important to suspect and investigate for a vasculitic process early on. Usually, patients present with rather acute onset of pain in a single peripheral nerve or nerve root distribution followed

TABLE 19.2 Etiologic Clues in Peripheral Neuropathy

Differential for Autonomic Neuropathy	Differential for Acute Neuropathy
Diabetes mellitus	Guillain-Barré
Amyloidosis	syndrome
Autoimmune autonomic	Vasculitis
neuropathy	Critical illness
Paraneoplastic neuropathy	polyneuropathy
Vitamin B_{12} deficiency	Porphyria
HIV	Toxic exposure
Sjögren syndrome	Nutritional deficiency
Prior chemotherapy	(e.g., thiamine)
Heavy metal toxicity	
Hereditary neuropathies	

Differential for Mononeuropathy Multiplex	Differential for Motor-Predominant Neuropathy
Vasculitis	Chronic inflammatory
Amyloidosis	demyelinating polyne
Diabetes mellitus	uropathy (CIDP)
Multifocal acquired	Multifocal motor
demyelinating sensory	neuropathy (MMN)
and motor neuropathy	Hereditary neuropathy
(MADSAM)	(Charcot-Marie-Tooth
MMN	disease)
Hepatitis B and C	Paraneoplastic
Lyme disease	neuropathy
Leprosy	Lead toxicity
Compressive/traumatic	Porphyria
neuropathies	Diphtheria
Hereditary neuropathy with	
liability to pressure	
palsies	
(HNPP)	

by weakness shortly afterwards. If multiple nerves become affected over time, symptoms and exam findings become more confluent and can be challenging to distinguish from a length-dependent polyneuropathy. Even in such cases, a subacute onset, slight asymmetry of exam findings, and/or subtle non–length-dependent findings can serve as a clue and should not be ignored.

Modalities to Examine

In a patient with suspected neuropathy, examination should at least include assessment of motor function, sensory function, and the deep tendon reflexes. In

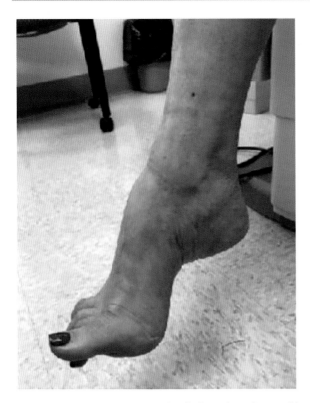

Fig. 19.1 Common lower-extremity findings in patients with hereditary neuropathy. High-arched feet (pes cavus), hammertoes, and atrophy of the distal calf—all evident in this patient with neuropathy—are common in patients with Charcot-Marie-Tooth disease (CMT). Hereditary neuropathy is an important, common, and underrecognized consideration in patients presenting with distal symmetric polyneuropathy. Patients present with disproportionately more weakness and atrophy relative to the degree of sensory involvement. CMT is the most common form of hereditary neuropathy. (From Doughty CT, Seyedsadjadi R. Approach to peripheral neuropathy for the primary care clinician. Am J Med. 2018;131(9):1010–1016.)

addition to testing for specific muscle weakness, the motor examination should also identify the presence of muscle atrophy that can be seen in chronic neuropathy affecting motor fibers. Distal calf and extensor digitorum brevis muscle atrophy, hammertoes, and pes cavus (high-arched feet) are characteristics of a longstanding neuropathy, often seen in hereditary neuropathies (Figure 19.1). When motor deficits are comparable to or greater than sensory deficits, demyelinating disorders such as chronic inflammatory demyelinating polyneuropathy (CIDP) or hereditary neuropathies

must be considered (Table 19.2). CIDP should also be considered if non–length-dependent motor or sensory deficits are identified, such as prominent proximal weakness.

The sensory examination should test both large fiber modalities (vibration and/or proprioception) and small fiber modalities (pain and/or temperature). Proprioceptive deficits can manifest as sensory ataxia, mimicking cerebellar dysfunction. The Romberg sign is an effective screening tool for sensory ataxia. The patient stands with their feet directly together and then closes their eyes; the patient must rely on sensory information alone to maintain balance. If the patient is steady with eyes open but sways and takes a step to steady themselves with eyes closed, the test is positive.

Deep tendon reflexes may be diminished in a length-dependent pattern, with unobtainable ankle reflexes. Diffuse areflexia should prompt investigation for CIDP or hereditary neuropathy. Asymmetric reflexes—for example, if only one ankle reflex is absent—may suggest a superimposed mononeuropathy or radiculopathy. Accentuated deep tendon reflexes or extensor plantar responses are not seen in neuropathy; this finding would instead suggest a central nervous system disorder such as cervical myelopathy or vitamin B_{12} deficiency.

Isolated small fiber neuropathy is less common than typical DSP. Pain and allodynia are particularly common in patients with small fiber neuropathy. However, the only detectable exam abnormalities will be loss of pain and/or temperature sensation. Large fiber function will be normal, and reflexes will be preserved.

Screening for Neuropathy in Asymptomatic Patients

History alone may be insufficient to exclude a neuropathy in high-risk patients, such as those with diabetes. Many patients have only mild negative symptoms that go unnoticed but still put them at risk for injuries or foot ulcers. The lifetime risk of foot ulcers in patients with diabetic neuropathy, for example, is 15%–25%. The American Diabetes Association recommends that patients with diabetes be screened for signs of neuropathy annually. The highest yield bedside screening tests for large fiber sensory dysfunction are use of a 10-g Semmes-Weinstein monofilament or testing vibratory sensation with a 128-Hz tuning fork. The monofilament is pressed against the skin and designed to buckle when

10-g of force is applied, allowing for a consistent and quantifiable stimulus. Single modality testing can miss up to 25%–50% of patients with diabetic neuropathy, however. The combination of both tests is about 90% sensitive and 85%–89% specific for peripheral neuropathy in diabetic patients. Testing of pinprick sensation should also be considered, as such patients with isolated small fiber neuropathy will not be identified if only monofilament and vibratory sensation testing are carried out.

Finally, it is important to note that some aspects of the neurologic examination are expected to change with normal aging. In particular, many older adults will have reduced vibration sense in the toes and reduced or absent Achilles tendon reflexes. These patients often have no symptoms of neuropathy and no signs of neuropathy on electrodiagnostic testing. This emphasizes that these screening tests on examination are only the beginning of the diagnostic process; the findings still need to be put into the context of the patient's history and eventual workup.

IDENTIFYING A PHENOTYPE

After a history has been taken and the suggested neurologic examination has been performed, the information that was gathered can be used holistically to (1) ensure that peripheral neuropathy remains the most likely diagnostic category and (2) classify a specific phenotype for the neuropathy. Realistically, a trained neurologist may be best suited for this exercise. However, careful attention from a primary care provider can go a long way toward triaging those cases that truly require the expertise of a neurologist. When the history and examination reveal symmetric, length-dependent signs and symptoms suggesting DSP, the differential diagnosis includes either lumbosacral radiculopathy or myelopathy (process affecting the spinal cord). We have already provided some pearls in the history of exam that can identify these mimics. Low back pain, pain radiating into the legs, or bladder or bowel dysfunction may suggest radiculopathy. Hyperreflexia, spasticity, or sensory deficits in the trunk occur in myelopathy.

When it comes to classifying a neuropathy phenotype, a simple paradigm utilizing just four questions can be used:
1. What is the time course?
2. Are symptoms and signs on examination symmetric?
3. Are symptoms and signs on examination length-dependent?
4. Which modalities (e.g., motor, large fiber sensory, small fiber sensory, autonomic) are involved?

DSP is a chronic process leading to symmetric, length-dependent, sensory-predominant (large and small fiber) deficits. This pattern can be readily identified in the primary care setting. Our tips for diagnosis and management that follow will largely focus on this phenotype. If the answers to any of these questions deviate from the prototype of DSP, then the workup and management may need to change. This is where involvement of a neurologist, or at the very least some additional diagnostic testing (usually nerve conduction studies and/or electromyography), can be of higher yield.

DIAGNOSING NEUROPATHY

Symptoms alone (e.g., burning feet) have poor diagnostic accuracy for neuropathy. Neurologic examination findings such as distal sensory loss or absent ankle jerks are more sensitive and specific. In one cohort, the presence of two out of three suggestive symptoms, abnormal temperature sensation, or diminished ankle reflexes was 87% sensitive and 91% specific for neuropathy. Neuroimaging is not routinely indicated in patients with neuropathy. Spinal imaging, however, should be considered when the neurologic examination suggests a concurrent myelopathy or when the diagnosis of neuropathy is not firmly established and lumbosacral radiculopathy remains in the differential diagnosis.

The most reliable diagnosis of neuropathy rests on the combination of symptoms, the neurologic exam, and confirmatory findings on nerve conduction studies and electromyography. It is debatable whether all patients with suspected neuropathy require electrodiagnostic evaluation (EDX). This does not occur in current clinical practice; a study utilizing a database of Medicare patients demonstrated that only 20% underwent EDX within 6 months of their initial diagnosis of neuropathy. If multiple symptoms and exam findings suggest DSP, EDX may indeed be low yield. In a sample of patients over age 65 with a high prevalence of diabetes, for example, EDX led to a change in diagnosis or management in <1% of patients. By contrast, in samples of patients referred to academic medical centers for evaluation of neuropathy, EDX led to a change in diagnosis in 24%–43% of patients.

BOX 19.1   **Symptoms and Exam Findings That Should Prompt Electrodiagnostic Studies and/or Neurologic Consultation**

Acute onset
Asymmetry
Non–length-dependent weakness and/or sensory loss
Diffuse areflexia
Pure or predominant motor symptoms
Pure or predominant autonomic symptoms
Mononeuropathy multiplex

Guidelines put forward by the American Association of Neuromuscular and Electrodiagnostic Medicine state that EDX is likely to be low yield in those patients in whom symptoms and physical exam findings are mild, the findings are symmetric and both distal- and sensory predominant, there is little suspicion of a coexisting nerve disorder (e.g., carpal tunnel syndrome), and there is a known cause of the neuropathy. There are certain features in the history or physical exam, however, that should always prompt further neurologic consultation and possible EDX (Box 19.1). These features either raise the possibility that the neuropathy is demyelinating in nature or, when confirmed, change the differential diagnosis for the causative process in a significant way. EDX is the primary method by which a neuropathy is determined to be axonal or demyelinating in nature. Some findings in the history and physical examination can clue the clinician into a demyelinating neuropathy—diffuse areflexia, for example—but there is no definitive way to distinguish based on the history and exam alone. Recognition of demyelination is of critical importance because the differential diagnosis shrinks considerably, with CIDP or its variants and hereditary neuropathy being the primary considerations. It is especially important to recognize CIDP because it is amenable to treatment with immunosuppressive therapies; this can not only stabilize but also improve patient's deficits. The most common presentation of CIDP is subacute, progressive, non–length-dependent weakness and sensory loss.

Of note, patients with primarily small fiber neuropathy will have normal findings on EDX, as it evaluates motor and large sensory fiber function. Skin biopsy with measurement of the intraepidermal nerve fiber density (IENFD) has become the de facto gold standard for

diagnosis of small fiber neuropathy, with an estimated specificity of 95%–97%, and can be performed in the office. In a study of 14 patients presenting with burning feet found to be due to spondylotic cervical myelopathy, for example, none of the patients were found to have an abnormal IENFD.

Autonomic function testing (AFT) can be a useful adjunct to document autonomic nervous system involvement in patients with peripheral neuropathy. Patients with small fiber neuropathy will very commonly have abnormalities that are demonstrable on the Quantitative Sudomotor Axon Reflex Test (QSART), which measures the integrity of postganglionic autonomic nerve fibers mediating sweating. QSART may help to differentiate central causes of autonomic dysfunction (e.g., pure autonomic failure or multiple system atrophy) from a neuropathy affecting autonomic fibers. AFT should probably not be used in isolation in diagnosing a neuropathy, however, as it is less sensitive than skin biopsy for detecting small fiber neuropathy.

FINDING A CAUSE

Initial Workup

Once a diagnosis of neuropathy has been made, the focus should shift toward finding the underlying etiology. The type of neuropathy identified should guide the diagnostic workup, as the highest yield tests will vary. The workup for a subacute demyelinating neuropathy and that for a chronic small fiber neuropathy, for example, will differ considerably. In cases of DSP, the search for a cause can be particularly daunting, given the plethora of known causes (Box 19.2). Sending off an extensive, indiscriminate panel of tests is unnecessary and can be counterproductive. For example, in a sample of patients with cryptogenic neuropathy in which 58% of patients were found to have a laboratory abnormality, only 9% of these abnormalities were ultimately felt to be etiologically relevant. An organized approach can be applied to minimize unnecessary testing and efficiently reach a diagnosis (Box 19.3).

Review of the medical history, medications, and occupational exposures may reveal the cause of neuropathy in a substantial proportion of patients. Particular focus should be paid to the patient's current and previous medications, especially chemotherapy, as numerous medications have been associated with the development

BOX 19.2 Causes of Distal Symmetric Polyneuropathy

Autoimmune	**Toxic**
Connective tissue disease	Ethanol
Vasculitis	Heavy metals
Inflammatory bowel disease	Organic solvents
Sarcoidosis	**Medications**
Celiac disease	Chemotherapy
Cancer associated	Ado-trastuzumab emtansine
Paraprotein associated	Brentuximab vedotin
Monoclonal gammopathy of	Eribulin,
unknown significance (MGUS)	Ixabepilone
Multiple myeloma	Etoposide
Waldenstrom	Ifosfamide
macroglobulinemia	Platinums
Lymphoma	Proteasome
AL amyloidosis	inhibitors (e.g.,
Paraneoplastic	bortezomib)
Endocrine/metabolic	Taxanes
Diabetes mellitus	Thalidomide,
Prediabetes	lenalidomide,
Hypothyroidism/	Pomalidomide
hyperthyroidism	Vincristine
Chronic renal failure	Amiodarone
Liver disease	Chloroquine
Infectious	Colchicine
HIV	Disulfiram
Human T-cell lymphotropic virus 1	Ethambutol
Leprosy	Hydralazine
Inherited	Isoniazid
Charcot-Marie-Tooth disease	Leflunomide
Familial amyloidosis	Metronidazole
Nutritional	Nitrofurantoin
Vitamin B_{12}	Nucleoside reverse
deficiency	transciptase
Vitamin B_1 deficiency	Inhibitors
Vitamin B_6 deficiency or toxicity	Phenytoin
Postgastric bypass	

BOX 19.3 Suggested Initial Etiologic Workup of Distal Symmetric Polyneuropathy

Detailed review of medical and family history, current and prior medications
Hemoglobin A1c and/or oral glucose tolerance test
Vitamin B_{12}
Methylmalonic acid
Serum protein electrophoresis (SPEP) with immunofixation (IFE)
TSH
Comprehensive metabolic panel
Complete blood count

---

of peripheral neuropathy. Asking patients about vitamins and supplements is also important; vitamin B_6 toxicity, for example, is known to cause neuropathy. Likewise, occupational exposures should be explored. Heavy metals—lead, arsenic, thallium, and mercury—and industrial agents such as acrylamide and volatile solvents have all been associated with neuropathy. Screening patients for alcohol abuse is essential, given the common association between longstanding alcohol overuse and neuropathy.

Hereditary neuropathy is an important and under-recognized consideration in patients presenting with DSP. Hereditary neuropathies such as Charcot-Marie-Tooth disease (CMT) are fairly common, with an estimated prevalence of 1:2500 in the general population. Patients commonly present with disproportionately more weakness and atrophy relative to the degree of sensory involvement. A careful family history is also crucial, as many patients with CMT either are not aware of affected family members' symptoms or have never connected them with their own symptoms. Specifically asking about family members with high arches, unexplained gait trouble, or unexplained pain may reveal previously unrecognized affected family members. In patients with cryptogenic neuropathy without either a classic phenotype (e.g., pes cavus and hammertoes) or a suggestive family history, the yield of genetic testing is unknown, so routine testing is not currently recommended.

The American Academy of Neurology (AAN) published guidelines in 2009 identifying blood glucose, vitamin B_{12} and metabolites (methylmalonic acid [MMA] and/or homocysteine), and serum protein electrophoresis (SPEP) with immunofixation (IFE) as the highest yield laboratory tests for evaluation of DSP. A comprehensive metabolic panel and complete blood count are also commonly done as part of the initial laboratory evaluation. We also advocate for routine testing of TSH in patients with DSP, as it is a readily treatable cause and the fourth most common identified in some cohorts. A similar standardized workup was applied to a cohort of 138 patients with DSP in the primary care setting. SPEP with IFE, B_{12},

TSH, and an oral glucose tolerance test (OGTT) were tested in all patients; MMA was also tested in patients with B_{12} levels between 200 and 300 pg/mL. Select patients had SS-A and SS-B antibodies and vitamin B_6 tested. An etiology was found in 69% of these patients. Despite such evidence, there remains poor adherence to screening recommendations. Callaghan and colleagues found that hemoglobin A1c was tested in <20% of patients with neuropathy, vitamin B_{12} in 41%, and SPEP in 19%.

Most Common Causes

Diabetes is the most common cause of neuropathy and specifically DSP. Testing patients with unexplained DSP reveals abnormalities in blood glucose in approximately 11% of patients. The prevalence of polyneuropathy among diabetic patients increases with longer disease duration. In a cohort of patients with type 1 diabetes mellitus, the prevalence of neuropathy was 18% in patients <30 years old and 58% in patients ≥30 years old. In a cohort of patients with type 2 diabetes mellitus (T2DM), the prevalence of neuropathy was 8.3% shortly after diagnosis and 41.9% after 10 years. Poor glycemic control has also been shown to correlate with an increased risk of developing neuropathy. It is important to remember that diabetes is not always the cause of neuropathy in a patient with diabetes. Metformin, for example, can reduce serum B12 levels. In one cohort of 278 patients with T2DM, 9 patients were found to have polyneuropathy that was thought to be due to a cause other than diabetes.

Epidemiologic studies have suggested that patients with prediabetes and specifically impaired glucose tolerance may also have increased prevalence of neuropathy. The American Diabetes Association uses a hemoglobin A1c of 5.%–6.4% to define prediabetes and blood glucose of 140–199 mg/dL on 2-hour 75-g OGTT to define impaired glucose tolerance. Obesity, dyslipidemia (particularly hypertriglyceridemia), and the metabolic syndrome have been implicated as additional risk factors for neuropathy, suggesting that it may be a confluence of risk factors that is responsible for development of neuropathy in these patients.

Approximately 10% of patients with chronic sensorimotor neuropathy have an associated serum paraprotein. This is in contrast to 1% of the general population, though the presence of paraproteinemia does increase with age, reaching a prevalence of 10% in those above the age of 80. Testing IFE is recommended in addition to SPEP, as it is more sensitive. Two-thirds of neuropathy

cases are associated with a monoclonal gammopathy of unknown significance (MGUS), but neuropathy can also be seen in patients with multiple myeloma, Waldenstrom macroglobulinemia, amyloidosis, and other hematologic malignancies. Patients with MGUS have a 1% annual risk of developing hematologic malignancy, and patients with concurrent neuropathy are at slightly higher risk, so these patients are best comanaged with a hematologist or oncologist.

Paraproteinemia has been associated with multiple types of neuropathy, including both DSP and CIDP. A phenotype of demyelinating neuropathy known as distal acquired demyelinating sensory neuropathy has been associated with IgM MGUS. Two-thirds of these patients will harbor antibodies against myelin-associated glycoprotein (anti-MAG) in serum. This phenotype resembles DSP, but characteristic demyelinating EDX findings (performed in those patients who have an identified paraprotein) allow for distinction. Autonomic symptoms and pain are common in the neuropathy associated with amyloidosis. In patients with an unexplained autonomic neuropathy and negative SPEP/IFE, genetic forms of amyloidosis should also be considered.

Vitamin B_{12} deficiency can be found in approximately 2.2%–8% of patients with DSP. Testing metabolites that become elevated when B_{12} is deficient, namely, MMA and homocysteine, increases sensitivity. MMA is more sensitive and specific than homocysteine; in one study, testing MMA together with B_{12} increased diagnostic yield from 2% to 8%. If not tested routinely, MMA should be considered when B_{12} levels are borderline (200–500 pg/mL). Patients with vitamin B_{12} deficiency may be found to have hyperreflexia, as vitamin B_{12} deficiency can also cause subacute combined degeneration of the spinal cord.

Second-Tier Workup

If the diagnosis remains uncertain after initial workup, additional testing can be considered tailored to the clinical situation. Many clinicians routinely test markers of inflammation and rheumatologic disease. In a cohort of patients with multiple types of idiopathic neuropathy, however, rheumatologic testing only led to a change in management in patients with known rheumatologic disease, symptoms suggestive of a rheumatologic disorder, or atypical features such as an acute or asymmetric presentation. Two exceptions may be Sjögren syndrome and celiac disease, in which neuropathy may either precede or be the sole manifestation of the disease. Rheumatologic testing may be of higher yield in patients with isolated small fiber neuropathy.

In patients with weight loss or gastrointestinal illness, testing for nutritional deficiencies is reasonable. If a patient has never been previously screened for HIV infection, this could also be considered. Hereditary TTR amyloidosis should be considered in patients with a positive family history, heart failure, and/or prominent autonomic symptoms (e.g., gastrointestinal involvement, early satiety, weight loss, and IBS-like symptoms), since early treatment may slow and even stop disease progression.

Even after a complete laboratory workup, a specific cause will not be found in 18%–26% of patients with DSP. More invasive testing is rarely indicated. CSF analysis offers low diagnostic yield except in cases of demyelinating polyneuropathy. Nerve biopsy should not be pursued simply because the cause of neuropathy remains uncertain. Although it is a minor procedure, permanent sensory loss in the distribution of the biopsied nerve is common, and other adverse effects do occur. In one cohort of 67 patients who underwent sural nerve biopsy, 29.8% had chronic pain in the sural nerve distribution, and 46.8% had persistent dysesthesia.

MANAGEMENT

Depending on the specific characteristics and etiology of the neuropathy, the treatment can be guided by the referring provider or neurology teams. Treatment of underlying infectious or metabolic causes may stop or reverse progression of the secondary neuropathy. Certain inflammatory neuropathies, such as CIDP, may respond to immunotherapy. Toxic neuropathies such as ethanol and chemotherapy-induced neuropathies often improve to a variable degree once toxic exposure is discontinued. Despite treatment of the underlying cause, patients typically continue to experience residual neuropathic symptoms, including positive sensory phenomena, paresthesia or dysesthesia, sensory ataxia, and imbalance and weakness.

Counseling is very important for patients who have been diagnosed with neuropathy. Patients with sensory loss in the feet need to be educated about routine foot care and surveillance for wounds and injuries. The American Diabetes Association recommends annual comprehensive foot evaluation to identify risk factors for

ulceration and amputation. Nonpharmacologic measure to help prevent injury include appropriate comfortable socks and shoes. Patients should inspect their feet daily for any breaks in skin and injuries and inspect their shoes daily for anything that may cause injury. They should also be counseled to avoid walking barefoot. Walking on the beach can be especially perilous, as patients may not appreciate the heat of the sand and may not recognize when they have stepped on sharp objects such as shells.

Patients with sensory ataxia are at risk of falls. Other factors such as foot pain, orthostatic hypotension, and medication side effects (e.g., dizziness) can compound this risk. Proactively suggesting modifications in the home can be helpful to reduce the risk of fall. Handlebars can be installed in the shower and around the toilet. Nightlights should be used for the path from the bed to the bathroom. Slip-resistant surfaces for outdoor decks and nonslip bathmats are important as well. Depending on the degree of weakness and imbalance, patients may benefit from physical therapy with emphasis on balance training and core-strengthening exercises. Ground reaction ankle foot orthotics (AFOs) may be considered to help with gait and balance and reduce fall risk in patients with ankle dorsiflexion weakness.

Patients with neuropathic pain may require symptomatic treatment. The first consideration is ensuring that the patient's complaints are due to neuropathic pain, as discomfort can result from other causes, including joint deformities or arthropathic pain, foot ulcerations, or restless leg syndrome. Importantly, negative symptoms, such as numbness and coldness, and non-neuropathic symptoms usually do not respond to neuropathic medications. Second, before embarking on treatment trials with medications, it can be useful to keep in mind other modifiers of pain perception. Treating frequently comorbid conditions, such as major depression and obstructive sleep apnea, may have an important impact on pain management as well.

Four classes of medication should be considered first line for the treatment of neuropathic pain in patients with neuropathy: gabapentinoids (e.g., gabapentin and pregabalin), tricyclic antidepressants (TCAs; e.g., amitriptyline and nortriptyline), serotonin-norepinephrine reuptake inhibitors (SNRIs; e.g., duloxetine and venlafaxine), and sodium-channel blockers (e.g., oxcarbazepine, valproic acid, lacosamide, lamotrigine) (Table 19.3). It is very important to know that every individual is different with regard to what medications or what combinations of

TABLE 19.3   Pharmacologic Agents for the Management of Neuropathic Pain in Patients With Neuropathy[a]

Name	Instructions for Starting	Goal Dose	Max. Dose	Good for Patients With:	Consider Alternatives If:	Common Side Effects
Gabapentin	100 mg TID or 300 mg at bedtime	300 mg TID	3600 mg/d	Seizure disorder	Renal insufficiency	Dizziness, sedation, gait disturbance, confusion, peripheral edema
Pregabalin	75 mg BID	150 mg BID	600 mg/d	Seizure disorder	Renal insufficiency	Dizziness, sedation, gait disturbance, confusion, peripheral edema
Amitriptyline/ nortriptyline	10–25 mg at bedtime	50–100 mg at bedtime	150 mg/d	Insomnia Migraine	Cardiac disease, arrhythmia, other serotonergic medications	Dry mouth (more common with amitriptyline), sedation, dizziness, confusion, QT prolongation, orthostatic hypotension
Duloxetine	30 mg daily	60 mg/d (daily or split BID)	120 mg/d	Depression, anxiety, fibromyalgia	Hepatic failure, other serotonergic medications, anticoagulants	Nausea, dyspepsia, constipation, sedation, dry mouth, dizziness, hyperhidrosis, sexual dysfunction
Venlafaxine	37.5 mg daily (XR)	150 mg daily (XR)	225 mg/d	Depression, anxiety	Uncontrolled hypertension, other serotonergic medications	Nausea, dyspepsia, sedation, dizziness, nervousness, insomnia, hypertension, sexual dysfunction
Oxcarbazepine	150 mg BID	300–600 mg BID	900–1200 mg BID	Seizure disorder	History of Stevens-Johnson syndrome, hyponatremia, or renal impairment	Hyponatremia (serum sodium should be checked after initiation), blood dyscrasias, allergic reactions including Stevens-Johnson syndrome, dizziness, ataxia, fatigue

[a]There is no evidence that efficacy differs for medications within the same class. This table is not exhaustive for all options within the four first-line classes of neuropathic pain medications but instead focuses on commonly used examples in each class.

medications might work best. An initial first-line agent may be chosen from the four classes listed above based on the patient's comorbidities, drug interactions, and cost. For example, oxcarbazepine might be a good choice in a patient with both epilepsy and neuropathic pain, whereas amitriptyline might be better in a patient with both migraines and neuropathic pain. A patient who is already on an SSRI should probably avoid a tricyclic antidepressant or SNRI, so gabapentin might be favored. Unless there are prohibitive side effects, it is essential to increase the therapeutic dose before concluding that a medication trial has failed. In clinical trials, more than 9% of patients stopped taking each of the suggested first-line medications due to perceived adverse effects. If a medication is ineffective or not tolerated, trialing a medication from another class is appropriate. Combination therapy may be more effective than monotherapy, so this can be considered before trying second-line agents.

A meta-analysis examining the treatment of neuropathic pain in both central and peripheral nervous system disorders calculated the number needed to treat to achieve 50% reduction in pain in one patient: 3.6 for TCAs (most studies were of amitriptyline), 6.4 for SNRIs (duloxetine and venlafaxine), 7.2 for gabapentin, and 7.7 for pregabalin. Given the paucity of head-to-head trials, Griebler and colleagues performed a comparative effectiveness network meta-analysis for painful diabetic neuropathy in 2014; Waldfogel and associates updated the analysis with recent trials in 2017. For each trial that was included, a standardized mean difference (SMD) reflecting the effectiveness of each medication was calculated, allowing for comparisons between agents. The analysis concluded that pregabalin, TCAs, and SNRIs were effective when compared to placebo. In contrast to the studies above, the analysis concluded that gabapentin was not more effective than placebo. Based on calculated SMDs, SNRIs were found to be significantly more effective than pregabalin. No significant difference in effectiveness was found between TCAs and either pregabalin or SNRIs.

Hoffman et al. recently examined the use of opiates in the treatment of neuropathy. Neuropathy patients receiving opioids were more likely to use gait assist devices and had worse functional status. Opiate use did not improve functional status but rather was associated with higher rates of depression, opiate dependence, and opiate overdose. Waldfogel's network analysis also concluded that typical opiates were not effective for treating painful diabetic neuropathy. Atypical opiates—tramadol and tapentadol—have evidence supporting their use and are better alternatives to consider should first-line therapies fail. If pain is localized, topical agents are appealing second-line agents because of their lack of significant drug interactions and low rates of systemic adverse effects. Options include capsaicin cream or patches, lidocaine patches, percutaneous electrical nerve stimulation, and botulinum toxin. Alpha lipoic acid supplementation, taken by mouth at 600 mg daily or 300 mg twice a day, can also be considered as an adjunctive therapy. This has been best studied in patients with diabetic polyneuropathy. Among nonpharmaceutical compounds, ginkgo biloba has the best evidence from clinical trials. Acupuncture also has positive evidence, but cost may be a barrier.

Finally, educating patients about the natural history of neuropathy can be very impactful. Newly diagnosed patients may worry that they will someday require a wheelchair or an amputation, which can cause stress and affect mood and sleep. There is reason to strike an optimistic tone with patients, however. In patients with an identified etiology, progression of neuropathy will depend on ongoing exposure to the inciting cause. In idiopathic neuropathies, very slow progression over many years is the norm. In one case series, 85% of patients had no discernible progression over the course of 1 year of follow-up. In another study, patients who were followed for as long as 9 years maintained independent ambulation. Finally, in yet another series 35 out of 127 patients who were followed eventually required a gait aid (e.g., cane, adjusted shoes, AFOs, or walker), but none stopped walking entirely.

CONCLUSION

Although the presentations of peripheral neuropathy are diverse, a standardized approach to taking a history and the neurologic examination allow the clinician to easily recognize many forms of neuropathy. Applying a standardized approach to the workup of neuropathy allows for the efficient recognition of the etiology in most patients with minimal testing. Offering supportive care to limit disability, prevent foot ulcers and falls, and ameliorate neuropathic pain is an essential task for the primary care clinician.

"For the full bibliography list, please use the pincode on the inside front cover to access the electronic version of the text at ebooks.health.elsevier.com."

20

Motor Neuron Disease*

Mohammad Kian Salajegheh and Manisha Thakore-James

INTRODUCTION

Motor neuron diseases are the result of dysfunction of upper motor neurons in the precentral gyrus of the frontal lobe and/or lower motor neurons in the ventral horn of the spinal cord. In general, they cause weakness without notable sensory symptoms or pain. The most common motor neuron disease is amyotrophic lateral sclerosis (ALS), which is the primary focus of this review. Other motor neuron diseases include hereditary spastic paraparesis, spinobulbar muscular atrophy, and infectious motor neuron diseases including polio and West Nile virus. Spinal muscular atrophy (SMA) is a genetic motor neuron disease with advances in therapy, including the antisense oligonucleotide nusinersen, which was approved in 2016. While adult-onset SMA exists, SMA more often affects infants and toddlers and is therefore not discussed further in this review. Motor neuron disease mimics, including multifocal motor neuropathy, are also briefly discussed because disease-modifying therapy is available for them.

AMYOTROPHIC LATERAL SCLEROSIS

ALS is the most common motor neuron disease with an incidence of about 2 in 100,000. Although the average age of onset is in the seventh decade, ALS can present at a wide range of ages. The pathophysiology of ALS is

unknown. Current theories include dysregulation of microRNA, changes in ion channels resulting in cellular excitotoxicity, and endoplasmic reticular and mitochondrial stress, among others. Areas of current research are ongoing to identify serologic/cerebrospinal fluid markers, genetic tests, and other biomarkers to better stratify patients to determine whether one or more of these factors are involved in the pathophysiology of disease in individual patients. Expansion of information in this area will help to identify better treatments for ALS. Interestingly, an increased incidence of ALS in the veteran population has been reported. While the exact etiology for this has not been identified, environmental exposure, strenuous exercise, and potential head injuries have all been postulated as potential causes. Some reports have suggested that athletes who experience repeated head trauma are more likely to develop ALS; however, more rigorously controlled studies have failed to demonstrate a clear correlation between head trauma and ALS. Additionally, pathologic evaluation of ALS patients with head trauma were not significantly different from evaluations of those without head trauma.

Clinical Features

The hallmark of ALS is a combination of upper motor neuron (UMN) and lower motor neuron (LMN) involvement with progression of weakness over time. The degree of UMN and LMN involvement varies among patients, and since UMN and LMN findings are common in neurologic disease, there are many mimics for ALS, particularly when patients present early in the disease process, at which time UMN and LMN features may not be present simultaneously. The initial symptom in ALS is often painless extremity weakness, manifested

---

* Based on Foster LA, Salajegheh MK. Motor neuron disease: pathophysiology, diagnosis, and management. *Am J Med.* 2019;132(1):32–37. ISSN 0002-9343. https://doi.org/10.1016/j.amjmed.2018.07.012.

as difficulty writing, turning keys in locks, raising the arm overhead, or tripping due to foot drop. Patients may or may not notice muscle atrophy, stiffness, or fasciculations in this stage, and fasciculations, which are one of the hallmark findings of ALS, may not be present in every case. About 80% of patients present with this limb-onset disease, with the remaining 20% presenting with dysarthria and dysphagia, the so-called bulbar-onset. A small group of patients may present with isolated respiratory symptoms at the onset, without clear involvement of limb or bulbar muscles. In the following months and years, extremity weakness progresses gradually, resulting in impaired mobility and difficulty with activities of daily living (ADLs). Progressive dysphagia results in inadequate caloric intake and weight loss. ALS itself may also change metabolism, contributing to weight loss. Many patients with ALS develop dysarthria, which impedes communication. Respiratory symptoms in ALS are important to be screened for and recognized, since frank dyspnea is a late symptom and may be missed, given limited patient mobility. Symptoms that may suggest respiratory involvement include overall fatigue and mental slowness, morning headaches, and dyspnea on exertion and even with lying down (orthopnea). Most patients who do not opt for vent/tracheostomy die 3–5 years after symptom onset as a result of pneumonia and/or hypoxia related to bulbar dysfunction and respiratory failure. A small minority of patients may present with primary lateral sclerosis (PLS) or progressive muscular atrophy (PMA), which are considered the extreme cases of upper motor neuron–predominant and lower motor neuron–dominant disease, respectively. The prognosis for PLS is comparatively longer (8–10 years median survival) than that for PMA. Both PLS and PMA may transition to ALS in time, with progression to having both upper and lower motor neuron features. At present, methods to prognosticate a clinical course for individual patients remain obscure.

Physical examination is used to verify the upper motor neuron signs (spasticity, hyperreflexia) and lower motor neuron signs (flaccid weakness, fasciculations, and diminished reflexes). Weakness is mostly asymmetric, and its pattern, in time, extends beyond a single nerve distribution and appears to be myotomal. For example, a "split hand" results in atrophy of the abductor pollicis brevis and first dorsal interosseous on the radial aspect of the hand, while the bulk and strength of the abductor digit minimi may be relatively preserved,

suggesting T1>C8 myotome involvement. Conversely, an isolated ulnar neuropathy would involve the first dorsal interosseous and abductor digiti minimi but not the abductor pollicis brevis. The absence of sensory loss in the distribution of nerves and roots is further supportive of involvement of motor neurons rather than other possibilities. Reflexes may be increased in the case of upper motor neuron involvement and decreased in the case of lower motor neuron involvement. A preserved reflex in an atrophied and weak limb may be indicative of both upper and lower motor neuron involvement.

Cognitive and behavioral impairment can occur with ALS. Cognitive impairment in the form of frontotemporal dementia most often is characterized by executive dysfunction—impaired attention, working memory, organization, and planning—while typical behavioral features include personality changes, obsessions, and disinhibition. Because patients may have communication impairment and fatigue, specialized screening instruments such as the Amyotrophic Lateral Sclerosis Cognitive Behavioral Screen are favored over traditional comprehensive neuropsychiatric evaluation.

Symptoms that are notably absent in ALS are diploplia, sensory symptoms, and urinary/fecal incontinence. The presence of these symptoms should suggest an alternative diagnosis.

Diagnostic Workup

The diagnosis of ALS is mainly based on history and examination. A laboratory workup and imaging are done to exclude other potential etiologies (Table 20.1). Most importantly, these studies are used to exclude diseases that mimic ALS but have treatments and/or to identify diseases with a more favorable prognosis.

The differential diagnosis for ALS varies based on the presenting symptoms. It is helpful to identify the differential diagnosis/diagnostic workup based on how the patient is presenting:

A. UMN

B. LMN

C. UMN and LMN

D. Bulbar

For patients who present with UMN-predominant symptoms, important mimics are vitamin B12 deficiency (subacute combined degeneration), copper-deficiency/zinc toxicity, hereditary spastic paraplegia, cervical spinal stenosis, autoimmune disease with spinal cord involvement (multiple sclerosis,

TABLE 20.1   Workup of Motor Neuron Disorders

	Workup	Diseases Being Considered
UMN	Labs: B12, MMA, copper/zinc, ESR, CRP, ANA, HIV, HTLV I+II, Lyme serology (endemic areas) Imaging: MRI brain, cervical, thoracic spine EMG/NCS (for subclinical LMN findings) Consider: Lumbar puncture for cells, protein, glucose, stain and culture IgG synthesis rate, OCB VLCFA, genetic testing HSP and ALS	Vitamin deficiencies, autoimmune disorder, infections, demyelinating disease, genetic disorders (adrenoleukodystrophy, hereditary spastic paraplegia), neurodegenerative diseases such as corticobasal degeneration, PSP
LMN	Labs: ESR, CRP, CMP, TSH, serum electrophoresis, serum immunofixation, ganglioside panel, Lyme serology (endemic areas), West Nile virus, and enterovirus antibodies MRI spine if polyradiculopathy is suspected EMG/NCS Consider CPK, aldolase, anti-IBM Ab, muscle-specific autoantibodies Consider: Lumbar puncture for cells, protein, glucose, stain and culture, cytology, viral Ab's CT chest, abdomen/pelvis muscle biopsy, genetic testing for ALS and myopathies	Renal dysfunction, endocrine dysfunction, hematologic malignancy, monoclonal gammopathy, polyneuropathy, polyradiculopathy, myopathy, Lyme disease, W. Nile infection, post-polio syndrome, multifocal motor neuropathy, CIDP variants, vasculitis, cancer cachexia
UMN and LMN	Labs: ESR, CRP, ANA, RPR, HIV, HTLV I+II, Lyme serology (endemic areas), serum ACE Imaging: Cervical spine Consider brain and thoracic spine imaging EMG/NCS Consider genetic testing ALS, HSP	Cervical spondylosis, systemic lupus erythematosus, sarcoid, Lyme disease, HIV, HSP
Bulbar	Labs: AchR Ab binding/modulating, MUSK, LRP 4 Ab, VGCC Ab Imaging: Brain MRI EMG/NCS to include repetitive nerve stimulation or SFEMG Consider: ENT referral, genetic testing ALS, OPMD, Kennedy disease	Myasthenia gravis/Lambert-Eaton myasthenic syndrome, stroke, neurodegenerative diseases such as PSP, genetic disorders (OPMD, Kennedy disease)

AChR Ab, Acetylcholine receptor antibody; *ANA,* antinuclear antibodies; *CBC,* complete blood count; *CIDP,* chronic inflammatory demyelinating neuropathy; *CMP,* comprehensive metabolic panel; *CPK,* creatine phosphokinase; *CRP,* c-reactive protein; *EMG/NCS,* electromyography/nerve conduction studies; *ESR,* erythrocyte sedimentation rate; *HIV,* human immunodeficiency virus; *HSP,* hereditary spastic paraparesis; *HTLV,* human T-lymphocytic virus; *IBM,* inclusion body myositis; *LMN,* lower motor neuron; *LRP 4,* low-density lipoprotein receptor related protein 4; *MMA,* methylmalonic acid; *MRI,* magnetic resonance imaging; *MUSK,* muscle-specific kinase; *OCB,* oligoclonal bands; *OPMD,* oculopharyngeal muscular dystrophy; *PSP,* progressive supranuclear; *SFEMG,* single-fiber electromyography; *TSH,* thyroid-stimulating hormone; *UMN,* upper motor neuron; *VLCFA,* very long chain fatty acids.

sarcoid, etc.), or degenerative CNS disorders (PSP). Obtaining brain and spinal imaging with MRI is an important part of the workup for ALS to exclude these possibilities.

For patients who present with LMN-predominant symptoms, the most important differential diagnosis is multifocal motor neuropathy, Lyme disease, West Nile encephalitis, and other viruses affecting motor neurons, post-polio syndrome, and spinal muscular atrophy. Multifocal motor neuropathy is an important diagnosis to identify, since the weakness that is seen in this condition is completely reversible with immunotherapy. Occasionally, diseases such as inclusion body myositis or some hereditary myopathies may present with asymmetric patterns of weakness and exhibit widespread fibrillation potentials and positive sharp waves on needle electromyography (EMG), mimicking the EMG findings that are seen in ALS.

For patients who present with a combination of UMN and LMN findings, the most important differential diagnostic considerations are cervical spondylosis with cervical stenosis and neural foraminal narrowing. Conversely, patients with ALS may coincidentally have cervical spinal stenosis, and it is important to correlate the areas with profound weakness with findings on spine imaging to prevent patients from having unnecessary spinal surgery. Systemic disorders that can involve the peripheral and central nervous systems, such as Lyme disease, sarcoid, systemic lupus erythematosus, and HIV, should also be considered in patients with this type of presentation. Occasionally, malignancy seeding the CNS and meninges may present in a similar manner, mimicking ALS.

For patients who present with bulbar symptoms, important differential diagnostic considerations include myasthenia gravis, foramen magnum tumors, degenerative CNS disorders, and cerebrovascular disease. Since cerebrovascular disease is common and may be incidentally seen on brain imaging, it is important to review the history of the onset of bulbar symptoms for correlation with the time of prior stroke. In ALS the bulbar symptoms are insidious in onset, whereas in stroke the onset is sudden. In patients with myasthenia gravis, the bulbar symptoms fluctuate and are worse after a long conversation or meal and can improve with rest. Kennedy's disease is an X-linked lower motor neuron condition presenting with atrophy/fasciculations of facial, bulbar, and limb muscles associated with gynecomastia. This disorder has a much more favorable prognosis compared to bulbar ALS and is therefore important to recognize.

Electromyography

Nerve conduction studies support the diagnosis by demonstrating intact sensory studies and motor conduction velocities in the presence of decreased compound muscle action potential amplitudes (depending on the myotomes that are involved). Fibrillation potentials and reduced recruitment of motor units on needle EMG suggest acute denervation; and tall, long motor units suggest chronic reinnervation changes. Fasciculation potentials are less specific but, in the appropriate clinical context, are suggestive of lower motor neuron dysfunction. EMG findings can be notably absent in cases in which UMN findings are predominant. The diagnostic criteria for ALS are mainly for research purposes and are designed to minimize a false positive diagnosis. The categories are based on how many of the four body regions (bulbar, cervical, thoracic, and lumbosacral) are involved. Diagnostic certainty increases with the number of body regions affected.

Biomarkers and Genetic Testing

The study of biomarkers for ALS is an ongoing area of research, and biomarkers are not yet available commercially or reliable for testing. Genetic testing can play an important role in diagnosis in ALS. However, given the complexity of these tests, they should be performed in consultation with a genetics and ALS expert. It is typically pursued in patients who have a family history of motor neuron disease or frontotemporal dementia or those who are particularly young at disease onset (less than 50 years old). However, this is an evolving topic as precision medicine expands, for example, the approval of tofersen for superoxide dismutase (SOD1)-associated ALS. *C9orf72* is the most common genetic mutation in the United States, present in about 40% of cases of familial ALS and 7% of cases of sporadic ALS. This genetic mutation is also associated with frontotemporal dementia. *SOD1*, *FUS*, and *TARDBP* are the other most common genetic mutations that have been identified. At present, identification of a genetic mutation will change management only for patients with SOD1 genetic mutation. However, genetic testing may be useful for family-planning purposes and, in some cases, inclusion in clinical trials.

Primary care physicians should consider the diagnosis of ALS, and referral to a neurologist, for patients who develop painless progressive weakness without sensory changes, particularly if accompanied by muscle atrophy and hyporeflexia or hyperreflexia, dysarthria, dysphagia, or dyspnea. Delay in diagnosis can lead to patient distress, and misdiagnosis can lead to unnecessary procedures (e.g., cervical laminectomy). Rarely, patients are first diagnosed with ALS during a hospitalization for respiratory failure. Intensivists should consider motor neuron disease as a possible etiology for inability to wean patients from a ventilator, particularly if they have a history of prehospitalization muscle weakness. In this case, additional history about symptoms of respiratory insufficiency in the weeks prior to hospitalization should be sought (dyspnea on exertion, orthopnea, morning headaches).

Management

Although ALS is not a curable disease, there are several treatment options. These treatments can be divided into disease-modifying therapies and symptomatic management. The goal of treatment interventions is to focus on maximal function and independence while reducing pain and suffering. It is important to provide patients with information and strategies to help preserve their dignity and autonomy.

Disease-Modifying Therapy

Currently in the United States there are four disease-modifying therapies for ALS (Table 20.2). Each of these therapies targets different processes of neural degeneration. Since there are currently no markers to identify which pathophysiology is playing a role in individual ALS patients, the current standard of care in the United States is to utilize three of these agents for all patients with ALS. In the pivotal trials leading to approval of these agents, patients were in early stages of the disease (i.e., <2–3 years from diagnosis, no respiratory symptoms, ambulating), with the thought that early initiation of these agents is likely to yield the most benefit.

Riluzole was approved in 1995 and is administered orally twice daily. While the exact mechanism of action is unknown, its neuroprotective effect has been attributed to inhibition of glutamate release, inactivation of voltage-gated sodium channels, and interference with intracellular response to excitatory receptor activation.

TABLE 20.2 Disease-Modifying Treatment for Amyotrophic Lateral Sclerosis		
Medication	**Administration**	**Side Effects**
Riluzole	50 mg orally twice daily	GI symptoms (abdominal pain, nausea, diarrhea), hepatotoxicity
Edaravone intravenous	Initial cycle: 60 mg IV daily for 14 days, then 14 days drug free Subsequent cycles: 60 mg IV daily for 10 days out of 14, then 14 days drug free	Anaphylaxis, headache
Edaravone oral	Initial cycle: 105 mg/5 mL orally/NGT daily for 14 days, then 14 days drug free Subsequent cycles: 105 mg/5 mg orally/NGT daily for 10 days out of 14, then 14 days drug free	Anaphylaxis/hypersensitivity reaction, gait abnormalities
Tofersen	100 mg (15 mL) intrathecally q 14 days for 3 doses, then q 28 days thereafter	Common: arthralgias, pain Serious: meningitis, radiculitis, myelitis, raised intracranial pressure

GI, Gastrointestinal; *IV*, intravenous; *NGT*, nasogastric; *q*, every.

It has been shown to increase survival by 2–3 months. The most common side effect of riluzole is gastrointestinal upset. Liver enzymes are monitored routinely to evaluate for hepatotoxicity.

The second medication, edaravone, was approved in 2017. Edaravone is a free radical scavenger that is believed to prevent motor neuron degeneration by reducing oxidative stress. It was originally available as an intravenous infusion but now is available as an oral formulation. In a select patient population ≤2 years from the first ALS symptom, minimal respiratory involvement, and minimal disability based on the Amyotrophic Lateral Sclerosis Revised Functional Rating Scale (ALSFRS-R), edaravone was associated with slower decline over 6 months compared with placebo.

The third medication, AMX0035 is a combination therapy of sodium phenylbutyrate and taurursodiol that is designed to reduce neuronal death through blockade of key cellular death pathways originating in the mitochondria and endoplasmic reticulum. This medication, which was a once promising therapeutic option, was found to be ineffective in a follow-up study.

Tofersen is an antisense oligonucleotide that mediates the degradation of SOD1 messenger RNA to reduce SOD1 protein synthesis. This drug is the first approved by the FDA for use in the United States for ALS patients with a genetic form of ALS associated an SOD1 genetic mutation.

Tofersen 100 mg (15 mL) is administered intrathecally every 14 days for three doses, then every 28 days for maintenance therapy. Although the pivotal trial did not meet its primary endpoint measure, in a 52-week open-label extension follow-up, treatment with tofersen was associated with reduced progression of ALS by several measures, including slower declines in ALSFRS-R scores, vital capacity, and grip strength.

Symptomatic Management

While the medications described previously can modestly increase survival, the mainstay of ALS treatment is symptom management (Table 20.3). This can be divided into two main categories: pharmacologic and nonpharmacologic interventions.

Interestingly, many of the pharmacologic treatments for ALS embody the principles of palliative care. Palliative care physicians routinely manage pain, constipation, sleep issues, depression/anxiety, dyspnea, and secretion management. Although there are no well-established guidelines, several articles suggest that

TABLE 20.3   Symptomatic Treatment of Amyotrophic Lateral Sclerosis

Symptom	Pharmacologic Treatment	Nonpharmacologic Treatment
Spasticity	Baclofen, tizanidine, botulinum toxin injections	Stretching exercises
Cramps	B-complex, magnesium, mexiletine	Stretching exercises, adequate hydration, salt intake, nutrition
Pain	Acetaminophen, NSAIDs, opioids	Physical therapy, range of motion exercises, massage
Dyspnea	Opioids	Noninvasive ventilation, invasive ventilation, nebulizer treatments
Dysphagia		Dietary modifications, gastrostomy tube
Sialorrhea	Scopolamine patch, glycopyrrolate, atropine, papaya enzyme, salivary gland botulinum toxin injections	Oral care
Constipation	Laxatives, fiber supplements	Hydration, exercise
Dysarthria		Augmentative and alternative communication (letter board, text-to-speech applications, eye-gaze devices)
Pseudobulbar affect (involuntary emotional expression disorder)	Dextromethorphan, SSRIs	Education and expectation setting

NSAIDs, Nonsteroidal antiinflammatory drugs; *SSRIs,* selective serotonin reuptake inhibitors.

exploration of palliative care strategies in the management of ALS patients makes sense.

Rehabilitation medicine concepts offer nonpharmacologic tools for symptom management in ALS outlined in the article by Majmudar et al.

Multidisciplinary Clinics

Patients who are followed in a multidisciplinary ALS clinic have been shown to have increased survival. The focus of these multidisciplinary clinics is to provide anticipatory guidance and symptom management regarding issues that increase morbidity and mortality, such as falls, aspiration risks, and respiratory distress. The multidisciplinary team structure can vary but usually includes a physician (often a neurologist or physiatrist), physical therapist, occupational therapist, speech/language pathologist, nutritionist, and social worker, among others. The effectiveness of this approach is likely due to the team approach, which allows for delivery of disease-modifying therapies, rehabilitation strategies, and palliative care strategies during the continuum of the disease by providers who have developed expertise in the care of ALS patients.

The symptomatic management of ALS varies based on how patients are presenting and how advanced the disease is. For this reason, it is useful to stratify patients into arbitrary stages of disease. This concept is outlined in the review by Majmudar et al., which describes the role of rehabilitation in ALS at different stages of the disease.

Early in the disease, the goals of treatment interventions include maintenance of independence. Patients with difficulty performing ADLs can utilize occupational health referrals for education on the use of equipment and exercise strategies to maintain independence. Patients with lower extremity weakness may need bracing and fall risk management. A physical therapist can provide education on maintaining safety and independence. Patients with bulbar symptoms may need secretion management, a voice amplifier, and talk-to-text strategies to aid with communication. Early intervention with nutrition consultation and supplements to prevent weight loss can improve weight and energy levels. Weight loss in ALS has been identified as a predictor of poor prognosis and is a potentially modifiable risk factor. In the early stages of the disease, it is important to involve a social worker to review advanced directives. Advocacy groups such as the ALS Association and

Compassionate Care ALS, referral to VA-based ALS clinics for veterans, and so forth can assist with education about the disease and information on services and how to access durable medical equipment. Early conversations about long-term goals are important, since home modifications to make the home accessible may take time, funding, and planning. Early involvement with palliative care is helpful initially for symptom management of secretion management, depression and anxiety, sleep issues, constipation, and pain management with gradual transition to understanding the long-term goals of care. Discussions about goals of care evolve over time with ALS patients. Understanding what is important to the patient paired with education helps to reduce fear and empower patients to maintain some degree of control in decision-making regarding different aspects of care. It is important to begin goals-of-care discussions early, since issues such as aspiration pneumonia, DVT, and mucous plugging can cause an acute decline in functional status. Understanding the patient's views on life-sustaining treatments is important in maintaining dignity and some sense of control in decision-making in end-of-life goals. This is particularly important in patients who are losing their ability to speak, since these conversations can be extremely difficulty with loss of voice. Although communication devices are helpful, they are difficult to use for long conversations in later stages of the disease.

As the disease progresses, patients with increasing upper extremity loss of function and inability to perform ADLs may need home health support. This type of assistance can help to reduce caregiver burden. Similarly, patients with lower extremity weakness with loss of ability to transfer and walk will need to discuss the use of a walker, cane, and/or lift devices and addition of home health services. Early introduction of these tools can help to reduce the pain in the patient that is incurred by difficult transfers and can reduce injury to caregivers. As patients, become more sedentary due to mobility issues, it is important to screen for deep vein thrombosis and skin breakdown issues. Rehabilitation strategies such as passive range of motion exercises, stretching exercises, and offloading strategies can reduce musculoskeletal pain and minimize risk for these serious and potentially fatal complications.

For patients with bulbar onset disease who are unable to maintain weight via oral intake due to increasing difficulty in chewing and swallowing, discussion of the role of a gastrostomy tube to supplement nutrition and hydration is recommended. Gastrostomy tube placement can also be considered in patients when mealtime is prolonged due to difficulty using the hands. For most patients, placement of a gastrostomy does not preclude eating. With close monitoring and education with a speech/language pathologist and nutritionist, most patients with ALS can continue to eat small amounts of food. Risk mitigation strategies include education on safe foods, textures. and amounts that are least likely to cause aspiration. Generally, placement of a gastrostomy tube under fluoroscopic guidance is preferred over an endoscopic procedure, which on retrospective study was shown to increase risk of aspiration and lead to longer hospitalization. Gastrostomy placement should occur before there is advanced respiratory decline, preferably when functional vital capacity is above 50% predicted. The neurology report of the Quality Standards Subcommittee of the American Academy of Neurology titled "Drug, Nutritional, and Respiratory Therapies: An Evidence-based Review" is an excellent resource for further details on this topic. For dysarthria, devices ranging from letter boards to brain-computer interfaces help to maintain communication ability. Early consultation with a speech/language pathologist is needed to customize equipment for ease of use and for potential voice banking. For respiratory insufficiency, noninvasive ventilation, including continuous positive airway pressure, is the mainstay of treatment. Studies have shown that initiation of noninvasive ventilation can prolong survival even in patients with bulbar ALS.

As the disease progresses, there can be increased needs regarding pain management, constipation, increasing fear and depression, more episodes of shortness of breath, increasing difficulty with secretion management, and risk for aspiration. It can be more cumbersome to go to the hospital for every new symptom that can evolve. At this time, introducing hospice care can greatly reduce tiresome trips to the hospital and allow for in-home evaluation and treatment of uncomfortable but manageable symptoms. This often aligns with the patient's goal of minimizing time in the hospital and spending more time at home with loved ones.

Some patients choose tracheostomy and mechanical ventilation; however, diaphragmatic pacing has been shown to decrease survival and is not recommended.

The primary care physician, hospitalist, and intensivist play important roles in the management of noted symptom of ALS as well as chronic diseases, such as hypertension and diabetes, in these patients. Patients and their medications may need to be monitored more frequently as their nutritional status and activity level change with disease progression. In the setting of acute or chronic respiratory failure (e.g., pneumonia or mucus plugging), it is important to temporarily suspend anticholinergic medications if they are being used to treat sialorrhea. Patients may also develop infections (urinary tract infections, decubitus ulcers) related to immobility that need to be treated. Bowel obstructions and deep venous thromboses are also common and require monitoring and therapy.

PRIMARY LATERAL SCLEROSIS

Primary lateral sclerosis (PLS) is a motor neuron disorder, at one end of the spectrum for ALS, in which only upper motor neuron signs are present. Patients present with a spastic paraplegia, with slowness and stiffness of gait with or without slowness of arm movement. Some patients develop spastic bulbar symptoms such as spastic dysarthria. This disease can mimic hereditary spastic paraplegia Examination shows increased tone, UMN pattern weakness in the upper extremities (with extensors weaker than flexors) and lower extremities (with flexors weaker than extensors) and hyperreflexia. Since some patients with ALS initially present with these symptoms and signs early on, these two diseases cannot be distinguished right away. If spasticity develops without development of lower motor neuron signs within a 3-year period, a diagnosis of PLS is suspected. No biomarkers are currently available to distinguish the two disorders.

The differential diagnosis of PLS is outlined in Table 20.1 in the UMN section. These include diseases that preferentially involve the corticospinal tracts.

The diagnosis of PLS is important to recognize, since the prognosis of PLS is significantly better than that of ALS.

Currently, the treatment for ALS can be used for PLS. Spasticity management is one of the mainstays of treatment for this patient group.

PROGRESSIVE MUSCULAR ATROPHY

Progressive muscular atrophy (PMA) is a motor neuron disorder at the other end of the spectrum for ALS, in which only lower motor neuron signs are present. Patients present with atrophy, fasciculations, and weakness. However, none of the typical UMN signs that are traditionally seen in ALS develop. Since some patients with ALS initially present with these symptoms and signs early on, these two diseases cannot be distinguished right away. No biomarkers are currently available to distinguish these two disorders.

The differential diagnosis of PMA is outlined in Table 20.1 in the LMN section. These include diseases that preferentially involve the anterior horn cells and the axonal component of peripheral nerves. This includes a wide differential of autoimmune, infectious, and neurodegenerative diseases.

The prognosis in PMA is variable. At times, the progression is relentless, similar to traditional ALS. However, there is a subset of patients with PMA who have a longer course and a better prognosis. No clear identifiers exist to distinguish the prognosis in individual patients.

Currently, the treatment for ALS can be used for PMA.

SPINOBULBAR MUSCULAR ATROPHY

Spinobulbar muscular atrophy, or Kennedy's disease, is an X-linked motor neuron disease that affects middle-aged males; it is caused by a CAG trinucleotide repeat in the androgen receptor gene. A greater number of repeats is associated with earlier disease onset, although age at presentation varies widely. The prevalence of spinobulbar muscular atrophy is estimated at about 3 per 100,000, but there are regions with prevalence as high as 7 per 100,000.

Clinical Features

The most prominent symptoms of Kenney's disease are in the bulbar region, resulting in dysarthria and dysphagia. In addition, patients develop proximal limb weakness, sensory neuronopathy presenting with gait imbalance and/or foot numbness, and paresthesias. Chin fasciculations and even myokymia are unique features of this disease. Myokymia is an involuntary muscle movement that is often described as wormlike or continuous rippling movements seen under the skin. Life expectancy from symptom onset is typically decades. Since this is typically years longer than in typical bulbar ALS, it is important to recognize Kennedy's disease.

Diagnostic Workup

Nerve conduction studies demonstrate axonal sensory neuronopathy. Findings suggestive of motor neuron disease are also present, such as decreased compound muscle action potential amplitudes, fasciculation and fibrillation potentials, and motor unit remodeling with reduced recruitment pattern. Genetic testing is commercially available.

Management

At present, there is no definitive disease-modifying therapy for Kennedy's disease, and treatment focuses on symptomatic management. Genetic counseling is recommended.

HEREDITARY SPASTIC PARAPARESIS

Hereditary spastic paraparesis is a group of disorders whose defining feature is increased extensor tone in the lower extremities. The age of onset varies widely from childhood onset to onset in the 70s. The prevalence is about 4 per 100,000. Many genetic causes have been identified, but the pathogenesis of common phenotypes remains unknown.

Clinical Features

Patients with uncomplicated hereditary spastic paraparesis have symmetric lower extremity spasticity and may also have pes cavus foot deformities, mild sensory loss, and mild urinary symptoms. Complicated hereditary spastic paraparesis, by definition, causes other associated symptoms, such as peripheral neuropathy, ataxia, visual impairment, cognitive changes, seizures, deafness, and cataracts. Neurologic examination demonstrates increased tone in the lower extremities with hyperreflexia (lower more than upper limbs), and extensor plantar responses. Loss of vibratory sense; mild weakness in the lower extremity hip, knee, and ankle flexors (upper motor neuron pattern); and distal atrophy may be present. Symptoms are gradually progressive over decades.

Diagnostic Workup

MRI of the brain and spine is recommended to investigate alternative causes of spasticity, such as multiple sclerosis or spinal cord compression. Other workup includes ruling out noncompressive causes of myelopathy, such as B12 deficiency, zinc toxicity, autoimmune and inflammatory disorders of the brain and spinal cord. Genetic testing is commercially available and can involve either a panel of genes associated with hereditary spastic paraparesis or testing that is more targeted based on presenting features and inheritance pattern.

Management

Treatment is supportive. Medications that are used to treat spasticity include baclofen, tizanidine, dantrolene, and benzodiazepines. These may paradoxically worsen gait by unmasking weakness. If systemic side effect of sedation is dose-limiting, then intrathecal administration of medication could be pursued. While botulinum toxin injections may be useful in managing focal spasticity early in the disease, the affected muscular regions in later stages are generally too large to make botulinum toxin injections feasible as a long-term solution.

ACUTE FLACCID PARALYSIS ASSOCIATED WITH VIRAL INFECTION

The prototypical example of acute flaccid paralysis is poliomyelitis, caused by the polio enterovirus. A polio vaccine was developed in the 1950s and has essentially eradicated the disease except for a few cases in some countries. Other enteroviruses that are associated with acute flaccid paralysis include Coxsackie virus A and B and Enterovirus-D68 and -A71. The flaviviruses Japanese encephalitis, tick-borne encephalitis, and West Nile virus may also cause acute flaccid paralysis. The incidence of acute flaccid paralysis worldwide is estimated at 4 per 100,000, and in many cases, the virus remains unidentified.

The retroviruses HIV and HTLV-1 can cause weakness mimicking that of motor neuron disease, but pathologic evaluation has not shown preferential involvement of motor nerves.

Clinical Features

Weakness is typically preceded by a viral prodrome of fever, malaise, myalgia, nausea, vomiting, and/or diarrhea. Some patients also develop confusion and obtundation, which is attributed to concomitant encephalopathy. Respiratory failure from diaphragm weakness may require intubation. Physical examination is notable for extremity weakness and hyporeflexia. Sensation is typically intact, although some viruses are also associated with transverse myelitis, which is associated with loss of sensation and bladder or bowel dysfunction.

Diagnostic Workup

MRI of the spinal cord is neither sensitive nor specific but is recommended to evaluate for the alternative etiology of cord compression. In some cases, T2-signal hyperintensity is evident in the region of the anterior horn cells ("owl eyes"). Enhancement may also be present in the acute phase. Cerebral spinal fluid analysis typically reveals a lymphocytic pleocytosis and elevated protein. Viral polymerase chain reaction may help identify the cause within the spinal fluid in the first 5 days. IgM antibodies in cerebral spinal fluid are indicative of central nervous system infection because these antibodies cannot cross the blood-brain barrier. IgG antibodies, if present in ratio greater than 100:1 compared to the serum, may also be suggestive of production of antibodies within the central nervous system and hence evidence if prior primary central nervous system infection. Viral polymerase chain reaction can also be tested on a respiratory or stool sample, in some cases.

Management

Currently, no antivirals are approved for treatment of enteroviruses and flaviviruses, so treatment is supportive. An immune response may be contributing to symptoms in some cases, so steroids are recommended for some patients with severe neurologic deficits. If spinal cord swelling is significant, then a short course (5–7 days) of high-dose intravenous steroids may be indicated in selected cases. Consultation with infectious disease specialist for the most updated diagnostic and treatment recommendations can be useful when infectious causes are suspected.

MOTOR NEURON DISEASE MIMICS

Several conditions have overlapping features with motor neuron disease and warrant consideration. The most common mimic is radiculopathy due to disc herniation or facet arthropathy. If a cervical radiculopathy is associated with spinal cord compression, both upper and lower motor neuron signs may be present; however, upper motor neuron signs will be caudal to the region of lower motor neuron signs, so one should have high suspicion for ALS when upper motor neuron signs are cranial to the lower motor neuron signs, even when there is spinal stenosis. Physical examination and electrodiagnostic finding will be limited to a myotome (or myotomes if multiple levels are involved), and imaging of the neural axis, such as MRI, should demonstrate mechanical compression corresponding to the level on examination.

While typical chronic inflammatory demyelinating polyradiculoneuropathy has prominent sensory features, its motor variant affects only motor nerves and presents with relatively symmetric proximal and distal weakness without sensory changes as described in the European Academy of Neurology/Peripheral Nerve Society Task Force updated guidelines (2021). Patients with multifocal motor neuropathy also have pure motor involvement and present with multiple motor mononeuropathies (a common feature is wrist and finger drop due to involvement of the radial nerve) without sensory involvement. Patients rarely have bulbar or respiratory involvement. The diagnosis for both is made based on the presence of demyelinating features on motor nerve conduction studies with normal sensory responses. Treatment is typically with IVIG immunotherapy.

Some inherited and inflammatory myopathies can also cause progressive focal weakness and atrophy. For example, inclusion body myositis typically involves the finger flexors and knee extensors asymmetrically early in the disease course. Facioscapulohumeral muscular dystrophy, a hereditary myopathy, causes asymmetric involvement of muscles of the face, shoulder blades, and upper arms. Hereditary motor neuropathies such as distal hereditary motor neuropathies and porphyria can also present with pure motor weakness. On examination, however, upper motor neuron signs are absent, distinguishing them from ALS but not clearly from LMN-predominant ALS. Typically, in these conditions, disease progression is gradual over many years.

Myasthenia gravis and Lambert-Eaton myasthenic syndromes are neuromuscular junction disorders that can present with weakness without sensory symptoms. Myasthenia gravis can present with bulbar symptoms. These symptoms are often worse with activity such as eating and talking and may improve with rest. Serologic testing can distinguish these disorders from ALS.

CONCLUSION

A clinician should suspect motor neuron disease when a patient develops progressive painless muscle weakness and atrophy without sensory changes, particularly in the setting of hyperreflexia and bulbar involvement. Referral to a neurologist for diagnosis and treatment is recommended. For patients with the most common motor neuron disease, ALS, symptom management is beneficial, as is management of unrelated medical conditions (e.g., hypertension, diabetes) that may change quickly as the patient's condition declines.

"For the full bibliography list, please use the pincode on the inside front cover to access the electronic version of the text at ebooks.health.elsevier.com."

21

Demyelinating Disease*

Danielle M. Howard and Jonathan Zurawski

INTRODUCTION

In 1868 Jean-Martin Charcot provided the first detailed anatomic illustrations of "la sclérose en plaques," characteristic periventricular white matter lesions that are now appreciated as a pathologic hallmark of multiple sclerosis (MS), the most common autoimmune demyelinating disease of the central nervous system (CNS). Although MS is traditionally characterized by relapsing and progressive stages, the disease may be best understood as heterogeneous, with considerable overlap between stages. This is hypothesized as being due to a complex immune response whereby the adaptive immune system drives pathology in the early stages of the disease, then wanes and is overtaken by other disease processes mediated by the innate immune system, involving mitochondrial dysfunction, microglial activation, glutamate toxicity, and reduced compensatory ability, among other mechanisms, leading to gradual disability accumulation in older age. Treatment of MS remains a clinical challenge, being the most frequent cause of permanent disability in young adults, with annual healthcare costs totaling more than $10 billion in the United States.

EPIDEMIOLOGY

An estimated 727,000 people in the United States (309 people per 100,000) and 2.3 million people worldwide

are affected by MS. The mean age of diagnosis is 31 years, though patients may present from the first to the seventh decades of life. MS affects females disproportionately, with an estimated female-to-male incidence ratio of 2.8:1, skewing further toward female predominance in more recent studies. Some have speculated that the changing social status of females during the past century contributed to increased rates of MS diagnosis, and several observations point to the important underlying role of hormones: (1) Increased female MS risk develops around age 11 years (near puberty onset); (2) earlier menarche correlates with earlier MS onset in multicenter case-control studies of pediatric MS; (3) females with MS may experience clinical worsening around the time of menopause. MS was historically thought to affect people of Northern European descent at higher rates, though recent studies have shown MS prevalence in Black Americans to be nearly as high as that in their White counterparts, with fewer people of Asian and Hispanic descent being affected.

MS is not typically considered to be a strongly genetic disorder; however, there is evidence of heritability, and genetic susceptibility is complex and multifactorial. Twin studies demonstrate a 25% concordance rate among monozygotic twins and a 5.4% concordance rate among dizygotic twins. A growing number of genes have been linked to MS risk, with recent genome-wide studies identifying over 100 alleles of significance with immune function that alter disease risk. Perhaps the best-studied genetic association is the link between MS and major histocompatibility complex class I and class II alleles, particularly HLA-DRB1. Recent work has characterized protective and risk alleles, although no combination can

*Based on Zurawski J, Stankiewicz J. Multiple sclerosis re-examined: essential and emerging clinical concepts. *Am J Med*. 2018;131(5):464–472. ISSN 0002-9343. https://doi.org/10.1016/j.amjmed.2017.11.044.

be used to definitively predict the development of MS, and genetic testing is not clinically available.

MS prevalence increases the farther one moves from the equator; this finding is hypothesized to be related to differences in genetic background, infection exposure, and vitamin D levels. In many countries with a high prevalence of MS (United States, Northern Europe, Russia, Canada, and New Zealand) there is a latitude gradient of MS risk; however, in regions with lower prevalence this relationship does not always hold. Classic MS migration studies have shown that individuals moving from low-to high-prevalence regions after age 15 maintain the low risk of the area from which they migrated, whereas individuals migrating before this age assume the risk of the region to which they move.

The relationship between MS risk and latitude led to the hypothesis of vitamin D functioning as a key mediator of MS susceptibility. Vitamin D is predominantly synthesized in the skin in response to ultraviolet light. Its receptors are expressed ubiquitously on immune cells and function to reduce immune activation of autoreactive T and B cells in MS. There is a relationship between low vitamin D levels and increased risk of MS, clinical relapse/progression, and new magnetic resonance imaging (MRI) activity, although evidence is mixed as to whether supplementation of vitamin D leads to significant differences in MS clinical outcomes. Nonetheless, vitamin D is an important developmental immunomodulator that is involved in immune system maturation and self-antigen recognition during critical developmental windows.

Cigarette smoke exposure (both direct inhalation and secondhand smoke) has been associated with an increased risk of MS. Smokers have a 50% higher chance of developing MS than nonsmokers, regardless of age at smoking start. Increasing cumulative pack-year exposure is associated with a higher overall risk of MS. Studies show that there may be a reduction in elevated MS risk among patients who quit smoking, by approximately 5 years later. Tobacco smoking has been shown to affect other aspects of the MS disease course as well: smokers have a higher risk of conversion from relapsing-remitting MS (RRMS) to secondary progressive MS (SPMS), and a higher risk of development of neutralizing antibodies to certain disease-modifying therapies (DMTs), making them less effective.

Obesity in childhood and adolescence has been associated with increased risk in both pediatric- and adult-onset MS, and abdominal obesity has been associated with worsened disability in people living with MS. Early exposure to shift work may also increase the risk of developing MS, possibly related to the negative effects of inadequate sleep in adolescence. Caffeine and alcohol are not believed to strongly affect disease risk.

Epstein-Barr virus (EBV) exposure has long been a hypothesized trigger for the development of MS, with many early studies demonstrating nearly 100% seropositivity in MS patients, and in pediatric-onset MS there is an unexpectedly high rate of asymptomatic EBV seropositivity. Mononucleosis in adolescence has been associated with increased subsequent risk of MS (relative risk: 2.3, 95% CI: 1.7–3.0). Recently a large cohort study showed a 32-fold increase in risk of MS after EBV seroconversion, a risk adjustment that is not seen after infection with any other virus (including cytomegalovirus, which is transmitted similarly). EBV infection is likely necessary, though not sufficient, for the development of MS; this is hypothesized to be due to "molecular mimicry" via amino acid sequence homology between virus proteins and myelin basic protein causing autoreactivity and infection of B cells, which may mediate chronic inflammation in MS.

MULTIPLE SCLEROSIS PATHOPHYSIOLOGY

The acute MS lesion is the pathophysiologic end result of a highly coordinated cascade of inflammatory activity. Active blood-brain barrier breakdown is mediated by the recruitment of perivascular inflammatory infiltrates comprised of myelin-reactive T cells, B cells, and macrophages. The pathologic hallmark of acute MS is focal white matter demyelination and relative sparing of axons with a variable associated perivascular inflammation or gliosis. Areas that are commonly affected in MS include the periventricular and juxtacortical white matter (regions with dense perivenular topography), although lesions may occur throughout the CNS, including the optic nerves, cerebellum, and spinal cord.

MS is commonly described as a disease of focal white matter demyelination; however, histologic studies have revealed a more complex pathology. Apart from lesions, it is well established that there is diffuse microglial inflammation of the normal-appearing white matter in MS even at disease onset. Axonal degeneration is present in MS lesions at all ages, frequently in regions of active or acute demyelination. Cortical gray matter demyelination is prevalent in MS, with subpial (type III) cortical demyelinating lesions considered to be a unique, specific feature of the disease. Cortical demyelination is frequently widespread on postmortem analysis of progressive MS patients, accrues with disease duration (though it is found in early disease stages), and has a correlation with cortical microglia and leptomeningeal inflammation on histology. The meninges are hypothesized immunologic regulatory sites for the inflammatory response in MS, and meningeal B-cell follicles (present in 40% of patients with progressive MS and also found in early MS stages) may function to organize and sustain chronic inflammation of progressive disease. Additional mechanisms drive chronic MS inflammation in parallel, including cytokine production, microglia and astrocyte activation, complement activation, glutamate excitotoxicity, iron accumulation, nitrous oxide production by macrophages, ion channel redistribution and dysfunction, and oxidative/mitochondrial injury, among other processes.

MULTIPLE SCLEROSIS AND MAGNETIC RESONANCE IMAGING

MRI is used to confirm the presence of MS inflammatory lesions. Lesions are traditionally evaluated by T2-weighted fluid attenuation inversion recovery sequence (FLAIR), where they are visible as hyperintensities with distinct characteristics and spatial distribution. They are classically ovoid and oriented perpendicularly to the ventricles (Fig. 21.1), giving the impression of finger-like projections on the sagittal T2-FLAIR sequence (known as "Dawson fingers"). MS lesions are commonly found in the periventricular white matter and corpus callosum, although they can be evident throughout the white matter. When the spinal cord is involved in MS, lesions usually span a single vertebral body, occupy a fraction of the cord on axial cross section, and lack associated cord edema. Acute lesions show active gadolinium contrast extravasation on T1 post-gadolinium MRI sequence due to active blood-brain barrier disruption. Contrast enhancement usually resolves by 30–40 days from onset and rarely persists until 8 weeks; if they are present for a longer duration, a diagnosis other than MS should be considered.

MAKING THE DIAGNOSIS OF MULTIPLE SCLEROSIS

RRMS typically presents in young adulthood (average age: 31 years) with exacerbations of neurologic symptoms lasting more than 24 hours in duration that may include weakness, numbness/paresthesias, optic neuritis, brain stem dysfunction (intranuclear ophthalmoplegia and nystagmus being common), impaired balance, L'hermitte sign, or transverse myelitis. Fatigue, cognitive dysfunction, and mood symptoms are underappreciated facets of MS presentation that often coincide with physical symptoms. MS attacks usually present over the course of days, plateau over the course of days to weeks, and recover over the course of weeks to months.

Studies of MS natural history that predate the treatment era cite high rates of SPMS transition among untreated patients, with as many as two-thirds of RRMS patients becoming progressive after ~15 years, though more recent data since the evolution of effective MS therapy have shown a lower risk of SPMS and longer disease duration prior to SPMS transition.

Secondary progressive transition is often contrasted with primary progressive MS (PPMS), which is rarer (10%–15% of patients) and is characterized by gradual disability accumulation from disease onset. Progressive MS (regardless of whether PPMS or SPMS) is often described in terms of worsening ambulatory dysfunction, though symptom progression may involve many symptoms that are attributable to RRMS, including fatigue, cognitive dysfunction, bowel/bladder dysfunction, mood/affective disturbances, sleep disturbances, sexual dysfunction, and spasticity. There is evidence to suggest that progressive MS may exist along a continuum rather than as a distinct transition point. Progressive disease (primary or secondary) begins around the same absolute age (41), and once progression begins, the rate of disability accrual is essentially identical, likely reflective of a common pathology at these stages. More recently, there has been effort to classify progressive MS by terminology that may better reflect the pathologic underpinnings of the progressive stage. Patients who have clinical relapses and/or MRI activity in the progressive MS stage (defined as active progressive MS), are viewed as a unique subpopulation of MS patients and may have better response to traditional MS DMTs compared to nonactive progressive MS patients. Treatment of nonactive progressive MS remains one of the major challenges in the field, as this stage is driven by

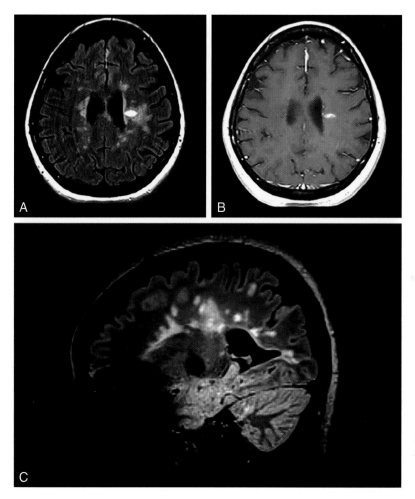

Fig. 21.1 Magnetic resonance imaging brain lesions that are typical of multiple sclerosis. (A) Axial T2-FLAIR (fluid attenuation inversion recovery sequence) imaging shows multiple hyperintensities that are ovoid and perpendicular to the ventricles. The most hyperintense lesion in the left frontal white matter enhances on (B) a postgadolinium T1 weighted image. (C) A sagittal T2-FLAIR shows similar hyperintensities in the typical "Dawson's Fingers" appearance adjacent to the corpus callosum. (From Zurawski J, Stankiewicz J. Multiple sclerosis re-examined: essential and emerging clinical concepts. Am J Med. 2018;131(5):464–472.)

processes that are not substantially affected by currently available therapies.

The McDonald criteria, most recently revised in 2017, are the standardized criteria used to diagnose MS. They outline requirements for dissemination in space and dissemination in time that can be met by a combination of clinical history and MRI. Dissemination in space requires that characteristic MRI lesions be present in at least two of four areas of the CNS (periventricular, cortical/juxtacortical, infratentorial, or spinal cord). Dissemination in time criteria can be met by the simultaneous presence of enhancing and nonenhancing lesions on contrasted MRI,

by the development of new typical lesions on subsequent MRIs, or occasionally by the presence of oligoclonal bands in the cerebrospinal fluid (CSF) (Table 21.1). Oligoclonal band testing is positive in 95% of patients with clinically definite MS and doubles the risk of progression to MS among patients with clinically isolated syndrome. Evoked potentials, optical coherence tomography, or prospective monitoring can provide additional evidence to support a diagnosis of MS but are not part of the formal diagnostic criteria.

For the diagnosis of PPMS, patients need to display a progressive worsening of symptoms over the course of

TABLE 21.1   2017 McDonald Criteria

Relapsing-Remitting Multiple Sclerosis

	Number of Lesions	Additional Data Needed for Diagnosis
≥2 clinical attacks	≥2	None
≥2 clinical attacks	1	Need dissemination in space: 1. A reported history of a previous attack involving a second CNS location OR 2. The development of another attack involving a second CNS location OR 3. The development of additional T2 lesion(s) on MRI in at least 2 MS-typical regions: periventricular, cortical/juxtacortical, infratentorial, spinal cord
1 clinical attack	≥2	Need dissemination in time: 1. The presence of both enhancing and nonenhancing lesions on MRI[a] OR 2. The development of another attack involving a second CNS location OR 3. The development of additional T2 lesion(s) on MRI in at least 2 MS-typical regions: periventricular, cortical/juxtacortical, infratentorial, spinal cord OR 4. The presence of CSF-specific oligoclonal bands
1 clinical attack	1	Clinically isolated syndrome Need dissemination in space: 1. The development of another attack involving a second CNS location OR 2. The development of additional T2 lesion(s) on MRI in at least 2 MS-typical regions: periventricular, cortical/juxtacortical, infratentorial, spinal cord AND Need dissemination in time: 1. The development of another attack involving a second CNS location OR 2. The development of additional T2 lesion(s) on MRI in at least 2 MS-typical regions: periventricular, cortical/juxtacortical, infratentorial, spinal cord OR 3. The presence of CSF-specific oligoclonal bands
Primary Progressive Multiple Sclerosis At least 1 year of disability progression without a history of clinical attacks		At least two of the following: 1. ≥1 characteristic MRI lesion in a periventricular, cortical/juxtacortical, or infratentorial region 2. ≥2 T2 hyperintense MRI lesions in the spinal cord 3. The presence of CSF-specific oligoclonal bands

CNS, Central nervous system; CSF, cerebrospinal fluid; MRI, magnetic resonance imaging; MS, multiple sclerosis.
[a]Note that if lesions are all enhancing or all nonenhancing, this can also meet diagnostic criteria for clinically isolated syndrome until dissemination in time criteria are met.

1 year with no history of clinical relapses. For diagnosis, patients also require at least two of the following: (1) at least one characteristic MRI brain lesion, (2) at least two MRI spinal cord lesions, (3) the presence of oligoclonal bands in the CSF (see Table 21.1).

Patients who have a single clinical attack corresponding to either a single lesion or multiple enhancing lesions without the presence of nonenhancing lesions are said to have Clinically Isolated Syndrome (CIS) (see Table 21.1). Clinicians assess clinical status and MRI lesion burden in CIS to determine whether to recommend treatment, but often treatment is initiated and justified based on approximately a 60%–75% rate of conversion to MS over 15 years. Risk factors for conversion from CIS to MS include increased number of initial MRI lesions, younger age at presentation, and the presence of CSF-specific oligoclonal bands.

Occasionally MS-typical lesions are incidentally found among patients obtaining an MRI for other reasons, such as headaches, trauma, etc., though they have never had symptoms of an MS clinical attack. These patients are said to have Radiologically Isolated Syndrome (RIS), which carries an approximate 30% risk of conversion to clinically   definite MS at 5 years and ~50% at 10 years after the initial MRI. Risk factors for conversion to MS include the presence of CSF-specific oligoclonal bands and/or spinal cord lesions on initial MRI. Treatment is not routinely started in RIS stage, although in high-risk cases can be a consideration.

Nonspecific white matter lesions on MRI brain are one of the most common cause for MS misdiagnosis, as a differential diagnosis list includes normal variant (such as enlarged perivascular spaces), migraines, small-vessel ischemic changes (secondary to smoking, hypertension, or hyperlipidemia), infections, neoplasms, and leukodystrophies. MRI lesion features/topography along with history and physical exam help narrow the differential diagnosis list. One potentially helpful diagnostic imaging tool to evaluate nonspecific white matter lesions is T2* imaging for central veins which can be visualized in demyelinating disease at 3 T and 7 T MRI ('central vein sign'). While not yet widely clinically available, the ultra-high-field 7 T MRI platform affords high sensitivity for detection of central veins to assess demyelinating etiology, with recent data suggesting that a >40% central vein sign cutoff distinguishes lesions typical of MS from non-MS cases.

THE DIFFERENTIAL DIAGNOSIS OF MULTIPLE SCLEROSIS: IMPORTANT CONSIDERATIONS RELATED TO CLINICAL PRESENTATION AND DIAGNOSTIC MIMICS

Multiple sclerosis can present with a wide variety of clinical symptoms depending on the location of inflammation, although typical MRI lesions can help to narrow the differential diagnosis. However, two common clinical presentations—optic neuritis and spinal cord myelitis—can occur in the absence of MRI brain lesions and have unique differential diagnoses to consider.

Optic Neuritis

Optic neuritis is the presenting attack in 15%–20% of MS patients, and ~40% of patients with first-time optic neuritis go on to be diagnosed with MS in the next 10 years. Symptoms typically include a subacute loss of vision associated with painful movements of the eye. Neuritis can be unilateral or bilateral but is more commonly unilateral in MS. Optic neuritis can sometimes be seen as T2 hyperintensity of the affected optic nerve on orbital MRIs (often with associated contrast enhancement) and often show signs of optic disc swelling on ophthalmologic evaluation. Ophthalmologic evaluation is highly recommended if a patient is suspected to have optic neuritis, as the symptoms overlap heavily with other disorders of the eye.

Optic neuritis is not specific to MS and is often seen in other neurodemyelinating disorders. Neuromyelitis optica (NMO) and myelin oligodendrocyte glycoprotein antibody disorder (MOGAD) are two neuroinflammatory diseases that can present similarly to MS and should also be high on the differential when a patient presents with optic neuritis. Other considerations, such as infections, neoplasms, and ischemic changes, can be seen in Table 21.2. In fact, optic neuritis has so many potential causes that clinical relapses of optic neuritis, per the 2017 McDonald criteria, are not sufficient to meet dissemination in space criteria.

Myelitis

The terms "myelitis" and "transverse myelitis" are often used synonymously to denote inflammation of the spinal cord, although the term "transverse myelitis" specifically refers to an inflammation that covers an

TABLE 21.2   Differential Diagnosis of Optic Neuritis and Transverse Myelitis

Optic Neuritis Specific	Transverse Myelitis Specific

• Ischemic optic neuropathy
  • Vascular disease
  • Temporal arteritis
  • Postsurgical complications
• Infection
  • Bartonella (cat-scratch disease)
  • West Nile Virus
  • Herpes Simplex Virus
• Neoplastic compression
• Thyroid eye disease
	• Metabolic abnormalities
	  • B12 deficiency
	  • Copper deficiency
	  • Zinc toxicity
	  • Nitrous oxide abuse
	• Infection
	  • Tuberculosis
	• Vascular Disease
	  • Spinal cord infarction
	  • Dural arteriovenous fistula
	• Spinal cord tumors

Either
- Autoimmune disorders
  - Multiple sclerosis
  - Neuromyelitis optica
  - Myelin oligodendrocyte glycoprotein antibody disorder
  - Sarcoidosis
  - ADEM
  - Behcet disease
  - Lupus
  - Sjögren
  - Paraneoplastic syndromes
- Infections
  - Syphilis
  - Lyme disease
- Genetic disorders
- Idiopathic

ADEM, Acute disseminated encephalomyelitis.

entire transverse section of the cord. The myelitis that is encountered in MS is rarely transverse, as it tends to affect the spinal cord in an eccentric pattern, as can be seen by T2 hyperintense lesions on MRI. As with optic neuritis, NMO and MOGAD can cause myelitis similar to that seen in MS; particularly when myelitis involves the cervical spine, these diagnoses should be high on a differential. There are multiple causes of spinal cord lesions that should be considered when these abnormalities are seen on MRI (see Table 21.2).

Neuromyelitis Optica

Clinical Features

Neuromyelitis optica (also known as Devic disease) was first described by Dr. Eugene Devic in Paris in 1894. Due to NMO's similar pattern of relapses of demyelination, specifically with episodes of optic neuritis and transverse myelitis, it was considered a variant of MS until the identification of the NMO-specific pathologic antibody Aquaporin-4 (AQP4) IgG in 2004. NMO affects mostly females, with a female-to-male ratio of ~9:1 and an average age of onset of 40 years. NMO is more common in East Asians (prevalence 3.5/100,000) and Blacks (prevalence 1.8–10/100,000) than in Whites (1/100,000).

AQP4-IgG targets the water channels in the endfeet of astrocytes, which activates the complement pathway and secondarily damages oligodendrocytes, causing demyelination. NMO relapses occur more frequently than MS relapses (annualized relapse rate of 0.82) and tend to be more severe with impaired recovery after attacks.

Although the formal diagnostic criteria for NMO are beyond the scope of this chapter, NMO, like MS, requires the presence of a clinical relapse with MRI changes and exclusion of alternative causes in order to make a diagnosis. Although most patients who are diagnosed with NMO have AQP4 antibodies, these are not required for diagnosis, with about 20%–30% being AQP4 negative. NMO lesions tend to be both larger and less well defined on MRI than in MS.

Eighty-five percent of patients with NMO present with either optic neuritis or transverse myelitis, which can make it difficult to distinguish NMO from MS. However, there are clinical, laboratory, and MRI characteristics that can help to differentiate these diagnoses (Table 21.3). Optic neuritis in NMO is more likely to be bilateral, and both the vision loss and pain tend to be more severe. On MRI the optic nerve lesions tend to be longitudinally expansive and involve the posterior optic nerve or optic chiasm, in comparison to the short-segment lesions that are seen in MS. This is also seen in NMO transverse myelitis, which tends to be large (covering more than half of the transverse section of the spinal cord) and longitudinally extensive (covering at least three vertebral bodies) in comparison to the small, peripheral lesions that are associated with MS (Fig. 21.2).

TABLE 21.3 Comparison of Clinical, Laboratory, and Magnetic Resonance Imaging Characteristics of Multiple Sclerosis (MS), Neuromyelitis Optica (NMO), and Myelin Oligodendrocyte Glycoprotein Antibody Disorder (MOGAD)

	MS	NMO	MOGAD
Average age of onset	20–40	30–50	Bimodal: • 1–10 • 31–40
Female:male ratio	2.8:1	9:1	1:1
Clinical course at onset	• 85% Relapsing-remitting • 15% Progressive	Relapsing	• Frequently relapsing • Up to 50% monophasic
Optic neuritis features	• Typically unilateral • Short-segment lesions anywhere in the optic nerve	• Often bilateral • Longitudinally extensive lesions, typically of the optic chiasm or posterior optic nerves	• Often bilateral • Longitudinally extensive lesions, typically of the anterior optic nerves • Optic nerve sheath enhancement
Transverse myelitis features	• Small lesions, <1 vertebral body in length • Peripherally located, usually in the dorsal or lateral columns	• Longitudinally extensive lesions, ≥3 vertebral bodies in length • Involve more than half the cross-sectional area of the spinal cord	• Longitudinally extensive lesions, ≥3 vertebral bodies in length
CSF oligoclonal bands	Persistently seen in 95% of patients with clinically definite MS	Transiently seen in <20%	Transiently seen in <20%
CSF white blood cells	Normal to mildly elevated	>50/µL in 13%–35%	>50/µL in 35%

CSF, Cerebrospinal fluid.

Disease Management and Prognosis

Treatment of acute NMO relapses should be initiated as soon as possible. Acute relapses of NMO are initially treated similarly to MS relapses, with high-dose intravenous steroids for 3–7 days. However, unlike in MS, plasma exchange (PLEX) can be considered a first-line therapy instead of or in conjunction with steroids, and it often has better outcomes than steroids alone. In cases in which steroids and/or PLEX have failed, intravenous immunoglobulin (IVIG) can be beneficial.

Until 2019 treatments for NMO were off-label and consisted of steroids, azathioprine, mycophenolate mofetil, methotrexate, and rituximab, along with other immunomodulators/immunosuppressors. However, since then, four treatments have been FDA approved for use in AQP4-positive NMO: eculizumab (a C5 complement inhibitor administered intravenously every 2 weeks after initial loading doses), inebilizumab (an anti-CD19 monoclonal antibody administered intravenously every 6 months after initial loading doses), satralizumab (an IL-6 receptor antagonist administered subcutaneously every 4 weeks after initial loading doses), and ravulizumab (a C5 complement inhibitor administered intravenously every 8 weeks after initial loading doses).

Living with NMO poses multiple challenges. Although most disability is accrued during relapses, with little to no progression occurring between attacks, recovery is often slow and incomplete, and many symptoms persist. Eighty-three percent of patients report pain as a very frequent symptom, and 30%–70% endorse cognitive changes. Prior to the recent development of FDA-approved drugs for NMO, by around 6 years of disease duration, 18% of patients had permanent bilateral visual disability, 34% had permanent motor disability, and 23% had become wheelchair dependent. Hope remains that with increasing use of newly developed drugs, the prognosis for people diagnosed with NMO will improve.

Myelin Oligodendrocyte Glycoprotein–Associated Disorders

Clinical Features

Myelin oligodendrocyte glycoprotein (MOG) is expressed on the outer surface of myelin only within the CNS, and as a result, MOGAD can present as a variety of demyelinating disorders. This is likely why many MOGAD patients were misdiagnosed as having MS or NMO prior to 2018, when cell-based assays for IgG1-MOG antibody became clinically available.

In contrast to MS and NMO, MOGAD does not have a gender predilection, occurring equally often in males and females. MOGAD can be diagnosed at any age but has a bimodal age distribution, occurring most often in children ages 1–10 years, followed by young adults ages 31–40 years. Presenting symptoms vary by age, with children more likely to present with acute disseminated encephalomyelitis (ADEM) and adults more likely to present with optic neuritis or transverse myelitis. Other epidemiologic data for MOGAD is limited due to the relative novelty of the diagnosis.

MOGAD, much like MS and NMO, presents with clinical attacks that are attributed to inflammatory demyelination; these attacks are often very similar to those in MS and NMO. With the exception of ADEM in children, the most common presentations of MOGAD are optic neuritis and transverse myelitis. As in NMO, in addition to the presence of MOG-specific antibodies, there are clinical, laboratory, and MRI factors that can help to differentiate MOGAD from these similar disorders (see Table 21.3).

White matter lesions in MOGAD tend to be less well defined than in MS, are not as frequently contrast enhancing, and are unique in that they tend to fully resolve with treatment. Optic neuritis in MOGAD is, as in NMO, more often bilateral and longitudinally extensive than in MS and on MRI is specifically associated with anterior optic nerve involvement and optic nerve sheath enhancement, features that are not typically seen in MS or NMO (although optic nerve sheath enhancement is not specific to MOGAD and can be seen in multiple other disorders, such as sarcoidosis, tuberculosis, and neoplasms). As in NMO, MOGAD more often presents with longitudinally extensive lesions in both the optic nerve and the spinal cord that are unlike those seen in MS (see Fig. 21.2).

Disease Management and Prognosis

As in MS and NMO, the first-line treatment of an acute relapse of MOGAD is high-dose intravenous steroids. However, unlike MS and NMO, MOGAD has a tendency to rebound after cessation of steroids, so a prolonged taper is recommended. For patients who do not respond to steroids, either PLEX or IVIG can be used.

As up to 50% of patients may have a monophasic course of MOGAD with a single clinical attack, maintenance therapy is not recommended until a relapsing course has been proven. There are no FDA-approved medications for the long-term management of relapsing MOGAD, but multiple immunomodulators/immunosuppressors have been used off label, including rituximab, azathioprine, mycophenolate mofetil, tocilizumab, and IVIG. Unfortunately, despite long-term treatment, some patients continue to have high relapse rates.

The long-term prognosis for MOGAD remains unclear. Most patients diagnosed with this disorder have good outcomes after attacks, but there are not yet good predictors for disease course or outcomes. Younger patients and those with fewer attacks tend to have better outcomes than older patients with more frequent attacks, but other demographic and disease factors have not been associated with disability accumulation. Many patients with positive MOG-IgG1 antibodies will become antibody negative over the course of their disease, but there remains equipoise about whether this has any impact on relapse risk. As with many of the diseases discussed in this chapter, more time is needed to better study these outcomes.

MANAGEMENT OF ACUTE EXACERBATIONS OF MULTIPLE SCLEROSIS

Acute MS exacerbations are treated with glucocorticoids, typically with a course of 3–5 days of intravenous methylprednisolone 1000–1250 mg daily without subsequent oral prednisone taper. A noninferior alternative regimen with equivalent bioavailability is oral prednisone 1250 mg daily for the same duration. Both formulations restore the blood-brain barrier as assessed by resolution of contrast enhancement on MRI. Glucocorticoids at the doses and durations that are used to treat MS flares have minimal side effects, though caution should be used in patients with recurrent infections, gastric reflux,

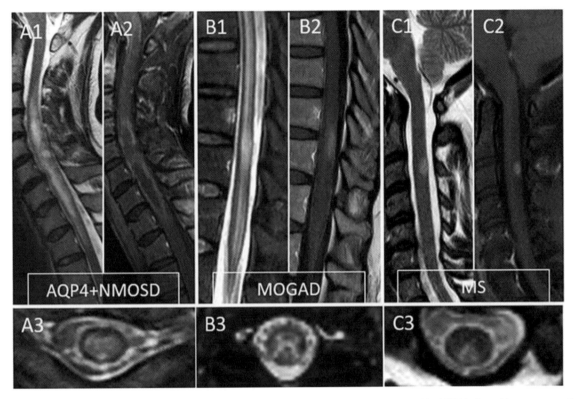

Fig. 21.2 Typical magnetic resonance imaging findings in patients with myelitis associated with AQP4-IgG-positive neuromyelitis optica spectrum disorder (AQP4+NMOSD), MOG-IgG associated disease (MOGAD), and multiple sclerosis (MS). A typical longitudinally extensive T2 lesion affecting the cervical spinal cord in a patient with AQP4+NMOSD is evident on sagittal images (A1), with peripheral enhancement after gadolinium administration—"elongated ring" enhancement (A2). Axially, the T2 lesion involves the majority of the spinal cord (A3). In patients with MOGAD myelitis, involvement of the conus medullaris by the longitudinally extensive T2 lesions (B1) is significantly more common compared to NMOSD or MS, with accompanying patchy or nonspecific enhancement in about half of cases (B2). On axial T2 images, a predominant involvement of the central gray matter is common forming an "H-sign" (B3). MS myelitis T2 lesions are typically short, spanning a single vertebral body on sagittal images (C1) and peripherally located along the dorsal (C3) or lateral columns axially. After gadolinium administration, lesion enhancement can be nodular (C2) or ring-like. (Adapted from Fadda G, Flanagan EP, Cacciaguerra L, Jitprapaikulsan J, Solla P, Zara P, Sechi, E. Myelitis features and outcomes in CNS demyelinating disorders: Comparison between multiple sclerosis, MOGAD, and AQP4-IgG-positive NMOSD. *Front Neurol.* 2022;13:1011579.)

or psychiatric history. Retreatment with steroids is commonly attempted for refractory flares, though patients who are experiencing more severe recurrent demyelinating events may benefit from plasmapheresis.

MULTIPLE SCLEROSIS MAINTENANCE THERAPY

Management of MS has become increasingly complex, as there are now 26 FDA-approved DMTs for MS (Table 21.4). MS medications can be broadly classified into three groups: (1) early injectable medications

(beta-interferons and glatiramer acetate); (2) oral medications (sphingosine-1-phosphate modulators, fumarates, teriflunomide, and cladribine); and (3) infusion therapies/monocloncal antibodies (natalizumab, CD20-inhibitors, mitoxantrone, and alemtuzumab).

First-line injectable MS therapies, administered via either intramuscular or subcutaneous injection, have dosing schedules that range from once daily (glatiramer acetate 20 mg) to every 2 weeks (pegylated beta interferon-1a). Beta-interferon is a cytokine that alters the autoreactive environment in MS. Glatiramer acetate is a mixture of amino acids with antigenic similarity to myelin basic protein that alters T-cell activation. Injectable drugs were the first medications historically available, and most MS experts believe that they are less efficacious than oral or infused drugs based on trial data, though they have a comparatively favorable safety profile and are not considered immunosuppressive. Intolerance of injections or associated side effects, however, may necessitate switching to another class of medication in many instances.

Oral medications offer easier administration but have unique side effect and safety profiles. Dimethyl fumarate is a twice-daily oral pill with immunomodulating activity that depletes autoreactive lymphocytes, though it has possible side effects of gastrointestinal upset, facial flushing, lymphopenia, and, rarely, progressive multifocal leukoencephalopathy (PML). Several similar fumarate medications have come to market in the past several years. In 2019 diroximel fumarate was approved for use in MS. It and dimethyl fumarate are both metabolized into the same active metabolite—monomethyl fumarate—which itself was approved in 2020 for use in MS. The three share similar efficacy.

Fingolimod is a once-daily oral sphingosine-1-receptor (S1P) modulator that alters lymphocyte migration. Because sphingosine receptors are also found on cardiac myocytes and in the eye, bradycardia and macular edema can occur. Prior to initiation of fingolimod, an electrocardiogram and dilated eye examination are recommended, and patients should have an observed first dose. Lymphopenia should be monitored, and there is rare risk of PML. In the last decade, three other S1P receptor modulators have been approved for use in MS: siponimod, onzanimod, and ponesimod. Because these more recent drugs are more specific for the S1P receptor relative to fingolimod, they do not all require first-dose monitoring, although their side effect profiles are otherwise similar. Teriflunomide is a once-daily oral option that causes inhibition of pyridine-related T-cell activation. Its efficacy is in line with that of the injectable medications (tier I), while the fumarates and S1P receptor modulators are considered a second tier of efficacy. Teriflunomide side effects include hair thinning, diarrhea, and abnormal liver function tests, though the medication is generally well tolerated. It is known to be teratogenic in animals and is pregnancy category X, limiting its use in females of childbearing age. A single case of PML following natalizumab has been reported with this drug. Finally, cladribine is a high-efficacy oral nucleoside metabolic inhibitor

that cytotoxically depletes B and T cells. It is given in two courses: the first course consists of a 5-day cycle of once-daily pills followed 23–27 days later by a second 5-day cycle. The second course occurs approximately 1 year after the first. Although cladribine is considered highest tier of efficacy, it comes with potentially more serious side effects of sustained lymphopenia and increased infection and malignancy risk, so it is most typically used after other DMTs have failed.

Currently available FDA-approved infusions for MS treatment are in the highest (third) tier of efficacy. Natalizumab, a monthly integrin α-4 antibody infusion, has excellent efficacy in the treatment of active inflammatory MS, but this comes with a significant risk of PML. Duration of treatment (>24 months) and prior exposure to immunosuppression increase risk, and a JC virus antibody index may be obtained from the serum to stratify at-risk patients (ranging from a 1:10,000 risk of PML among antibody-negative patients to an approximately 1:100 risk among those with JC antibody titers >1.5 who are treated for longer than 24 months).

Ocrelizumab is an anti-CD20 antibody infusion that was approved in 2017 and has become widely used for MS. Phase III clinical trial data show high efficacy in RRMS and reduced disability progression in PPMS patients. After two introductory half doses 2 weeks apart, ocrelizumab is administered once every 6 months. Infusion reactions can occur but these are generally mild, and risk is highest with initial doses. Rates of certain infections (respiratory infections, herpesvirus) were slightly increased in ocrelizumab-treated patients. In phase III trials there were slightly more breast cancer cases in ocrelizumab-treated patients compared with placebo- or interferon-treated groups, though the long-term malignancy risk with ocrelizumab is unclear, and subsequent studies have not found increased risk of breast cancer or other malignancies in ocrelizumab-treated patients compared to the general population. Rare cases of PML have been noted with ocrelizumab use, although a majority of these were patients who were transitioned to ocrelizumab from natalizumab or fingolimod. Given the pharmacologic similarity of ocrelizumab to rituximab (both are anti-CD20 monoclonal infusions), PML risk in ocrelizumab would be expected to be similar to that of rituximab in rheumatoid arthritis, in which the risk is estimated at 1:25,000. Since ocrelizumab's approval in 2017, there have been two other anti-CD20 drugs approved for use in MS. Ofatumumab, approved in 2020, is a once-monthly injection that can be done at home, and ublituximab, approved in 2022, is a twice-yearly infusion. These medications have similar efficacy, though they offer advantages of self-administration or faster infusion time, respectively.

Alemtuzumab, a monoclonal antibody that targets CD52-reactive immune cells is also considered to be in the highest (third) tier of efficacy. It is infused in two separate courses, 12 months apart. Dosing of the drug can precipitate autoimmune side effects, including thyroid disease (seen in 30% of patients at 5 years), immune thrombocytopenia (~2%), and, rarely, antiglomerular basement membrane kidney disease. Increased risk of infection, bone marrow suppression, and malignancy (thyroid cancer, melanoma, lymphoproliferative disease) have also been associated with the drug. The severity of the side effects means that alemtuzumab is typically reserved for aggressive or refractory MS. Mitoxantrone is an every-3-month infusion of a topoisomerase II inhibitor, though due to its severe cardiac risks, it is not often used.

Historically, limited therapy choices in MS resulted in a widespread de facto "escalation" treatment strategy. Patients were routinely placed on injectable medications as first-line treatment, and failure dictated cessation or use of strong immunosuppressants with unfavorable side effects. As a wider variety of treatment options became available in the 2000s, patients were transitioned to alternatives that offered improved efficacy and administration but had less favorable safety profiles. There remains an ongoing debate in the MS community as to whether an "escalation" or "early efficacy" approach to treatment initiation is optimal, though recent advances in the characterization of MS suggest that subtle disease pathology can begin early, can be widely disseminated, and is not well detected by conventional clinical MRI, clinical examination, or randomized clinical trials. Recent real-world data have shown benefit in the early use of high-efficacy therapies in reducing MS relapses and MRI activity and delaying the onset of progressive stage. There is also an ongoing randomized clinical trial to evaluate the impact of early aggressive treatment versus traditional treatments for MS on prevention of disability accumulation (Traditional versus Early Aggressive Therapy for Multiple Sclerosis Trial [TREAT-MS]; clinicaltrials.gov identifier NCT03500328). With so many beneficial therapies that can be used to manage MS, treatment decisions are not one-size-fits-all. Choice of DMT requires joint patient-provider decision-making that incorporates

careful risk-benefit calculation, consideration of immune side effects and patient preference, awareness of the impact of early high-efficacy therapy, and willingness to treat assertively when circumstances warrant.

SPECIAL POPULATIONS IN MULTIPLE SCLEROSIS

MS can present at nearly any age and is a lifelong illness. While guidelines and treatments are applicable to most patients over 18 years old, there exist a few notable populations for whom data are limited and management varies: the pediatric population, patients who are pregnant or planning a family, and the elderly. While a full discourse on these populations is beyond the scope of this chapter, we will address some of the most important factors surrounding management of these groups.

Pediatric Multiple Sclerosis

Fewer than 10% of people with MS become symptomatic before age 16 years, and fewer than 1% become symptomatic before age 10. Pediatric-onset MS (POMS) patients are nearly exclusively of the relapsing MS subtype, and relapses are more frequent than in adult-onset MS. The 2017 McDonald criteria are 71% sensitive and 95% specific for the diagnosis of MS in children, although they should not be applied to children who present with acute demyelinating encephalomyelitis (ADEM) and should be used in caution in children under age 11 years. In general, a broad differential diagnosis should be kept, as only ~20% of pediatric patients presenting with an acquired demyelinating syndrome are later diagnosed with pediatric MS. The disease is fairly similar in pediatric and adult patients, although POMS patients typically reach disability milestones earlier than their adult-onset MS counterparts and have faster cognitive decline. Early treatment of pediatric MS is encouraged. While only fingolimod has been FDA-approved for treatment of POMS in the United States, patients are often treated off label with other MS therapies (see Table 21.4).

Pregnancy

Given that MS most typically affects females of childbearing age, questions from patients regarding family planning and pregnancy are extremely common. Pregnancy does not pose a specific relapse risk for patients with MS. Historically, relapse rates were reported to increase during

TABLE 21.4   Summary of the Disease-Modifying Treatments for Multiple Sclerosis

Drug	Year FDA Approved for MS	Dosing	Proposed Mechanism of Action	Notable Side Effects
Injectable DMTs				
Interferon β-1b		Three-times-weekly injection	Unknown; thought to bind interferon β-1b receptors producing antiproliferative and immunomodulatory effects	• Injection site reactions • Transient flu-like symptoms
(Betaseron)	1993			
(Extavia)	2009			
Interferon β-1a		Injection, weekly Three-times-weekly injection	Unknown; thought to bind interferon β-1a receptors, producing antiproliferative and immunomodulatory effects	• Injection site reactions • Transient flu-like symptoms
(Avonex)	1996			
(Rebif)	1998			
Glatiramer acetate		Daily injection OR Three-times-weekly injection	Unknown; thought to augment the activity of suppressor T cells	• Injection site reactions • Lipoatrophy with prolonged use
(Copaxone)	1996			
(Glatopa)	2015			
(generic)	2017			
Pegylated Interferon β-1a (Plegridy)	2014	Every 2 weeks injection	See above, interferon β-1a	See above, interferon β-1a
Oral DMTs				
Sphingosine-1-phosphate receptor modulators		Oral, daily	Binds sphingosine-1-phosphate receptors, alters lymphocyte migration into the CNS	• First-dose bradycardia, heart block, hypertension • Macular edema • Lymphopenia • Rare risk of PML • Rare but increased risk of skin malignancies
Fingolimod (Gilenya)	2010			
Siponimod (Mayzent)	2019			
Ozanimod (Zeposia)	2020			
Ponesimod (Ponvory)	2021			
Fingolimod (generic)	2022			
Teriflunomide		Oral, daily	Inhibits pyrimidine-dependent lymphocyte activation	• Hepatotoxicity • Alopecia • Nausea/diarrhea • Teratogenicity • Rare risk of PML
(Aubagio)	2012			
(generic)	2023			
Fumarates		Oral, twice a day	Activates nuclear-factor-like-2, resulting in modulation of oxidative stress and reduced activation of autoreactive T cells	• Nausea/diarrhea • Skin flushing • Lymphopenia • Rare risk of PML
Dimethyl Fumarate[a] (Tecfidera)	2013			
Diroximel fumarate[a] (Vumerity)	2019			
Monomethyl fumarate[a] (Bafiertam)	2020			
Dimethyl fumarate[a] (generic)	2020			

TABLE 21.4 **Summary of the Disease-Modifying Treatments for Multiple Sclerosis—cont'd**

Drug	Year FDA Approved for MS	Dosing	Proposed Mechanism of Action	Notable Side Effects
Cladribine (Mavenclad)	2019	Oral, daily for 5 days, followed 3 weeks later by another cycle of oral, daily for 5 days. Repeat course after 1 year	Cytotoxically depletes B cells and T cells by acting as a nucleoside metabolic inhibitor	• Increased risk of malignancies • Lymphopenia • Increased infection risk, including rare risk of PML
Infusible DMTs/Monoclonal Therapies				
Mitoxantrone (Novantrone)	2000	IV infusion, every 3 months	Inhibits topoisomerase II, causes DNA breakage, inhibits RNA crosslinking	• Serious cardiac toxicity, cardiomyopathy • Cytopenia, secondary leukemia
Natalizumab (Tysabri)	2004	IV infusion, monthly	Monoclonal antibody, binds integrin receptors on leukocyte cell walls and alters migration into the CNS	• Potentially high risk for PML dependent on JCV status, requires routine serum monitoring • Infusion reactions
Alemtuzumab (Lemtrada)	2014	IV infusion, two infusions, the first lasting 5 days and the second lasting 3 days, separated by 12 months	Monoclonal antibody, binds CD52 cell surface glycoprotein resulting in B cell, T cell, NK cell, and macrophage lysis	• Autoimmune diseases: thyroid disorders, immune thrombocytopenia • Serious infusion reaction risk • Malignancy risk: thyroid cancer, melanoma, lymphoproliferative disorders • Increased infection risk
Anti-CD20 Antibodies			Monoclonal antibody, binds B-lymphocyte CD20 surface antigen	• Infusion/injection reactions • Increased infection risk, including rare risk of PML
Ocrelizumab (Ocrevus)	2017	IV infusion, every 6 months		
Ofatumumab (Kesimpta)	2020	Injection, monthly		
Ublituximab (Briumvi)	2022	IV infusion, every 6 months		

CNS, Central nervous system; *DMTs*, disease-modifying therapies; *JCV*, JC virus; *MS*, multiple sclerosis; *PML*, progressive multifocal leukoencephalopathy.
[a]Both dimethyl fumarate and diroximel fumarate are metabolized to monomethyl fumarate.

pregnancy, but data actually demonstrate lower-than-average relapse rate in the second and third trimesters, with a relative increase in risk postpartum. Patients with MS may be at higher risk for pregnancy complications; recent data show that patients with MS had higher rates of premature labor, infectious complications, cardiovascular disorders of pregnancy, and congenital fetal abnormalities than their non-MS counterparts.

MS that is well controlled in the year leading up to pregnancy is associated with stability in the partum and postpartum periods. Generally, DMTs are discontinued in patients who are planning a family; the exact timing of DMT discontinuation depends on the therapy in question. Only glatiramer acetate is pregnancy Category B, though many providers also consider natalizumab until the end of the second trimester, as it has shown to be safe in this period (and to avoid rebound disease caused by abrupt discontinuation in anticipation of pregnancy). Of special note is teriflunomide, which is pregnancy Category X (contraindicated in pregnancy or in females of childbearing age who are not on contraception) and so is generally avoided in favor of safer DMT options in this population and should be discontinued with an accelerated drug elimination procedure prior to family planning.

Breastfeeding has been shown to be protective against MS relapses early in postpartum, and most patients and providers prefer to continue off DMTs for this time, although there are some DMTs that may be safe during lactation, and several studies are ongoing to determine safety. Once patients have completed breastfeeding, a rapid restart of MS therapy is encouraged.

Older Patients with Multiple Sclerosis

Fewer than 10% of MS cases present after age 50, termed "late-onset MS" (LOMS) and less than 5% after age 60, termed "very-late-onset MS" (VLOMS). These patients commonly present with motor impairment and progressive disease courses.

The average age of people living with MS has increased, from ~40 years in the 1990s to ~60 years in the early 2010s. This is likely secondary to improved diagnostics and treatment options; however, the seminal trials for most MS DMTs exclude older and more disabled patients. It can be difficult to determine optimal treatment for older patients with LOMS and VLOMS, as some studies have suggested that DMT risks may outweigh benefits, and there is uncertain risk of MS activity/progression off treatment in this population. Current recommendations encourage treatment of MS patients with active disease (defined as recent clinical relapse or evidence of MRI activity), regardless of age. In practice, treatment decisions in this group are made with careful attention to risks and benefits, taking into account individualized prognostic factors, MRI, and patient preference and risk tolerance.

MULTIPLE SCLEROSIS PROGNOSIS

The estimated lifespan of MS patients is marginally less than that of healthy controls (estimated 5 years), and the data do not yet reflect the impact of recent advances in therapy. Positive predictive factors associated with benign MS include female sex and younger age at onset. Poorer prognosis has been linked to incomplete recovery

after ther initial attack, a short time interval between the first two attacks, and African American race. Initial MS flare symptoms do not strongly affect prognosis, with the exception of early bowel/bladder involvement, which correlates with a worse disease course. Smoking history is related to poor prognosis, namely, a faster onset of progressive disease and more rapid accumulation of MRI lesion burden.

CONCLUSION

In *Multiple Sclerosis: A History of Disease*, historian T. Jock Murray recounts the words of a 30-year-old British man who in 1919 died from an illness that is believed to have been MS: "It would be nice if a physician from London, one of these days, were to gallop up hotspur, tether his horse to the gait post, and dash in waving a reprieve—the discovery of a cure!" Over a century later, the race for a cure for MS continues. Strategies for curing MS are currently focused on (1) stopping disease activity and progression, (2) reversing fixed neurologic deficit (remyelination), and (3) disease prevention. While new high-efficacy disease-modifying medications address the first of these aims, treatment of progressive MS presents a continued challenge. Remyelination and disease prevention are the subjects of continued study. With new diagnostic tools and emerging treatments, however, the field of MS research continues to make strides toward that ultimate goal of a cure.

CLINICAL SIGNIFICANCE

- Multiple sclerosis (MS) is the most common demyelinating disease of the central nervous system.
- MS is an autoimmune-mediated condition with a genetic basis. However, environmental factors more strongly influence disease development.
- Diagnosis of MS requires specific magnetic resonance imaging and clinical criteria.
- MS consists of relapsing and progressive phases driven by distinct pathophysiology.
- There are 26 FDA-approved therapies for relapsing MS, but treatment of progressive MS remains a challenge, and there is no cure.

"For the full bibliography list, please use the pincode on the inside front cover to access the electronic version of the text at ebooks.health.elsevier.com."

22

Autonomic Disorders*

Peter Novak, Sadie P. Marciano, and Alexandra Knief

ANATOMIC AND PHYSIOLOGIC REMARKS

The principal role of the autonomic nervous system (ANS) is the maintenance of homeostasis by regulating and integrating the activities of essentially all organs. The ANS has been divided into the central autonomic system also called central autonomic network (CAN) or the preganglionic system, and the peripheral or postganglionic system, which includes the parasympathetic, sympathetic, and enteric systems. ANS regulates internal organs and controls heart rate, blood pressure, sweating, digestion, respiration, pupillary reactivity, urination, and sexual arousal.

The ANS has three main branches: the sympathetic nervous system, the parasympathetic nervous system, and the enteric nervous system. The sympathetic and parasympathetic systems have opposite actions (Table 22.1). The sympathetic system is the "fight or flight" system, while the parasympathetic is the "rest and digest" system. The enteric nervous system controls gut functions, and although it is relatively autonomous, it has numerous connections with the central nervous system.

Autonomic fibers are small, lightly myelinated Aδ fibers and unmyelinated C fibers. Sympathetic preganglionic fibers originate in the intermediolateral nucleus of the spine at the T1–L2 level. The fibers synapse at the sympathetic ganglia, which send the postganglionic (postsynaptic) fibers to the effector organs. Parasympathetic preganglionic fibers originate in the cranial nuclei and at the sacral portion of the spine.

*Based on Novak P. Autonomic disorders. *Am J Med.* 2019;132(4):420–436. ISSN 0002-9343. https://doi.org/10.1016/j.amjmed.2018.09.027.

The CAN is composed of structures dispersed throughout the central nervous system. CAN structures include the insular cortex, cingular gyrus, amygdala, hypothalamus, thalamus, brain stem nuclei, and ventrolateral medulla. Integration centers are composed of neurons with autonomic and nonautonomic functions. For example, the periventricular nucleus of the hypothalamus integrates autonomic functions with the energy balance.

The CAN controls autonomic functions and at the same time modulates a number of other functions, including emotional, attentional, behavioral, endocrine, respiratory, vestibular, sexual, and pain responses. The CAN is connected with all organs through the parasympathetic and sympathetic nerves innervations. Many CAN centers are defined by their function rather than by distinct anatomic or histologic landmarks. For example, the reticular formation in the brain stem is a complex network of nuclei that integrate and coordinate many vital brain systems without having precise boundaries of nuclei. Most structures of the CAN are bilaterally and reciprocally interconnected, and usually a bilateral lesion is needed to produce a well-defined and lasting effect.

NEUROTRANSMITTERS AND NEUROMODULATORS

The main excitatory neurotransmitters in the ANS are amino acid glutamate and aspartate, and the inhibitory neurotransmitter is γ-aminobutyric acid. These transmitters elicit fast, short-lasting responses mediated specific ion channel receptors. The neurotransmitters that are characteristic for ANS functions are catecholamines

TABLE 22.1   **Main Autonomic Functions**

Organ/System	Sympathetic (Fight or Flight)	Parasympathetic (Rest and Digest)
Pupil	Dilatation	Constriction (CN III)
Salivary gland	Inhibition	Stimulation (CN VII, IX)
Heart	Increases	Decrease (CN X)
Vessels	Constricts most vessels except dilates vessels of the skeletal muscles during exercise	Minimal or no effect
Sweat glands	Stimulates sweating	No innervation
Bronchi	Relaxation	Constriction (CN X)
Digestion	Inhibition (CG), decreased activity of glands and muscles of digestive system, vasoconstriction and sphincter contraction	Stimulation (CN X). Increased motility and secretion in the digestive system, relaxes sphincter
Liver	Stimulation of glucose production (CG)	No effect
Adrenal glands	Stimulation	
Bladder	Relaxation of bladder (detrusor muscle, IMG) Contraction of bladder neck (IMG)	Contraction of detrusor (sacral)
Penis	Ejaculation (IMG)	Erection (sacral)
Vagina, clitoris	Contraction	Erection
Coagulation		Increases
Fat tissue		Stimulates lipolysis

Sacral: the sacral S2–S4 portion of the spine. *CG*, Celiac ganglion; *CN*, cranial nerve; *IMG*, inferior mesenteric ganglion.

(norepinephrine and epinephrine) and acetylcholine. Preganglionic sympathetic and parasympathetic neurons utilize acetylcholine. Postganglionic neurons of the parasympathetic nervous system utilize acetylcholine via cholinergic fibers. Postganglionic neurons of the sympathetic nervous system release norepinephrine upon activation via adrenergic fibers. The adrenal medulla is the major source of epinephrine, which is released into the blood. A number of additional, especially peptidergic neurotransmitters were described in the central autonomic network with a profound effect upon autonomic functions. Many of these transmitters interact with the principal transmitters and modulate autonomic responses, through G protein–coupled specific receptors.

NOMENCLATURE REMARKS

Neuropathy is a broader term that signifies damage to the whole neuronal system. Neuronopathy is a form of neuropathy that results from a degeneration of the neuronal cell body. Ganglionopathy is a neuronopathy with damage to the ganglionic cells, either sensory or autonomic.

Malfunction of the autonomic system is called autonomic dysfunction or dysautonomia. The term "dysautonomia" is an umbrella term that covers any type of autonomic dysfunction. Autonomic failure is a type of dysautonomia that manifests clinically as autonomic hypoactivity. By definition, the isolated failure of one system leads to unopposed action of the other. For example, isolated damage of the parasympathetic "rest" system leads to unopposed action of the sympathetic "fight" system with a net effect of sympathetic overactivity, such as hypertension. Thus the term "autonomic failure" is used when the autonomic hypofunction dominates. A typical example of autonomic failure is neurogenic orthostatic hypotension (NOH). In autonomic hyperactivity, the net effect of the lesion is parasympathetic or sympathetic overactivity, such as in several types of hypertension. Dysautonomia can be continuous or paroxysmal (intermittent); acute, subacute or chronic; and preganglionic (affecting the central nervous system), postganglionic (peripheral), or mixed, affecting both central and peripheral nervous system.

Many small sensory fibers are located in close proximity to autonomic fibers and are frequently damaged together with autonomic fibers; therefore sensory and autonomic symptoms accompany each other, as is seen in mixed small fiber neuropathies. If the pain prevails, the term "painful small fiber neuropathy" is used; for predominantly autonomic symptoms, the term "autonomic neuropathy" is used. Probably the most common are mixed small fiber neuropathies with variable proportion of sensory and autonomic complaints.

AUTONOMIC SYMPTOMS

The ANS acts unconsciously via efferent (motor) fibers; therefore autonomic dysfunction manifests as an organ malfunction. For example, damage of vasomotor fibers may result in neurogenic orthostatic hypotension (OH). In contrast, activity of sensory small fibers can be felt, and thus their dysfunction may result in a variety of neuropathic complaints including pain or burning sensation.

Dysautonomia is associated with numerous symptoms. They can be divided into orthostatic, nonorthostatic, and diffuse (Box 22.1). Orthostatic symptoms are typically associated with cerebral hypoperfusion (typically manifesting as lightheadedness and dizziness) and/or sympathoexcitation (typically manifesting as palpitation and restlessness). Frequent nonorthostatic symptoms include gastrointestinal and urinary problems, cold or hot intolerance, excessive sweating or loss of sweating, and erectile dysfunction in males. Common additional nonspecific complaints include fatigue, headaches, brain fog, and insomnia. The majority of patients present with a combination of orthostatic and nonorthostatic symptoms.

SENSORY SYMPTOMS

Damage of small sensory fibers is typically associated with burning pain on the feet or hands and less frequently with lightning-like or lancinating pain, aching, or uncomfortable paresthesia (dysesthesias) or with pain to nonpainful stimuli (allodynia). Chest pain and dyspnea are also frequent.

BOX 22.1 Autonomic Symptoms

Orthostatic
Lightheadedness or dizziness
Syncope
Impending fainting sensation (presyncope)
Palpitations
Sense of weakness
Restlessness
Tremulousness
Nausea
Shortness of breath
Pallor,
Vertigo
Chest pain
Exacerbation by heat, exercise, meals, menses
Visual loss
Exercise intolerance
Neck pain

Nonorthostatic
Dysphagia, odynophagia, heartburn, reflux
Nausea, vomiting
Early satiety, bloating
Diarrhea, constipation
Abdominal pain
Bladder symptoms: incomplete emptying, incontinence
Pupillary symptoms
Dry eyes or mouth
Impotence, erectile dysfunction
Changes in skin color and texture
Hair loss
Hyperemia, cold, pale feet
Excessive sweating
Loss of sweating
Cold or hot intolerance
Erectile dysfunction

Diffuse
Fatigue
Sleep disturbances
Migraine
Brain fog

EXAMINATION

History Taking

Guidelines for taking a medical history and performing a medical examination should be followed. A careful past medical history and a detailed review of medications are necessary. Dysautonomia due to medication effect is very common in elderly people; therefore a detailed review of the use of any medication that can interact with the ANS is of utmost importance. Many medications interact with the ANS, including common drugs used for therapy for depression and pain with anticholinergic effect and antihypertensive/urinary medications with antiadrenergic effect.

The onset of the presenting problem is important diagnostically and must be documented (sudden, gradual, insidious) as well as the duration (acute, subacute, chronic), progression (rapidly or slowly progressive, static, regressive), and severity (mild, moderate, severe) of illness. Patients need to be questioned about the use of drugs, alcohol, diet, supplements, toxic exposures, history of Lyme disease, and history of travel and risk behavior. Dysautonomia features include the simultaneous involvement of multiple organ systems, fluctuations of symptoms from day to day or from position to position, history of hypermobility, multiple allergies, poor healing, or frequent infections. The patient's voiding and gastrointestinal history and any voiding or gastrointestinal complaints can be helpful for assessment of neurogenic bladder and gastric motility disorders.

Physical Examination

Specific features of the autonomic examination are postural variations in the blood pressure and heart rate, pupillary light reactions, skin temperature and color, and patterns of sweating. The dryness of the skin or excessive sweating, cold distal limbs, and pupillary changes point to dysautonomia. The blood pressure and heart rate must be measured with the patient in the supine position, preferentially after at least 10 minutes of rest, and during standing. The vital signs should be obtained at the first minute and third minute at a minimum. If postural tachycardia syndrome or delayed OH is suspected, the heart rate and blood pressure should be checked up to the 10th minute or longer of standing. Ideally, both blood pressure and heart rate should be checked every minute of standing. This approach can detect OH, which can occur at any time during standing. OH without a compensatory rise in heart rate usually indicates autonomic failure. A reduced or elevated core temperature may indicate central dysautonomia with abnormal hypothalamic functions. Dry mouth and dry eyes are common in dysautonomia affecting the sudomotor system. Pupillary abnormalities are also common in autonomic neuropathies.

The neurologic evaluation should assess the function of the small fibers, which transmit pain and temperature sensation. Pain and temperature sensation in the distal leg are abnormal in small fiber neuropathy (SFN). Sensation to light touch can be affected, but it is nonspecific, since it is carried by both large and small fibers. Vibration sense and proprioception, modalities that are transmitted by large fibers, should be normal in small fiber neuropathies unless there is concomitant involvement of large fibers. Deep tendon reflexes should be normal, and there should not be a muscle weakness in SFN.

Laboratory Evaluation

Laboratory evaluation complements the history and physical examination. Patients with suspected dysautonomia might benefit from a thyroid function test, 12-lead electrocardiogram, hematocrit, 24-hour ambulatory blood pressure monitoring, transthoracic echocardiogram, exercise stress testing, and carotid sinus massage. If orthostatic vital signs are normal and the clinical suspicion of orthostatic intolerance is high, autonomic testing can be considered.

Established autonomic cardiovascular reflex function tests include deep breathing, Valsalva maneuver, and the tilt test. The deep breathing test evaluates parasympathetic cardiovagal function. The Valsalva maneuver and tilt test measure predominantly sympathetic adrenergic function. Monitoring of cerebral blood flow with end-tidal CO_2 during the tilt tests is essential for differential diagnosis of postural tachycardia syndrome (POTS), hypocapnic cerebral hypoperfusion(HYCH), orthostatic cerebral hypoperfusion syndrome (OCHOS), and syncope. A neuronal autoimmunity panel (Table 22.2) may be ordered for suspected autoimmune dysautonomia or SFN.

Postganglionic sudomotor functions can be evaluated by the quantitative sudomotor axon test (QSART), electrochemical skin conductance (ESC), or sympathetic skin response (SSR). Skin biopsies can be used for direct evaluation of small nerve fiber damage. Epidermal nerve fiber density (ENFD) evaluates sensory fibers and sweat gland nerve fiber density (SGNFD) evaluates autonomic sudomotor fibers. Gastroenterology motility studies can be considered for evaluation of gastric motility disorders when enteric neuropathy is suspected. Urodynamic studies may be used to assess neurogenic bladder.

TABLE 22.2   Antibodies Associated With Small Fiber Neuropathy

Antibody	Underlying Tumor Disease Autonomic Syndromes
NMO/AGP4	Devic disease, neuromyelitis optica Variable
Anti-Hu/ANNA-1	Small cell lung carcinoma Sensory and autonomic neuropathy, autonomic ganglionopathy, enteric neuropathy
ANNA-2	Bladder and cervical cancer Unclear
ANNA-3	Small cell lung carcinoma Autonomic neuropathy?
AGNA-1	Autonomic neuropathy, pseudoobstruction
CRMP-5/Anti-CV2	Small cell lung carcinoma, thymoma Autonomic neuropathy, enteric neuropathy
Anti-Yo/PCA-1	Ovarian, breast cancer, cerebellar degeneration, Gastrointestinal dysmotility
PCA-2	Small cell lung carcinoma Autonomic neuropathy
PCA-TR	Hodgkin lymphoma Unclear
CRMP-5 IgG	Small cell lung carcinoma
Antiamphiphysin	Lung or breast cancer, stiff person syndrome, Variable autonomic dysfunction
P/Q-type voltage-gated calcium channel	Small cell lung carcinoma, Lambert-Eaton myasthenic syndrome Variable
N-type voltage-gated calcium channel	Small cell lung carcinoma, Lambert-Eaton syndrome, Sensory and autonomic neuropathy
Ganglionic (α3) acetylcholine receptor	Small cell lung carcinoma, Postural tachycardia syndrome, gastrointestinal dysmotility, autonomic ganglionopathy
Muscarinic (M3) acetylcholine receptor	Sjögren syndrome Variable
VGKC	Thymoma, limbic encephalitis Autonomic hyperactivity
CASPR2	Variable
LGIi (glioma inactivated 1 protein-IgG)	LGIi Variable
TS-HDS	Painful small fiber neuropathy
FGFR3	Sensory small fiber neuropathy
Striated muscle antibody	Thymoma, myasthenia, Lambert-Eaton myasthenic syndrome, small cell lung carcinoma, breast carcinoma Variable
GAD65	Thymoma, renal cell carcinoma, breast cancer, colon adenocarcinoma variable

CASPR2, Contactin-associated protein-2-IgG; *VGKC*, voltage-gated potassium channel.

Consultations With Specialists

A consultation with a specialist is warranted if a patient presents with a severe dysautonomia that had an acute or subacute onset and/or is rapidly progressing. A referral for autonomic testing is also recommended for patients with established diagnoses whose symptoms are responding poorly to therapy.

CLASSIFICATION OF AUTONOMIC AND RELATED DISORDERS

There are several classification schemes, but from the clinical point of view, dysautonomia can be conceptually divided into orthostatic intolerance syndromes, central dysautonomia, and small fiber neuropathies. According to another classification system, primary dysautonomia includes orthostatic intolerance syndromes, small fiber neuropathies with autonomic involvement, and pure autonomic failure (PAF). Secondary dysautonomia includes a number of other conditions in which dysautonomia coexists with other symptoms or signs.

ORTHOSTATIC INTOLERANCE SYNDROMES

The term "orthostatic intolerance" is a broad term but has a specific meaning in autonomic neurology. It is used to describe symptoms that occur upon standing, and are relieved by recumbence that cannot be explained by other disorders, such as cardiovascular or pulmonary disease. Orthostatic symptoms that may occur with cardiovascular, respiratory, metabolic, or systemic disorders are not considered part of orthostatic intolerance syndromes. Common orthostatic intolerance syndromes are presyncope, neurally mediated syncope, NOH, postural tachycardia syndrome, hypocapnic cerebral hypoperfusion, and orthostatic cerebral hypoperfusion syndrome (Table 22.3 and Fig. 22.1).

Presyncope

Presyncope, also known as near syncope, is a sensation of feeling faint, lightheaded, or dizzy without fainting. Presyncope is a very common and poorly understood syndrome. Dysautonomia is among multiple potential causes of presyncope, including cardiac and noncardiac.

Neurally Mediated Syncope

Syncope is a transient loss of consciousness due to global cerebral hypoperfusion (Table 22.3).

Syncope is very common, with a lifetime cumulative incidence of 35%, affecting more females, in 66% of cases of the neurally mediated subtype. Neurally mediated (reflex) syncope is triggered by still poorly understood reflex associated with a withdrawal of sympathetic traffic, resulting in vasodilation, a reduction in peripheral resistance, venous return, and preload, resulting in systemic hypotension and reduced cardiac output. Neurally mediated syncope can be further divided into cardiovagal (vasovagal, cardioinhibitory), vasodepressor, and the most common mixed type of syncope. Evaluation is focused to rule out cardiac syncope because of the difference in treatment and prognosis of cardiac syncope. Isolated neurally mediated syncope has good prognosis except when associated with autonomic failure and OH. Treatment of neurally mediated syncope includes both nonpharmacologic and pharmacologic approaches (Box 22.2). Proamatine can be effective in preventing vasovagal syncope. Cardiac syncope may be life threatening.

Postural Tachycardia Syndrome

POTS is one of the most common forms of orthostatic intolerance, and it is estimated to affect up 3 million Americans. POTS affects more females (female-to-male ratio: 5:1) and ages from adolescence (>15) to adulthood (<50 years). POTS is associated with the orthostatic intolerance and the presence of excessive tachycardia upon standing (Table 22.3).

POTS has been associated in a subset of patients with mast cell disorders including hereditary tryptasemia, hypermobile Ehlers-Danlos syndrome, and hypermobility spectrum disorder.

Nonorthostatic symptoms are common in POTS, including gastrointestinal, insomnia, impaired cognitive functions, depression, and anxiety. POTS is a syndrome with multiple causes, including neuropathy, hypovolemia, and hyperadrenergic state. POTS can be diagnosed at the office by observing symptomatic excessive tachycardia in the standing position without OH. Autonomic testing can be used to get a more detailed evaluation of POTS, including its subtypes. Therapy for POTS is complex and includes education and a variety of nonpharmacologic approaches (Box 22.3). Pharmacotherapy is usually reserved for more advanced POTS.

Neurogenic Orthostatic Hypotension

OH is defined as a decrease in systolic blood pressure of ≥20 mm Hg or a decrease in diastolic blood pressure

TABLE 22.3 Orthostatic Syndromes

Name	Definitions
POTS	1. Symptoms of orthostatic intolerance (>6 months) 2. Sustained and exaggerated heart rate increment ≥30 beats per minute (bpm) during the 10 minutes of head-up tilt test or active standing exceeding 120 bpm in the absence of OH Autonomic testing usually shows decline in orthostatic cerebral blood flow velocity associated with hypocapnia Forms: hyperadrenergic (plasma norepinephrine ≥600 pg/mL while standing), neuropathic, central, autoimmune, hypovolemic, associated with deconditioning
HYCH	Orthostatic decline in cerebral blood flow velocity due to hypocapnia (similar to that in POTS) but without OH HYCH subjects phenotypically resemble patients with POTS
Syncope, neurally mediated	Loss of consciousness due to global cerebral hypoperfusion Triggers: orthostasis, deglutition, defecation, micturition, cough, exercise. Types: cardiovagal, vasodepressor, mixed.
Presyncope	Probably common and poorly understood syndrome that may correspond to incomplete syncope, HYCH, or OCHOS.
Neurogenic OH	Orthostatic decline in systolic/diastolic blood pressure by 20/10 mm Hg or more Forms: Neurogenic nonneurogenic, initial (within the first minute of the tilt or standing), transient, delayed (after 3 minutes of the tilt test or standing), compensated, uncompensated. Compensated OH is defined as OH with stable orthostatic cerebral blood flow due to preserved cerebral autoregulation with normal compensatory orthostatic cerebral vasodilation. Patients are usually asymptomatic. Uncompensated OH is defined as OH with abnormally reduced orthostatic cerebral blood flow due to (1) either abnormal cerebral autoregulation with loss of compensatory orthostatic cerebral vasodilation or (2) a decline in orthostatic blood pressure below the autoregulatory range, which is typically 60 mm Hg of mean systemic blood pressure. Patients are usually symptomatic.
OCHOS	Orthostatic decline in cerebral blood flow velocity without OH and without hypocapnia
IST	A symptomatic mean resting HR >100 bpm during the daytime hours or with a mean 24-hour heart rate >90 bpm not due to primary cause and/or a rapid stable symptomatic increase in resting HR ≥30 bpm when moving from a supine to a standing position or in response to physiologic stress Can mimic POTS
PST	A transient and exaggerated heart rate increment ≥30 bpm occurring before the third minute of the tilt test or active standing. OH is absent.
Orthostatic hypertension syndrome	A postural increase of systolic blood pressure by at least 20 mm Hg or above 120% where the supine baseline is equal to 100%
Psychogenic pseudosyncope	Apparent loss of consciousness without global cerebral hypoperfusion
Baroreflex failure	Can be caused by neck trauma or surgery, usually results from the lesions of the afferent limb of baroreflex at the carotid sinus or medulla Signs: orthostatic intolerance Symptoms: labile hypertension, episodic or orthostatic tachycardia, bradycardia, OH (mild)

HYCH, Hypocapnic cerebral hypoperfusion; *IST*, inappropriate sinus tachycardia; *OCHOS*, orthostatic cerebral hypoperfusion syndrome; *OH*, orthostatic hypotension; *POTS*, postural tachycardia syndrome; *PST*, paroxysmal sinus tachycardia.

of ≥10 mm Hg (Table 22.3). Although OH is common (prevalence: 5%–30%) and has numerous causes, OH is rare. It results from impaired sympathetic vasoconstriction. OH is associated with sympathetic and parasympathetic failure, which can be confirmed by an autonomic testing. OH can be seen in Parkinson disease (37%–58%), multiple system atrophy (75%), PAF (100%), diabetic (7.4%–8.4%) and nondiabetic small fiber neuropathies,

and acute dysautonomia. Box 22.4 and Table 22.4 summarize nonpharmacologic and pharmacologic treatment of OH and related postprandial hypotension.

Hypocapnic Cerebral Hypoperfusion

HYCH is a form of orthostatic intolerance with reduced orthostatic cerebral blood flow velocity due to hypocapnia but without excessive tachycardia or OH (Table 22.2).

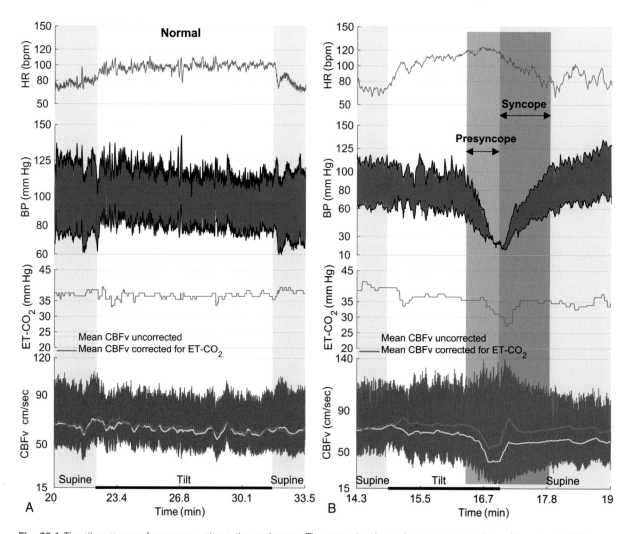

Fig. 22.1 The tilt patterns of common orthostatic syndromes. The normal orthostatic response consists of heart rate (HR) increment of (A) 10–30 bpm and stable blood pressure (BP), end-tidal CO_2 (ET-CO_2), and cerebral blood flow velocity (CBFv). (B) Neurally mediated syncope of vasodepressor type. Syncope is associated with reduced BP, a decline in ET-CO_2, and a decline in mean CBFv. Widening of transcranial Doppler signal (difference between systolic and diastolic CBFv) indicates compensatory cerebral vasodilation and functioning cerebral autoregulation. HR did not change immediately before (designated as presyncope) or during syncope (heart rate started to decline after the patient was placed in the supine position), which is consistent with the vasodepressor type of syncope. The presyncope onset is associated with a decline in BP and widening of the CBFv. Many patients are able to abort syncope in the presyncopal stage.

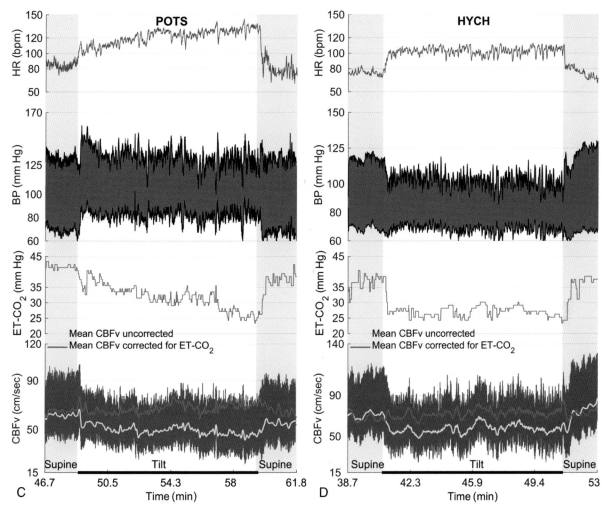

Fig. 22.1 cont'd (C) Postural tachycardia syndrome (POTS) is associated with exaggerated orthostatic tachycardia but stable BP. Orthostatic CBFv is reduced in POTS due to vasoconstrictor effect of hypocapnia (reduced ET-CO$_2$). Mean CBFv corrected for the ET-CO$_2$ is stable. Reduced orthostatic CBFv is associated with cerebral hypoperfusion and orthostatic symptoms in POTS. (D) Hypocapnic cerebral hypoperfusion (HYCH) is associated with reduced orthostatic CBFv due to vasoconstrictor effect of hypocapnia, similarly in POTS. Mean CBFv corrected for the ET-CO$_2$ is stable. Reduced orthostatic CBFv is associated with cerebral hypoperfusion and orthostatic symptoms in HYCH. POTS can be a subset of HYCH with orthostatic tachycardia. Orthostatic hypotension (OH) can be compensated

Clinical presentations are similar to that of POTS except that the postural tachycardia is absent. HYCH affect predominantly females of age <50 years, and typical complaints are orthostatic dizziness, shortness of breath, chronic fatigue, and a variety of other autonomic symptoms. Autonomic testing shows similar patterns in HYCH and POTS except that excessive tachycardia is absent in HYCH. Therefore HYCH and POTS may represent a spectrum of the same disorder. Treatment of HYCH is similar to POTS therapy with a combination of nonpharmacologic and pharmacologic approaches (Box 22.3). Pyridostigmine and selective serotonin reuptake inhibitors may improve shortness of breath.

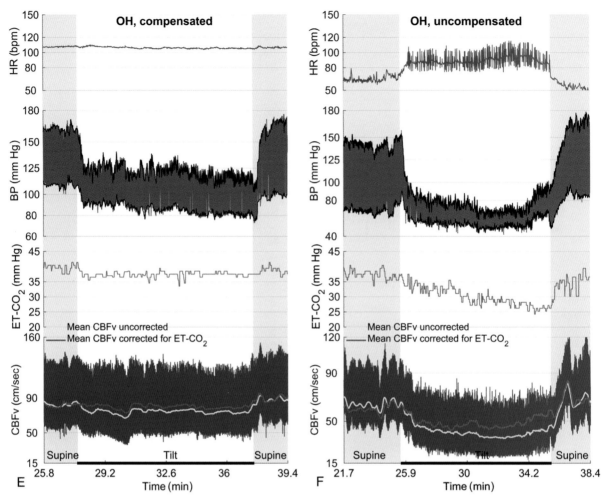

Fig. 22.1 cont'd (E) and uncompensated (F). Compensated OH is associated with stable orthostatic CBFv (E) since functioning cerebral autoregulation keeps CBFv stable by compensatory cerebral vasodilation. Uncompensated OH is associated with a decline in CBFv, and patients are symptomatic. A decline in CBFv in part F is due to both OH and hypocapnia, since even the corrected orthostatic CBFv is lower than the supine CBFv. Compensated OH is much more common than uncompensated, as the majority of OH patients are asymptomatic. OH due to autonomic failure is usually associated with lack of HR increment to tilt (fixed HR) as seen in part E. (From Novak P. Autonomic disorders. *Am J Med.* 2019;132(4):420–436.)

Orthostatic Cerebral Hypoperfusion Syndrome

OCHOS is associated with orthostatic intolerance and reduced orthostatic cerebral blood flow velocity without OH, bradycardia, hypocapnia, and excessive tachycardia (Table 22.3). OCHOS may result from abnormal cerebral arteriolar vasoconstriction associated with cerebral autoregulatory failure. OCHOS has been described in postacute sequelae of COVID-19 and Long COVID

disease. Our approach to therapy of OCHOS is the use of calcium channel blockers or angiotensin-converting enzyme blockers for patients with hypertension or pre-hypertension and volume expansion with salt, fluids, fludrocortisone, or the use of pressor medications in patients with low blood pressure.

Inappropriate Sinus Tachycardia

Inappropriate sinus tachycardia (IST) resembles POTS except that there is a persistent tachycardia (>100 bpm)

BOX 22.2 Treatment of Syncope

Nonpharmacologic
Education about the condition
Avoidance of precipitating factors in situational syncope
Physical therapy
Countermaneuvers: crossing, squatting or tensing of lower extremities at the onset of prodromes

Pharmacotherapy
Proamatine is modestly effective for vasovagal syncope
Conflicting results have been shown for beta-blockers or fludrocortisone
Paroxetine for patients with concurrent psychiatric illness

Permanent Dual-Chamber Pacing
Usually reserved for patients with severe asystole

BOX 22.3 Treatment of Postural Intolerance Syndrome (POTS)

Nonpharmacologic
Education about the condition
Avoidance of precipitating factors
Diet:
Daily >8 g of sodium (not for hyperadrenergic variant with elevated blood pressure)
(1 g of salt = 0.4 g of sodium)
Daily >1.5 L of fluids
Compression stockings, pantyhose size, pressure 20–40 mm Hg
Compression garment (leggings)
Corset
Graded exercise training
Physical therapy
Reclined exercise, such as swimming, reconditioning program
Countermaneuvers
Stress management

Pharmacotherapy
Beta-blockers:
Hypovolemic form: fludrocortisone
Vasoconstrictors
Proamatine
Droxidopa
Pyridostigmine
Ivabradine
Hyperadrenergic form:
Clonidine 0.1–0.2 mg po twice a day or patch, can cause drowsiness
Alpha methyl dopa 125–250 mg po bid po, can cause drowsiness
Immunomodulation (IVIG) for autoimmune form

BOX 22.4 Treatment of Neurogenic Orthostatic Hypotension

Nonpharmacologic
Education about the condition
Avoidance of precipitating factors/triggers
Diet:
Bolus ingestion of 500 mL water
Small frequent meals
Daily >8 g of sodium (1 g of salt = 0.4 g of sodium)
Daily >1.5 L of fluids
Compression stockings, pantyhose size, pressure 20–40 mm Hg
Compression garment (leggings)
Corset
Physical therapy
Physical countermaneuvers: leg crossing, squatting, tip-toeing, bending forward
Physical maneuvers: Squatting, genuflection-contraction, knee flexion, toe raise, neck flexion, abdominal contraction, thigh contraction, combination
Sleeping with head-up tilt 30 degrees

Pharmacotherapy
Fludrocortisone, proamatine, pyridostigmine, droxydopa, yohimbine, atomoxetine, ephedrine, erythropoetin

at rest even in a supine position (Table 22.3). Exercise or an upright position may induce exaggerated ("inappropriate") tachycardia. The treatment of IST includes beta-blockers and ivabradine. Drug-refractory patients may need ablation. The long-term outcome is benign for most patients.

Paroxysmal Sinus Tachycardia

Paroxysmal sinus tachycardia is associated with a transient increase in the heart rate ≥30 bpm usually at the beginning of the tilt and can be due to underlying anxiety disorder (Table 22.3).

DYSAUTONOMIA IN NEURODEGENERATIVE DISORDERS

Typical neurodegenerative disorders associated with prominent dysautonomia are multiple system atrophy (MSA), Parkinson disease, and PAF (Table 22.5). Postprandial hypotension can be part of dysautonomia in neurodegenerative disorders.

TABLE 22.4	Medication for Neurogenic Orthostatic Hypotension
Name	**Main Features**
Proamatine Proamatine (Midodrin)	Alpha-1 adrenergic agonist, peripherally acting A prodrug, requires liver metabolism for active compound Potent short-acting peripheral vasoconstrictor, no central effect FDA approved in 1996 Dose: start a trial dose 2.5 mg, tid po, last dose not later than 6 pm Can be titrated up to 40 mg/day. Can induce congestive heart failure (CHF) and renal failure, patients taking midodrin should avoid spending time in a supine position to reduce supine hypertension
Fludrocortisone (Florinef)	Synthetic mineralocorticoid At small doses, sensitizes vessels to norepinephrine At larger doses, retains sodium and expands volume Full pressor effect after 1–2 weeks Dose: start 0.1 mg daily or twice a day, can titrate in 0.1-mg increments at 1–2 weeks typically to 0.4 mg/day, maximal dose 1 mg/day Fluid retention > expected weight gain of 2–5 pounds, may develop benign pedal edema Sit can cause supine hypertension, CHF, hypokalemia is common Hypomagnesemia (50%) headache in young patients Diarrhea, bradycardia
Pyridostigmine (Mestinon)	Acetylcholine esterase inhibitor Enhances sympathetic ganglionic transmission Suggested for treatment of supine hypertension + orthostatic hypertension Dose: 30–60 mg bid-tid, Side effects: diarrhea, bradycardia
Droxydopa (Northera)	Synthetic precursor of norepinephrine Crosses the blood-brain barrier Potent centrally and peripherally acting vasoconstrictor FDA approved in 2014 for treatment of neurogenic orthostatic hypotension Dose: start 100 mg tid po, last dose 3 h, maximal dose 600 mg tid po Number of side effects such as supine hypertension, headache, dizziness, nausea, fatigue
Atomoxetine	A selective norepinephrine (noradrenaline) reuptake inhibitor 18 mg daily
Ephedrine	a nonspecific direct and indirect a- and b-adrenoceptor agonist 25–50 mg tid
Erythropoietin	Stimulates red cell mass production and increases circulating blood volume

All are off label except proamatine and droxydopa.

Parkinson Disease

Parkinson disease (PD) affects more than 1 million Americans and is the second most common neurodegenerative disease after Alzheimer dementia. PD has average onset at approximately 60 years of age and survival of 15 years. Dysautonomia manifesting as a small fiber polyneuropathy is a frequent nonmotor complication, correlates with decreased activities of daily living and poor quality of life, and may indicate disease progression in PD. PD is associated with a generalized autonomic failure of variable severity. SFN affects all autonomic branches, including the adrenergic, the parasympathetic, and the sudomotor functions, including cardiac and sympathetic denervation. The most severe symptom of PD is OH due to adrenergic failure. OH affects about 58% of PD patients and is a major risk factor for falls and cognitive decline. OH can be associated with failure of

TABLE 22.5 Neurodegenerative Disorders Associated With Dysautonomia

Disorders	Comments
Parkinson disease	Mixed central and peripheral dysautonomia Symptoms: early anosmia Signs: orthostatic hypotension in 40% of patients
Multiple system atrophy	Central dysautonomia due to degeneration of brain stem and spinal autonomic nuclei Symptoms: Autonomic failure: erectile dysfunction, urinary incontinence Signs: combination of cerebellar syndrome, parkinsonism, and autonomic failure
Pure autonomic failure	Central dysautonomia Symptoms: impotence, dizziness on standing, urinary problems Signs: orthostatic hypotension, neurogenic bladder, sympathetic and parasympathetic failure

TABLE 22.6 Medication for Postprandial Hypotension

	Administer before meals
Acarbose	Alpha-glucosidase inhibitor, used for treatment of diabetes 100 mg
Voglibose	Alpha-glucosidase inhibitor 200 µg
Octreotide	Somatostatin analog, inhibits growth hormone, glucagon, and insulin 1 µg/kg, contraindicated in diabetes Has a number of gastrointestinal side effects, hyperglycemia, supine hypertension
Caffeine	250 mg

cerebral autoregulation and reduced brain perfusion during standing up.

Multiple System Atrophy

MSA is an alpha-synucleinopathy with rapidly progressing symptoms that span multiple neurologic systems, including cognitive, autonomic, cerebellar, and both pyramidal and extrapyramidal motor pathways. The average age of onset is earlier than that of PD (58–61 years), and average survival is shorter (6.2–7.5 years). An early, prominent, and severe dysautonomia is characteristic of MSA and can precede motor symptoms by years. Autonomic symptoms are widespread and include sphincter dysfunction (urinary incontinence, constipation), erectile dysfunction, OH, respiratory stridor, and sweat gland dysfunction. Cognitive impairment is common and primarily affects the frontal/executive, visuospatial, memory, and emotional regulatory systems.

Pure Autonomic Failure

Pure autonomic failure (PAF) is a rare alpha-synucleinopathy that affects <0.003% of the population and has a good prognosis, with survival >20 years. PAF affects primarily autonomic fibers, without motor involvement. The

most common manifestation is OH due to denervation of adrenergic postganglionic fibers, but parasympathetic fibers are also involved. A diagnosis of PAF should be considered in patients with chronic OH but mild or no neurologic or motor symptoms. Other presentations may include mild incoordination, supine hypertension, postprandial hypotension, constipation acral venous pooling, anhidrosis, urinary and sexual dysfunction, and anemia.

Orthostatic Hypotension Management

OH, a marker of more advanced autonomic failure, poses a serious risk to the brain due to failure of cerebral autoregulation and cerebral hypoperfusion and also poses a risk of ischemic injury to other organs. Management of OH includes nonpharmacologic and pharmacologic approaches (Box 22.4, Table 22.4). Table 22.6 shows treatment modalities for postprandial hypotension.

PAROXYSMAL SYMPATHETIC HYPERACTIVITY

Paroxysmal sympathetic hyperactivity, formerly called central autonomic storm, is a form of sympathoexcitation that occurs in some patients with severe traumatic brain injury. Excessive hypothalamic stimulation of the sympathetic system can results in brief episodes of tachycardia, hypertension, hyperthermia, posturing, dystonia, tachypnea, and diaphoresis. Treatment is focused at minimizing triggers and pharmacologic management of adrenergic hyperactivity.

BAROREFLEX FAILURE

Baroreflex failure is a rare form of labile blood pressure. Baroreflex failure occurs when afferent baroreceptive nerves or their central connections become impaired. The consequent loss of buffering ability results in labile hypertension in which episodes of severe hypertension are followed by periods of symptomatic hypotension and eventually syncope. Baroreflex failure caused by a lesion to the afferent or efferent portion of the baroreflex arc most commonly occurs during the neck surgery, tumors, or radiation therapy to the neck. Valsalva maneuver is commonly used to assess the baroreflex-mediated heart rate responses. Treatment should be done in specialized centers.

AUTONOMIC DYSREFLEXIA

Autonomic dysreflexia is a form of paroxysmal autonomic adrenergic overactivity due to disinhibited spinal reflexes in spinal cord injury above the T6 level. Autonomic dysreflexia is typically associated with hypertensive episodes provoked by painful or innocuous stimuli below the level of injury, such as distended bladder, constipation, or a pressure sore. Regular bladder and bowel care are mainstays in preventing episodes of autonomic dysreflexia. Hypertensive medication can be used if the episodes of dysreflexia cannot be prevented.

SMALL FIBER NEUROPATHY

SFN is a generic term for neuropathies that affect small fibers of various types and causes (Table 22.5). SFN is very common; it is estimated that at least 4 million Americans have some form of SFN. SFN can coexist with large fiber neuropathies, can be idiopathic, or can be secondary due to other disorders (Tables 22.7 and 22.8). The autonomic neuropathies are a group of disorders in which the small autonomic nerve fibers are

TABLE 22.7	Classification of Small Fiber Neuropathies (SFNs)	
SFN CLASSIFICATIONS		
Classifier		**Comments**
Coexisting large fiber involvement	Yes	Mixed large and small fiber neuropathy.
	No	Restricted small fiber neuropathy
Type	Mixed	Both sensory and autonomic fibers are affected, the most common form
	Autonomic	Isolated autonomic neuropathy
	Sensory	Isolated small fiber sensory neuropathy
Distribution	Length dependent	
	Non–length dependent	
	Patchy	
Mechanisms	Primary (idiopathic)	The cause unknown
	Secondary	The cause is known
Autoimmune	Seropositive with systemic autoimmunity	Positive underlying systemic autoimmunity, for example Sjögren syndrome
	Seropositive with neuronal autoimmunity	Known neuronal antibody, for example acetylcholine receptor antibody
	Seronegative	Neuronal antibody unknown or systemic autoimmunity is absent but clinically course is highly suggestive of autoimmune cause
Duration (weeks)	Acute	≤ 4
	Subacute	4–8
	Chronic	≥ 8

TABLE 22.8 Acute Autonomic Neuropathy (Duration ≤4 Weeks)

Name	Prominent Clinical Features
Autoimmune autonomic ganglionopathy (acute autoimmune neuropathy, acute/subacute pan/autonomic neuropathy/pandysautonomia)	Generalized autonomic failure with sympathetic adrenergic and cholinergic failure
Acute polyneuropathy (autonomic, sensory and motor)	Autonomic failure of variable severity with sensory symptoms and weakness
Acute sensory and autonomic neuropathy	Generalized autonomic failure with sensory dysfunction
Acute adrenergic ganglionopathy/neuropathy	Sympathetic adrenergic failure: orthostatic hypotension, recurrent syncope
Acute cholinergic ganglionopathy/neuropathy	Parasympathetic cholinergic failure = gastrointestinal dysfunction, loss of pupillary constriction (Adies pupils), bladder atony, reduced salivation and sweating, erectile failure

Classification based on the affected systems.

predominantly affected. The most common type of SFN is mixed, affecting both sensory and autonomic fibers, as many patients with painful SFN have evidence of dysautonomia.

Idiopathic Small Fiber Neuropathies

In about 20%–50% of patients with SFN, no cause will be found. Treatment is supportive and symptom-oriented. A variety of pain medications can be used to treat the pain associated with SFN (Table 22.9).

Secondary Small Fiber Neuropathies

A number of disorders are associated with SFN (Table 22.10), including toxin-related disorders (Box 22.5).

Diabetic Neuropathy

Neuropathy associated with diabetes is the most common complication of diabetes and the most common form of neuropathy in the developed world. Diabetic neuropathy is a heterogeneous condition that can affect large and small fibers, both sensory and autonomic. The most common form is distal sensory or sensory motor polyneuropathy, which affects both large and small fibers. Patients typically present with s combination of positive (burning, stabbing pain) and negative (numbness, weakness, sensory loss) signs. Some patients, however, may be asymptomatic. In contrast, painful SFN with s burning sensation occurs in 10%–26% of diabetic patients. Diabetic autonomic neuropathy (DAN) can coexist with other neuropathies in diabetes or can be isolated. DAN can be widespread, affecting the cardiovascular (OH, exercise intolerance, resting tachycardia), urogenital (erectile dysfunction), gastrointestinal (gastroparesis, diarrhea, constipation), pupillomotor, thermoregulatory, and sudomotor (loss of sweating) systems in variable combination. Table 22.9 summarizes the treatment of pain, and Box 22.4 and Table 22.4 summarize the treatment of OH due to autonomic failure.

Inflammatory Small Fiber Neuropathy

Acute and subacute autonomic neuropathies and ganglionopathies. Acute autonomic neuropathies are relatively common (Table 22.8). They are characterized by a sudden onset of dysautonomia of variable severity. There are several forms, with signs and symptoms ranging from mild restrictive dysautonomia to severe generalized autonomic failure. Acute autonomic neuropathies are probably ganglionopathies, since experimental evidence and clinical experiences indicate that the primary pathophysiology affect autonomic sympathetic and sensory ganglia rather than small fibers. Perhaps the most common is a usually clinically mild cholinergic neuropathy associated with cholinergic dysfunction and with nausea, vomiting, and hypohidrosis or hyperhidrosis. On the other side of clinical spectrum is autoimmune autonomic ganglionopathy associated with a sudden onset of OH, loss of sweating, gastrointestinal and urogenital symptoms, and/or pain. Autoimmune neuropathies and ganglionopathies can be associated with neuronal antibodies (Table 22.2).

TABLE 22.9   Commonly Used Medication for Burning Pain Associated With Small Fiber Neuropathy

Name	Main Features
Pregabalin (Lyrica)	Anticonvulsant Dose: initial 25–75 mg, 1–3 times/day, effective 300–600 mg/day Side effects: somnolence, dizziness, seizures, suicidal thoughts
Gabapentin (Neurontin)	Anticonvulsant Dose: initial 100–300 mg, 1–3 times/day, effective 900–3600 mg/day Side effects: somnolence, dizziness, seizures, suicidal thoughts
Topiramate (Topamax)	Anticonvulsant Dose: initial 25 mg, 1–2 times/day, effective 25–100 mg/day, may titrate up 400 mg/day Side effects: somnolence, dizziness, suicidal thoughts
Duloxetine (Cymbalta)	Serotonine and norepinephrine reuptake inhibitor Dose: initial 20–30 mg, 1 time/day, effective 60–120 mg/day Side effects: somnolence, dizziness, cardiac arrhythmia, seizures, hypertension, suicidal thoughts
Venlafaxine (Effexor)	Serotonine and norepinephrine reuptake inhibitor Dose: initial 37.5 mg, 1 time/day, effective 75–225 mg/day Side effects: somnolence, dizziness, hypertension, suicidal thoughts
Amitriptyline (Elavil)	Tricyclic antidepressant Dose: initial 10–25 mg, 1 time/day, effective 25–150 mg/day Side effects: somnolence, dizziness, suicidal thoughts
Nortriptyline (Pamelor)	Tricyclic antidepressant Dose: initial 25–50 mg, 1 time/day, effective 25–150 mg/day Side effects: somnolence, dizziness
Tapendatol (Nucynta)	Opioid Dose, immediate release: initial 50–100 mg, 4–6 times/day, 300–700 mg/day Dose, extender release: initial 50 mg, 2 times/day, 50 mg 2 times/day Side effects: somnolence, dizziness, hypertension
Tramadol (Ultram)	Opioid Dose: initial 25–75 mg, 1–3 times/day, effective 300–600 mg/day Side effects: somnolence, nausea, vomiting, depression, hypertension, seizures
Capsaicin (Qutenza)	8% patch, apply for 30 min Side effects: burning pain at site of application

From Djaldetti R, Lev N, Melamed E. Lesions outside the CNS in Parkinson's disease. *Mov Disord.* 2009;24:793–800.

Acute autonomic neuropathies have variable prognoses and variable impacts on the patient's quality of life. In general, these disorders should be promptly recognized and treated. Autonomic testing is very important, as other conditions may mimic autonomic neuropathies. Treatment is symptomatic in milder cases. Severe autoimmune neuropathies may require immunotherapy. Depending on the type of neuropathy, patients may benefit from steroids, intravenous immunoglobulins, plasma exchange, chemotherapy, or their combination.

Inflammatory small fiber neuropathy with systemic autoimmunity. Chronic SFN with systemic autoimmunity includes Sjögren syndrome, celiac disease, sarcoidosis, vasculitis, Churg-Strauss syndrome, rheumatoid arthritis, lupus, psoriatic arthritis, and others. It is important to identify SFN associated with systemic autoimmunity, since immunomodulatory therapy can be effective.

Inflammatory small fiber neuropathy with positive neuronal autoimmunity. This group of SFN includes both acute and chronic SFN with positive antibodies targeting the neural elements. The most widely studied are ganglionic acetylcholine receptor antibodies, although other antibodies have been reported (Table 22.2).

TABLE 22.10 Chronic Secondary Small Fiber Neuropathy (SFN)

Classifier		Comments
Idiopathic	Mixed	
	Autonomic	
	Sensory	
Secondary	Impaired glucose tolerance, diabetes	Usually mixed SFN
	Metabolic syndrome	
	Thyroid dysfunction	
	B12 deficiency	
	Infectious	HIV, Lyme disease,
	Toxic	
	Connective tissue disorders	Ehlers-Danlos syndrome spectrum
	Neurotoxic medication	
	Paraproteinemia, amyloidosis	Variable dysautonomia
	Paraneoplastic syndromes	Variable dysautonomia
	Alcohol abuse	Variable dysautonomia
	Dyslipidemia	Variable dysautonomia, usually mild
	Neuronal autoimmunity with known antibodies	Chronic inflammatory SFN with known neuronal antibodies, may respond to immunomodulatory therapy
	Neuronal autoimmunity with unknown antibodies	Chronic inflammatory SFN with unknown neuronal antibodies, may respond to immunomodulatory therapy
	Systemic autoimmunity	Examples are rheumatoid arthritis, Sjögren syndrome, psoriasis, systemic lupus erythematosus. SFN and related dysautonomia are variables
	Porphyria	
	Mast cell disorders	Mast cell activation disorder, mastocytosis Associated with paroxysmal dysautonomia, including sympathoexcitation
Familiar	Fabry disease	Mutations of α-galactosidase A, X-linked
	Transthyretin-related familial amyloidosis	A point mutation within the TTR gene, autosomal dominant
	Pompe disease	Glycogen storage disease type 2, lysosomal storage disorder Acid alpha-1,4-glucosidase mutation, autosomal recessive
	HSAN type I	Affected gene: SPTLC1, RAB7A, DNMT1
	HSAN type II	Affected gene: HSN2
	HSAN type III	Affected gene: ELP1 (formerly IKBKAP)
	HSAN type IV	Affected gene: NTRK1
	HSAN type V	Affected gene: NGFb
	Painful SFN	Affected gene: SCN9A. Encode the voltage-gated sodium channels Na_v 1.7
	Painful SFN	Affected gene: SCN10A, Encode the voltage-gated sodium channels Nav 1.9

BOX 22.5	**Toxic Small Fiber Neuropathies**

Toxin
Organic
Acrylamide
Heavy metals
Organic solvents
Vacor
Vinca alkaloids
Platinum derivatives
Taxanes
Epotilones
Bortezomib
Cytosine arabinoside
Perhexiline maleate
Podophyllin
Gold
Pentamidine
Amiodarone
Doxorubicin
Lenalidomide
Thalidomide
Alcohol
Statins

Small fiber neuropathy with negative neuronal auto-immunity but with suspected autoimmune cause. This group includes SFN (acute or chronic) in which the clinical course is indicative of inflammatory mechanisms (history of trigger) but known antibodies are negative and the clinical workup does not reveal the cause.

DYSAUTONOMIA IN MYALGIC ENCEPHALOMYELITIS/CHRONIC FATIGUE SYNDROME

Myalgic encephalomyelitis/chronic fatigue syndrome (ME/CFS) is a debilitating disease with unknown causes; the estimated prevalence in the United States ranges from 800,000 to 3.4 million Americans. ME/CFS is characterized by profound fatigue, postexertional malaise, cognitive impairment, and sleep problems. ME/CFS is accompanied by cardiovascular dysregulation with deficits in cerebral blood flow, platelet and endothelial dysfunction, impaired venous return, and impaired peripheral oxygen extraction. There are a number of associated comorbidities of ME/CFS, including POTS. There is a symptom overlap between ME/CFS and long COVID. Treatment remains a challenge. Careful management of activity is important to prevent postexertional malaise and worsening of ME/CFS.

DYSAUTONOMIA IN GUILLAIN-BARRÉ SYNDROME

Guillain-Barré syndrome (GBS) is an acute inflammatory disease that is often preceded by a viral infection or vaccine, usually affecting the myelin of peripheral nerves and presenting with symmetric ascending weakness and sensory loss. Autoimmunity is believed to underlie the disease, since the majority of cases are triggered by preceding (1–3 weeks) infection. Treatment should be done in an intensive-care setting and includes immunomodulation with intravenous immunoglobulins or plasma exchange. Up to two-thirds of patients with GBS experience autonomic dysfunction. GBS causes parasympathetic failure and activation of the sympathetic noradrenergic and adrenergic systems. This can result in fluctuations in blood pressure, abnormal sweating, arrythmias, and gastrointestinal dysmotility. Elevated catecholamines and excessive sympathetic outflow can damage the myocardium, leading to left ventricular dysfunction and cardiomyopathy. This may, along with baroreflex impairment, contribute to the blood pressure abnormalities. Autonomic involvement in GBS typically improves with routine treatment for GBS with immunomodulation. However, severe autonomic instability requires close monitoring and can lead to life-threatening cardiovascular complications such as cardiac arrest

DYSAUTONOMIA IN HYPERMOBILE EHLERS-DANLOS SYNDROME

Ehlers-Danlos syndrome (EDS) is a clinically and genetically heterogeneous spectrum of connective tissue disorders characterized by joint hypermobility, skin hyperextensibility, and visceral dysfunction, with an estimated prevalence of about 1 in 5000 births. Hypermobile EDS (hEDS) is the most common (90%) subtype of EDS; the diagnosis is based on clinical evaluation, as the genetic phenotype of hEDS is unknown.

Autonomic complaints are common in hEDS and include orthostatic intolerance and bladder, gastrointestinal, secretomotor, and pupillomotor complaints. Cardiovascular autonomic manifestations in hEDS are POTS, neurocardiogenic syncope, and OH.

Musculoskeletal and neuropathic pain due to SFN is an important feature of hEDS. Treatment is complex, typically including multiple specialties with a focus on rehabilitation therapy.

DYSAUTONOMIA IN MAST CELL DISORDERS

Mast cell disorders comprise a wide spectrum of syndromes caused by mast cells' degranulation. Release of mast cell mediators, which have proinflammatory activities, may result in a variety of allergic, hypersensitivity, and toxic reactions, including anaphylaxis. The presentation of mast cell disorders may include urticaria, pruritus, angioedema, rhinitis, flushing, sweats, fever, asthma, and diarrhea. Most common disorders are mast cell activation syndrome (MCAS) and hereditary alpha tryptasemia (HAT). The estimated prevalence of MCAS is 17%. HAT is a genetic trait and may affect over 5% of the Caucasian population. Neurologic symptoms in mast cell disorders are common and heterogeneous and include orthostatic intolerance, palpitations, dyspnea, chronic fatigue and pain, brain fog, and other cognitive complaints. There is considerable overlap between mast cell activation and autonomic complaints, which may render the correct diagnosis difficult. Symptoms of MCAS and HAT can be managed by blockade of mediator receptors (H1 and H2 antihistamines, leukotriene receptor blockade), inhibition of mediator synthesis (aspirin, zileuton), mediator release (sodium cromolyn), anti-IgE therapy, or their combination.

DYSAUTONOMIA IN TRAUMATIC BRAIN INJURY

Autonomic dysfunction following traumatic brain injury apparently arises from dysfunction of central autonomic network. Symptoms vary from patient to patient. Paroxysmal sympathetic hyperactivity is an example of central autonomic network dysfunction. Patients with this syndrome experience tachycardia, tachypnea, and hypertension, often in the setting of dystonic posturing. Concussion, a milder form of traumatic brain injury, can be associated with acute autonomic symptoms, which often fade away or may become persistent in some cases (postconcussion syndrome). Common complaints include exercise intolerance, brain fog, fatigue, dizziness, orthostatic tachycardia, and nausea. POTS can also accompany traumatic brain injury. These symptoms may arise from damage to a functional connectivity among some parts of the central autonomic network and may be variable and persistent. An individualized exercise program is recommended for patients with dysautonomia.

DYSAUTONOMIA IN PREGNANCY

Pregnancy is a well-described POTS trigger, and patients who report autonomic symptoms or orthostatic intolerance during or after pregnancy should be evaluated for POTS and other autonomic syndromes.

Although POTS is common and affects predominantly females of childbearing age, the studies on POTS and pregnancy are limited. Symptoms of POTS appear to be variable throughout pregnancy with a tendency toward improvement during pregnancy. Most pregnant females (60%–68%) with POTS experienced either stable or improved symptoms, while 30%–40% experiencing worsening of symptoms. The improvement in symptoms, particularly in the second and third trimesters, is thought to be due to the increase in blood and plasma volumes and increased cardiac output. POTS may present a challenge during labor and delivery, due to the potential for exaggerated tachycardia and hemodynamic instability triggered by pain. Early utilization of anesthetic management during labor is recommended for pregnant females with POTS.

Nevertheless, dysautonomia and POTS are frequently comorbid with migraine, hypermobile EDS, CFS, syncope, MCAS, and autoimmune disorders. The comorbidities may have an important impact on pregnant POTS/dysautonomia patients and may affect maternal and fetal outcomes.

Preeclampsia, a life-threatening obstetric complication, occurs in 2%–10% of pregnancies and is a major risk factor for maternal morbidity and mortality. Preeclampsia is a multisystem disease that is associated with sudden-onset hypertension and proteinuria and maternal organ dysfunction driven by a dysfunctional placenta. Autonomic dysfunction is common; 94% of females with preeclampsia have autonomic cardiovascular dysfunction consisting of reduced parasympathetic and increased sympathetic activity. Tests of cardiovascular autonomic function might be helpful to identify females who are at risk and to monitor disease progression. However, the role of dysautonomia in preeclampsia remains to be determined.

A common question is whether the POTS and dysautonomia affect the pregnancy. In general, common dysautonomia and POTS are not a contraindication to pregnancy. For example, pregnancies do not trigger the deterioration of autonomic nervous function and development of autonomic neuropathy in diabetic females. However, there are several autonomic conditions that are associated with high-risk pregnancies due to blood pressure lability, for example, as in familial dysautonomia requiring multidisciplinary approach.

Management of dysautonomia during pregnancy can be challenging, as the medications that are typically used to treat symptoms should be avoided in pregnancy and breastfeeding, since no FDA class A safe medication for pregnant females is used in POTS or dysautonomia therapy. Under the guidance of a multidisciplinary team, including obstetrics, neurology, and cardiology, autonomic patients who become pregnant are often tapered off medications, including fludrocortisone, proamatine, pyridostigmine, droxidopa, and beta-blockers, with a transition to nonpharmacologic management. Sodium supplementation is generally considered safe unless hypertension occurs. For patients with severe symptoms, such as syncope and impaired functioning, low doses of category B or C medications may be considerable but are not ideal and require a discussion of risks versus benefits and collaboration with the obstetrician. Discontinuation of all medications before conception is preferable, and medical leave should be considered for patients who experience inability to perform job functions prior to consideration of medications.

DYSAUTONOMIA IN TICK-BORNE ILLNESS

Acute Lyme disease caused by *Borrelia burgdorferi* and other tick-borne illnesses can be associated with acute neurologic manifestations, with both central (meningitis, encephalitis) and peripheral (cranial or radicular neuritits, mononeuritis, demyelinating and axonal polyneuropathy) manifestations. The acute neurologic complications of Lyme disease usually respond to antibiotic therapy.

In a minority of patients, symptoms can persist for months following completion of therapy. A constellation of fatigue, cognitive dysfunction, and musculoskeletal pain persisting beyond 6 months has been termed posttreatment Lyme disease syndrome (PTLDS) and/

or chronic Lyme disease, the latter vaguely attributed to presumed persistent *Borrelia burgdorferi* infection. The role of coinfection in chronic disease is not clear. Quantitative autonomic testing has shown that PTLDS is associated with SFN and widespread but mild-to-moderate dysautonomia in a small cohort. A variety of therapies have been described, including prolonged use of antibiotics, symptomatic therapy, and therapy directed at decreasing the inflammatory response by the immune system, including intravenous immunoglobulin. Chronic problems that persist after antibiotic treatment for Lyme disease remain a challenge in infectious medicine and should be studied more.

DYSAUTONOMIA IN AMYLOIDOSIS

Although amyloidosis is a rare disease, it is important to recognize the association between dysautonomia and amyloidosis because the therapy can be effective. Peripheral autonomic neuropathy is commonly seen in hereditary transthyretin (ATTR) amyloidosis and the most common type of systemic amyloidosis, primary immunoglobulin light chain–derived (AL) amyloidosis. OH, amyloid cardiomyopathy with heart failure, and urinary and/or fecal incontinence can develop in ATTR amyloidosis. In AL amyloidosis, a monoclonal immunoglobulin light chain is produced in excess by clonal or malignant plasma cells. The AL amyloid is deposited mainly in the heart, kidneys, and gastrointestinal tract. OH and sensory-dominant polyneuropathy are characteristic of AL amyloidosis. Recommended laboratory evaluations include TTR gene analysis and Tc-99m pyrophosphate myocardial scintigraphy for TTR amyloidosis and serum free light chain assay and serum and urine immunofixation electrophoresis for AL evaluation. TTR amyloidosis can be treated with tafamidis, which binds to transthyretin and inhibits the formation of amyloid fibrils, and patisiran, an antisense oligonucleotide drug that blocks the production of hepatic TTR mRNA. Both tafamidis and patisiran slow the progression of TTR amyloidosis. AL amyloidosis is treated by chemotherapy. It is recommended that amyloidosis evaluations and treatment be done the specialized centers.

DYSAUTONOMIA IN PORPHYRIA

Porphyrias are rare hereditary disorders that affect fewer than 200,000 children and young people 15–45 years old in the United States; it is more common in females. Porphyrins and their precursors fail to convert into hemoglobin, increasing iron levels and accumulating in the liver and bone marrow. Porphyrins are excreted the urine, which becomes dark during an attack. There are several types of porphyria, and symptoms vary, depending on the type of porphyria. Porphyrias manifest in the nervous system as mental disturbances and extreme sensitivity of the skin to light.

DYSAUTONOMIA IN MULTIPLE SCLEROSIS

Multiple sclerosis (MS) is the most common progressive autoimmune neurologic disorder of younger adults age 20–40 years old, affecting 0.03% of people worldwide and about 1 million in the United States. The life expectancy of people with MS is about 5–10 years lower than average, and females are affected 2.8 times more than males. Symptoms reflect central and spinal cord lesions and include fatigue, difficulty walking, poor balance, blurred vision, poor bladder control, difficulty learning and planning, and executive dysfunction. Neuroinflammation affects both sympathetic and parasympathetic systems. The most common complaints are urinary bladder dysfunction, affecting up to 80% of patients; erectile dysfunction in up to 70% of males; and vaginal dryness in females. Other symptoms include gastrointestinal complaints, palpitations, and thermoregulation dysfunction with heat and cold sensitivity. Dysautonomia may be related to disease activity. Treatment includes steroids and a variety of immunomodulatory therapies.

DYSAUTONOMIA IN LONG COVID

Long COVID, also referred to as postacute sequelae of SARS-CoV-2 infection (PASC), stands for a wide range of new, returning, or ongoing health problems that people experience after having been infected with the SARS-CoV-2 virus that causes COVID-19. Based on a conservative estimate, at least 10% of infected people have Long COVID. Long COVID is a multisystem disorder with a wide spectrum of clinical manifestations consistent with pulmonary, cardiovascular, endocrine, hematologic, renal, gastrointestinal, dermatologic, immunologic, psychiatric, or neurologic disease.

Autonomic and other neurologic or related complaints, such as brain fog, chronic fatigue, and pain,

are major feature of Long COVID. Objective testing showed widespread mild-to-moderate dysautonomia, cerebrovascular and respiratory dysregulation, and SFN. POTS, HYCH, and OCHOS. OCHOS associated with cerebral autoregulatory failure and related cerebral hypoperfusion can be responsible for such disabling symptoms as chronic fatigue and brain fog. Limited evidence exists to date on the potentially multiple overlapping pathophysiologic mechanisms of Long COVID; immune dysregulation, endothelial dysfunction, hypercoagulability with fibrinoid microclot formation, and oxidative stress may play a role. COVID-19 vaccination may reduce risk of developing long COVID. Dysautonomia is commonly comorbid with ME/CFS in Long COVID. The treatment of dysautonomia in Long COVID is based on symptoms, using the same principles as for other dysautonomia, as there are currently no validated effective treatments.

SPECIFIC AUTONOMIC SYNDROMES

Primary Hyperhidrosis

Primary hyperhidrosis is defined as excessive, nonthermoregulatory sweating due to predominantly emotional stimuli in body regions that are controlled by the anterior cingulate cortex. The estimated prevalence of primary hyperhidrosis is up 3%, and it significantly affects the patient's quality of life. Usually, the axillae, palms, and soles are affected the most. The diagnosis is based on the patient's history, signs of excessive sweating, and ruling out secondary causes of hyperhidrosis, particularly due to medication effects. Treatment of hyperhidrosis includes topical application of aluminum chloride, oral anticholinergic agents, beta-blockers, water iontophoresis, and/or sympathectomy. Focal injections of botulinum toxin (BTX) are probably the most effective therapy. BTX blocks neuronal acetylcholine release in the cholinergic autonomic neurons, resulting in reversible local chemodenervation.

Neurogenic Bladder

Neurogenic bladder is defined as an abnormal control of bladder due to brain, spinal cord, or nerve damage. Neurogenic bladder affects 90% of patients with spinal cord injury, 50%–80% of patients with multiple sclerosis, and 95% patients with spina bifida. Neurogenic bladder is also frequently seen in diabetes and after stroke.

TABLE 22.11	Neurogenic Bladder Classification
Name	**Comments**
Uninhibited bladder	Lesion: above the pontine micturition center Signs: reduced awareness of bladder fullness, incontinence may occur.
Upper motor neuron bladder (Detrusor-sphincter dyssynergia)	Lesion: between the pontine micturition center and sacral cord Signs: Detrusor is usually spastic, simultaneous detrusor and urinary sphincter contractions increase pressures in the bladder, can lead to vesicoureteral reflux that and renal damage. Incontinence may occur.
Mixed type A bladder	Lesion: sacral cord lesion at the detrusor nucleus with sparring of the pudendal nucleus Signs: the detrusor muscle is flaccid, bladder is large, external urinary sphincter is spastic, incontinence uncommon
Mixed type B bladder	Lesion: sacral cord lesion at the pudendal nucleus with sparring of the detrusor nucleus Signs: The bladder is spastic, and the external urinary sphincter is flaccid. Incontinence is common.
Lower motor neuron bladder	Lesion: sacral cord or sacral root while the thoracic sympathetic outflow to the lower urinary tract is preserved Signs: The bladder is large and hypotonic, incontinence is uncommon.
Detrusor hyperactivity with impaired bladder contractility	Lesion: unclear Signs: frequent but weak involuntary detrusor contraction with incontinence

Normal micturition depends on the interplay between the somatic system and the ANS and therefore is both reflex and voluntary. Micturition involves the filling and emptying of the bladder. Functionally, the bladder problems can be divided into failure to store (overactive bladder), failure to empty (underactive flaccid bladder), or a combination of the two (Table 22.11). The type of neurogenic bladder depends on the lesion site. A neuro-urologic evaluation should include obtaining a history of voiding complaints (dysuria, urgency, hesitancy, nocturia, incontinence) and voiding pattern. Management of neurogenic bladder includes nonpharmacologic, pharmacologic, and/or surgical procedures (Box 22.6). Usually, the urologist plays a dominant role in providing care with neurogenic bladder.

Gastrointestinal Motility Disorders

Gastrointestinal motility disorders are associated with abnormal movements of the digestive system. Motility of the GI system is controlled by the enteric nervous system (ENS). Interestingly, the ENS comprises both motor and sensory neurons in addition to interneurons. Since ENS is part of the ANS, many disorders associated with dysautonomia also result in motility disorders. A careful history may be helpful in localizing gastrointestinal motility disorders (Tables 22.12 and 22.13). Diabetic gastroparesis is particularly common, affecting 25% of diabetics. Table 22.13 and Box 22.7 summarize common motility disorders and their treatment.

Chronic Idiopathic Anhidrosis

Chronic idiopathic anhidrosis is an isolated clinical syndrome with loss of sweating and a good prognosis.

Autoimmune Autonomic Ganglionopathy

Autoimmune autonomic ganglionopathy (AAG) is a rare form of dysautonomia. Approximately 100 patients are diagnosed with AAG yearly. AAG is typically associated with generalized autonomic failure with disabling NOH, recurrent syncope, fixed and dilated pupils, dry mouth and dry eyes, widespread anhidrosis, bowel and bladder hypomotility, and erectile dysfunction. The onset may be acute, subacute, or gradual. AAG may be progressive and debilitating.

BOX 22.6 Treatment of Neurogenic Bladder

Nonpharmacologic
Education, fluid schedule, timed voiding, nursing support, Crede maneuver, incontinence pads, condom catheters for males with incontinence and significant functional impairment
Intermittent catheterization—preferred for partial or complete urinary retention, part of self-care
Indwelling Foley catheter for severe incontinence
Suprapubic catheter

Pharmacologic
Anticholinergic antimuscarinic agents
First line in treatment of neurogenic detrusor overactivity
Reduce reflex involuntary detrusor activity by blocking muscarinic receptors
Antimuscarinic agents:
Nonselective: may produce cognitive impairment
Oxybutinin, Tolterodine, Trospium
Selective: fewer side effects
Solifenacin, Darifenacin, Fesoterodine
Tricyclic antidepressant—second line due to side effects
Imipramine reduces bladder tone, increases internal sphincter tone, reduces urinary urgency and frequency in uninhibited bladder
Amitriptyline: Similar to imipramine, has less anticholinergic effect
Cholinergic agonists
Urecholine: promote muscle contractions in mixed type A or lower motor neuron bladder
Alpha-2 adrenergic agonists
Relaxes internal urinary sphincter and reduces bladder outflow resistance
Useful for detrusor-sphincter dyssynergia in upper motor neuron bladder lesion
Clonidine, Tizanidine
Alpha-1 adrenergic antagonists
Reduce urinary outflow resistance
Dibenzyline, terazosin, tamsulosin, alfuzosin, and doxazosin
Benzodiazepines (GABA-A agonists)
Potentiate the effects of the inhibitory neurotransmitter GABA (gamma aminobutyric acid).
Useful in treatment of external sphincter spasticity from upper motor neuron or mixed type A
GABA-B agonists
Similar to GABA-A agonists, less dependence
Baclofen—Useful in treatment of external urinary sphincter spasticity; can be administered intrathecally for refractory spasticity
Botulinum toxin
Blocks cholinergic transmission across the neuromuscular junction and prevents the excitatory effects of nerve growth factor on bladder function.
Injections into the bladder detrusor result in improvement of detrusor overactivity
Vanilloids
Intravesical administration of capsaicin reduces detrusor overactivity

Surgical
Sacral nerve root stimulation, dorsal rhizotomy, pundendal nerve stimulation, enterocystoplasty, appendicovesicostomy, anastomosis
Sphincterotomy, urethral stents and balloon dilatation, artificial urinary sphincter, sling procedures

TABLE 22.12 **Gastrointestinal Complaints Associated With Motility Disorders**	
Name	**Comments**
Esophagus	Complaints: dysphagia, odynophagia, heartburn and reflux Diagnostic tests: barium swallow, endoscopy, esophageal motility and manometry studies
Stomach and small intestine	Complaints: nausea, vomiting, anorexia, bloating and abdominal pain Diagnostic tests: endoscopy
Colon and rectum	Complaints: abdominal pain, diarrhea, constipation and/or fecal incontinence Diagnostic tests: colorectal motility studies

TABLE 22.13 **Classification of Gastrointestinal Motility Disorders**	
Name	**Comments**
The esophagus	Gastroesophageal reflux disease dysphagia Achalasia Signs: dysphagia, chest pain, and regurgitation Comments: due to denervation of the intrinsic nervous system of the esophagus, with loss of nitric oxide–containing neurons Diffuse esophageal spasm Nutcracker esophagus Isolated hypertensive lower esophageal sphincter Idiopathic hypotensive lower esophageal sphincter Ineffective esophageal motility Functional chest pain
The stomach	Delayed gastric emptying (gastroparesis) 20% due to diabetes 50% idiopathic Rapid gastric emptying (dumping syndrome) Functional dyspepsia discomfort or pain centered in the upper abdomen, often associated with negative symptoms of fullness, bloating, or early satiety Cyclic vomiting syndrome
Small intestine	Intestinal dysmotility, Intestinal pseudoobstruction Signs: abdominal pain, vomiting, bloating, constipation, and diarrhea Primary (neuropathic, myopathic, or mesenchymopathic), Secondary (collagen vascular disease, endocrine, neoplastic, neurologic), idiopathic Small bowel bacterial overgrowth
Large intestine—colon	Constipation Diarrhea Hirschsprung disease Irritable bowel syndrome
Anorectum and pelvic floor	Fecal incontinence Hirschsprung disease Outlet obstruction type constipation (pelvic floor dyssynergia)

BOX 22.7   Treatment of Gastrointestinal Motility Disorders

Gastroparesis
Lifestyle modifications
Diet:
Low fiber—to prevent bezoar formation
Low fat, as fat delays gastric emptying
Liquids should be emphasized over solid foods.
Walking after eating may improve gastric emptying in some patients.
Drugs:
Antiemetic drugs: phenothiazines 5-HT3 receptor antagonist
Benzodiazepines cannabinoids
Prokinetic agents:
Metoclopramide, FDA approved
Erythromycin
Domperidone
Tegaserod
Chronic intestinal pseudoobstruction:
Erythromycin
Neostygmine
Pyridostigmine
Gastric resection
Gastric electrical stimulation

Irritable Bowel Syndrome (IBS)
Loperamide—for diarrhea-predominant IBS
Tegaserod, a 5-HT4 agonist—with constipation prominent IBS
Renzapride, a mixed 5-HT4 receptor agonist/5-HT3 receptor antagonist, accelerates colonic transit in constipation-predominant IBS patients
Psychotherapy
Smooth muscle antispasmodics
Cimetropium bromide, pinaverium bromide, octylonium bromide, trimebutine, and mebeverine
Tricyclic antidepressants
Serotonin reuptake inhibitors
Probiotics are a potential new therapy for the treatment of IBS; they may normalize the ratio of antiinflammatory to proinflammatory cytokines.
in the gastrointestinal system
Constipation:
Lactulose, a nonabsorbable synthetic disaccharide
Tegaserod, a 5-HT4 agonist
polyethylene glycol, a nonabsorbable, chemically inert polymer that acts as an osmotic agent to retain water in the stool
Lubiprostone, a bicyclic fatty acid that opens chloride channels (CIC-2) in GIU tract
Mosapride, a 5-HT4 agonist with 5-HT3 antagonist properties
Alvimopan, orally, a μ-opioid receptor antagonist
Transplant surgery for severe intestinal pseudoobstruction—transplantation
Biofeedback may be effective for constipation due to pelvic floor dyssynergia

Patients who are refractory to symptomatic treatment may benefit from immunomodulatory therapy. Patients with suspected AAG should be referred to specialists.

"For the full bibliography list, please use the pincode on the inside front cover to access the electronic version of the text at ebooks.health.elsevier.com."

23

Gait Disorders*

Jessica M. Baker

INTRODUCTION

Walking is an extraordinarily complex task requiring integration of the entire nervous system, making gait susceptible to a variety of underlying neurologic abnormalities. Gait disorders are common and contribute significantly to morbidity through falls. Abnormal gait is particularly prevalent in the elderly, affecting approximately one in three community-dwelling individuals older than 60 years. Gait disorders in this population are associated with diminished quality of life and nursing home placement and may be an indicator of progression to dementia in individuals with mild cognitive impairment. Prompt recognition, examination, and classification of gait disorders are therefore of paramount importance.

In this review, we offer a pragmatic approach to examining gait and discuss clinical features of common gait disorders and their underlying etiologies. A careful examination of gait may yield clues to diseases occurring at all locations of the nervous system, making the examination of gait one of the most complex and high-yield components of the neurologic examination.

Gait disorders may be broadly classified as neurologic and nonneurologic in origin. Among the neurologic gait disorders, we review abnormal gaits due to sensory ataxia, parkinsonism, frontal lobe dysfunction, and cerebellar ataxia as well as gaits due to lesions of motor systems (spasticity and neuromuscular weakness). We

discuss the remarkably diverse phenomenology of functional (psychogenic) gait disorders and briefly touch on more rare causes of gait disorders, such as stiff person syndrome and hyperkinetic movement disorders. We offer a pragmatic approach to the diagnosis and management of neurologic gait disorders, because prompt recognition and intervention may improve quality of life in affected individuals.

PHYSIOLOGY AND THE GAIT CYCLE

Normal gait requires precise control of limb movements, posture, and muscle tone, an extraordinarily complex process that involves the entire nervous system. Specialized groups of neurons in the spinal cord and brain stem generate rhythmic activity and provide output to motor neurons, which in turn activate muscles in the limbs. The cerebral cortex integrates input from visual, vestibular, and proprioceptive systems; additional input is received from the brain stem, basal ganglia, cerebellum, and afferent neurons carrying proprioceptive signals from muscle stretch receptors (which may be damaged in peripheral neuropathy). Together, these systems allow individuals not only to walk in a straight, unencumbered line but also to adapt their gait to avoid obstacles and adjust their posture to maintain balance. Abnormalities of any portion of the nervous system can therefore give rise to a gait disorder.

The gait cycle (Fig. 23.1) begins when one heel (illustrated here as the right heel) strikes the ground. Supported by the stance of the right leg, the person's body weight shifts forward as the left leg flexes at the hip and knees and swings forward, eventually striking the left heel on the ground. The weight then shifts forward

*Based on Baker JM. Gait disorders. *Am J Med*. 2018;131(6):602–607. ISSN 0002-9343. https://doi.org/10.1016/j.amjmed.2017.11.051.

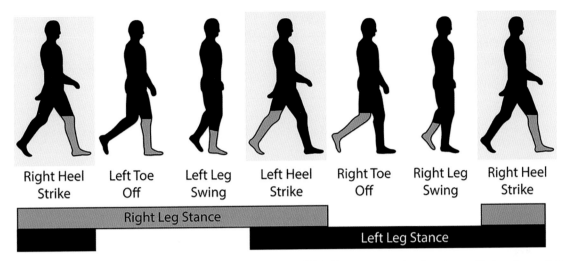

Fig. 23.1 The gait cycle. The right leg is shaded gray. The gait cycle is divided into stance and swing phases. During stance, the body weight shifts forward on the supporting leg while the opposite leg swings forward, eventually making contact with the ground via the heel. Overlapping shaded boxes indicate periods of double support, during which both the left and right legs make contact with the ground. (From Baker JM. Gait disorders. *Am J Med.* 2018;131(6):602-607.)

on the left leg while the right leg swings forward and again strikes the ground. Thus, while one leg is in *stance* phase, the opposite leg is in *swing* phase. Periods of double support, during which both legs make contact with the ground, normally comprise approximately 10% of the gait cycle but increase as compensation for unsteadiness in many abnormal gaits.

EXAMINATION OF GAIT

Individuals with a gait disorder may complain of unsteadiness on their feet, imbalance, or numbness, or weakness in the legs or may present with a history of falls. Evaluation of a suspected gait disorder begins with a comprehensive neurologic exam, with attention to confrontational strength testing and sensation in the lower extremities, deep tendon reflexes, and tone. The Romberg sign is tested by asking patients to stand still with feet together and eyes closed and is considered positive (abnormal) if eye closure provokes a fall. Other findings (e.g. tremor, dysmetria in the limbs) may also hint at the underlying cause of a gait disorder.

The examination of gait begins with observing a patient as he or she walks from the waiting area to an examination room. The ideal setting for a formal gait examination is a long, uncluttered hallway that provides enough distance to reach a comfortable walking speed

with good arm swing. The hands should be free except for necessary assistive devices. The gait examination provides significant insight into an individual's functional status, and much will be missed if the assessment is limited to the examination room. Observe individuals as they walk in a straight line, but also note any difficulty rising from a chair, initiating gait, turning, or walking through narrow spaces. Make note of velocity (distance covered in a given time) and cadence (steps per minute). Stride length measures the distance covered by the gait cycle; step length measures the distance covered during the swing phase of a single leg. Step width or base is the distance between the left and right feet while walking (Fig. 23.2). Also make note of posture, arm swing, the height of each step, leg stiffness, or side-to side lurching. Test tandem gait by asking the patient to take at least 10 steps touching heel-to-toe, as if walking on a tightrope. Heel or toe walking can unmask subtle distal weakness that might be missed by direct confrontational testing.

Examination of gait is particularly high-yield during telemedicine encounters, during which it may be impossible to directly test strength, muscle tone, sensation, and deep tendon reflexes. An accompanying person (ideally with a mobile device) can easily train the camera on a patient walking up and down a hallway or other open space, providing information not only on gait but also on functional status in the patient's home environment.

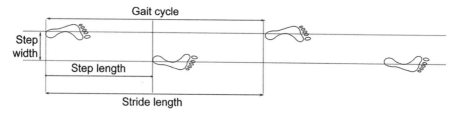

Fig. 23.2 Terminology describing the gait cycle. (From Pirker W, Katzenschlager R. Gait disorders in adults and the elderly: a clinical guide. *Wien Klin Wochenschr.* 2017;129:81–95.)

CLINICAL FEATURES AND ETIOLOGY OF GAIT DISORDERS

Gait disorders may be neurologic or nonneurologic in origin. Common nonneurologic causes of abnormal gait include osteoarthritis of the hip and knee, orthopedic deformities, lumbar spinal stenosis, and visual loss. Individuals may reduce the stance time of the affected limb to reduce pain, and range of motion around the affected joint may be limited, resulting in an asymmetric antalgic gait.

Mildly shortened step length, decreased velocity, slightly widened base, and increased double support time are seen as a response to perceived instability, either intrinsic (e.g., disequilibrium) or extrinsic (e.g., walking on ice). Individuals may walk with hands outstretched in an attempt to steady themselves. This cautious gait is nonspecific but may herald an underlying neurologic gait disorder.

The cause of gait disorders in older adults is often multifactorial. Many features of the cautious gait, particularly diminished step length, widened base, and decreased velocity, are present as a feature of normal aging. Inability to compensate rapidly for slight perturbations increases the risk of falls. Osteoarthritis of the hip and knee are particularly common in this age group and contribute to the changes in gait that are so commonly seen in older adults. Decline in gait speed and impaired dual-task walking are increasingly recognized as early signs of dementia in older adults. Note that polypharmacy is a potentially modifiable cause of falls in older adults; antidepressants, antipsychotics, antihypertensives, and benzodiazepines are common culprits.

Common neurologic causes of abnormal gaits are listed in Table 23.1 and are described in further detail in the following subsections.

Sensory Ataxic Gait

Sensory ataxia is among the most common neurologic gait disorders in older adults. Impaired proprioception (limb and joint position sense) limits one's ability to sense the position of the feet relative to the ground, resulting in an unsteady gait. The stance is wide based, with a shortened, often irregular step length and a stomping quality as the foot hits the ground. Joint position and vibratory sense are diminished in the lower extremities; Romberg sign is abnormal. Visual cues may partially compensate for proprioceptive deficits, so affected individuals often look down at their feet while walking. Gait therefore worsens dramatically in the dark or with eyes closed, a feature that is useful for differentiating sensory from cerebellar ataxia.

Sensory ataxic gaits are commonly caused by lesions of peripheral nerves (e.g., sensory polyneuropathy) or the dorsal columns of the spinal cord, such as with syphilis, compression of the spinal cord, or multiple sclerosis. Loss of reflexes in the ankles or knees suggests the presence of a peripheral neuropathy, which can be confirmed by electromyography with nerve conduction studies. Imaging of the spine (typically with magnetic resonance imaging [MRI]) is warranted if there is concern about dorsal column dysfunction.

Subacute combined degeneration is caused by vitamin B12 deficiency and may present with a prominent sensory ataxia due to degeneration of the dorsal columns. Paresthesias are typically present. Weakness and spasticity occur due to involvement of the corticospinal tract. If subacute combined degeneration is suspected, serum levels of vitamin B12, methylmalonic acid, and homocysteine should be checked.

Treatment should be directed at the underlying cause of sensory ataxia. Many patients improve with physical therapy targeting gait and balance. Fall risk can be

TABLE 23.1 Prevalence of Neurologic Gait Disorders (GDs) in 117 Community-Dwelling Adults

Neurologic GD	Number (%)[a]	Total Number[b]	Causes (Number)
Single Neurologic GD	81 (69.2%)		
Sensory ataxic	22 (18%)	46	Peripheral sensory neuropathy (46)
Parkinsonian	19 (16.2%)	34	Parkinson disease (18), drug-induced parkinsonism (8), other (8)
Frontal	9 (7.7%)	31	Vascular disease (20), normal pressure hydrocephalus (1), dementia (7), other (3)
Cerebellar ataxic	7 (6.0%)	10	Stroke (3), multiple sclerosis (1), essential tremor (3), chronic alcohol abuse (1), other (2)
Cautious	7 (6.0%)	7	Idiopathic (7)
Paretic/hypotonic	6 (5.1%)	14	Lumbar spinal stenosis (7), peripheral nerve injury (5), other (3)
Spastic	6 (5.1%)	7	Ischemic stroke (3), intracerebral hemorrhage (3), congenital (1)
Other	5 (4.3%)	10	Vestibular disease (6), dyskinetic (4)
Multiple Neurologic GD	36 (30.8%)		
Total	117		

[a]Percentage represents individuals with a single gait disorder as a proportion of the entire study population.
[b]Total number of individuals with each gait disorder, including individuals with multiple causes of gait disorders. For example, 22 of 117 individuals had an isolated sensory ataxic gait disorder, and 24 individuals had sensory ataxia and an additional neurologic gait disorder. From Mahlknecht P, Kiechl S, Bloem BR, Willeit J, Scherfler C, Gasperi A, et al. Prevalence and burden of gait disorders in elderly men and women aged 90-97 years: a population-based study. *PLoS ONE.* 2013;8:e69627.

reduced by the use of assistive devices and modification of the home environment, such as the use of floor-directed lighting at night.

Parkinsonian Gait

The classic "shuffling" appearance of the parkinsonian gait is caused by a decrease in both step length and height. In Parkinson disease, the base is narrow to normal, posture is stooped, and arm swing is reduced (Fig. 23.3B). An asymmetric parkinsonian (resting) tremor may activate during walking; arm swing and step length are diminished more on the affected side. Asymmetric shuffling can often be heard as scuffing of one foot more than the other. En bloc turns are characterized by simultaneous rotation of the head, trunk, and pelvis; in normal individuals, the head rotates first, followed by the trunk and then the pelvis.

Freezing of gait and festination are features of more advanced Parkinson disease. Freezing is defined as "an episodic inability (lasting seconds) to generate effective stepping" despite the intention to walk. Affected individuals feel as if their feet are stuck to the floor, often associated with alternating trembling of the legs. Freezing is commonly seen while initiating gait, turning, or approaching a destination but can also be provoked by features of the environment, such as narrow hallways, doorways, or even large crowds. Freezing is a major contributor to fall risk. The term "festination" refers to a phenomenon in which steps become increasingly rapid and short such that gait takes on the appearance of running. The center of gravity moves forward. Festination may precede freezing but also occurs independently and further contributes to fall risk.

Parkinson disease remains a clinical diagnosis; imaging of the brain is warranted with atypical features (e.g., prominent and early gait disorder) or if there is a concern regarding cerebrovascular disease. Treatment of Parkinson disease is primarily with dopaminergic therapies, such as levodopa. Step length, velocity, arm swing, and turning speed improve with dopaminergic

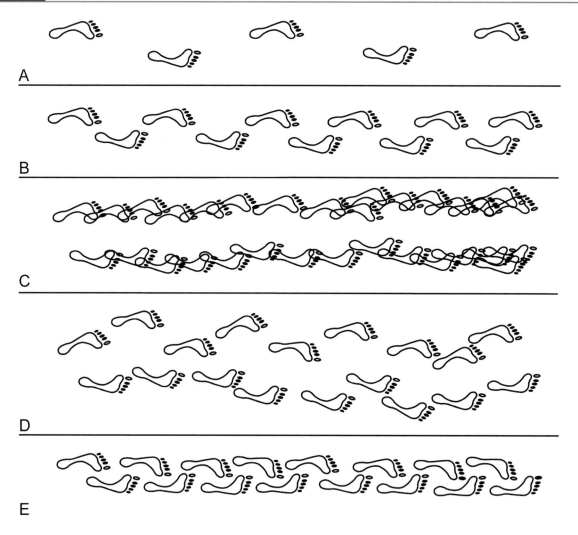

Fig. 23.3 Graphic representation of classical gait disorders. (A) Normal step length and width. In the parkinsonian gait (B), step length is diminished, with a normal to narrow base. In frontal gait disorders (C), step width is widened; step length is decreased and variable. Cerebellar ataxic gaits (D) are variable in both step length and base, often with side-to-side veering. Bilateral spastic gaits (E) are characterized by shortened step length and a very narrow base. See text for details. (From Pirker W, Katzenschlager R. Gait disorders in adults and the elderly: a clinical guide. *Wien Klin Wochenschr.* 2017;129:81–95.)

treatment. Freezing of gait may improve with optimization of dopaminergic medications, particularly if occurring during the "off" state in individuals with motor fluctuations. If freezing persists despite medication adjustment, symptoms often improve with visual or auditory cueing. For example, individuals may avoid or overcome freezing by consciously stepping over a line on the floor or marching to the beat of a metronome. A laser line produced by an attachment to a cane or walker may be a particularly effective intervention.

Treatment with antidopaminergic therapies (Table 23.2) may cause a syndrome that mimics Parkinson disease, though it is typically more symmetric with less prominent tremor. The associated gait disorder generally improves over a short number of months with discontinuation of the offending drug. Quetiapine and clozapine are less potent antagonists of the D_2 dopamine receptor and less likely to cause parkinsonism as a side effect, hence their utility in treating psychosis in Parkinson disease. The antiemetics metoclopramide and prochlorperazine are underrecognized causes of drug-induced parkinsonism.

Though relatively rare, atypical, neurodegenerative parkinsonian syndromes can present with gait abnormalities similar to those of Parkinson disease. Progressive supranuclear palsy presents with relatively symmetric parkinsonism and an early, prominent gait disorder, characterized by frequent falls, often backwards, and at times freezing of gait. In contrast to the stooped posture of Parkinson disease, individuals with progressive supranuclear palsy tend to stand more upright, and retropulsion is apparent on pull testing. Abnormalities of vertical gaze, prominent dysarthria, and dysphagia serve to further differentiate this disorder, though in practice there is significant phenotypic overlap. Atrophy of the midbrain may be apparent on imaging. Levodopa is of limited benefit in most patients, and falls contribute significantly to morbidity and mortality.

Strokes of the cerebral peduncle, affecting the substantia nigra, can cause relatively rapid onset of parkinsonism affecting the contralateral side of the body. The somewhat controversial term "vascular parkinsonism," describing a "lower body parkinsonism" with prominent gait disorder and MRI findings of leukoaraiosis (white matter changes), is discussed in the next subsection.

Frontal Gait

Higher-level gait disorders encompass a class of gaits that are not caused by lesions of the corticospinal tract, basal ganglia, cerebellum, or neuromuscular systems. Among the most common higher-level gait disorders are frontal gait disorders, which are caused by lesions of the frontal lobes (see Fig. 23.3C). Impaired balance is a core feature, and as in cerebellar and sensory ataxia, step width is widened. Step length is decreased and variable, and step height is diminished. Failure to initiate gait is a prominent feature; the feet may appear glued to the floor when an individual attempts to begin walking. Freezing with turns is common. These features lead to the classic description of this gait as "magnetic." Frontal release signs, brisk reflexes in the lower extremities, cognitive impairment, and urinary incontinence are common exam findings in individuals with a frontal gait disorder.

Common causes of frontal gait disorders are listed in Table 23.3. The term "vascular parkinsonism" typically describes a symmetric, wide-based, shuffling gait that is associated with microvascular ischemic changes in the frontal lobes. In contrast to Parkinson disease, response to levodopa is limited. Imaging of the brain is warranted in suspected frontal gait disorders. For individuals with frontal gaits from disorders other than normal pressure

TABLE 23.2 Medications Associated With Drug-Induced Parkinsonism

Class	Examples
First-generation (typical) antipsychotics	Haloperidol Chlorpromazine Fluphenazine Pimozide Perphenazine
Second-generation (atypical) antipsychotics	Risperidone Olanzapine Ziprasidone Lurasidone Paliperidone Aripiprazole[a]
Dopamine depleters (VMAT2 Inhibitors)	Tetrabenazine Deutetrabenazine Valbenazine
Antiemetics	Metoclopramide Prochlorperazine

Note: This list is not comprehensive.
[a]D_2 dopamine receptor partial agonist.

TABLE 23.3 Common causes of frontal gait disorders

Vascular disorders	Microvascular ischemic disease Stroke
Neoplasms	Meningiomas Gliomas
Neurodegenerative disorders	Alzheimer disease Frontotemporal dementia
Other	Normal pressure hydrocephalus Traumatic brain injury

hydrocephalus, physical therapy and assistive devices may improve ambulation and decrease fall risk.

Normal pressure hydrocephalus deserves special attention, given the relative frequency of incidental ventriculomegaly identified on imaging of the brain in older adults presenting with falls. Normal pressure hydrocephalus classically presents with the triad of a gait disorder, urinary incontinence, and cognitive impairment. Presentation without the complete triad is common; moreover, these symptoms are highly prevalent in older adults, necessitating a high degree of suspicion to identify patients with suspected normal pressure hydrocephalus. The gait disorder of normal pressure hydrocephalus is typically wide based, with shortened step length and height. Freezing of gait is variably present.

Differentiating normal pressure hydrocephalus from other causes of gait impairment is challenging. Imaging with MRI of the brain should reveal ventriculomegaly out of proportion to global cerebral atrophy. The term "hydrocephalus ex vacuo" describes ventriculomegaly caused by cerebral atrophy, as with poststroke encephalomalacia or neurodegenerative disorders, such as Alzheimer disease. It is crucial to differentiate this from the disproportionate ventriculomegaly of normal pressure hydrocephalus. Imaging findings suggestive of normal pressure hydrocephalus include disproportionately enlarged subarachnoid space hydrocephalus and a lower callosal angle (Fig. 23.4).

Definitive treatment is with ventriculoperitoneal shunt placement. However, appropriate patient selection is of the utmost importance. Because imaging features may not predict response to shunting, trial of cerebrospinal fluid drainage with a large-volume lumbar puncture (removing 30–40 mL) and/or lumbar drain trial should be pursued before considering shunt placement. In addition to the subjective report of the patient, objective evaluation of gait should be performed before and after the procedure, including video recording of gait and a timed 10-meter walking test. Ideally, these procedures should be deferred until other confounding variables (e.g., osteoarthritic pain of the knees, metabolic encephalopathy) have been addressed, typically on an outpatient basis or elective inpatient admission in the case of a lumbar drain trial.

Patients with a prominent gait disorder, shorter duration of symptoms (<6 months), and positive response to cerebrospinal fluid drainage tend to have a more favorable response to shunt placement, whereas

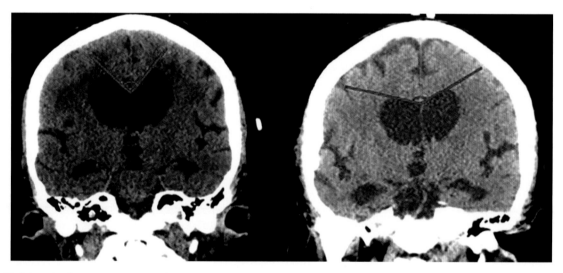

Fig. 23.4 Imaging features suggestive of normal pressure hydrocephalus. In normal pressure hydrocephalus (left), there is crowding of the high convexity sulci with enlargement of the Sylvian fissure, named disproportionately enlarged subarachnoid space hydrocephalus. Also on the left, a relatively low callosal angle (angle of the corpus callosum in the coronal plane, outlined in red) differentiates normal pressure hydrocephalus from hydrocephalus ex vacuo (right). (From Simon J, Jusue-Torres I, Prabhu V, Anderson D, Schneck MJ. Chapter 12: Normal pressure hydrocephalus. In: Tubbs RS et al., eds. *Cerebrospinal Fluid and Subarachnoid Space.* Volume 2: Pathology and Disorders. Academic Press; 2022.)

prominent dementia and onset of gait disorder after dementia should give clinicians pause before pursuing shunt placement. Unfortunately, nonspecific response to shunting can be seen early in the course of neurodegenerative diseases, and a certain proportion of patients will ultimately be diagnosed with a parkinsonian syndrome, such as progressive supranuclear palsy.

Cerebellar Ataxic Gait

Lesions of the cerebellum cause irregular, uncoordinated movements called ataxia. Ataxia of the limbs (appendicular ataxia, as might be assessed with finger–nose–finger testing) is typically caused by lesions of the cerebellar hemispheres, whereas ataxia of gait is caused by midline lesions of the cerebellar vermis. In its mildest form, the cerebellar ataxic gait may manifest only as difficulty with tandem gait; individuals may sway or fall when asked to walk heel-to-toe. In more severe forms, the gait is wide based (to compensate for instability), step length is variable, turns are unsteady, and there is frequent side-to-side lurching or deviation (Fig. 23.3D). Symptoms do not worsen substantially with eye closure, helping to differentiate cerebellar ataxia from the sensory ataxic gait. Eye movement abnormalities, such as gaze-evoked nystagmus and hypermetric saccades, often accompany cerebellar gait disorders, in addition to incoordination in the limbs.

The broad differential diagnosis of cerebellar ataxia may be narrowed by the time course of symptom onset: acute, subacute, or chronic. Stroke is a common cause of acute ataxia; autoimmune or other inflammatory disorders are often subacute, and neurodegenerative conditions or alcohol use causes chronic cerebellar ataxia. Laboratory testing and imaging of the brain are warranted. If available, MRI is preferred over computed tomography (CT) due to bone artefact in the posterior fossa. Table 23.4 lists common causes of cerebellar ataxia and suggested initial evaluations.

Alcohol use is a common cause of cerebellar ataxia across the spectrum of acuity. Alcohol intoxication causes an acute cerebellar syndrome. Wernicke encephalopathy is caused by thiamine deficiency and presents relatively acutely with altered mental status, ophthalmoplegia, and gait ataxia, though only 10% of individuals present with the complete triad. Though most commonly associated with alcohol use, Wernicke encephalopathy may occur in individuals with any cause of nutritional deficiency, such as bariatric surgery, hyperemesis gravidarum, or

TABLE 23.4 Common Causes of Cerebellar Ataxia and Suggested Initial Evaluation

Time Course	Common Causes	Suggested Investigations
Acute (minutes to hours or days)	Stroke Toxic ingestions (alcohol, lithium, phenytoin, etc.) Infectious and postinfectious cerebellitis Wernicke encephalopathy	MRI brain with imaging of cerebral vasculature Toxicology screen Serum levels of prescribed therapeutic medications Lumbar puncture
Subacute (days to weeks)	Neoplasms Paraneoplastic cerebellar degeneration Miller Fisher syndrome (variant of Guillain-Barré syndrome) Multiple sclerosis	MRI brain with and without contrast Lumbar puncture Paraneoplastic and ganglioside antibody panels
Chronic (months to years)	Alcohol use Vitamin deficiencies Multiple system atrophy Hereditary neurodegenerative disorders – Spinocerebellar ataxias, episodic ataxia (AD) Friedreich ataxia, Wilson disease (AR) Fragile X-associated tremor ataxia syndrome	MRI brain with and without contrast Social and family histories History suggestive of REM sleep behavior disorder or autonomic dysfunction (e.g., orthostatic hypotension) TSH, PTH Vitamin B12, B1, and E levels Copper, ceruloplasmin Genetic testing

Note that substantial overlap exists in terms of acuity of presentation (acute, subacute, chronic) for many of these conditions.
AD, Autosomal dominant; *AR*, autosomal recessive; *PTH*, parathyroid hormone; *TSH*, thyroid stimulating hormone.

malignancy. MRI of the brain may reveal abnormalities in the mammillary bodies, dorsomedial thalamus, and periaqueductal grey matter.

Wernicke encephalopathy is primarily a clinical diagnosis, and treatment should be started promptly in suspected cases, typically with high-dose intravenous thiamine, followed by long-term oral thiamine supplementation. Diagnostic testing (e.g., imaging) should not delay treatment in suspected cases of Wernicke encephalopathy. With treatment, improvement in ophthalmoplegia may occur over days to weeks. Improvement in mental status and gait ataxia is more variable and often incomplete. Left untreated, most patients with Wernicke encephalopathy will go on to develop Korsakoff syndrome, which is characterized by permanent cognitive impairment, with prominent deficits in memory and at times confabulation.

Cerebellar degeneration may occur as a consequence of chronic alcohol consumption, causing atrophy of the cerebellar vermis and disproportionate effects on gait. Presentation is typically insidious, with impaired gait and incoordination of the legs, though incoordination in the arms and slurred speech also occur. Alcohol cessation should be encouraged, though deficits are not typically reversible. Coexisting peripheral polyneuropathy due to chronic alcohol consumption may also contribute to gait disorders in this population.

Miller Fisher syndrome is a variant of Guillain–Barré syndrome and represents an immune-mediated cause of cerebellar ataxia. The typical presentation is one of subacute ataxia, ophthalmoplegia and absent deep tendon reflexes. Lumbar puncture typically reveals albuminocytologic dissociation (elevated protein with normal cell counts). Nerve conduction studies can further support the diagnosis, though it may be normal early in the disease course. Anti-GQ1b antibodies are present in the vast majority of cases. Treatment is with intravenous immunoglobulin (IVIG).

Multiple system atrophy is a sporadic neurodegenerative disorder characterized by cerebellar ataxia and/or parkinsonism with early and prominent dysautonomia. Anterocollis (dystonic forward flexion of the neck) may be apparent while walking. Cognitive impairment is rare. Dream reenactment, or rapid eye movement (REM) sleep behavior disorder, is a prodromal feature of multiple system atrophy (and other synucleinopathies, such as Parkinson disease) and may precede the onset of motor symptoms by years. Treatment is supportive; response to levodopa is limited. Orthostatic hypotension can be treated with nonpharmacologic measures (e.g., compression socks), discontinuation of exacerbating medications (e.g., antihypertensives), and, if needed, medications such as fludrocortisone and midodrine. Survival is variable, typically 5–10 years after diagnosis. A "hot cross bun" sign may be seen on MRI of the brain (Fig. 23.5).

Genetic forms of ataxia may be inherited in an autosomal dominant, autosomal recessive, or X-linked fashion.

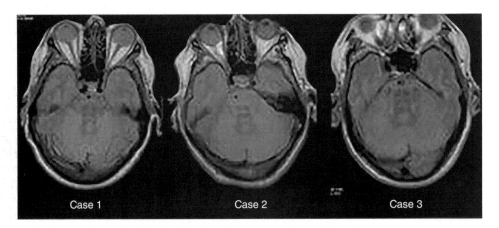

Case 1　　Case 2　　Case 3

Fig. 23.5 "Hot cross bun" sign in multiple system atrophy. The cross-shaped hyperintensity seen on axial MRI imaging is due to degeneration of pontocerebellar fibers, and has also been reported in other causes of cerebellar degeneration. (From Bermejo MR, Muñoz SN, Martínez BE, Aveleira CM, Ruiz RG. "Hot-cross bun sign" in multiple system atropy: a presentation of 3 cases. *Neurologia (English Edition)*. 2012;27:314–315. © Sociedad Española de Neurología.)

The spinocerebellar ataxias are a heterogeneous group of autosomal dominant inherited neurodegenerative disorders, with onset typically in early or mid-adulthood, though this is highly variable. Progressive cerebellar ataxia is a core feature, involving not only gait but also eye movements and limb coordination. Certain features may serve to distinguish the various spinocerebellar ataxias on clinical grounds (Table 23.5), though there is significant phenotypic overlap, and ultimately, genetic testing is required for a definitive diagnosis. Other neurologic features, such as parkinsonism, spasticity, or neuropathy, are variably present. Features of the most common spinocerebellar ataxias are listed in Table 23.5. Genetic testing is warranted in suspected cases of inherited forms of cerebellar ataxia, including those without a positive family history whose clinical picture fits that of a spinocerebellar ataxic syndrome. Genetic testing is most commonly obtained through a commercially available panel; the most common spinocerebellar ataxias are due to repeat expansions that may not be identified on whole-exome sequencing. At-risk family members may benefit from genetic counseling.

Spinocerebellar ataxia type 3 (SCA3, Machado Joseph disease) is one of the most common types of spinocerebellar ataxia worldwide. The phenotype can vary significantly, even within families. Features may include rigidity, muscle cramps, and peripheral neuropathy. Spinocerebellar ataxia type 2 (SCA2) is particularly prevalent in Cuba, though it is also relatively common worldwide. Slowed saccadic eye movements may distinguish SCA2 from other types of spinocerebellar ataxia. Spinocerebellar ataxias types 5 and 6 tend to present as relatively pure cerebellar syndromes, with few other neurologic signs or symptoms. Vision impairment due to retinopathy is a unique feature of spinocerebellar ataxia type 7. Though rare, spinocerebellar ataxia type 17 can present with prominent chorea, at times mimicking Huntington disease.

The prognosis of the spinocerebellar ataxias is variable. Spinocerebellar ataxia type 1 tends to progress relatively rapidly, with most patients wheelchair-bound 15 years after symptom onset, whereas spinocerebellar ataxia type 6 tends to progress more slowly. Longer CAG repeat lengths are associated with more rapid progression. Treatment is generally supportive, though the oral antioxidant riluzole may be considered in select cases. Mobility and ability to perform activities of daily living can be supported by physical and occupational therapy, respectively. Dysarthria and dysphagia should prompt referral to a speech/language pathologist. Periodic screening for cognitive disorders should be performed as clinically indicated.

Friedreich's ataxia is the most common autosomal recessive cause of cerebellar ataxia. Onset is typically in childhood or young adulthood. Notable comorbidities include diabetes and heart failure. Heart failure is the cause of death in a substantial number of patients. The antioxidant medication omaveloxolone was recently approved for the treatment of Friedreich's ataxia.

Fragile X tremor–ataxia syndrome (FXTAS) is seen in adults who carry a premutation in *FMR1*, pathogenic expansions in which cause fragile X syndrome in males. FXTAS presents with progressive ataxia and action tremors, at times with cognitive changes and parkinsonism. A family history of intellectual disability or

TABLE 23.5 Clinical Features of the Most Common Spinocerebellar Ataxias

Type	Gene	Clinical Features
SCA1	*ATXN1*—CAG repeat expansion	Pyramidal findings (brisk reflexes, spasticity)
SCA2	*ATXN2*—CAG repeat expansion	Slow saccadic eye movements, prominent cerebellar atrophy on imaging
SCA3	*ATXN3*—CAG repeat expansion	Parkinsonism, muscle cramps, neuropathy, facial/tongue fasciculations, ophthalmoplegia
SCA5	*SPTBN2*—Point mutation/deletion	Pure cerebellar syndrome, slowly progressive
SCA6	*CACNA1A*—CAG repeat expansion	Pure cerebellar syndrome, slowly progressive, down beat nystagmus
SCA7	*ATXN7*—CAG repeat expansion	Vision loss in adults (retinopathy), prominent anticipation
SCA8	*ATXN8 OS*—CTG/CAG expansion	Variable penetrance
SCA10	*ATXN10*—Intronic ATTCT expansion	Seizures

premature ovarian failure should heighten suspicion for this condition. Hyperintensities of the middle cerebellar peduncles may be seen on MRI of the brain. The diagnosis can be confirmed with genetic testing. Treatment is supportive; tremors may improve with medications that are used for essential tremor (e.g., propranolol, primidone), though response is variable.

Treatment of cerebellar ataxia is focused on the underlying disorder. Physical therapy and use of assistive devices such as a walker may decrease the risk of injury due to falls.

Neuromuscular Gaits

Weakness of muscles of the lower extremities may manifest as a gait disorder. The waddling gait can be seen in cases of proximal muscle weakness, such as myopathy. In normal gait, the gluteal muscles serve to stabilize the pelvis, elevating the non-weight-bearing side with each step. With weakness of these muscles, particularly the gluteus medius, instability of the weight-bearing hip instead causes the non–weight-bearing side to drop (Trendelenburg sign). This leads to excessive side-to-side trunk motion, giving the gait a waddling appearance (Fig. 23.6). Individuals

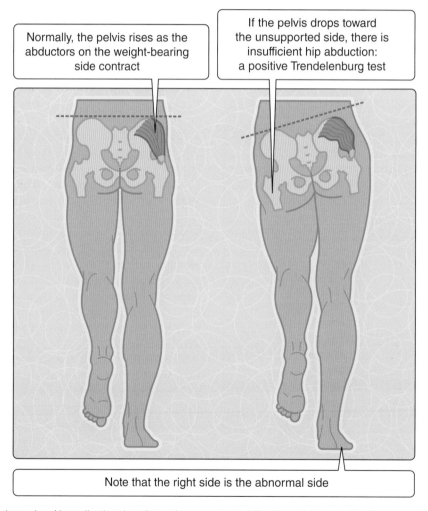

Normally, the pelvis rises as the abductors on the weight-bearing side contract

If the pelvis drops toward the unsupported side, there is insufficient hip abduction: a positive Trendelenburg test

Note that the right side is the abnormal side

Fig. 23.6 Trendelenburg sign. Normally, the gluteal muscles serve to stabilize the pelvis, elevating the non–weight-bearing side of the pelvis with each step (left). With weakness of the gluteal muscles, the non–weight-bearing side drops, leading to excessive sway and, with repeated steps, a waddling appearance (right). (From Keighley MRB, Bhangu AA. 59 – Hip examination. In: *Flesh and Bones of Surgery*; 2007. Image Identifier pii:B9780723433767500590/f59-01-9780723433767.)

with proximal muscle weakness often have difficulty rising from a chair without using their arms.

The steppage gait is caused by weakness of ankle dorsiflexion, also known as a foot drop. Individuals with a steppage gait lift the swinging leg higher to compensate for the toes' inability to clear the ground with each step; the foot landing often has a slapping quality. Weakness of ankle dorsiflexion may be appreciated by direct testing on physical examination, though more subtle weakness may be elicited when an individual is asked to walk on the heels. Foot drop may be bilateral, as can be seen in peripheral polyneuropathy, or unilateral. Common causes of unilateral foot drop include an L5 radiculopathy or peroneal neuropathy, which can be differentiated from the former by preservation of ankle inversion on physical examination. Electromyography with nerve conduction studies may aid in diagnosis. Individuals with foot drop may benefit from ankle foot orthoses, which stabilize the ankle in a neutral position.

Spastic Gait

Spastic gaits are caused by lesions in the corticospinal tract at any level and may be unilateral or bilateral. When the spastic gait is unilateral, the affected leg is held in extension and plantar flexion; the ipsilateral arm is often flexed. There is circumduction of the affected leg during the swing phase of each step. Common causes include stroke or other unilateral lesions of the cerebral cortex. If bilateral, the spastic gait may appear stiff-legged or scissoring, owing to increased tone in the adductor muscles, such that the legs nearly touch with each step (Fig. 23.3E).

Imaging of the brain or spine, typically with MRI, is warranted. Common causes of bilateral spastic gait (spastic paraparesis) include cerebral palsy, cervical spondylotic myelopathy, and multiple sclerosis, among many others, and are often accompanied by signs of myelopathy, such as bowel and bladder dysfunction, increased reflexes in the lower extremities, and positive Babinski signs. Antispasticity agents such as baclofen or tizanidine are variably effective in improving gait but may reduce painful spasms. Botulinum toxin injections may be useful in cases of focal spasticity.

Functional Gait Disorders

Functional gait disorders frequently co-occur with other functional neurologic disorders and are common in clinical practice. Though their presentation is heterogeneous, functional gait disorders are typically abrupt in onset, fluctuate over time, and are both suggestible and easily distractible. Common patterns include excessive slowing of gait or buckling of the knees, usually without falls. Abnormal twisting or muscle contractions may superficially resemble dystonia. The term "astasia-abasia" describes an inability to stand or walk without support, despite the ability to otherwise use the legs normally. Inefficient postures that appear unsteady yet do not result in falls are another feature of functional gait disorders. Mood disorders are present in a substantial number of patients but are not required for diagnosis.

The diagnosis of a functional gait disorder is made not purely by exclusion of organic disease but by positive identification of internal inconsistencies or distractibility. For example, functional gait disorders or postural instability may normalize when an individual is asked to walk while talking on the phone. Sharing these inconsistent features with the patient highlights their potential reversibility and may be therapeutic. Communicating the diagnosis should focus more on positive features than diseases that have been excluded and emphasize mechanism over etiology. The metaphor of "a problem with the software, not the hardware" may be particularly effective. Treatment often involves a multidisciplinary team of neurologists and psychiatrists; consensus-based guidelines for physical therapy have been published.

Other Neurologic Gait Disorders

Individuals with vestibular dysfunction report unsteadiness and imbalance while walking, often associated with a sense of movement and a compensatory wide-based and slow gait. Oscillopsia, the perception that one's environment is moving from side to side, may occur.

Stiff-person syndrome is an immune-mediated disorder characterized by progressive rigidity, stiffness and spasms of axial muscles. Gait is wide based with exaggerated lumbar lordosis. Antibodies to GAD65 are often positive; treatment is with benzodiazepines and/or immunomodulatory therapies such as IVIG.

Gait disorders also occur in individuals with hyperkinetic movement disorders. Dystonia involves patterned, sustained muscle contractions that often result in twisting or abnormal sustained postures with walking, such as foot/ankle inversion. Hemibody dystonia involving gait may be an early sign of Parkinson disease, particularly in younger adults.

Huntington disease is an inherited neurodegenerative disorder in which chorea (involuntary, irregular flowing movements) is the predominant movement disorder. Affected individuals often have substantial neuropsychiatric comorbidities. Gait is characterized by random, irregular movements of the limbs, trunk, neck, and head, at times creating a dance-like appearance.

CONCLUSIONS

Gait disorders are a major source of disability, morbidity, and mortality in individuals of all ages, particularly the elderly. Gait disorders may be neurologic or nonneurologic in origin. When neurologic in origin, gait disorders arise from lesions in any part of the nervous system. This review has provided an overview of the clinical features of various gait disorders, emphasizing clinical features that allow for prompt recognition, offering an opportunity for intervention and improvement in quality of life.

ACKNOWLEDGMENTS

I thank Dr. Lewis Sudarsky for insightful comments on an early draft of this review.

"For the full bibliography list, please use the pincode on the inside front cover to access the electronic version of the text at ebooks.health.elsevier.com."

24

Epilepsy*

Tracey A. Milligan and Manisha G. Holmes

EPILEPSY: A CLINICAL OVERVIEW

The diagnosis and treatment of seizures and epilepsy are common tasks of the physician. Approximately 1 in 10 people will have a seizure during their lifetime. Epilepsy, which is the tendency to have unprovoked seizures, is the fourth most common neurologic disorder, affecting 1 in 26 people in the United States and 65 million people worldwide. Evaluation of a patient presenting with a seizure involves excluding an underlying neurologic or medical condition, classifying the seizure type, and determining whether the patient has epilepsy. Proper treatment requires accurate diagnosis of the epilepsy type and syndrome and use of a medication that is effective and does not have adverse effects. Most patients can achieve complete seizure control with medication, but if medication is unsuccessful, surgical treatment with resection or neuromodulation devices can be an option. Special situations in the care of people with epilepsy include status epilepticus, women with epilepsy (WWE), the older adult, and safety issues. The rapid expansion of epilepsy treatment in the last 20 years presents a number of options with increased tolerability, improved efficacy, and decreased invasiveness compared to the past.

INTRODUCTION

The word "epilepsy" is derived from the Greek word *epilepsia*, meaning "to seize or attack." Seizures and epilepsy are common disorders and have been documented since the earliest recordings of humans. Initially, epilepsy was believed to be a spiritual disease, and the oldest detailed account of epilepsy was in 2000 BCE. It was not until the fifth century BCE that epilepsy was described as a brain disease (as Hippocrates identified it in "On the Sacred Disease"). In most cultures, epilepsy has continued to be stigmatized. It is only in the past few decades that there have been more organized efforts to counter the stigma, secrecy, and discrimination that are often associated with epilepsy.

Epilepsy is the tendency to have recurrent nonprovoked seizures. A seizure is a brief, excessive discharge of electrical activity in the brain that transiently alters behavior. Neurons communicate through chemical and electrical signals and form networks with other neurons. In most seizures, a relatively small number of abnormal neurons cause changes in other neighboring or networked neurons. During a seizure there is a progressive recruitment of other neurons in the network, resulting in a pattern of hypersynchrony. This abnormal propagation occurs due to insufficient inhibition and/or excessive excitation within the neuronal network. This abnormal neuronal hypersynchrony can be congenital or may develop at any time during life.

Epilepsy is defined as a disorder of the brain characterized by an enduring predisposition to generate epileptic seizures and by the neurobiologic, cognitive, psychological, and social consequences of this condition. This definition emphasizes that epilepsy consists not only of the neurobiology of seizures but also of the associated neuropsychosocial comorbidities. The most recent definition of epilepsy requires the occurrence of at least one epileptic seizure. After a single seizure, epilepsy can be diagnosed if the seizure was unprovoked (e.g., unrelated to drugs,

*Based on Article— Milligan TA. Epilepsy: a clinical overview. *Am J Med*. 2021;134(7):840–847.

alcohol, hyponatremia, or glucose abnormality) and the patient has a greater than 60% chance of having another unprovoked seizure. Epilepsy is fully defined as follows:

Epilepsy is a disease of the brain characterized by any of the following conditions: (1) At least two unprovoked (or reflex) seizures occurring >24 hours apart; (2) one unprovoked (or reflex) seizure and a probability of further seizures similar to the general recurrence risk (at least 60%) after two unprovoked seizures, occurring over the next 10 years; (3) diagnosis of an epilepsy syndrome.

Epilepsy affects more than 3.4 million people in the United States (1.2% of the US population). The lifetime prevalence rate is 3%. Epilepsy affects people of every age and background but most commonly starts before the age of 1 year and increases again after the age of 50, with the highest incidence after the age of 75. The annual cost of epilepsy in the US is over 12.5 billion dollars. Only 44% of American adults with epilepsy reported having their seizures controlled. However, approximately 70% of patients might become seizure free with appropriate treatment. The remaining 30% of patients have drug-resistant epilepsy (DRE), which is the failure of adequate trials of two tolerated, appropriately chosen and used antiseizure medication (ASM) schedules to achieve sustained seizure freedom.

CLASSIFICATION OF SEIZURES AND EPILEPSY

There are distinct types of epileptic seizures. The classification of seizure type has important consequences for determining the etiology, best treatment and overall prognosis. Seizures are classified based on the appearance of the seizure and parts of the cerebral cortex involved in the seizure. The 2017 classification system for seizures and epilepsy builds on the original classification system but emphasizes updated terms with the goal of being more understandable (Fig. 24.1).

The first step in classification of seizures is to identify whether the seizures are focal in onset (involving a localized network of neurons) or generalized in onset (rapidly engaging a bilaterally distributed neuronal network). Focal seizures are due to a small group of neurons that have enhanced excitability and the ability to occasionally spread that activity to neighboring regions, thereby causing a seizure. A seizure can begin in any lobe of the brain, but the most common lobe is the temporal lobe, particularly the mesial temporal lobe

containing the amygdala and hippocampus. The clinical manifestations of focal seizures will depend on the normal function of the region of cortex that is involved in the seizure (Table 24.1).

During a focal seizure, there may be preservation of consciousness and full awareness throughout the seizure. In the older nomenclature this type of seizure was referred to as a simple partial seizure or aura. In the 2017 classification system, this type of seizure is more precisely termed a focal aware seizure. During a focal aware seizure, the patient is alert and able to respond and remembers the seizure. This type of seizure is synonymous with an aura. Focal seizures can either progress to altered awareness or begin with altered awareness, during which time the patient has altered responsiveness and memory. This type of seizure is called a focal seizure with impaired awareness and in the older classification system was called a complex partial seizure. Automatisms are common during focal seizures with impaired awareness and can include the eyes (blinking), mouth (lip smacking, chewing), hands (fumbling, picking), vocalizations (grunts, repetition of words or phrases), or more complex acts (walking, attempting to use a cellphone). This type of seizure generally lasts from 30 seconds to 2 minutes and is followed by a brief period of confusion and fatigue. A focal seizure can spread to involve networks in both cerebral hemispheres, leading to tonic-clonic movements. This process is called focal to bilateral tonic-clonic. This term distinguishes convulsions that begin focally and spread, focal to bilateral tonic-clonic, from primary generalized tonic-clonic seizures, which have a different mechanism and etiology.

Primary generalized seizures involve bilaterally distributed networks at onset. The different seizure types include myoclonic, absence, atonic, tonic, clonic, and tonic-clonic seizures. Myoclonic seizures are very quick shock-like jerks of a muscle or group of muscles and typically involve the upper extremities without altered level of awareness. In contrast, the other forms of generalized seizures involve loss or alteration in consciousness. Absence seizures consist of brief episodes (2–15 seconds) of sudden onset and offset staring, impaired responsiveness, and eye fluttering and do not have a postictal confusion (in contrast to focal seizures with impaired awareness). Tonic and atonic seizures consist of sudden changes in muscle tone lasting seconds and often leading to falls. Tonic-clonic seizures are commonly referred to as convulsions or grand mal seizures.

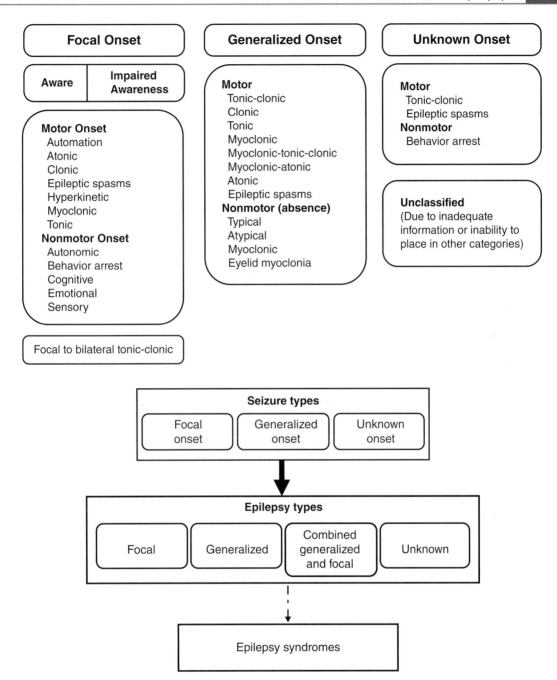

Fig. 24.1 2017 International League Against Epilepsy seizure and epilepsy classification systems.

They begin with loss of consciousness. The tonic phase can lead to falls and an epileptic cry caused by air forced through contracted vocal folds. The clonic phase consists of jerking of the upper and lower extremities with cyanosis, tongue biting, foaming at the mouth, and incontinence. Following the tonic-clonic seizure, the patient is lethargic and confused and may become agitated as consciousness is regained.

TABLE 24.1	Seizure Semiology
Localization	Signs and Symptoms
Mesial temporal (amygdala, hippocampus)	Déjà vu, jamais vu, depersonalization, derealization, olfactory hallucinations, oral and manual automatisms, behavioral arrest, sweating, pallor, piloerection, epigastric sensations, anxiety, fear
Temporal lobe	Auditory hallucinations, aphasia (left)
Frontal lobe	Contralateral tonic and/or clonic movements, contralateral gaze deviation, contralateral versive head movement, bizarre appearing hypermotor movements
Parietal lobe	Contralateral tingling and other somatosensory phenomena
Occipital	Visual hallucinations (simple— colors, shapes), more complex visual hallucinations (temporo-occipital), vision loss

TABLE 24.2	Common Causes of Epilepsy
Age Group	Common Causes
Infants	Perinatal hypoxia, metabolic disorders, intracranial hemorrhage, genetic disorders, developmental and congenital maldevelopment
Children	Perinatal anoxia, injury at birth or later, infections, vascular, metabolic, cortical malformations, genetic disorders
Teens and young adults	Trauma, infection, genetic disorders, brain tumors, congenital
Adults	Stroke, trauma, brain tumor, infection
Older adults (over 60 years)	Stroke, dementia, brain tumor, infection, trauma

Some forms of epilepsy can be classified as an epilepsy syndrome. Epilepsy syndromes are types of epilepsy in which a clear demographic, seizure type(s), electroencephalography (EEG) pattern, and prognosis are known. Increasingly, the etiology is also known, and it is often genetic. Examples of epilepsy syndromes include infantile spasms (West syndrome), Lennox-Gastaut syndrome, childhood absence epilepsy, and juvenile myoclonic epilepsy.

ETIOLOGY

Seizures have different causes, of which epilepsy is one. A diagnosis of epilepsy requires that the seizures are not provoked. Epilepsy also has a wide variety of etiologies. The most likely cause depends on the age of onset (Table 24.2). Often, despite extensive diagnostic testing, the etiology cannot be determined.

DIAGNOSIS

The diagnosis of epilepsy requires the occurrence of at least one unprovoked seizure and the likelihood of >60% that the patient will have another unprovoked seizure. The likelihood of having a subsequent seizure can be determined by etiology and EEG. However, the initial step in diagnosis is to determine whether the event was in fact a seizure and to explore the possibility that the seizure was provoked. Convulsive syncope and psychogenic nonepileptic seizures (PNES) can appear like epileptic seizures and are often mistaken for epileptic seizures. Syncope, PNES, and epileptic seizures account for 90% of transient loss-of-consciousness episodes and have features that can help to differentiate between them. Syncope often has prodromal symptoms of tunnel vision, dizziness, and palpitations and can have triggers such as fear, micturition, or Valsalva. Episodes are usually brief and do not have disorientation following. PNES can involve crying, hip thrusting, side-to-side head movements, bilateral shaking with preserved awareness. In general, these events are less stereotyped, more prolonged (lasting 5–30 minutes), and often associated with feelings of panic. It is important to note some patients may have both epileptic and nonepileptic seizures. Other seizure mimickers are listed in Table 24.3. Once a seizure has been determined to be an epileptic seizure, consider whether it was provoked. Illicit and prescription drugs, alcohol withdrawal, and glucose and electrolyte abnormalities are common reasons for provoked seizures (Box 24.1). The International League Against Epilepsy offers an educational website for the diagnosis of epilepsy, which illustrates seizure types and provides video and EEG examples (https://www.epilepsydiagnosis.org).

The diagnosis of epilepsy is made by history, examination, neuroimaging, and EEG. Risk factors for the development of epilepsy include complications of

TABLE 24.3 Differential Diagnosis of Seizures and Seizure Mimickers

Seizure
Syncope (convulsive)
Psychiatric disturbance (psychogenic nonepileptic seizure)
Migraine
Cerebral ischemia (transient ischemic attack)
Movement disorder
Sleep disorder
Metabolic disturbance

BOX 24.1 Common Causes of Provoked Seizures

Metabolic (hyponatremia, hypoglycemia, hyperthyroidism, nonketotic hyperglycemia, hypocalcemia, hypomagnesemia, renal failure, porphyria)
Medications (benzodiazepine withdrawal, barbiturate withdrawal, phenothiazines, bupropion, tramadol)
Substance abuse (alcohol withdrawal, cocaine, amphetamine, phencyclidine, methylenedioxymethamphetatime ["ecstasy"])
Acute neurologic insults (within 1 week of injury)
Eclampsia

pregnancy and childbirth; history of febrile seizures; family history of epilepsy; developmental delay or autism; history of traumatic brain injury, brain infection, or other structural lesion of the cerebral cortex; and dementia. Physical examination for causes of provoked seizures and epilepsy includes blood pressure and other vital signs; skin exam for stigmata of systemic or neurologic disease (café au lait spots seen with neurofibromatosis or adenoma sebaceum seen with tuberous sclerosis); extremity examination for smaller limbs or a smaller thumbnail, which can indicate early life injury to the contralateral cerebral cortex; physical examination for signs of cancer or infection; and a full neurologic examination assessing for cognitive dysfunction and focal abnormalities.

EEG is a necessary component in the evaluation of epilepsy. EEG can help in determining whether the seizure was focal or generalized in onset, which can assist in choosing the appropriate ASM for treatment. If the seizure was focal, EEG can also help to determine the location of the seizure onset. Ambulatory EEG monitoring has increased sensitivity and can be performed at home for several days at a time. In general, interictal EEG sensitivity is only 20%–55%, with only about one-third of initial routine EEGs being abnormal in a patient who is later diagnosed with epilepsy. Sensitivity improves to 80%–90% if EEGs are repeated over time. EEGs with sleep deprivation can reveal epileptiform discharges in 13% of patients who had no epileptiform activity on standard EEG. Thus it is imperative to remember that a normal EEG does not negate a diagnosis of epilepsy. If an EEG does show epileptiform activity, assuming a pretest probability of 50%, patients with epileptiform discharges on routine EEG after a first unprovoked seizure have a 66%–77% probability of having a second seizure and should be started on an ASM to prevent further seizures.

Video EEG is helpful when it remains unclear whether the event in question is an epileptic seizure, especially when events continue despite treatment. Video EEG allows correlation of the event to electrical changes consistent with a seizure on EEG. This is often done in an epilepsy monitoring unit (EMU), where seizures can be provoked by weaning medication in a safe, closely monitored setting. While electroclinical correlation is the gold standard for diagnosis, many patients do not have access to a hospital with an EMU; even if they do, up to one-third of patients may not have an event captured in the time during which they are in the unit. These days, an easier and often more practical option is the use of smartphone video to assist in diagnosis. Studies have shown that videos of events can be taken safely and review of the semiology by a neurologist specializing in seizures can lead to accurate diagnosis even when EEG is not available. Neuroimaging is important in the evaluation of seizures and epilepsy. In nonacute settings, magnetic resonance imaging (MRI) is the preferred imaging modality. MRI can assess for the etiology of the seizure and help to determine the risk of recurrence after a first-time seizure. Typically, MRI brain protocol for epilepsy involves thin cuts through the temporal lobes and can be done with contrast when there is a high suspicion of a mass or infections process as the etiology. Neuroimaging reveals the cause of a first-time seizure approximately 28% of the time and is most sensitive in patients with focal seizures. Neuroimaging can reveal mesial temporal sclerosis, neurocystercercosis, brain tumors, and some neurodevelopmental abnormalities, such as cortical dysplasia, as well as other structural abnormalities. Detection of potentially epileptogenic MRI lesions is generally considered to be associated with a high seizure recurrence risk (>60%). Concordant localizing data, in which seizure semiology, EEG findings, and/or MRI lesions localize to the same region have the most value in establishing a diagnosis of epilepsy after a single seizure.

TREATMENT OF EPILEPSY

Antiseizure Medication

Once a diagnosis of epilepsy has been made, an ASM should be initiated. The goal of selecting an ASM is to find a medication that is fully efficacious and to which the patient has no side effects, ideally with monotherapy, though polytherapy is often required. About 70% of patients will have seizures controlled with one of the first two medications that are trialed. The best chance of choosing an ASM that controls seizures with no side effects is to choose one that fits the patient's epilepsy type and seizure frequency and is likely to be best tolerated, considering the patient's age, gender, comorbidities, drug interactions, compliance, and ability to obtain the medication. Medications vary in cost, time necessary to achieve therapeutic doses, drug-drug interactions, and teratogenicity.

ASMs are divided into narrow-spectrum and broad-spectrum agents. This is the initial deciding point in choosing an ASM. If the epilepsy type is unknown, a broad-spectrum agent is necessary. Narrow-spectrum ASMs work only for specific types of seizures and may be ineffective with other types of seizures or even worsen them. Narrow-spectrum focal ASMs include carbamazepine, oxcarbazepine, gabapentin, pregabalin, tiagabine, and eslicarbazepine. These ASMs can exacerbate myoclonic and absence seizures. Broad-spectrum ASMs have some efficacy for a wide range of seizures (focal, absence, generalized tonic-clonic, and myoclonic) and include ASMs such as levetiracetam, valproic acid, lacosamide, and clobazam.

Currently, no ASM has been proven to be more effective than another, which makes safety and tolerability of high consideration in choosing and ASM. Adverse reactions can include those that are idiosyncratic, dose related, teratogenic, and worsening of comorbidities. The newer ASMs generally have fewer side effects than

the older agents. Potential side effects that common to all ASMs include fatigue, gastrointestinal side effects, mood changes, and cognitive side effects. The older-generation ASMs have more side effects and tend to be strong hepatic inducers which result in increased drug-drug interactions and can affect hormone and vitamin D levels. These include phenytoin, carbamazepine, and phenobarbital. They are associated with an increased rate of fractures due to osteopenia. Bone density screening is recommended for anyone who has taken one of these agents for 5 years or longer: phenytoin, phenobarbital, primidone, valproate, or carbamazepine. The ASMs with the least drug–drug interactions include levetiracetam and lacosamide. Some side effects, especially those that are dose related and reflect the peak effect of drug concentration, may have improved tolerability from extended-release formulations.

Some ASMs can be loaded or at least initiated at immediate therapeutic doses; others require a gradual titration over weeks. Depending on the patient's seizure frequency, an ASM with a faster ability to reach therapeutic doses may be necessary and part of the consideration in choosing an ASM. Often, when an ASM has been initiated, many clinicians choose to check serum concentrations to determine whether the dose is adequate. However, it is important to remember that reference levels are not representative of efficacy, and doses should be adjusted according to patient response. After initial titration to the lowest therapeutic dose, doses are increased until seizure control is achieved, side effects are present, or further escalation in dose is unlikely to produce increased efficacy. With polytherapy, it is important to consider drug interactions between ASMs.

Ease of availability can affect adherence, which will affect efficacy. Considerations include cost, prior authorizations for insurance coverage, and release of controlled substances. Fig. 24.2 depicts a flowchart for choosing an ASM.

In addition to maintenance medication, rescue medication should be considered. Benzodiazepines such as clonazepam, diazepam, and midazolam can be prescribed and delivered orally, rectally, or intranasally for use at home when needed for prolonged seizures or clusters of seizures. Intranasal formulations allow for quick, easy, and safe delivery even when the person is unconscious, and they have been shown to be of equivalent in efficacy to intravenous lorazepam. Early delivery of rescue medication can help to prevent status epilepticus.

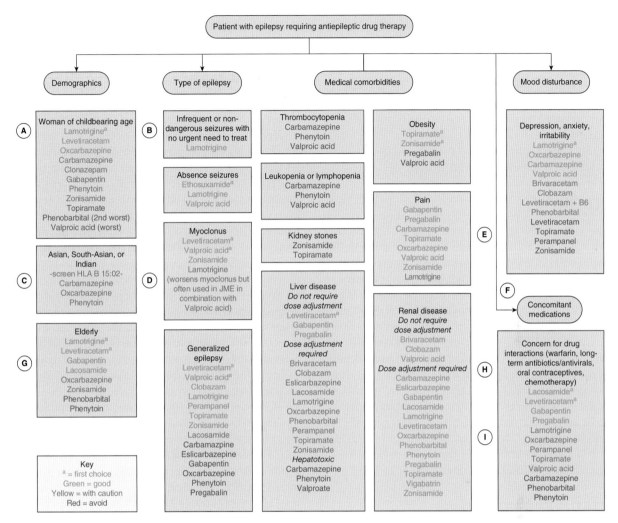

Fig. 24.2 Flowchart for the treatment of a patient with epilepsy requiring antiepileptic drug therapy. (From Cucchiara B, Price RS. *Decision-Making in Adult Neurology.* Elsevier; 2020.)

WOMEN WITH EPILEPSY

Many WWE have increased seizures associated with their menstrual cycle (catamenial epilepsy). WWE also have a higher rate of anovulatory cycles and polycystic ovarian syndrome. Folate supplementation, 0.4–1 mg daily, is recommended for all women of childbearing potential, as it decreases the risk of neural tube defects. Some ASMs, particularly those that are inducers, reduce the efficacy of hormonal contraception. Hormonal contraception reduces the level of lamotrigine, placing women who take lamotrigine at risk of breakthrough seizures with the addition of hormonal contraception

unless the dose is appropriately increased. Long-acting reversible contraceptives (progestin implant) or intra-uterine devices are recommended for WWE on medications that decrease the efficacy of oral contraceptives. WWE can have safe and healthy pregnancies when they are monitored closely by a neurologist and an obstetrician. The two ASMs with the most safety data for women during pregnancy are levetiracetam and lamotrigine, and they are currently the preferred agents for use during pregnancy. Levels of both can drop during pregnancy, and serum levels can be monitored with doses adjusted as needed during pregnancy and lowered following delivery. Close follow-up throughout the pregnancy and during the postnatal period with a neurologist/epileptologist is advised. Though ASMs can pass through breast milk to infants, women are encouraged to breastfeed if they choose to, as studies have shown increased IQ of children at 6 years of age of breastefed children compared to children who were not breastfed in WWE on ASMs. The agents with the highest known teratogenicity are valproic acid, phenobarbital, and topiramate, and they should be avoided if possible and women counseled accordingly.

ELDERLY

The risk of developing epilepsy is at its highest after the age of 65 and increases in risk with older age. The metabolism of ASMs slow down, and a given dose of an ASM results in a higher serum level. A low dose of an ASM with no or limited drug–drug interactions is preferred. There has been one randomized controlled study of ASM efficacy and tolerability in the elderly, which compared carbamazepine, gabapentin, and lamotrigine. Lamotrigine was the most efficacious and best tolerated of the three. The dose in that study was 50 mg bid titrating up as needed. Levetiracetam has also been compared to carbamazepine and lamotrigine and was shown to be efficacious and well tolerated. Levetiracetam has the advantage of having no drug-drug interactions and being easily titrated, but that needs to be balanced against side effects of irritability and poor mood.

STATUS EPILEPTICUS

Status epilepticus, which is a life-threatening neurologic emergency, is defined as a state of continuous seizures without interval recovery. The most recent definition of status epilepticus recognizes two points in time. For convulsive seizures, the first-time point at 5 minutes is when the patient should be clinically diagnosed and treated for status epilepticus, and the second time point at 30 minutes is when neuronal damage is likely to occur. Status epilepticus is treated with benzodiazepines given intravenously, intramuscularly, or intranasally and ASMs delivered intravenously. Refractory status epilepticus requires intubation for airway protection; continuous EEG monitoring, given the increased risk of nonconvulsive seizures once convulsive status epilepticus has resolved; and use of an anesthetic agent such as midazolam, propofol, ketamine, or pentobarbital. The

prognosis of status epilepticus is primarily determined by the etiology of the status epilepticus.

SURGICAL MANAGEMENT OF EPILEPSY

All patients with drug-resistant epilepsy should receive evaluation for possible surgical treatment. There is Level 1 evidence that for patients who are candidates for temporal lobectomy, epilepsy surgery is superior to medical therapy. At 1 year, 58% of surgically treated patients were seizure free versus only 8% in the medically treated group. The presurgical workup involves capturing habitual seizures on video EEG to localize and lateralize onset and brain MRI to assess for structural lesions that may be contributing to the etiology. Often, other ancillary testing, such neuropsychological testing to assess baseline cognitive function, brain positron emission tomography to assess for metabolic dysfunction, functional MRI to assess for language lateralization, and Wada testing to assess for language and memory lateralization, are employed to help assess the risk of deficits with resection. The goal of surgical resection is to remove the seizure focus without any deficits. When there is a question of overlap with eloquent cortex, intracranial electrodes are placed either as subdural electrodes or as depth electrodes to more accurately localize seizure onsets and test brain function in the EMU. This can be done via open craniotomy or with techniques such as stereo EEG (SEEG), which involves placement of depth electrodes via burr holes. SEEG allows for a less invasive option. The most common surgical approach is open resection of the epileptogenic cerebral cortex, but a new method of MRI-guided laser ablation is increasingly being used that is less invasive with a quicker recovery, as it does not require a craniotomy.

When seizures have broad or multiple regions of onset or the onset overlaps with eloquent cortex, neuromodulation devices are options that have shown improved outcomes in DRE versus medication alone. There are now three FDA-approved neuromodulation devices for epilepsy: the responsive neurostimulator (RNS), the vagal nerve stimulator (VNS), and the deep brain stimulator (DBS). Overall, these devices have shown 50%–75% reduction in seizure frequency over time but lower rates of seizure freedom compared to surgical resection. VNS approved in 1997 for ages >4 years, used for focal and generalized epilepsies provides open-loop stimulation (stimulation at constant intervals) to the vagus nerve with a generator implanted in the chest. Common side effects include hoarseness and coughing that can often be improved by adjusting parameters during programming. Additional stimulation can be provided by swiping a magnet over the generator during a seizure, and newer models can be programmed to detect changes in heart rate that may be associated with seizures to trigger additional stimulation. DBS was approved in the United States in 2018 for ages 18 years and over with focal epilepsy; it provides open-loop stimulation to bilateral anterior nuclei of the thalamus with a generator in the chest. The target in the thalamus for DBS in epilepsy is different from that used for Parkinson disease. DBS allows for some programming to be done remotely. Outcomes thus far have been best in focal epilepsies with onsets in the frontotemporal regions. There can be mood side effects with DBS. Finally, RNS was approved in 2013 for ages 18 years and over with focal epilepsy; it involves implantation of two to four electrode strips or depths in the areas of seizure onset with a generator placed in the skull. Unlike the other two devices, RNS provides closed-loop stimulation (stimulating only when it detects a pattern concerning for a seizure) and chronic electrocorticography recordings, allowing for individualized seizure detection and information regarding seizure patterns. Stimulation is not felt by patients. Patients with any of these devices can receive selective MRIs if necessary, but the devices must be turned off and placed in MRI mode for safety.

DIETARY TREATMENT OF EPILEPSY

The ketogenic diet (KD) and the modified Atkins diet (MAD) are the most established diets for the treatment of epilepsy. Both primarily restrict carbohydrates and increase fat (KD > MAD) and can effectively reduce seizures, with 33%–47% of patients having a >50% seizure reduction and up to 27% having >90% seizure reduction at 1 year when combined with medication. However, especially the KD is challenging for many people, as it may not be palatable and requires strict adherence. The low-glycemic-index diet is also being used in the treatment of epilepsy.

SAFETY ISSUES

People with epilepsy have an increased risk of injuries and accidents, particularly drowning, burns, poisoning, adverse effects of medication, and traumatic brain injury. The risk of sudden unexpected death in epilepsy (SUDEP) is approximately 1 per 1000 adults a year and 1 per 4500 children a year. The risk factors for SUDEP include convulsive seizures and uncontrolled seizures.

Counseling regarding safety issues is a vital component of the treatment plan. It is temporarily illegal to drive after a seizure. Discussions about driving are an important topic. The role of the physician in both reporting and determining the amount of time the patient must be seizure free before driving varies from state to state from physician discretion to 3 months to more than a year. The law of each state can be found at epilepsy.com/driving-laws.

DEPRESSION

There is a bidirectional relationship between epilepsy and depression. Patients with major depressive disorder have a fourfold to sevenfold increased risk of an unprovoked seizure. Patients with epilepsy have a higher rate of depression, with about 30% of people with DRE developing clinically significant depression. There is an increased risk of suicide in people with epilepsy, particularly at the time of diagnosis and in individuals with a history of depression. Treatment with selective serotonin and norepinephrine reuptake inhibitors is considered safe in people with epilepsy when used at therapeutic doses and there is no concern for bipolar disorder. Bupropion is one antidepressant that should be avoided if possible, as it can provoke seizures.

WITHDRAWING MEDICATIONS

Once patients have been seizure free for a certain period of time (typically 4–5 years in adults), it is important to reassess whether or not medication can be withdrawn through a tapering process. Abrupt cessation is unsafe, and the longer the patient has been seizure free, the better their prognosis for successful withdrawal of ASM. The seizure recurrence rate is 34% on average but varies depending on the history of the individual patient. Recent nomograms have been published as tools to estimate the risk of seizure recurrence after ASM withdrawal. Important negative predictors for seizure freedom include longer duration of epilepsy, an abnormal neurologic examination, an abnormal EEG, and lesion on MRI of the brain, and certain epilepsy syndromes (e.g., juvenile myoclonic epilepsy) are known to increase the risk of recurrence.

Patients with acute symptomatic seizures (seizures typically occurring within 7 days after a brain insult, such as traumatic brain injury or stroke) have a lower incidence of recurrent seizures compared to those with a remote symptomatic etiology. Many patients can discontinue ASM sooner following acute symptomatic seizures. Similarly, ASMs that are started as seizure prophylaxis following neurologic surgery can typically be weaned soon after surgery, as patients do not have a diagnosis of epilepsy.

CONCLUSION

Epilepsy is a common disorder that is encountered in both inpatient and outpatient settings and affects people of all ages and backgrounds. A knowledge of the types of seizures and manifestations of seizures, diagnostic workup, and treatment options is of critical importance to physicians. The overall goal of care is to precisely diagnose the type and cause of seizure before calling it epilepsy and then, after diagnosis of epilepsy, to provide treatment that prevents seizures, tailoring this treatment to prevent side effects and maximize quality of life. High-quality care of patients with epilepsy also includes screening for and treating depression and referring any patient with uncontrolled seizures to an accredited epilepsy center.

"For the full bibliography list, please use the pincode on the inside front cover to access the electronic version of the text at ebooks.health.elsevier.com."

25

Dizziness*

Gregory T. Whitman

INTRODUCTION

The term "dizziness" can be used to refer to vertigo, lightheadedness, disorientation, presyncope, confusion, generalized weakness, or postural instability. Given this multiplicity of definitions, the differential diagnosis of dizziness is correspondingly broad. A deliberate and careful clinical assessment of the symptoms and signs associated with a chief complaint of dizziness is an effective strategy in the production of a successful diagnostic approach.

Anatomically, the vestibular system has peripheral and central parts. Critical for normal posture and gait, the vestibular system also supports clear vision during head movements, due to its contribution to the vestibulo-ocular reflex (VOR). The VOR uses head position and motion information derived from the inner ears to direct eye position and achieve gaze stability.

The peripheral vestibular system consists of the vestibular nerve, plus the inner ear balance organs, namely, the three semicircular canals and two otolith organs called the utricle and the saccule. The inner ear is protected within the petrous temporal bone. The semicircular canals—each side having one horizontal, one anterior, and one posterior canal—occur in pairs, called the right anterior left posterior (RALP) and left anterior right posterior (LARP) canal pairs. The two horizontal semicircular canals detect rotation in horizontal planes. This bilaterality and pairing of canals provides redundancy that enables recovery after vestibular system

insults. Such recovery is called vestibular compensation. The central vestibular system is less well defined, including but not limited to the brainstem vestibular nuclei and cerebellum.

Vestibular function is inherently multisensory. The neural pathways from the sensory organs of the inner ear, the visual pathways from the eye to the brain, afferents from the neck muscles, the joints of the spine, and the peripheral sensory organs and nerves of the limbs, together provide the brain with redundant cues about movement, that is, acceleration, velocity, and position relative to various reference frames, including position relative to gravity. The outputs of the vestibular system involve the combined function of the brain, spinal cord, peripheral nerves, muscles, and neuromuscular structures. There is also growing interest in processing of vestibular signals in the brain, for example, the role of the brain in determining the threshold above which motion can be detected by the inner ear. Additionally, spatial memory has been reported to be mediated, in part, by projections between brainstem vestibular nuclei and medial temporal lobe limbic structures, such as the entorhinal cortex. This raises the possibility of two-way causal connections between traditional vestibular disorders and temporal lobe diseases such as Alzheimer disease.

APPROACH TO HISTORY TAKING

It is good to begin by asking about the patient's subjective experience. Sometimes, the patient will not be able to describe what "dizziness" means, for it can be difficult to put into words. It is crucial to outline all evident aggravating and alleviating factors. The

*Based on Whitman GT, Dizziness. *Am J Med*. 2018;131(12): 1431–1437. ISSN 0002-9343. https://doi.org/10.1016/j.amjmed. 2018.05.014.

circumstances in which dizziness is aggravated often represent clues to one or more correct diagnoses. It is often helpful to explicitly ask about how dizziness is modified with, or whether it is induced by, motion or positional change. Peripheral vestibular hypofunction, particularly if bilateral, may cause oscillopsia, that is, instability of images during head motion, for example, while looking out the window of a moving vehicle or while walking. During the interview, begin to develop hypotheses about the differential diagnosis. By the end of the history, and potentially before any formal examination, the clinician should already have a fairly good differential diagnosis. This differential diagnosis can then be weighted by the objective findings of a physical examination.

APPROACH TO THE EXAMINATION

In taking vital signs, it can be helpful to add an orthostatic vital sign test, in which the patient is asked to stand reasonably motionless for a period of at least 3 minutes. Heart rate and blood pressure are traditionally recorded in this standing position. While the patient is standing motionless, they should be observed for complaints of escalating dizziness or blurred vision, as well as alterations of speech and cognition, and note should be made of any marked degradation of postural stability. It is conventional for abnormal orthostatic vital signs to be defined in terms of a large drop in blood pressure or a marked rise in heart rate after the patient moves to an upright position. One must note, however, that blood pressures in the standing position, though they may not reflect a major change from those in the sitting or supine position, may still be significant if they are low. For example, a standing diastolic blood pressure of 55 is a risk factor for dizziness even if the supine blood pressure is not much higher.

Otoscopy may disclose cerumen, a large quantity of which may help explain hearing loss. Middle ear disease, particularly the infrequent but important finding of a middle ear tumor, may be disclosed. All of the tools of the neurological examination have the potential to be useful in the evaluation of the dizzy patient. The methods of the neurological examination are beyond the scope of this review, but selected signs will be described here.

Some observations about mental status should be noted, including attention, which is critical for normal balance and gait. Abnormalities of visual acuity or visual fields may disturb balance and should be observed. Patients should be asked about double vision. In testing eye alignment, the alternate cover test is performed by covering one eye with something opaque while the other eye fixates on the examiner. The covered eye is then quickly uncovered, and the other eye is covered. In a positive test, an eye moves when it is uncovered, indicating a tendency toward misalignment or phoria. To detect strabismus the cover-uncover test is performed by covering one eye with something opaque and observing the uncovered eye for movement. Next, the covered eye is uncovered. In considering these two tests, the alternate cover test is more sensitive, and the cover-uncover test is more specific for detection of misalignment. Vertical misalignment of the eyes, especially if large, strongly favors a localization to the posterior fossa of the brain, though more subtle hypertropia can be seen with acute inner ear disease, possibly due to involvement of the utricle or its nerve.

Smooth pursuit is tested by asking the patient to follow a visual target, such as the examiner's finger that is slowly moving from right to left and then up and down. The examiner observes the breakdown of smooth pursuit into saccades. The evenness of smooth pursuit depends on frequency and/or the speed of target motion. If the patient is able to follow the examiner's finger from the midline all the way to the right, then all the way to the left, then back to the midline in less than 3 seconds without saccades, then smooth pursuit is likely normal. The prevalence of saccadic pursuit in older people is high, rendering bedside smooth pursuit less useful with increasing patient age.

During smooth pursuit testing, spontaneous and gaze nystagmus can be recorded. Nystagmus consists of involuntary oscillating eye movements; and the most common type of nystagmus, that is, jerk nystagmus, has well-defined slow and fast phases. In practice, nystagmus is most often coarser with eye deviation and gaze holding in the direction of fast phases. Gaze-holding, direction-switching nystagmus, for example, fast phases to the right with gaze to right and fast phases to the left with gaze to left, is a central sign. Gaze-holding downbeat nystagmus is another central sign that suggests a disturbance of the cerebellum or craniocervical junction. In cerebellar disorders, one may observe positional nystagmus that persists as long as the patient remains in one position, that is, static positional nystagmus.

The clinical head impulse test, which is now commonly performed in emergency rooms, is intended to test the horizontal angular VOR. In this test, the patient is first asked to fixate, for example, on the examiner's nose or eyes. The patient's head is then gently turned back and forth about 10–20 degrees to the right or left of midline; then, in an unpredictable fashion, the examiner suddenly turns the patient's head from an eccentric position to the midline, or past the midline, through a total angle of about 20 degrees, using reasonable caution to avoid injury. In an abnormal result, when the head is suddenly, impulsively turned toward a damaged peripheral vestibular system, the eyes move with the head and then make a corrective saccade away toward the intended direction of fixation.

A dynamic visual acuity test can be performed at the bedside. The patient is asked to view the near vision card while the examiner passively oscillates the patient's head in the yaw/axial plane at about 2 Hz. If near vision worsens from baseline by more than two lines of vision, the test is abnormal. This usually indicates bilateral vestibular hypofunction. Many patients with unilateral vestibular hypofunction readily report that dynamic visual acuity is less good during the half cycles when the head is being turned toward the affected side, for example, toward the left in a patient who has recently had acute left vestibular neuritis. The Dix-Hallpike positional test is discussed in the next section. Limb coordination can be tested by past pointing tests in which a patient with eyes closed extends both arms and repeatedly touches the examiner's fingers from above or below. The Romberg sign indicates excessive dependence of balance upon vision and can be caused by a variety of lesions. One cause of a Romberg sign is myelopathy. The walking Romberg test is sensitive to compressive cervical myelopathy and is performed by asking the patient to walk with eyes closed, noting any significant unsteadiness. In the Fukuda stepping test, the patient marches in place with the arms stretched out in front for about 1 minute or 50 steps; turning toward the right or left by more than 20 degrees is abnormal. This test is most useful when strong turning is noted in a particular direction on multiple trials. Gait dysfunction associated with central nervous system lesions frequently features excessively variable step length. In contrast, peripheral nerve lesions in the limbs, such as entrapment neuropathy, may cause abnormalities that repeat, machine like, from one gait cycle to the next. Patients who are able should be asked to walk up and down a hallway so that arm swing, axial stability, foot dorsiflexion, step width, step length, gait velocity, and other features of gait can be assessed and recorded.

Due to the reliance of normal balance and gait function on cognition, particularly attention, one can often bring out deficits through using dual-task paradigms that are intended to introduce a cognitive load during gait tests. For example, a patient can be asked to count backwards while walking, and if the gait velocity declines by more than 20% with the cognitive load, that would be suggestive of a gait disorder associated with limited cognitive reserve and the possibility of a brain disorder.

BENIGN PAROXYSMAL POSITIONAL VERTIGO

Benign paroxysmal positional vertigo (BPPV) is a disorder in which freely floating debris is trapped within and thus disturbs the function of one or more semicircular canals. The utricular macula is invested with calcium- and protein-containing complexes called otoliths. Otoliths can break down, releasing otolith debris that can migrate into the semicircular canals, most commonly the posterior semicircular canal. Head position changes, such as when the patient with BPPV lies down, rolls in bed, or looks up, may place the freely floating debris in a position from which it can move under the influence of gravity, leading to semicircular canal dysfunction and dizziness. A typical patient reports waves of vertigo with changes in position and may, in addition, have other, milder forms of dizziness, such as nondescript dizziness or imbalance while upright. Patients with BPPV are typically able to describe a latency between the position change and the onset of dizziness and may, for example, say something like "I lie down, and then after a second, I feel a big wave of dizziness."

A diagnosis of BPPV can be made at the bedside with the Dix-Hallpike test. While the patient is sitting, the head is turned 45 degrees toward the right or left. The patient is then laid back supine with the neck extended back 20 degrees. One observes the eyes for 30 seconds, looking for a burst of paroxysmal nystagmus. Depending on the examination environment and the patient's neck range of motion, it may be appropriate to achieve neck extension by placing a pillow under the upper back. Some patients with severe nausea may benefit from pretreatment with a vestibular suppressant, such as meclizine, before the Dix-Hallpike test is performed. Of note, immediate repetition of the Dix-Hallpike test may lead to a reduction in the intensity of the paroxysmal nystagmus, that is, the nystagmus may be fatigable. This raises some concern about whether the fatigable nature of the nystagmus might cause one to miss the diagnosis. Therefore, if the history strongly suggests BPPV but the Dix-Hallpike test is negative, one should examine again, allowing a longer time in each position, or consider reexamining on a different day.

In the most common form of BPPV, that is, posterior semicircular canal BPPV, the Dix-Hallpike test induces a burst of upbeat and torsional nystagmus. The torsional component is such that the upper poles of the eyes beat toward, that is, have fast phases directed toward, the ground. In the horizontal canal variant of BPPV, the nystagmus is mostly horizontal. In the anterior canal variant of BPPV, there is paroxysmal downbeat nystagmus.

For patients with pure vertical nystagmus, whether paroxysmal or not, the differential diagnosis of posterior fossa brain disease should be considered. Typically, positional nystagmus due to central nervous system disease is nonparoxysmal, in which case the term "static positional nystagmus" is used. Follow-up of patients with downbeat nystagmus of any type is critical to ensure correct diagnosis, and neuroimaging may be indicated.

The Epley maneuver (Fig. 25.1) is highly effective for the treatment of posterior canal BPPV. The goal should be stable resolution of all symptoms rather than incremental or incomplete improvement. In some cases, a prolonged course of physical therapy or multiple in-office particle repositioning maneuvers are necessary for symptom resolution. Adding mastoid vibration to the Epley maneuver remains unproven but anecdotally may occasionally be a reasonable adjunct to consider for

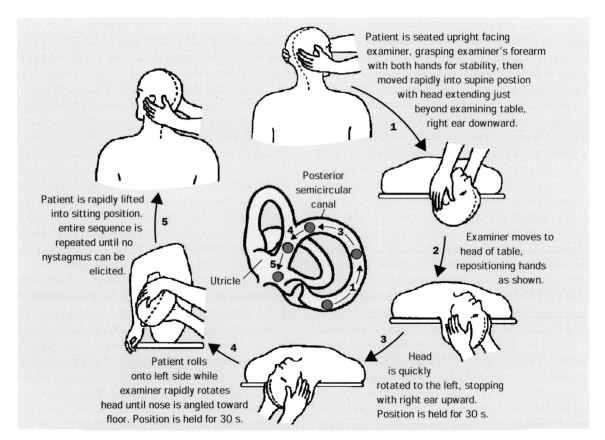

Fig. 25.1 The Epley maneuver for treatment of posterior semicircular canal benign paroxysmal positional vertigo. (From Baloh RW. Vertigo. *Lancet.* 1998;352:1841–1846.)

refractory cases in which the latency of the nystagmus is long.

In the horizontal canal variant of BPPV, the nystagmus is often seen in the Dix-Hallpike test, however, it is best elicited by having the patient lie supine and turning the patient's head toward the right or left. The nystagmus of the horizontal canal variant of BPPV is predominantly horizontal. It may be classified as geotropic—that is, beating toward the floor—or apogeotropic, beating away from the floor. The horizontal canal variant of BPPV can be severely symptomatic and refractory. An effective treatment for horizontal canal BPPV is the so-called log roll maneuver (Fig. 25.2). The supine patient is rolled toward one side or the other and continues to roll until they have made a 360-degree rotation around the long axis of the body. With careful instruction, this type of maneuver can often be successfully accomplished by the patient at home in bed. The anterior canal variant of BPPV may respond to a maneuver in which the patient is moved from sitting to supine and, in cases in which

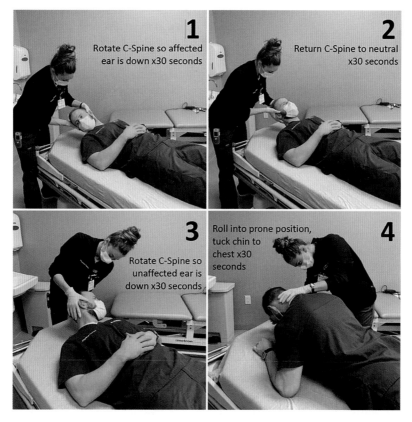

Fig. 25.2 Treatment of horizontal canal BPPV with the log roll maneuver, also known as the barbecue or Lempert maneuver: Record whether horizontal nystagmus is geotropic (toward the ground) or apogeotropic (away from the ground). For the patient with co-occurring posterior canal BPPV, the side of the affected horizontal canal is reasonably hypothesized to be the same as that of the affected posterior canal. Otherwise, one may hypothesize the following: for geotropic nystagmus, the affected side is that toward which turning induces brisker nystagmus; for apogeotropic nystagmus, the affected side is that toward which turning induces provokes weaker nystagmus. One must note that the rules for determining the affected and unaffected sides are imperfect. Thus, one often must adopt an empirical approach, e.g., treat as though the right side is affected on one or more days; and treat as though the left side is affected on different days. Note that after Step 4, as shown in the figure, the examiner turns the patient another 90 degrees, in the same direction and then moves the patient to the sitting upright position. (From Hwu V, Burris AK, Pavolko JR, Sawyer DT, Greenberg MR, Burmeister DB. Utilization of the lempert maneuver for benign paroxysmal positional vertigo in the emergency department. *Cureus.* 2022;14(4):e24288.)

it is deemed safe, hyperextends the neck while supine, in which position the patient stays for approximately 30 seconds before sitting back up.

After successful treatment of BPPV and resolution of nystagmus, some patients may experience a post-BPPV syndrome that consists of nonspecific dizziness and imbalance. This typically lasts for a period of weeks. The post-BPPV syndrome has been reported to be associated with utricular dysfunction. This is consistent with the fact that some patients with BPPV also manifest a head tilt and the fact that utricle stimulation varies with head tilted toward either side when the patient upright.

MÉNIÈRE DISEASE

Ménière disease, also known as Ménière syndrome, is defined by prolonged episodes of vertigo combined with fluctuating, single-sided or asymmetric, low-frequency-predominant sensorineural hearing loss (SNHL). Over time, many patients with Ménière disease develop progressive hearing loss that involves all frequencies of sound tested. The related Pathology term "endolymphatic hydrops" refers to dilation of inner ear spaces that contain endolymph. The overlap between clinical Ménière disease and hydrops is not one-to-one; however, recent magnetic resonance imaging (MRI) studies support the concept that many patients with clinical Ménière disease do indeed have hydrops. Ménière disease and hydrops are most often idiopathic and likely represent final common pathways of multiple different disease processes that cause inner ear dysfunction. Delayed endolymphatic hydrops may occur years after sudden SNHL.

The diagnosis of Ménière disease is typically made after an audiogram that is performed by an audiologist in a soundproof booth. During a pure tone audiogram, the patient is asked to signal when able to hear a series of frequencies of sounds, presented to each ear at gradually increasing volume starting below the perceptible volume, to identify a threshold above which the patient is able to hear. To distinguish between SNHL and conductive hearing loss, the audiologist looks for evidence of an air-bone gap, defined as a significant difference between the air conduction thresholds and bone conduction thresholds. Air conduction thresholds measure how well a person can hear using headphones or earphones that are inserted into the external ear canals.

Bone conduction thresholds measure how well a person can hear when sound is conducted through skull bones, and the stimulus is administered by a vibrating device placed over the mastoid bone behind the tested ear. Conductive hearing loss occurs when there is a disturbance in the conduction of sound information from the outside world through the middle ear. Middle ear function is affected by otosclerosis, otitis media, Eustachian tube dysfunction, and sinusitis. SNHL typically arises from a disorder of the cochlea or the cochlear nerve, though one must bear in mind the possibility of a retrocochlear lesion, in particular a cerebellopontine angle mass, as described later in this chapter.

First-line treatment for Ménière disease consists of limiting and smoothing out dietary sodium consumption over the course of each day. Consuming adequate amounts of water may also lead to a reduction in the frequency and severity of vertigo attacks. If dietary interventions fail, many providers prescribe diuretic medications. Although evidence for the effectiveness of diuretics is limited, most specialists who have treated patients with Ménière disease believe that diuretics are beneficial for at least some patients. The primary treatment goal in Ménière disease is to reduce the frequency and severity of vertigo attacks. Other symptoms of Ménière disease are less responsive to current interventions, and it is questionable whether any medical interventions favorably affect hearing, notwithstanding isolated reports that antiviral medication may reduce hearing loss and vertigo, an intriguing finding that unfortunately is not yet supported by randomized controlled trials. It is helpful for the patient with Ménière disease to have at least a small supply of vestibular suppressant medication available to use in case of a vertigo attack. For this purpose, lorazepam and meclizine are sometimes prescribed.

Although supported by only limited published evidence, intratympanic (IT) corticosteroid injection may be effective and offers the possibility of a sustained reduction in symptom frequency and severity potentially without the need for the long-term use of daily medication. Ablative surgery for Ménière disease is a last resort, appropriate for only a small proportion of patients with the disease. Likewise, ablative IT injection of the vestibular ototoxin, gentamicin, is reserved for refractory cases or patients with otolithic crises of Tumarkin. In otolithic crises, patients acutely lose balance and may suddenly fall, raising serious safety concerns. There is also some evidence suggesting that management of seasonal allergies may contribute to the effective management of Ménière disease.

VESTIBULAR MIGRAINE

In addition to meeting diagnostic criteria for migraine, patients with vestibular migraine experience episodes of dizziness, vertigo, or other vestibular symptoms. Migraine is defined primarily by a history of episodic headaches with nausea or photophobia. A close temporal association between vestibular symptoms and other migraine-associated symptoms, such as dizziness that occurs immediately before onset of headache and photophobia, increases the plausibility of a vestibular migraine diagnosis. The diagnosis of vestibular migraine relies on exclusion of other, better explanations. Although vestibular migraine and Ménière disease may both cause vertigo, it is unusual for migraine-related vertigo to last more than 30 minutes, while vertigo due to Ménière disease often lasts for hours. Many patients with Ménière disease also have migraine. Migraineurs frequently experience visual motion hypersensitivity or excessive sensitivity to optic flow, as while walking down a supermarket aisle lined with rows of items. Of note, BPPV often aggravates migraine, including vestibular migraine. This leads to cases in which patients with recent onset of BPPV present with a chief complaint of headache, nausea, photophobia, or spontaneous episodes of dizziness. This is unsurprising, given that vestibular testing, which induces dizziness, has been reported to trigger migraine symptoms.

Most interventions that are used for migraine headache have been anecdotally noted to be effective for patients with vestibular migraine, though there are insufficient data from randomized trials to guide therapy. Some patients with infrequent symptoms of vestibular migraine can be effectively managed by using as-needed vestibular suppressant medications, such as meclizine or promethazine. Benign paroxysmal vertigo (BPV) of childhood presents with episodic nonpositional dizziness. Many patients with BPV of childhood later develop migraine in adulthood. The approach to BPV resembles that used in the treatment of migraine. A fuller discussion of interventions for migraine can be found elsewhere in this book (see Chapter 11).

ACUTE UNILATERAL PERIPHERAL VESTIBULOPATHY INCLUDING VESTIBULAR NEURITIS

Acute unilateral peripheral vestibulopathy (AUPV) is associated with viral inflammation of the labyrinth and/or vestibular nerve. When AUPV is purely vestibular, the term "vestibular neuritis" is used, indicating acute unilateral failure of peripheral vestibular function. Analogously, a similar syndrome of acute unilateral failure of peripheral auditory function exists and is called sudden SNHL. When a patient has the acute signs and symptoms of both vestibular neuritis and sudden SNHL, the syndrome is called acute labyrinthitis. In Ramsay Hunt syndrome, inflammation related to varicella-zoster virus (VZV) involves the peripheral vestibular system, the peripheral auditory system, and the facial nerve. Ramsay Hunt syndrome generally presents with unilateral signs, including peripheral facial palsy, SNHL and tinnitus, dizziness, nausea, and blisters seen on the skin of the external ear. The incidence of Ramsay Hunt syndrome is expected to be lower in locations where a VZV vaccine, also known as the chickenpox vaccine, is available.

Vestibular neuritis causes a buildup, over hours, of acute, severe, and unrelenting vertigo; nausea; vomiting; and inability to walk normally. The clinical course may fluctuate considerably during the first few days after onset. The acute signs of AUPV persist for at least a few days. After this acute phase, more subtle signs remain for months. The persistence of the acute signs of AUPV for days allows one to distinguish AUPV from other disorders. The acute signs of AUPV include spontaneous, unidirectional, predominantly horizontal nystagmus with the fast phases of the horizontal component directed away from the involved ear, reflecting slow phases toward the affected ear. Head impulse testing with sudden, passive impulses delivered toward the affected ear induce corrective "catch-up" saccades, away from the affected ear toward the midline. The patient with AUPV who can walk typically falls or veers toward the affected ear.

Within several days, the spontaneous, unidirectional nystagmus of AUPV typically resolves and is replaced by nystagmus that is evident only upon gaze away from and beats away from the affected ear. This is an example of Alexander's law, which states that nystagmus is generally most evident upon gaze in the direction of the fast phases. Typically, in acute to subacute AUPV, the patient turns toward the affected ear on the Fukuda stepping test.

Comparable to many forms of neurological recovery, vestibular compensation proceeds over a period of months. For patients with AUPV who are recovering, residual dizziness and imbalance are most notable when the patient is tired. After AUPV, patients typically return to most of their activities of daily living within a month. Some experience prolonged, slow, or incomplete recovery, which can be severely frustrating. This type of frustration may be partially averted by counseling patients in advance about the possibility of incomplete recovery.

Recurrences of the full AUPV syndrome are rare. Months or years after recovery from AUPV, it is common for patients to continue to report mild, brief blurring of vision when the head is turned quickly toward the affected side, as when someone calls the patient's name. This type of mild gaze instability is typically one of the last features of AUPV to resolve and may be permanent. Additionally, some patients with AUPV develop BPPV, during the weeks following onset of the AUPV syndrome.

There is no consensus on the best acute treatment of AUPV. Anecdotally, early oral corticosteroids, such as high-dose prednisone, may accelerate recovery from AUPV but with uncertain long-term benefits. Most specialists consider initiating an oral corticosteroid medication during the first week after onset of AUPV, and multiple approaches to treatment are common in practice. Vestibular suppressant medications, such as meclizine and diazepam, provide temporary comfort. However, these should be stopped as soon as possible, ideally within the first week. Vestibular suppressant medications inhibit vestibular compensation and slow functional recovery. Vestibular physical therapy after AUPV likely speeds functional recovery. It is common practice to initiate vestibular physical therapy as soon as it is practical, and improvement may be expected to be faster once vestibular suppressant medication use has been discontinued.

FOCAL CEREBRAL ISCHEMIA

Cerebral ischemia produces multiple forms of dizziness, the nature of which depends on the sites of ischemia. Extracranial carotid artery ischemia, for example, may be oligosymptomatic, presenting with brief, nondescript lightheadedness and limb tingling. Cerebellar ischemia

may present with vertigo that is combined with other focal signs or symptoms. The labyrinthine artery is a branch of the anterior inferior cerebellar artery; therefore ischemia of the branches of this artery can cause audiovestibular dysfunction. Venous drainage of the labyrinth includes the petrosal veins, sigmoid vein, and jugular vein, raising the possibility of audiovestibular dysfunction from venous insufficiency. Almost any form of cerebral ischemia may be expected to come with a degree of postural instability albeit subtle in some instances. Differentiating between migraine and transient ischemic attacks can be challenging, especially for patients who experience a first-ever syndrome involving vertigo; in this instance, associated focal neurologic signs and symptoms further the diagnostic process. Transient ischemic attacks and stroke are covered in greater detail elsewhere in this book (see Chapter 5).

GLOBAL CEREBRAL HYPOPERFUSION

Global cerebral hypoperfusion typically presents with lightheadedness that is greatest in upright positions. It may be due to dysautonomia that involves the sympathetic nervous system and limits the effectiveness of venous return from portions of the body below the heart. The set of disorders that may contribute to dysautonomia includes vitamin B_{12} deficiency, hypothyroidism, diabetes mellitus, Lyme disease, obstructive sleep apnea, diffuse Lewy body disease, and Parkinson disease.

Dysautonomia should be suspected in patients who report lightheadedness upon standing up from a chair, even when lightheadedness is inapparent upon standing in the exam room. Dysautonomia-related dizziness often waxes and wanes, such that the patient has "good days and bad days." The first-line treatment for many patients with dysautonomia is maintenance of normal intravascular volume. Some medications cause hypotension, so a thorough review of the medication list is indicated.

ANXIETY DISORDERS

Dizziness is often a symptom of anxiety disorders. Complicating this is the fact that vestibular disorders may also present with or be complicated by the symptom of anxiety. Many patients with anxiety also report marked sensitivity to visual motion, for example, motion of patterns within one's vision. Persistent postural perceptual dizziness (PPPD) is a syndrome associated with anxiety that is defined by dizziness without spinning vertigo, aggravated by self-movement and complex visual environments. The criteria for PPPD include a requirement that the symptoms are not better explained by another disease or disorder. PPPD often presents after another acute vestibular disorder. Also notable is that patients with migraine or an anxiety disorder may be predisposed to development of PPPD. It has been hypothesized that PPPD is related to excessive dependence on visual cues, consistent with the development of PPPD after diagnosis of another vestibular disorder. In the setting of peripheral vestibular disorder, vision provides another potentially more reliable cue pertaining to position and motion, but it is conceivable that excessive reliance on vision as a cue may lead to dizziness. Based on this idea, vestibular physical therapy programs have been designed with an intent to reweight the brain's reliance on sensory cues and reduce overreliance on visual cues. Approaches to the treatment of anxiety-associated dizziness may include a combination of vestibular physical therapy, cognitive-behavioral therapy, and medication, such as selective serotonin reuptake inhibitors, though, as always, treatment must be careful individualized.

CERVICOGENIC DIZZINESS

Multiple forms of dizziness may be related to the neck. One well-defined example is compressive spondylotic cervical myelopathy, which frequently disturbs postural stability and gait. The term "cervicogenic dizziness," however, is typically reserved for nonmyelopathic dizziness attributed to altered proprioceptive input from the neck, for example, in the setting of facet arthropathy. The upper cervical spine musculoskeletal structures are invested with projections via cervical dorsal roots to the spinal cord and then the brainstem. Although normal subjects do not appear to rely extensively on neck afferents for balance, those with peripheral vestibular hypofunction manifest higher than normal cervico-ocular reflex gain, indicating greater reliance on cervical cues. This is an example of an instance in which the brain appears to take advantage of the multisensory nature of balance and then relies more on input from sensory channels that are more normal or less noisy, in the event that some sensory channels become less reliable. In support of the plausibility of the role of cervical

spine inputs in vestibular function, some pain specialists avoid injecting bilateral cervical facet joints due to the acute loss of bilateral vestibular input and the observation that bilateral deafferentation may cause dizziness or disequilibrium. Cervicogenic dizziness is often associated with neck pain or stiffness. Physical therapy, when deemed safe, is reasonable to consider, presuming that the intent is to improve function of the cervical spine.

MIDDLE EAR DISEASE

Many patients in Otoneurology subspecialty clinics report a sensation of fullness in one or both ears, raising the question of whether dizziness may be due to Eustachian tube dysfunction, which is a common cause of ear fullness. Unequal middle ear pressures cause vertigo in scuba divers, and a similar phenomenon may occur with continuous positive airway pressure (CPAP), when used for treatment of obstructive sleep apnea. Otosclerosis is a disease of the bones of the middle ear and causes conductive hearing loss. Less widely appreciated is that otosclerosis is associated with vertigo and vestibular dysfunction. This may be due to toxic metabolites derived from otosclerotic bones that penetrate the inner ear, leading to SNHL and vestibular dysfunction. Moreover, some patients with otosclerosis undergo stapedectomy, which is associated with a risk of dizziness and vestibular dysfunction.

THIRD MOBILE WINDOW DISORDERS

Given its location within the petrous temporal bone, the labyrinth is substantially isolated from external pressure changes with two notable exceptions: the round and oval windows. A pathologic third mobile window can be created by a superior semicircular canal dehiscence (SSCD), in which there is an absence or thinning of the bone covering the roof of the superior semicircular canal. Sound waves—the energy of which normally flows preferentially through the auditory portions of the labyrinth—instead travel excessively through the vestibular labyrinth. Loud sounds may trigger dizziness, that is, the Tullio phenomenon. Patients with SSCD report hearing the heart beating, eye movement, or other abnormally amplified sound, such as the sounds of feet on the floor. Audiometry reveals abnormally low thresholds for perception of bone-conducted sound, sometimes to such an extent that the patient can hear the sound of a tuning fork placed on an elbow or knee but not through the air at the same distance. Although the diagnosis is confirmed by a specially protocoled computed tomographic (CT) scan of the temporal bones, it is reasonable in some instances to first obtain an audiogram with air and bone stimuli.

BILATERAL VESTIBULAR HYPOFUNCTION

Patients with bilateral peripheral vestibular hypofunction present with oscillopsia or gait and balance dysfunction. Less commonly, vertigo may occur, presumably due to incremental, asymmetric loss of peripheral vestibular function. The head impulse test is abnormal bilaterally, as is the dynamic visual acuity test, and a Romberg sign may be present. Bilateral vestibular hypofunction is most often idiopathic, but it can be caused by gentamicin, tobramycin, syphilis, Lyme disease, bacterial meningitis, superficial siderosis, or autoimmune diseases. Patients with bilateral vestibular hypofunction are advised to avoid swimming alone because of the risk of underwater disorientation. Physical therapy may be beneficial, presumably in part because it capitalizes on preserved sensory channels.

VESTIBULAR PAROXYSMIA

Vestibular paroxysmia is a syndrome of sudden bursts of dizziness. These reportedly can be caused by injury or compression of the vestibular nerve, for example, by vascular loops or other focal disease adjacent to the vestibular nerve. The episodes of dizziness in vestibular paroxysmia have a sudden onset, are short lived, and are sometimes accompanied by lateropulsion. Anecdotally, these episodes are occasionally accompanied by paroxysmal auditory symptoms, and oxcarbazepine may be beneficial, though randomized trials of treatment of this condition are lacking.

OTHER FOCAL BRAIN DISEASES

A diverse array of focal central and peripheral neurological disorders may cause dizziness or imbalance. Examples of focal or multifocal central disorders include multiple sclerosis and brain tumors. Patients with Parkinson disease and related disorders may develop abnormal gait, falls, or dysautonomia with sympathetic failure that causes dizziness. Epilepsy occasionally causes dizziness but typically involves additional symptoms, for example, dizziness plus memory lapse. The patient with epilepsy is recognized by the presence of recurrent, paroxysmal, stereotyped, unprovoked behaviors or experiences that are referrable to the brain. Seizures and epilepsy are covered in greater detail elsewhere in this book (see Chapter 24).

Chiari malformations (types I and II) are readily visualized on brain MRI. Headache is the most common symptom. The eye movement exam may reveal saccadic smooth pursuit, downbeat nystagmus, and optokinetic nystagmus abnormalities.

In normal pressure hydrocephalus (NPH), gait dysfunction is an early sign. Deficits of cognition and bladder dysfunction typically develop later. Diagnostic tests may include a large-volume lumbar puncture or placement of a temporary lumbar drain. An uncommon cerebrospinal fluid–related condition, intracranial hypotension, can present with headache, dizziness, and balance dysfunction that improve in the supine position.

A vestibular schwannoma or other mass in the cerebellopontine angle may cause dizziness, though the most common first objective sign is asymmetric SNHL marked by a significant word recognition deficit. Balance dysfunction is a later sign, as the size of the tumor grows large enough to compress the brain. On examination, the patient has difficulty understanding whispered speech on the involved side. Significant asymmetric SNHL is an indication to rule out a vestibular schwannoma or other retrocochlear lesion, ideally through the performance of a contrast CT or MRI of the internal auditory canals. When an MRI of the internal auditory canals with contrast is impractical, for example, for patients who have a non-MRI compatible pacemaker, brainstem auditory evoked response tests may provide useful information. As an explanation of imbalance, one should also consider the differential diagnosis of peripheral neurological disorders, such as large fiber peripheral neuropathy due to vitamin B_{12} deficiency, diabetes mellitus, or excessive dietary consumption of vitamin B_6.

HEAD TRAUMA

Head trauma can cause dizziness, through multiple mechanisms. Persistent alteration of brain function that begins immediately after a head trauma may in some instances warrant a diagnosis of traumatic brain injury (TBI). TBI patients frequently report dizziness. When TBI is mild, the term "concussion" is sometimes used.

Subsequent symptoms may thus, in some instances, be viewed as a postconcussion syndrome. Diagnosis of TBI relies on documentation of altered brain function that begins soon after a head trauma. The head trauma can be either a blow to the head or a rapid acceleration. As is the case for most neurological disorders, a diagnosis of TBI requires that the clinician has reasonably excluded other, better explanations of the symptoms and signs. Head trauma may also cause labyrinthine concussion. It is well known that the labyrinth can be damaged in the setting of a temporal bone fracture. Additionally, head trauma in the absence of skull fracture can damage the labyrinth. Dizziness due to TBI is often aggravated by head motion. It may thus be necessary for physical therapists to reduce the intensity of balance-related exercises to improve their tolerability. TBI may also be a substrate for dysautonomia with sympathetic failure and orthostatic lightheadedness.

MAL DE DEBARQUEMENT SYNDROME

In mal de debarquement syndrome (MdDS), exposure to an unusual form of motion, such as an ocean cruise, a long road trip, or air travel, is followed by persistent sensations of rocking, frequently with associated gait and balance dysfunction. Symptoms may improve transiently, upon reexposure to the same type of motion that preceded the onset of the disorder. Some patients occasionally feel suddenly pulled in one direction or another while walking or report aggravation of imbalance when walking past large patterns on walls or floors.

It has reported that carefully selected paradigms involving full-field visual stimuli projected onto a curved wall in an otherwise dark or dim environment may have therapeutic efficacy in MdDS. The availability of this type of therapy remains limited to a handful of centers. Some patients with MdDS also have concurrent migraine that requires treatment. Anecdotally, patients with the MdDS may be less likely to experience a recurrence or aggravation of MdDS when they are treated with a benzodiazepine, such as clonazepam, concurrent with exposure to the same type of motion, for example, during air travel.

"For the full bibliography list, please use the pincode on the inside front cover to access the electronic version of the text at ebooks.health.elsevier.com."

26

Sleep Disorders*

Milena Pavlova and Elizabeth Benge

INTRODUCTION

Sleep is a universal function of living species, comprising one-third of human life. Poor quality or insufficient sleep has been associated with worsening function of most body systems, including endocrine, metabolic, higher cortical function, and neurologic disorders. Disorders of sleep can manifest as complaints of either a perceived need for excessive amount of sleep, insufficient sleep, or abnormal movements during sleep. Reproductive health and gender may differentially affect the presentation of sleep disorders as well as treatment.

MAJOR SLEEP DISORDERS

Insomnia: General Considerations

More than one-third of adults experience transient insomnia at some point in their life. In up to 40% of cases, insomnia can develop into a more chronic and persistent condition.

The diagnosis of insomnia is made when the patient reports dissatisfaction with sleep (sleep-onset or sleep-maintenance insomnia) as well as other daytime symptoms (e.g., sleepiness, impaired attention, mood disturbances). To be considered chronic, this condition occurs for at least three nights per week and last for more than 3 months. Although several insomnia subtypes have been delineated, diagnosis and treatment are similar.

*Based on Pavlova MK, Latreille V. Sleep disorders. *Am J Med*. 2019;132(3):292–299. ISSN 0002-9343. https://doi.org/10.1016/j.amjmed.2018.09.021.

The precise pathophysiologic mechanisms underlying insomnia have not been identified yet, but neurobiological and psychological models have been proposed. Known contributing factors may include emotional, behavioral, cognitive, and genetic factors. These are often conceptually classified into predisposing (genetic etc.), precipitating (often stress or illness), and perpetuating (maladaptive behaviors that lead to chronicity) factors.

Available treatments for insomnia include pharmacologic and nonpharmacologic therapies. The treatment plan should consider any comorbidities that could lead to sleep disruption. These include any primary sleep disorders (e.g., sleep apnea and periodic limb movement in sleep), medications, other comorbidities, and behavioral factors. Initial counseling and education about good sleep practices are usually helpful and are often sufficient to reduce insomnia symptoms. It is typically helpful to start by explaining, in comprehensible terms, the rationale and the concept that the duration of wakefulness and circadian rhythms both affect sleep onset independently and that specific substances (e.g., caffeine, medications, recreational compounds) as well as perpetual sleep-related stressors (e.g., activities performed in bed that do not involve intimacy or sleep) can affect sleep is a negative way. Thereafter, recommendation can be given to keep regular wake times, limiting time in bed to sleep time, use of bed for sleep and intimacy only, avoiding afternoon caffeine and limiting alcohol intake, and limiting daytime napping (otherwise, naps should be very brief, <30 minutes, and taken in the early afternoon at the latest). In cases of persistent insomnia, formal cognitive behavioral therapy programs may prove very helpful. In some reports, cognitive behavioral therapy for insomnia may have equal or better effect compared to pharmacologic treatment, and the effect may be longer lasting. However, use is often limited by insurance coverage, the availability of psychologists, and the necessary time commitments.

Pharmacologic therapy may be appropriate when treatment is anticipated to be short (e.g., insomnia in the setting of stress) or in addition to behavioral treatments. The choice of agent should consider (1) predominant type of complaints, whether sleep initiation or sleep maintenance; (2) frequency of insomnia symptoms (nightly versus intermittent); (3) length of treatment anticipated; and (4) age and comorbidities of the patient. Sleep initiation insomnia may respond well to short-acting medications, and these can be used as needed if the condition is intermittent; in this case the choice of hypnotics should depend on comorbidities. Nightly sleep maintenance insomnia may need nightly longer-acting medications, such as eszopiclone or suvorexant. Patients with comorbid anxiety or depressive symptoms may benefit from antidepressant treatment, such as mirtazapine or trazodone. A history of sleepwalking as a child should be considered a caution in using zolpidem and, to some extent eszopiclone, as they may increase the risk for complex behaviors in sleep. Other factors, such as the patient's age and gender, should also be considered before starting pharmacologic treatment for insomnia. In 2013 the FDA issued a warning, recommending that a lower dose of hypnotics be used to prevent next-morning impairment due to residual effects. Females appear to be more susceptible to this risk (Box 26.1). Orexin antagonists are a novel group of medications that have a favorable side effect profile. Their common mechanism is inhibition of the orexin A and B receptors in the lateral and posterior hypothalamus, which is responsible for the maintenance of wakefulness. The lack of direct action on GABA makes them attractive for treatment of individuals who are at risk of falls or those with concerns for any cognitive impairment.

Overall, the medications that are used most frequently in the treatment of insomnia include benzodiazepines, which have the advantages of being cheap and ubiquitous. However, they are associated with various problems, such as excessive sedation, high frequency of falls (due to nonselective GABA effects), hypotension, tendency to lose efficacy after longer use, muscle relaxant effect, and significant cognitive effects. Other treatments include hypnotic such as zolpidem, zolpidem XR,

---

BOX 26.1 FDA Recommendations Regarding Hypnotics

- Immediate-release products: *FDA is requiring the manufacturers of certain immediate-release zolpidem products (Ambien, Edluar, and Zolpimist) to lower the recommended dose. FDA has informed manufacturers that: (1) The recommended initial dose for women should be lowered from 10–5 mg, immediately before bedtime; (2) The drug labeling should recommend that health care professionals consider prescribing a lower dose of 5 mg for men. In many men, the 5-mg dose provides sufficient efficacy. (3) The drug labeling should include a statement that, for both men and women, the 5-mg dose could be increased to 10 mg if needed, but the higher dose is more likely to impair next-morning driving and other activities that require full alertness.*
- Extended-release products: *FDA is also requiring the manufacturer of extended-release zolpidem (Ambien CR) to lower the recommended dose. FDA has informed the manufacturer that: (1) The recommended initial dose for women should be lowered from 12.5–6.25 mg, immediately before bedtime; (2) The drug labeling should recommend that health care professionals consider prescribing a lower dose of 6.25 mg in men. In many men, the 6.25 mg dose provides sufficient efficacy.*

Intermezzo (zolpidem ultra-short-acting, 1.75–3 mg), zaleplon, and eszopiclone. The advantages of these hypnotics are that some are very short acting (Intermezzo, zaleplon) or are FDA approved for chronic insomnia treatment (eszopiclone, zolpidem CR). However, frequent problems include common side effects such as parasomnia and oversedation, and some also have a potential to lose efficacy. Other options for insomnia treatment include melatonin agonists (ramelteon), orexin antagonists (suvorexant, lemborexant, and daridorexant), antidepressants (mirtazapine, trazodone, amitriptyline), antihistamines, and other substances (herbal, etc.).

Circadian Rhythm Sleep Disorders

The timing of sleep and wakefulness is maintained on one end by homeostatic factors and on another by the endogenous circadian system. Normally, the sleep phase of the circadian rhythm occurs about 1–2 hours after the onset of melatonin secretion. It may occur later or earlier than society-driven scheduled sleep time, resulting in a delayed or advanced sleep-wake phase disorder.

Circadian rhythm sleep-wake disorders are common. In delayed sleep-wake phase disorder, sleep occurs systematically later than needed, whereas in advanced sleep-wake phase disorder, sleep occurs systematically earlier than needed. In both cases, sleep length is similar to that of healthy individuals, and patients feel refreshed when sleeping according to their naturally desired clock time. Delayed sleep-wake phase disorder is thought to account for 10% of patients with chronic insomnia and is particularly common in adolescents and young adults, occurring in 7%–16%. Advanced sleep-wake phase disorder is estimated to occur in 1% of middle-aged adults and even more commonly in older populations. Non–24-hour circadian rhythm disorder is thought to occur in >50% of blind individuals, and up to 80% of this population complains of sleep disturbances. Twenty percent of the workforce engages in shift work, and 10%–38% of this population is estimated to suffer from shift work circadian rhythm disorder.

The diagnosis and treatment of circadian rhythm sleep-wake disorders are sometimes difficult without an accurate assessment of the patient's circadian phase. In research conditions, plasma measurements of melatonin and core body temperature are commonly used. However, these are labor intensive and expensive, require special settings, and are therefore impractical for routine clinic use. More feasible assessment parameters include salivary and urine melatonin measures.

The evaluation of circadian sleep-wake disorders usually starts with a sleep log to assess typical sleep patterns. An objective measure, such as actigraphy, may provide supportive information about the pattern of rest and activity, though it does not necessarily coincide with the circadian phase for sleep. Knowledge of the circadian phase is important because light can have opposite effects on the circadian sleep phase depending on the time of exposure; bright/blue light in the "biological morning" can advance the sleep phase, while late light exposure delays it. Salivary measurement of dim light melatonin onset time (DLMO) may be feasible and convenient in regular clinical practice.

Despite their high prevalence, circadian rhythm sleep-wake disorders are commonly misdiagnosed as insomnia or, in some situations, hypersomnia. A recent study of patients diagnosed with primary insomnia demonstrated that 10%–22% had a bedtime that was out of phase with their circadian sleep time, suggesting a circadian etiology for their sleep problems. This misdiagnosis may lead to unsuccessful, expensive, and sometimes harmful consequences.

Treatment of circadian rhythm sleep disorders is based on timed bright or blue light (morning for delayed phase disorders and afternoon for advanced phase disorders) and melatonin (1 hour prior to required bedtime in delayed phase disorder). For non–24-hour sleep-wake phase disorders in blind individuals, tasimelteon has been recently found effective, but its side effects include elevated live enzymes. It is helpful to counsel patients that the accuracy of the timing of any interventions for delayed sleep-wake phase disorder may be crucial for successful treatment. As has been mentioned, the effect of light depends on the light spectrum/wavelength, intensity, prior light exposure, and, most important, timing. The same light intensity may delay the sleep phase of the circadian cycle if it is administered prior to the core body temperature minimum or advance it if administered after it. For the same reasons, administration of exogenous melatonin should also be timed by circadian phase. According to a recent study of exogenous melatonin in individuals with delayed sleep-wake phase disorder who also had a delayed DLMO, 0.5 mg melatonin administered 1 hour before the required sleep onset time (time the individual needs to be asleep to obtain a sufficient amount of sleep at the time they have to awaken for morning obligations) can be a safe and effective treatment option.

Sleep-Disordered Breathing: Obstructive Sleep Apnea and Central Sleep Apnea

Sleep apnea is a primary sleep disorder characterized by pauses of breathing during sleep. There are three main types of sleep apnea: obstructive sleep apnea, central sleep apnea, and complex sleep apnea. An obstructive apnea is defined as a cessation of airflow for at least 10 seconds and results from collapse of the upper airway during sleep. By contrast, during a central apnea, the interruption of airflow occurs when there is a lack of effort to breathe, usually arising from the brain respiratory centers to the muscles that control breathing. Some patients may have both obstructive and central apnea.

Sleep apnea can be diagnosed during polysomnography, in which the severity of sleep apnea is quantified by the number of respiratory events per hour of sleep.

Along with clinical symptoms, at least five events per hour (Apnea-Hypopnea Index ≥5) are required for a diagnosis of sleep apnea. According to prevalent criteria, an Apnea-Hypopnea Index between 5 and 14 is considered mild sleep apnea, an Index between 15 and 29 is considered moderate sleep apnea, and in Index of more than 30 events per hour is considered severe sleep apnea. Several screening scales for sleep apnea have been developed to identify at-risk patients. One of the most frequently used in clinic is the STOP-BANG questionnaire, which contains four yes-or-no questions that relate to clinical signs of sleep apnea (S: snoring; T: tiredness during daytime; O: observed apnea; P: high blood pressure) as well as four items related to the well-known sleep apnea risk factors (B: body mass index > 35; A: Age > 50 years; N: Neck circumference > 40 cm; G: male gender). A patient is at high risk of sleep apnea if three or more questions are answered positively.

In the general middle-aged population, moderate to severe sleep apnea can be found in about 30%–50% of males and 11%–23% of females. Clinical symptoms most often include loud snoring, choking and gasping, apneas witnessed by the bed partner, excessive sleepiness and fatigue, and morning headache. Sleep apnea has debilitating effects on the patient and their family's quality of life. When left untreated, sleep apnea can also have major negative health consequences; it increases the risk of hypertension, type 2 diabetes, and cardiovascular diseases. In a large cohort study, risk of stroke in males with moderate to severe obstructive sleep apnea increased incrementally with each unit of increased severity. Sleep apnea is also a well-known risk factor for cognitive deficits. The negative consequences of sleep apnea can be at least partially reversed by consistent and accurate treatment.

Several treatment options are available for sleep apnea. For mild cases of obstructive sleep apnea, conservative therapies such as weight loss and avoiding a supine position (for positional sleep apnea) can be helpful. The most widely used and currently first-line treatment for obstructive sleep apnea is positive airway pressure therapy. Continuous positive airway pressure is typically the initial treatment and consists of a continuous flow of air into the nose, while bilevel therapy provides a higher pressure on inspiration and a lower pressure on expiration. The latter is sometimes more comfortable with higher pressures. Autotitrating machines have been very helpful to expedite treatment.

Adaptive servoventilation can also be used to treat complex sleep apnea. Continuous positive airway pressure therapy in individuals with obstructive sleep apnea has been found to reduce subjective daytime sleepiness and improve cognitive functioning, as well as mood and quality of life. It also can improve blood pressure and glucose control. Oral appliances such as mandibular advancement devices may also help to improve mild to moderate cases of obstructive sleep apnea that are not associated with any significant risk factors or for patients who are intolerant to positive airway pressure therapy. Surgical treatment methods include most commonly soft palate surgery, nasal surgery, and maxillomandibular surgery. These may diminish sleep apnea severity, although they generally do not cure sleep apnea. In some situations, hypoglossal nerve stimulation can be considered in patients who cannot tolerate PAP therapy. Typically, individuals who are considered for this therapy undergo evaluation with endoscopy under anesthesia with direct visualization of the type of collapse of the upper airway. Those with concentric collapse or with pronounced anatomic abnormalities of the upper airway may not be ideal candidates, as the stimulation is not sufficiently helpful.

Hypersomnia Disorders, Narcolepsy, and Idiopathic Hypersomnia

In evaluating hypersomnia, the following issues should be considered:

1. Is there enough sleep opportunity? In adults, typical sleep need is more than 7 hours, with adequate, consistent timing.
2. Are there factors that impair sleep quality and, as a result, lead to insufficient or poor-quality sleep? These include medications, environmental factors, and primary sleep disorders, such as sleep apnea and sleep-related movement disorders.
3. Does the hypersomnia recur more than three times per week for more than 3 months?

Disorders causing central hypersomnia are rare. They include narcolepsy type 1 (with cataplexy), narcolepsy type 2 (no cataplexy), idiopathic hypersomnia (with long sleep time or without long sleep time), and recurrent hypersomnia (e.g., Kleine-Levin syndrome). Narcolepsy is a disorder of rapid eye movement (REM) sleep regulation. Classic symptoms include sleepiness, sleep paralysis, and hypnagogic hallucinations. Cataplexy in narcolepsy type 1 consists of a loss of muscle tone, provoked typically by positive emotions (classically, laughing or telling a joke). Occasionally, surprise or anger can be a trigger. For narcolepsy patients, all daytime naps are short (15–40 minutes) and refreshing. There is a common genetic association (DQB1*0602 haplotype), and patients with narcolepsy type 1 may also have lower orexin measured in cerebrospinal fluid.

The diagnosis is made first clinically; however, an objective documentation using the multiple sleep latency test is needed to confirm the sleepiness. This test is typically performed on the day after a polysomnography and consists of five nap opportunities. Most narcolepsy patients fall asleep within minutes if given the opportunity; therefore a short sleep latency (average of <8 minutes over the five nap opportunities) as well as REM sleep during these naps would be supportive of narcolepsy. Current criteria require that REM sleep is seen in two or more naps or that REM sleep is seen in one nap along with a REM latency of less than 15 minutes on the preceding polysomnogram. Cerebrospinal fluid measurements of hypocretin may help to establish the diagnosis of narcolepsy type 1 (with cataplexy); it became available in the United States in 2019.

The treatment of sleepiness often starts with wake-promoting medications. These can be modafinil or armodafinil. If these are not tolerated or are ineffective, stimulants (methylphenidate or amphetamine/dextroamphetamine) can be used. Cautions should include monitoring blood pressure and evaluating for arrhythmias, which can be worsened by these medications. Other medications that may be considered include solriamfetol, pitolisant, and oxybate (sodium oxybate or calcium, magnesium, potassium sodium oxybate). None of these have been approved for use in pregnancy. Cataplexy responds to antidepressants, typically selective serotonin reuptake inhibitors (SSRIs); sodium oxybate or calcium, magnesium, potassium, sodium oxybate; or pitolisant. Common comorbidities of narcolepsy include REM behavior disorder, which is present in as many as 10% of narcolepsy patients, as well as periodic limb movement of sleep. Both may be worsened by SSRIs, including the medications that are used for cataplexy treatment.

Hypersomnia can sometimes be seen after head trauma; in some reports, hypersomnia affects as many as half of patients with traumatic brain injury, and a quarter of these patients may have sleep-disordered breathing. Treatment of sleep-disordered breathing may be helpful, and use of any sedating medications should be judicious.

In rare conditions, hypersomnia can be idiopathic. Idiopathic hypersomnia condition typically presents with long, nonrefreshing naps as well as sleep inertia. Two types exist: (1) with a long sleep time and (2) without long sleep time. The criteria for diagnosis include the clinical presentation as well as supportive evidence from the multiple sleep latency test: a sleep latency <8 minutes and no sleep-onset REM. Treatment is often challenging. Modafinil or armodifinil at higher doses can be used, and sometimes other stimulants can be helpful. In another rare condition, Kleine-Levin syndrome, hypersomnia is recurrent. Kleine-Levin syndrome typically presents in adolescence or in the early 20s. It consists of periods that last for approximately 2 weeks, during which patients exhibit very long sleep (often 12–21 hours per day), and during the waking periods individuals exhibit cognitive abnormalities (i.e., major apathy, confusion, slowness, amnesia), dreamlike behavior, hyperphagia, or hypersexuality. Between episodes, individuals have a normal level of functioning. Treatment with lithium may decrease the frequency of episodes, while stimulants have a marginal effect during the events.

Non–Rapid Eye Movement Parasomnias

Parasomnias can be grouped by the type of behavior that is seen or may be based on the sleep stage in which they occur. The most common non-REM parasomnias include somnambulism, confusional arousals, and night terrors. These parasomnias are characterized by a wide variety of behaviors, but they mostly occur from slow-wave sleep, and as such, they typically arise in the first half of the night. They most commonly manifest with directed behaviors. They are not stereotypical and may have a variable duration. Upon awakening, the patient does not have any vivid dream recall. If any dream mentation is recalled, it is very brief. The pathophysiology of non-REM parasomnias is not well understood, although the hypothesis of dysregulated slow-wave sleep has been proposed.

Important steps in the diagnosis include (1) evaluation for comorbid sleep fragmenting disorders and (2) distinction from nocturnal seizures. A laboratory based polysomnogram is indicated in most cases to assess for comorbid sleep disorders, such as sleep apnea or REM behavior disorder. Consideration should be given to evaluation with an EEG, especially in adults. A routine EEG may be helpful to assess for any interictal epileptiform discharges, and if capturing events is needed, a 24- to 72-hour assessment may provide further information. If extended 10–20 EEG montage can be added during the polysomnogram, this may expedite evaluation.

Treatment of REM parasomnias may involve benzodiazepines or, in some cases, tricyclic antidepressants. Clinicians should be aware that some medications may induce somnambulism; according to a recent review, the strongest evidence for medication-induced sleepwalking was found for zolpidem and sodium oxybate. Counseling about safety of the sleep environment and treatment of comorbid sleep disorders provide relief for many patients.

Rapid Eye Movement Behavior Disorder

REM behavior disorder (RBD) is characterized by abnormal physical behaviors that emerge from REM sleep and can lead to injury and disturbed sleep. Most patients have frequent events—typically more than once per week. Abnormalities can be seen almost nightly and consist of intermittent loss of the normal atonia of REM sleep. This phenomenon is considered supportive of the diagnosis. Clinical screening for RBD includes clinical history and validated RBD questionnaires.

RBD has serious consequences for the health of the patient. Besides the risk of sometimes severe injury, a direct consequence of a violent nocturnal movement, it often leads to sleep disruption. Furthermore, it is commonly seen in association with Parkinson disease, and many experts in the field consider it a prodrome of neurodegenerative conditions. Other comorbidities may include a higher risk of cerebral hemorrhage as well as stroke. Multiple factors may contribute to the risk of RBD. Aside from neurodegenerative conditions, RBD is seen in association with disorders of REM sleep regulations, including narcolepsy, posttraumatic stress disorder, and the use of SSRIs. Though RBD prevalence is not known exactly, a few studies have estimated it to be approximately 0.5%–1.06% in the general population, with higher numbers among the elderly.

In healthy individuals, REM sleep is closely linked to circadian phase, with a peak a little after the nadir of the core body temperature; thus, it is also around the time when melatonin secretion is maximal. Studies using a forced desynchrony protocol suggest that the circadian system has a primary effect of REM sleep regulation with

a modifying effect from the homeostatic factors. Various other factors affect REM sleep, including complex interactions with the serotonergic system, primarily from the raphe nuclei in the medulla, which inhibit the REM-generating pontine tegmentum nuclei. Clinically, patients treated with antidepressants, particularly with serotonergic properties such as SSRIs, tend to suppress REM sleep; antidepressant use may also lead to REM sleep without atonia and/or trigger dream enactment events.

The melatonin MT_1 and MT_2 receptors likely both affect the NREM/REM ratio, with activation of the MT_2 leading to earlier and more abundant NREM sleep, while MT_1 receptor activation favors REM sleep. As was mentioned previously, RBD is common in patients with Parkinson's disease, and a reduced number of melatonin receptors have been found in the areas involved in neurodegeneration. A recent study found a depleted MT^1 receptor expression in the striatum and amygdala and depleted MT_2 receptor expression in the substantia nigra and amygdala. In addition to circadian phase shift, activation of MT_1 and MT_2 receptors has been implicated as a potential protective mechanism against multiple other progressive neurodegenerative disorders, while MT_2 receptors have been implicated in neurogenesis. Thus, REM suppression and/or disruption, as a result of the neurodegenerative process, that also involves impaired MT_1 and MT_2 receptor function may be a key mechanism for RBD pathophysiology and potential therapeutic target.

Treatment options for RBD are limited. The most commonly used agent is clonazepam, which must be used with caution in patients with dementia symptoms and has many potentially serious side effects. Due to the strong association with neurodegenerative conditions, RBD patients are likely to have contraindications for benzodiazepine treatment. Since the mechanism for RBD includes REM sleep disruption, much thought has been given to the question of whether improved REM sleep regulation can be a pathway to treat RBD.

Melatonin is the most common therapeutic alternative to clonazepam for RBD. Initial studies may have been partially prompted by its high clinical convenience, a very favorable side effect profile, and availability in the United States. It was first reported as effective in a case report in 1997 of a 64-year-old male who experienced improvement of his RBD symptoms after treatment with 3 mg melatonin, without any change in his REM proportion on polysomnography. Further studies have included open label case series. In one recent study, melatonin was found to be as effective as clonazepam for RBD treatment. However, studies have often been small, open label, and sometimes retrospective, and generally the timing of melatonin is not consistently reported.

The use of melatonin has several clinical challenges, since the medication is over the counter, not regulated, and dose and bioavailability can vary widely. It has therefore been proposed to also use melatonin agonists, which have a higher affinity to melatonin receptors, for treatment. Ramelteon has been reported to be successful in some cases. In 2013 Nomura et al. used 8 mg ramelteon in two patients who had polysomnography (PSG) confirmed RBD in association with parkinsonian syndromes. One of the patients had multisystem atrophy and could not tolerate clonazepam due to the lability of her blood pressure; the other had persistent symptoms despite clonazepam treatment. Both individuals experienced improvement in their RBD symptoms, including in the RBD severity scale, which is based on PSG recordings. Later, Esaki et al. treated 12 consecutive patients with idiopathic RBD in an open label trial, using 8 mg ramelteon given 30 minutes before bedtime, and reported a trend toward improvement. Another study examined the effect of ramelteon on motor and nonmotor symptoms in patients with Parkinson's disease, with or without RBD, and reported improvement in a variety of measures after treatment, including a statistically significant RBD improvement. Novel data (some in presentations at conferences) have recently emerged regarding the chronotherapeutic aspects of RBD, suggesting that there may be not only a potential for improved symptom control but also long-term benefit in terms of decreasing neurodegeneration. However, due to a large first-pass effect, the absolute bioavailability of ramelteon following an oral dose is less than 2%, and there is a large degree of intersubject variability in plasma concentration after exposure.

Other therapeutic targets may include sleep consolidation. Recent smaller-scale studies have explored treatment with sodium oxybate. A study of 12 participants with treatment-resistant RBD and 12 controls found some improvement of symptoms.

Restless Legs Syndrome and Periodic Limb Movements of Sleep

Restless legs syndrome is characterized by an uncomfortable sensation leading to an urge to move the limbs that occurs or worsens while at rest, has consistent evening predominance, is associated with dysesthesia, and is partially relieved by physical activity. Patients often describe the sensation as "creeping, crawling tingling" or shock-like feelings or simply as indescribable discomfort. Over the course of the disease, the sensations can spread to the arms or trunk. One of the major characteristics of restless legs syndrome is its worsening in the evening and at night, which results in difficulty initiating sleep, as patients often get up and pace around the room to relieve the discomfort. In turn, poor sleep often leads to fatigue and daytime sleepiness.

Restless legs syndrome is one of the most common sleep-related movement disorders, affecting about 15% of adults. Generally, it affects females more than males, and prevalence is higher with old age. The cause can be idiopathic or secondary. In its idiopathic form, there is no known cause, but most patients will have a family history of the syndrome. Secondary restless legs syndrome most often has a later onset course and is associated with various neurologic disorders (i.e., multiple sclerosis, Parkinson disease) iron deficiency (low ferritin level), or pregnancy.

The diagnosis is made by clinical review of the patient's medical history. Restless legs syndrome and periodic limb movement of sleep frequently cooccur; the latter is present in 80%–90% of patients diagnosed with restless legs syndrome. The presence of periodic limb movement of sleep is also supportive for the diagnosis of restless legs syndrome. Periodic limb movement of sleep can be diagnosed by clinical history, but a polysomnography may be useful to confirm the diagnosis, particularly in patients with unexplained symptoms of insomnia or hypersomnia.

Multiple studies highlight an important role of brain iron levels in the pathology of restless legs syndrome and periodic limb movement of sleep, but these are lower in patients with restless legs syndrome. Dysfunction of the dopaminergic system has also been demonstrated as a potential pathophysiologic mechanism for restless legs syndrome. Evaluation of the serum ferritin level is recommended. If the ferritin level is below 50 μg/L, replacement of iron should be considered via oral or intravenous supplementation. Otherwise, pharmacologic treatment of restless legs syndrome may start with either dopamine agonists or gabapentin or gabapentin enacarbil. Levodopa, ropinirole, pramipexole, cabergoline, and pergolide are all considered effective. The doses of dopamine agonists should be kept as low as possible to decrease the possibility of worsening symptoms over time (termed augmentation). Other effective medications include pregabalin and rotigotine. In more advanced disease, when other medications are no longer effective or in the setting of severe augmentation, opiates can be considered. Intravenous ferric carboxymaltose and pneumatic compression devices were reported to be likely effective in idiopathic restless legs syndrome. Clonidine and bupropion appear to have insufficient evidence for efficacy at this time.

A challenging long-term complication of restless legs syndrome is the development of augmentation. This phenomenon consists of earlier occurrence and worsening of the symptoms. For example, a patient who presented with typical symptom onset around bedtime (10:00–11:00 p.m.) and now reports that symptoms begin to occur in the early evening or afternoon likely suffers from augmentation. To decrease the likelihood of augmentation, initial treatment may consider gabapentin or gabapentin enacarbil instead of any dopamine agonists.

The occurrence of restless legs syndrome is notably higher in pregnant people compared to nonpregnant individuals, with prevalence reaching up to 16% during the third trimester. Pregnancy-associated restless legs syndrome is a transient condition. Risk factors include lower hemoglobin levels, iron and vitamin deficiencies, genetic factors, and smoking. Pregnant individuals who are affected by restless legs syndrome exhibit an elevated risk of preterm birth, poor quality of sleep, and depression during pregnancy. In considering treatment, nonpharmacologic approaches such as moderate exercise and yoga are recommended as initial steps. Iron replacement may be helpful as well. Other pharmacologic interventions remain controversial at this time.

SUMMARY AND CONCLUSIONS

Sleep is a vital function, universal for all living species, and it comprises roughly one-third of human lives. When sleep is disrupted or perturbed, there can be significant negative consequences on quality of life and daytime function. Therefore, sleep disorders should be promptly treated. When appropriate, a subspecialty referral should be considered.

"For the full bibliography list, please use the pincode on the inside front cover to access the electronic version of the text at ebooks.health.elsevier.com."

27

Pain Neurology*

Victor C. Wang and William J. Mullally

INTRODUCTION

Pain is an unpleasant sensory and emotional perception that is usually, but not always, the result of underlying tissue pathology. It is often the initial complaint that brings a patient to the physician's office and is the primary chief complaint in the emergency department. Clues to diagnosis will always begin with the history and exam of the patient but the history can sometimes be difficult to obtain, as pain can be difficult to describe for each patient. Accepted descriptions of pain in the medical literature can include "tingling," "numbness," "zinging," "dull," "sharp", "stabbing", "throbbing," and "aching." All of these descriptors carry different meaning to different patients, depending upon culture, language, or prior experiences. The temporal nature of pain further complicates the pain experience, whether pain is acute or chronic, or acute on chronic. Together these factors will change the description of pain in the patient's history.

Pain is a complex problem that is affected by physical and psychological factors. Further complicating the history taking, aside from the ability to describe pain, is the interpretation by the provider. Again, this is determined by culture, language, and prior pain experiences, but on the part of the provider. With no gold standard diagnostic test for pain, the interpretation really does depend upon this interaction between provider and patient. These challenges all contribute to the proper or improper diagnosis and treatment of the patient.

Patients in the current multidisciplinary healthcare model are often referred to specialists without a clear etiology for their pain. Referrals from specialists who are resigned to not knowing the cause of a patient's pain from diagnostic tests make it that much more difficult to ascertain the cause of pain with unknown etiology, and patients' expectations can sometimes add to the care burden. Pain can be seen as a neurologic problem, though neurologists are not specifically trained to treat pain. Neurology training is focused on acute stroke and eventually stroke prevention as well as chronic disease such as Parkinson disease, Alzheimer disease, and movement disorders. However, the nervous system becomes the conduit for recognizing pathology in the body; hence, unknown etiologies become a neurologic issue in the absence of a neurologic etiology.

The history of pain is complex, as it is related to the previously mentioned factors, which include experience, culture, language, anatomy, and actual neurologic lesions. However, pain has been a part of human history since ancient times; some civilizations have believed that pain was caused by evil spirits or demons and that it could be removed by rituals. With the inception of religious belief, pain was similarly attributed to punishment and sin. Hippocrates (460–377 BCE) argued that disease came not from a superstition or a god but rather was a natural process. Galen (CE129–216) believed that pain was an interconnected phenomenon between the mind/soul and the body. Descartes, during the 17th century, brought about the mechanistic model of pain by separating the body and the soul and medicalizing the pain condition. Not long afterward, Thomas Willis laid the foundation for neurology in the 17th century through his study and description of brain anatomy and the

*Based on Wang VC, Mullally WJ. Pain neurology. *Am J Med*. 2020;133(3):273–280. ISSN 0002-9343. https://doi.org/10.1016/j.amjmed.2019.07.029.

nervous system and explaining how sensory information, such as pain, is transmitted. Johannes Muller in the 1830s theorized that the perception of sensory stimuli was due not to the original stimuli, but to the activation of specific nervous structures and partially explained why different types of pain are perceived differently by the specific nervous system activation pattern. In the 1960s Wall and Melzack proposed the gate control theory, whereby the experience of painful stimuli is affected by the nonpainful stimuli through inhibition of the nervous system signal. The gate control theory has helped lead to treatment of pain through the use of technological devices such as spinal cord stimulators by which pain transmission is altered in the dorsal columns of the spinal cord.

Acute pain is typically short term and the result of an injury or a specific event. Chronic pain lasts for an extended period, usually more than 3 months and can be the result of an underlying medical condition, injury, or disease. Pain may be localized or radiating, spreading from its source to other areas of the body. Nociceptive pain is caused by activation of nociceptors, which are pain receptors in body tissue, and may be somatic, arising from skin, muscle, or joints, or may be visceral, related to internal organs. Neuropathic pain results from dysfunction or damage of the nervous system. Pain intensity can range from mild to severe, and various pain scales, such as the Numeric Rating Scale or the Visual Analog Scale, are used to assess and categorize pain based on severity. Referred pain is appreciated in an area that is removed from the source of the problem. An example is left arm pain occurring as a result of a heart attack.

When the primary complaint is pain, the history is often nonspecific, presenting a challenge to the clinician who is trying to determine whether the cause is benign or due to a serious illness. Obtaining a pain history includes location, duration (acute or chronic), exacerbating and relieving factors, and accompanying symptoms. Understanding the neurologic basis of pain is important in establishing a diagnosis and treatment plan. Knowing the different types of pain is important, as each pain requires a different treatment approach. This chapter aims to help rule out neurologic causes of pain and includes several of the most common presentations of pain that often prompt a neurology referral for further workup, focusing on common neurologic causes of pain seen in the primary care physician's office (Box 27.1).

> **BOX 27.1   10 Most Common Reasons for Visits to the Physician**
>
> 1. Skin problems
> 2. Joint pain and osteoarthritis
> 3. Back pain
> 4. Cholesterol (lipid metabolism)
> 5. Upper respiratory issues
> 6. Anxiety and depression
> 7. Chronic neurologic disorder
> 8. Hypertension
> 9. Headache and migraine
> 10. Diabetes

Diagnostic testing and an initial treatment for these disease pathologies will also be reviewed briefly.

LOW BACK PAIN

Low back pain is listed as one of the top 10 diseases in the population, and the prevalence is increasing with longer lifespans. It is one of the most common complaints in the primary care physician's office. Healthcare costs for low back pain are not insignificant, with low back and neck pain having estimated healthcare costs of over $87 billion in 2013, just behind ischemic heart disease. Referrals to neurologists and pain physicians are often made for chronic axial low back pain and lumbar radiculopathy. Common causes of low back pain are listed in Box 27.2.

The physical examination is extremely important in the evaluation of low back pain. Red flag symptoms include focal neurologic deficits such as motor weakness, bowel and/or bladder changes, saddle anesthesia, or asymmetry in reflexes and/or strength indicating a cauda equina syndrome where there is a dysfunction of multiple lumbar and sacral nerve roots at the end of the spinal cord referred to as the cauda equina due its resemblance to the tail of a horse. All of these symptoms mandate an expedited evaluation with magnetic resonance imaging (MRI) of the spine (Box 27.3). Initial workup may reveal disc herniation, causing severe spinal stenosis or more serious concerns, such as infection, compression fracture, and malignancy. Presentation of red flag symptoms can be acute or subacute in nature meaning from days to weeks, and patients may require surgical intervention in the first 48 hours. With regard

BOX 27.2 Common Causes of Low Back Pain

Muscle strain
Lumbar herniated disc
Degenerative disc disease
Facet joint pain
Sacroiliac joint disease
Spinal stenosis
Spondylolisthesis
Compression fracture

BOX 27.3 Red Flags Requiring Further Workup in Low Back Pain

Fever, chills, night sweats
Unexplained weight loss
Bowel or bladder changes
Intravenous drug use
Saddle anesthesia
Motor weakness in a lower extremity
Progressive neurologic changes
Asymmetric deficits
Trauma

to the characterization of pain, however, pain is defined as acute if it has been present for less than 3 months. Chronic low back pain, by contrast, is defined as pain lasting more than 3 months. Chronic pain affects 619 million people worldwide, according to the World Health Organization, with an estimated number of 843 million by 2050. These numbers are expected to increase due to the increasing global aging population and it is the leading cause of disability worldwide.

Nonspecific low back pain can be attributed to several causes, including the following:

- Degenerative disc disease: The intervertebral discs in the spine are under constant pressure. With age, they begin to decrease in thickness. These discs begin to lose their cushioning ability in the spine over time and can cause significant pain and stiffness in the low back and may lead to a decrease in motion.
- Herniated disc: The intervertebral discs begin to bulge with age and can put pressure on the spinal cord and spinal nerves. The disc is composed of an outer ring called the annulus fibrosus, which surrounds a gel-like center called the nucleus pulposus. A rupture in the disc is called a herniation, and the nucleus pulposus

can leak, causing irritation of the spinal nerve roots with resulting low back and/or sciatic pain.

- Spondylolisthesis: This is a condition in which a vertebra slips out of alignment of the spine, putting pressure on the spinal cord and/or nerve roots. Spondylolisthesis can also cause low back and/or sciatic pain, depending on the location of the compression.
- Arthritis: The facet joints in the spine provide flexibility and stability. With age and degenerative changes, the facet joints of the spine can become arthritic, causing pain anywhere along the spine, and can be a major contributor to low back pain with age. Interestingly, rib cage support is one reason that low back and neck pain are more prevalent than mid-back pain.
- Spinal stenosis: Narrowing of the spinal canal due to aging and arthritis. The narrowing can cause impingement of the nerve roots as well as compression of the spinal cord itself and again can cause low back or sciatic pain depending on the location. The pain, often referred to as neurogenic claudication, is intermittent and worsens with activities such as standing or walking. Sitting and bending at the waist tend to relieve the pain.
- Muscle strain: Any injury or strain of the back musculature can cause pain, stiffness, and decreased range of motion in the lower back.
- Osteoporosis: Decreased bone density with age increases the risk of spine compression fractures. Osteoporosis itself is not usually symptomatic until fractures occur, which can be extremely painful and debilitating.
- Psychological factors: Stress, anxiety, and depression all can exacerbate underlying pain diagnoses.

Treatment for chronic low back pain depends on the underlying etiology. For the primary care provider, the key decision is in referring for surgical treatment versus conservative therapy. In most cases, conservative therapy should be tried before proceeding to surgical intervention. These treatments include the following:

- Physical therapy (PT): Strengthening of the lumbar musculature helps to stabilize the spine and can increase the range of motion. PT can also help with conditions such as spinal stenosis, in which bending forward can relieve the pressure on the spinal cord.
- Ice and heat therapy: Ice therapy can be utilized for treatment of low back pain by decreasing inflammation of the lumbar musculature with ice. Heat can help with muscle loosening and relaxation.

- Transcutaneous electrical nerve stimulation (TENS): There is conflicting evidence as to the efficacy of TENS. TENS therapy consists of a low-voltage electric current applied by electrodes attached to the skin on the low back overlying the area of pain. The electric impulses can theoretically decrease pain by modifying the transmission of pain signals. Another theory is that TENS can increase the level of endorphin production in the body, thereby decreasing the pain levels. The therapy is sometimes used in conjunction with PT.
- Yoga: There is increasing evidence for yoga as a tool for decreasing low back pain. Like PT, yoga strengthens and stretches back muscles and can improve range of motion through stabilization of the spine.
- Massage therapy: Often combined with PT, massage therapy helps with improving tissue elasticity, reducing scar formation, decreasing inflammation, and increasing blood flow to tissues.
- Chiropractic treatment: While chiropractic treatment is controversial, some evidence does show that it can help with decreasing low back pain in several measures, such as pain intensity, disability, and decreased use of pain medicine.
- Acupuncture: Another less-accepted method of treatment, acupuncture has also shown some evidence for low back pain treatment. Acupuncture is thought to trigger release of endorphins as well as release of neurotransmitters in the brain, altering some of the pain pathways.
- Percutaneous injections: Percutaneous injection is a more accepted treatment of targeted steroid injections for reducing pain and inflammation at the joints or at the nerve roots, decreasing pain transmission at the source of the pain.
- Medication: Over-the-counter pain medications such as ibuprofen, naproxen, and acetaminophen are very effective at reducing inflammatory mediators. Muscle relaxants are another class of medications that can be used, especially in the case of myofascial pain. Some evidence has shown certain antidepressants such as the serotonin and norepinephrine reuptake inhibitors (SNRIs) to be effective at helping to control chronic pain.

Radiculopathy

Establishing the etiology of low back pain can be challenging, as there can be an extremely varied presentation. A patient can present with descriptions of pain that include dull aching pain, shooting pain, tingling, weakness, numbness, and sharp and stabbing pain. "Sciatica" is a common complaint for nerve pain, or radiculopathy, usually characterized as a shooting pain going down one or both legs because of the association with the sciatic nerve. Radiculopathy is not confined to the lower extremities and may emanate from the cervical spine, radiating down the arms or from thoracic pathology around the chest. These radiculopathies are named anatomically for the origin of the nerve impingement in the spine, with cervical radiculopathy for pathology coming from the neck, and thoracic and lumbar radiculopathies named by their respective spinal regions (Fig. 27.1).

The cause of nerve root impingement can result from anything that decreases the diameter of the neural foramen, causing nerve root compression. In most cases, this is caused by disc herniation, especially in older adults over age 65 years. Other causes can include osteophyte formation (bone spurs), facet hypertrophy, and ligamentous hypertrophy. All of these can cause impingement of the nerve root at the level of its exit from the spinal canal.

Treatment of radiculopathy in the absence of red flags includes initial conservative therapy with neuropathic medications such as gabapentin, and topiramate. Pregabalin has been shown in small studies to be effective in the treatment of radiculopathy, though a recent study found it to be ineffective in the treatment of sciatica. Referral for epidural steroid injections can be done for short-term relief. In intractable cases, surgery can be offered in the setting of imaging findings or in more serious cases with focal neurologic deficits. For intractable cases without clear imaging findings, newer technologies and medications have been explored. One of these technologies is spinal cord stimulation, which is a device consisting of a stimulating wire connected to a generator and implanted over the spinal cord preventing the pain signal from being sent from the spinal cord to the brain.

Other Causes of Low Back and Leg Pain

Other causes of pain radiating down the legs can include sacroiliac (SI) joint pain, greater trochanteric bursitis, or iliotibial band syndrome. Distinguishing between these disorders can be challenging; again, it begins with the history and physical exam. SI joint disease can present similarly to lumbar radiculopathy with pain starting in the low back and radiating down the posterolateral

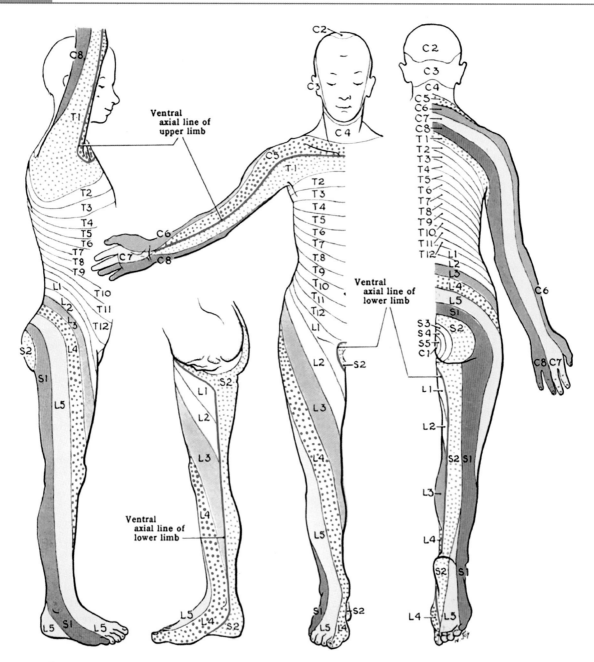

Fig. 27.1 Dermatomes of spinal sensory nerve roots (Boileau Grant JC. *Grant's Atlas of Anatomy*, 5th ed.; 1962.)

aspect of the upper thigh. Patients will usually localize most of the pain to the affected SI joint. Pain that is described more in the lateral hip can be attributed to greater trochanteric bursitis and/or iliotibial band syndrome, usually from repetitive use injury. Patients may have complaints of not being able to sleep on the affected side. Finally, axial low back pain without radiation can be characteristic of musculoskeletal changes, most often from degenerative changes in the spine and facet joints as well as from muscle weakness or injury.

Distinguishing between these pathologies starts with a thorough physical exam that should include commonly used provocative tests such as the straight leg raise (SLR), which is usually done in the evaluation of a patient's radicular pain with suspected disc herniation. It is performed with the patient supine and lifting the affected extremity off the exam table. Exacerbation of the sciatic pain between 30 and 70 degrees is considered a positive test. Sensitivity is reported to be 91% and specificity to be 26% in detecting a disc herniation, primarily at L5 or S1. Adjunct testing can help to increase the sensitivity of the SLR, such as the Bragard's sign, in which the patient's ankle is dorsiflexed on the affected side during the SLR. In the evaluation of other suspected pathologies of low back pain, the Patrick's test, also known as the FABER test (for flexion, abduction, external rotation), is used to evaluate SI joint and hip pathology. The patient is asked to flex the leg and then abduct the thigh externally, much in the same manner as sitting cross-legged. Ipsilateral anterior pain over the hip can indicate hip joint pathology, while contralateral posterior pain is more indicative of SI joint disease.

In equivocal cases in which the history and exam are not clear, further diagnostic study with imaging or electrodiagnostic testing may be warranted, though the current recommendation is that for symptoms lasting less than 6 weeks in the absence of red flags, computerized tomography (CT) and x-ray are usually done, due to lower cost and more rapid evaluation, though information is limited. MRI is more valuable in the evaluation of soft tissue, spinal, and nerve root compression. Electrodiagnostic testing includes nerve conduction studies and electromyography (EMG) and can be used when there is a question of chronicity and for help in distinguishing between central or more peripheral causes of nerve pain.

Initial treatment of chronic low back pain (greater than 12 weeks) includes conservative measures with oral analgesics such as nonsteroidal antiinflammatory drugs (NSAIDs), gabapentin, and muscle relaxers. A formal course of PT and adjunct therapies such as yoga and acupuncture have been found to be helpful in the treatment of chronic low back pain. For SI joint pain and hip pain, conservative management with NSAIDs and PT should be tried prior to more invasive options such as steroid injections or surgery.

NECK PAIN

Neck pain is a common, often debilitating condition and is the fourth leading cause of disability. Most acute episodes resolve spontaneously, but more than one-third of individuals will experience chronic discomfort that can interfere with their normal daily activities. The history and exam will help to determine whether the pain is mechanical-nociceptive or neuropathic and will also help to identify more serious pathology such as myelopathy or atlantoaxial subluxation. There are numerous causes of neck pain, including the following:

1. Musculoskeletal pain due to trauma from a fall or whiplash injury resulting in strain, sprain, or injury to muscles, ligaments, or joints in the neck.
2. Inflammatory disorders such as rheumatoid arthritis.
3. Nerve root compression resulting in radiculopathy due to a herniated nucleus pulposus or bone spur.
4. Degenerative changes such as cervical spondylosis.
5. Psychological factors that may contribute to the development of neck pain or exacerbate existing discomfort.

Chronic neck pain occurs when the brain becomes more sensitive to pain signals due to central sensitization amplifying the perception of pain. Changes in function and structure can then perpetuate the pain.

MRI of the cervical spine should be performed when there are focal neurologic symptoms or findings on exam or if the pain is refractory to standard treatment. A scan should also be obtained prior to interventional treatment. However, it should be noted that the imaging is characterized by a high prevalence of abnormal findings in asymptomatic individuals.

Effective management of neck pain requires a multidisciplinary approach. NSAIDs and muscle relaxants are effective for acute pain. There is strong evidence to support exercise treatment, with weaker evidence supporting acupuncture, massage, spinal manipulation, and yoga. There is weak evidence that supports epidural steroid injections and radiofrequency ablation for facet arthropathy and cervical radiculopathy. Surgery is more effective in the short term but not the long term in patients with radiculopathy or myelopathy. Younger patients with greater disease burden and small spinal canal tend to fare better with surgery than older patients with greater function and transverse spinal canal diameter. Cognitive behavioral therapy and relaxation for chronic neck pain can address psychological factors contributing to the pain and lifestyle modification can be beneficial.

COMMON NEURALGIAS IN THE PRIMARY CARE SETTING AND PERIPHERAL NERVE COMPRESSION

Entrapment neuropathies caused by compression is the most common cause of mononeuropathies. It is another common disorder in presentation in the primary care office setting, carpal tunnel syndrome being the most common. Other common entrapment neuropathies that are seen in the primary care setting include ulnar neuropathy and meralgia paresthetica. Cervical radiculopathy should also be considered here. For example, pain traveling down the upper extremity into the last two digits can present as either a C8 cervical radiculopathy or an ulnar neuropathy. C6 or C7 radiculopathy can present similarly to carpal tunnel syndrome. As was previously noted, along with a history and physical exam, EMG and/or cervical spine imaging can be helpful in determining peripheral causes of pain.

Carpal Tunnel Syndrome

Carpal tunnel syndrome is the most common entrapment neuropathy, affecting 3% of the adult population. Patients will present with pain, numbness, tingling, and paresthesias in the distribution of the median nerve, usually caused by a compression of the nerve at the wrist. Pain radiates outward from the wrist in the cutaneous distribution of the median nerve to include the palmar surface of the first three and a half digits and the distal aspect of the digits on the dorsal surface of the hand. The pain can awaken the patient from sleep and is usually described as tingling with burning, aching, and an electric sensation accompanied by numbness. It can be exacerbated with movements requiring wrist flexion, and one of the provocative tests for carpal tunnel is Phalen's test, in which the patient holds the dorsal surfaces of the hands together for 30–60 seconds. A positive Tinel's sign can be found with provocation test on examination in which symptoms are reproduced when the examiner taps on the wrist at the distal wrist crease. The Tinel's sign can be used for other compressive neuropathies by the same method of percussion at the point of suspected compression with reproduction of symptoms in the distribution of the peripheral nerve.

Electrodiagnostic testing is often included in the evaluation for carpal tunnel syndrome and can be especially helpful in ruling out more central causes of pain in the hand as in cervical radiculopathies or polyneuropathies. More recently, ultrasound has been used in the diagnosis of carpal tunnel syndrome with enlargement of the nerves at the site of compression.

Treatment for carpal tunnel syndrome starts usually with conservative therapy, using wrist splinting for a period of at least 6 weeks in mild to moderate cases. For patients who do not improve, an injection of a corticosteroid into the carpal tunnel may bring relief. Oral steroids can be helpful as well, though NSAIDs have not been shown to be effective. For severe or intractable cases, carpal tunnel release should be offered and has been shown to be effective long-term treatment.

Meralgia Paresthetica

Meralgia paresthetica is a mononeuropathy of the lateral femoral cutaneous nerve that manifests as pain, dysesthesias, and paresthesias over the anterolateral thigh. The pain is often described as tingling, numbness, coldness, sharp pain, and burning pain. The skin over the thigh is innervated by the lateral femoral cutaneous nerve, which travels down from the lumbar plexus into the anterolateral thigh. The nerve is susceptible to compression or stretching along the course by which it travels to the thigh. Sometimes, meralgia paresthetica can be misdiagnosed as a lumbar radiculopathy due to similarly overlying dermatomal pain distributions. Lumbar radiculopathy will be caused by a more proximal nerve lesion compared to the distal lesion of a peripheral nerve in meralgia paresthetica.

Patients can report an inability to wear tight clothing or belts. Not surprisingly, the risk for developing meralgia paresthetica is increased with diabetes, obesity, and/or pregnancy, due to tissue compression. Initial treatment of meralgia paresthetica begins with conservative measures that would include weight loss and wearing looser clothing. In intractable cases, a nerve block of the lateral femoral cutaneous nerve can be performed. Most cases of meralgia paresthetica will improve and resolve with symptomatic and supportive treatment.

Intercostal Neuralgia

Intercostal neuralgia is characterized by pain along the course of an intercostal nerve running between the ribs. Intercostal nerves provide sensation of the chest wall;

if they become damaged, compressed, or irritated, the result can be constant or intermittent burning, sharp, or stabbing pain in the chest or rib cage area. The pain may be accompanied by numbness and tingling, and movements such as breathing, twisting, and coughing may accentuate the discomfort. Common causes include trauma to the chest, resulting in rib fracture or bruising, herpes zoster infection, nerve root compression in the thoracic spine, and infections such as pneumonia or pleuritis. A diagnosis of idiopathic intercostal neuralgia is made when the exact cause cannot be identified.

Treatment will depend on the underlying cause. A nerve block with a local anesthetic can be used to alleviate the pain.

Trigeminal Neuralgia

There are several causes of intermittent facial pain. Commonly seen in the primary setting include trigeminal neuralgia and occipital neuralgia. Trigeminal neuralgia pain is usually described as short-lasting intermittent jabs or shocks in one of the three divisions of the trigeminal nerve, most commonly the mandibular and maxillary branches. It can be triggered by light touch, toothbrushing, eating, or even talking. The pain is often debilitating, and sometimes patients will present with a half-shaved face or partially applied makeup because of the inability to touch the affected side of the face without pain.

The trigeminal nerve is composed of three anatomic segments: the ophthalmic (V1), maxillary (V2), and mandibular (V3) divisions. More urgent diagnoses should be ruled out in evaluating a patient for facial pain and suspected trigeminal neuralgia. Other headache subtypes and, importantly, temporal arteritis can present similarly in the ophthalmic (V1) division of the trigeminal nerve (Fig. 27.2).

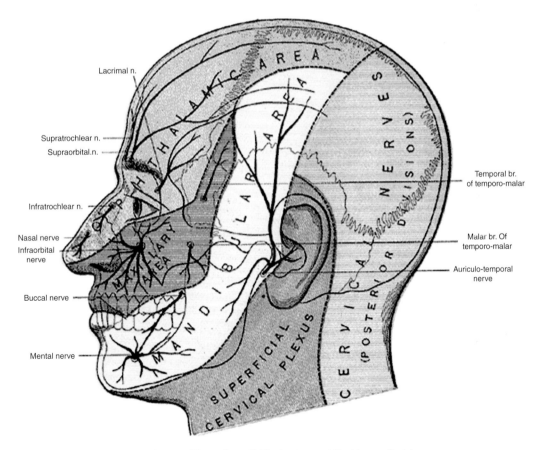

Fig. 27.2 Dermatomes of the trigeminal nerve (Henry Gray 1918 - Anatomy of the Human Body).

TABLE 27.1   Treatments for Trigeminal Neuralgia and Side Effects

Medication	Side Effects	Starting Dose
Carbamazepine	Dizziness, drowsiness, nausea, vomiting, headache. Leukopenia and aplastic anemia can occur. Must test for HLA-B*15:02 allele if considered for Asian patients	100 mg twice daily
Oxcarbazepine	Similar to carbamazepine	300 mg twice daily
Gabapentin	Dizziness, drowsiness, ataxia, fatigue, cognitive slowing	100–300 mg 1–3 times daily
Pregabalin	Dizziness, drowsiness, headache, fatigue, weight gain, peripheral edema, visual changes	25–150 mg daily or in 2 divided doses
Baclofen	Drowsiness, headache, confusion, nausea, vomiting	40 mg daily
Lamotrigine	Skin rash, nausea, drowsiness, insomnia	25 mg daily with slow titration

TABLE 27.2   Cranial Neuralgias

Neuralgia	Anatomy	Symptoms
Glossopharyngeal	Glossopharyngeal nerve	Unilateral stabbing pain on one side of the tongue or throat. Pain can extend to the ipsilateral ear.
Nervus intermedius	Branch of the facial nerve	Deep auditory canal pain.
Supraorbital and supratrochlear	V1 branches of the trigeminal nerve	Pain in the ipsilateral forehead and upper eyelid. Tenderness over the supraorbital notch.
Infraorbital	V2 branch of the trigeminal nerve	Pain below the ipsilateral eye.
Auriculotemporal	V3 branch of the trigeminal nerve	Pain anterior to the tragus of the ipsilateral ear.
Nasociliary	Branch of the V1 trigeminal nerve	Pain in the eyes, brow, and root of the nose.

Carbamazepine is usually the first-line treatment for trigeminal neuralgia (Table 27.1). Other medications include oxcarbazepine, baclofen, and lamotrigine. Medications that have shown some benefit in small studies include gabapentin, pregabalin, and topical lidocaine. For intractable cases, microvascular decompression (also known as the Jannetta procedure), gamma knife, injections, or radiofrequency ablation can be performed. Microvascular decompression involves performing a surgery in which the trigeminal nerve and offending vessel are visualized. The vessel is then mobilized away from the nerve, and a pad is placed between the vessel and nerve.

Other neuralgias of the face and neck that are not included here are described in Table 27.2. These diagnoses are relatively uncommon; for example, glossopharyngeal neuralgia has an incidence of 0.7 per 100,000 people per year. The other diagnoses have even lower incidence. Symptoms of the neuralgias usually follow a dermatomal pattern and can provide clues to the diagnosis. Treatment for the cranial neuralgias is similar to trigeminal neuralgia.

Occipital Neuralgia

Occipital neuralgia is often described as a shooting or burning pain that can be either continuous or intermittent, starting in the back of the head and radiating over the crown of the scalp, sometimes to the forehead. Patients also complain of pain behind the eyes, sometimes with photophobia. There may be tenderness over the affected distribution on the scalp and pain sometimes triggered by neck range of motion. The pain in occipital neuralgia is caused by irritation of the greater and lesser occipital nerves. The greater occipital nerve is formed by the C2 dorsal ramus, and the lesser occipital nerve is formed by the ventral rami of C2 and C3. Causes of pain can include neck tension, cervical osteoarthritis, prior neck injury, or lesions of the neck. Risk factors include gout, diabetes, and vasculitis.

Diagnosis of occipital neuralgia can be challenging, though treatments with occipital nerve blocks are both diagnostic and therapeutic. Other conservative treatments include PT, NSAIDs, muscle relaxants, and antiepileptics such as gabapentin. More invasive techniques, including high cervical blocks, have been used in intractable case. Current surgical interventions can be considered; these include microvascular decompression of the occipital nerves. Peripheral neurostimulation is yet another alternative that is sometimes used for intractable case.

Postherpetic Neuralgia

The human herpes virus-3, or varicella zoster virus (VZV), enters the nervous system during the acute phase of the infection, often during childhood, and can lie dormant in the dorsal root ganglia as well as in the geniculate or trigeminal ganglia. The virus can reactivate later in life and present as the characteristic painful rash of shingles in the dermatomal distribution of the nerve root. Pain can then persist where the rash occurred even after the lesions have healed. Postherpetic neuralgia is the most common complication that occurs after VZV infection and reactivation. Diagnosis technically requires that the pain persists for 90 days after the rash and can be severe in nature, usually described as burning or shock-like with hyperalgesia and/or allodynia.

Pain from postherpetic neuralgia can be very difficult to control and can significantly interfere with activities of daily living. Symptoms can persist for weeks to months to years. Treatment options are limited but include lidocaine patch and topical capsaicin. There is limited evidence for the use of both topical treatments. Oral medications include gabapentin and pregabalin, and both have been found to be somewhat effective compared to placebo. Finally, tricyclic antidepressants such as amitriptyline and nortriptyline have been used in the treatment of postherpetic neuralgia, though again evidence is somewhat limited in terms of the effectiveness of the medication.

MYOFASCIAL PAIN

Myofascial pain is a hyperirritable localized point of muscular pain. It has been associated with a tender taut band of muscle on examination, which is referred to as a trigger point and sometimes as muscle knots. Patients can present with localization of pain in one particular area of muscle that is alleviated by massage or by stretching. Unfortunately, the pain relief is usually only temporary.

Sometimes patients with myofascial pain will have complaints of being unable to find a comfortable position at rest due to the pain. A trigger point can also be a source of referred pain and may be associated with diagnoses such as migraine and tension-type headache. In these cases, the trigger point acts as a trigger for the other underlying diagnoses. Conversely, other musculoskeletal diagnoses, such as cervical radiculopathy, may be linked as a cause of myofascial pain, in which the primary diagnosis functions as a trigger for the pain. The primary cause of myofascial trigger points is unknown but possibly related to the inappropriate release of acetylcholine at the synaptic cleft, hence starting a cycle of increased metabolism and hypoxia at the muscle band, leading to sensitization of the muscle tissue. This sensitization may activate the autonomic system and potentiate an activation loop with continued acetylcholine release at the local contracture.

Treatment of myofascial pain includes regular massage, stretching, PT, and exercise. These therapies may serve to increase perfusion of the muscle and improve the pathophysiologic changes. Other treatment modalities that can be temporarily effective include trigger point injections, dry needling, transcutaneous electrical stimulation, and ultrasound therapy.

PAINFUL DIABETIC NEUROPATHY

Nerve damage due to diabetes mellitus can result in persistent severe burning, stabbing, or shooting pain primarily in the feet and occasionally the hands. The pain is accompanied by numbness and tingling and often hypersensitivity to touch. The neuropathic pain can be debilitating, interfering with sleep and normal daily activities. Afflicted individuals may experience depression.

Maintaining good blood glucose control is essential in the management of diabetic neuropathy. Medication options include tricyclic antidepressant medication such as amitriptyline or nortriptyline, pregabalin and gabapentin, and the serotonin-norepinephrine reuptake inhibitor duloxetine.

COMPLEX REGIONAL PAIN SYNDROME

Complex regional pain syndrome (CRPS) is a severe, painful condition that affects a limb (either an arm or a leg). CRPS is sometimes referred to as reflex sympathetic dystrophy or causalgia and usually occurs after injury to the limb, such as a fracture or surgery. CRPS has traditionally been separated into two types; type I is from an injury or prolonged immobilization (casting after fracture), and type II occurs after a known nerve injury in the limb. The two types are indistinguishable clinically with pain, allodynia, and hyperalgesia of the limb. The pain is described as being out of proportion to the initial injury. Other manifestations of CRPS include skin color changes, temperature changes, edema, and changes in hair growth and sweat patterns.

The current criteria that are used in the diagnosis of CRPS were initially proposed by the International Association for the Study of Pain (IASP) in 1994 and were revised in 2007 (IASP "Budapest criteria") for higher diagnostic specificity (Box 27.4).

BOX 27.4 Diagnostic Criteria for Complex Regional Pain Syndrome (Budapest Criteria)

To make the clinical diagnosis, the following criteria must be met:

- Continuing pain that is disproportionate to any inciting event.
- Must report at least one symptom in all four of the following categories:
  - Sensory: reports of hyperaesthesia and/or allodynia
  - Vasomotor: reports of temperature asymmetry and/or skin color changes and/or skin color asymmetry
  - Sudomotor/edema: reports of edema and/or sweating changes and/or sweating asymmetry
  - Motor/trophic: reports of decreased range of motion and/or motor dysfunction (weakness, tremor, dystonia) and/or trophic changes (hair, nail, skin).
- Must display at least one sign at the time of evaluation in two or more of the following categories:
  - Sensory: evidence of hyperalgesia (to pinprick) and/or allodynia (to light touch and/or temperature sensation and/or deep somatic pressure and/or joint movement)
  - Vasomotor: evidence of temperature asymmetry (>1°C) and/or skin color changes and/or asymmetry
  - Sudomotor/edema: evidence of edema and/or sweating changes and/or sweating asymmetry
  - Motor/trophic: evidence of decreased range of motion and/or motor dysfunction (weakness, tremor, dystonia) and/or trophic changes (hair, nail, skin)
- There is no other diagnosis that better explains the signs and symptoms.

Treatment of CRPS begins with early intervention and mobilization of the affected limb with PT and occupational therapy and patient education with psychological therapy. Limited evidence for pharmacologic management includes data showing some benefit of several drug classes such as NSAIDs, alpha-2-delta ligands (gabapentin and pregabalin), topical agents (lidocaine and capsaicin), and antidepressants. Referral for pain management may be helpful for sympathetic nerve blocks to help tolerate PT. There is limited evidence for more invasive procedures such as spinal cord stimulation and sympathectomy.

PHANTOM LIMB PAIN

Phantom limb pain occurs in most individuals who have undergone amputation of a limb and is a perception of pain in the limb that no longer exists. The pain fluctuates in intensity, may be intermittent or chronic, and varies from burning and shooting to cramping and squeezing. Patients often describe electric shock–like sensations and may experience itching or tingling. The etiology may be the result of central sensitization amplifying pain signals and residual activity of the nerve endings at the amputation site.

Treatment can be challenging, and PT and transcutaneous electrical nerve stimulation may provide relief. Antidepressant medication and antiepileptic drugs are sometimes prescribed. Advanced prosthetic devices may now include sensory feedback systems to reduce the phantom limb pain.

CHRONIC PAIN

Pain conditions that persist for more than 3 months are referred to as chronic pain and are not necessarily a chronologic extension of acute pain. Chronic pain is the principal symptom of several clinical conditions, such as headache, neuralgia, and fibromyalgia without clear tissue pathology. Chronic pain may also be a symptom of irreversible disease. Chronic pain is usually associated with anxiety, depression, and disability and represents a unique challenge to the primary care provider who is caring for the patient. The chronic pain sufferer often does not respond to medication, and in the past opioid analgesics became the treatment of choice for refractory patients, leading to overprescribing and the "opioid crisis." Medical management of chronic pain should consist of medication with the lowest risk of potentially toxic side effects, including antidepressants, anticonvulsants, muscle relaxants, and topical agents. Opioids should be used when indicated with strict limits and close monitoring. Complementary medicine treatment, including acupuncture, biofeedback, cognitive behavioral therapy, yoga, and tai chi, can often reduce the need for medication. Patients who have chronic pain usually require consultative care with a neurologist, a pain management specialist, and a behavior medicine practitioner.

CONCLUSION

The diagnosis and treatment of pain pose challenges that every primary care provider faces on a daily basis. Clinicians must have a basic knowledge of the common causes of pain and the ability to complete a cost-effective diagnostic workup, then deliver first-line treatment. The management of chronic pain often requires a multidisciplinary approach utilizing the skills of the neurologist, pain specialist, and behavioral health practitioner.

The future of pain treatment remains bright with the development of new technology such as nerve stimulation and brain stimulation techniques. As in other chronic diseases such as Alzheimer disease, the objectives of pain research will likely be improvements in the patient's quality of life rather than the complete resolution of pain. Accomplishing these goals will also reduce the economic burden of chronic disease and pain on society as a whole.

"For the full bibliography list, please use the pincode on the inside front cover to access the electronic version of the text at ebooks.health.elsevier.com."

INDEX

Page numbers followed by *f* indicate figures, *t* indicate tables and *b* indicate boxes.